CW00349359

Neoplastic Gastrointestinal Pathology

Neoplastic Gastrointestinal Pathology
An Illustrated Guide

Laura W. Lamps, MD
Professor and Vice-Chair for Academic Affairs
Department of Pathology
University of Arkansas for Medical Sciences
Little Rock, Arkansas

Andrew M. Bellizzi, MD
Clinical Associate Professor
Director of Gastrointestinal Pathology
Co-Director of Immunopathology Laboratory
Department of Pathology
University of Iowa Hospitals and Clinics
University of Iowa Carver College of Medicine
Holden Comprehensive Cancer Center
Iowa City, Iowa

Wendy L. Frankel, MD
The Kurtz Chair and Distinguished Professor
Chair and Director of Gastrointestinal Pathology
Department of Pathology
The Ohio State University Wexner Medical Center
Columbus, Ohio

Scott R. Owens, MD
Associate Professor of Pathology
Director, Division of Quality and Health Improvement
Department of Pathology
University of Michigan Health System
Ann Arbor, Michigan

Rhonda K. Yantiss, MD
Professor of Pathology and Laboratory Medicine
Chief, Gastrointestinal Pathology
Department of Pathology and Laboratory Medicine
Weill Cornell Medical College
New York, New York

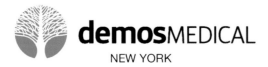
demosMEDICAL
NEW YORK

Visit our website at www.demosmedical.com

ISBN: 9781936287727
e-book: 9781617051210

Acquisitions Editor: Rich Winters
Compositor: Exeter Premedia Services Private Ltd

© 2016 Demos Medical Publishing, LLC. All rights reserved. This book is protected by copyright. No part of it may be reproduced, stored in a retrieval system, or transmitted in any form or by any means, electronic, mechanical, photocopying, recording, or otherwise, without the prior written permission of the publisher.

Medicine is an ever-changing science. Research and clinical experience are continually expanding our knowledge, in particular our understanding of proper treatment and drug therapy. The authors, editors, and publisher have made every effort to ensure that all information in this book is in accordance with the state of knowledge at the time of production of the book. Nevertheless, the authors, editors, and publisher are not responsible for errors or omissions or for any consequences from application of the information in this book and make no warranty, expressed or implied, with respect to the contents of the publication. Every reader should examine carefully the package inserts accompanying each drug and should carefully check whether the dosage schedules mentioned therein or the contraindications stated by the manufacturer differ from the statements made in this book. Such examination is particularly important with drugs that are either rarely used or have been newly released on the market.

Library of Congress Cataloging-in-Publication Data
Lamps, Laura W. (Laura Webb), author.
 Neoplastic gastrointestinal pathology : an illustrated guide / Laura W. Lamps, Andrew M. Bellizzi, Wendy L. Frankel, Scott R. Owens, and Rhonda K. Yantiss
     p. ; cm.
 Includes bibliographical references and index.
 ISBN 978-1-936287-72-7 — ISBN 978-1-61705-121-0 (e-book)
 I. Bellizzi, Andrew M., author. II. Frankel, Wendy L., author. III. Yantiss, Rhonda K., author. IV. Owens, Scott R., author. V. Title.
 [DNLM: 1. Gastrointestinal Neoplasms—diagnosis.   2. Gastrointestinal Neoplasms—pathology. WI 149]
 RC280.D5
 616.99′433—dc23
                                                                                                            2015008140

Special discounts on bulk quantities of Demos Medical Publishing books are available to corporations, professional associations, pharmaceutical companies, health care organizations, and other qualifying groups. For details, please contact:

Special Sales Department
Demos Medical Publishing, LLC
11 West 42nd Street, 15th Floor
New York, NY 10036
Phone: 800-532-8663 or 212-683-0072
Fax: 212-941-7842
E-mail: specialsales@demosmedical.com

Printed in the United States of America by Bradford & Bigelow.
15 16 17 / 5 4 3 2 1

To
Dr. Aubrey J. Hough, Jr.
Chairman, UAMS Dept. of Pathology, 1981–2002
Thank you for giving me the best job ever—LWL

To Sara May and Aidan, for standing by me through thick and thin; to Ed, Wendy, and Jason, for showing me how to be an academic surgical pathologist; to my students, especially Michael, Marty, Bryan, Tom, and Emily, for encouraging me to do great things—AMB

To my husband Brian Rubin for his endless patience—WLF

To Brendan, whose curiosity astounds me and whose precocious wisdom humbles me—SRO

For Madeleine and Zachary, my little loves—RKY

Contents

Contributors

Wei Chen, MD, PhD
Department of Pathology
The Ohio State University Wexner Medical Center
Columbus, Ohio

Matthew R. Lindberg, MD
Department of Pathology
University of Arkansas for Medical Sciences
Little Rock, Arkansas

Benjamin J. Swanson, MD, PhD
Department of Pathology
The Ohio State University Wexner Medical Center
Columbus, Ohio

Preface

"*Omnis cellula e cellula* (All cells come from cells)."
—Rudolph Virchow

Cancer remains one of the leading causes of mortality worldwide, and gastrointestinal malignancies (particularly colorectal, gastric, and esophageal) are responsible for a significant number of cancer deaths around the globe. In addition to the histologic criteria required for the diagnosis of gastrointestinal tumors, knowledge of ever-evolving staging parameters, immunohistochemical markers, and molecular testing for both prognosis and therapeutics is necessary. *Neoplastic Gastrointestinal Pathology: An Illustrated Guide* is intended to serve as an approachable and practical reference for pathologists that includes all of the information needed to evaluate and report these specimens in daily practice.

I am fortunate to have had the opportunity to create this book with a uniquely talented and dedicated group of co-authors; their contributions reflect both their diagnostic abilities and their passion for education. It is my hope that the organization of the book, combined with the extensive number and variety of illustrations, will prove to be a valuable reference companion for all aspects of neoplastic gastrointestinal pathology. We would also like to specifically acknowledge certain colleagues who provided invaluable help and support on this project. Rhonda Yantiss would like to acknowledge Dr. Wade Samowitz for sharing his seemingly endless funds of knowledge and patience. Wendy Frankel would like to thank Shawn Scully in the Department of Pathology at OSU for help with the figures. Personally, I would like to extend a special thanks to all of my residents, fellows, and colleagues who have contributed cases and photographs over the years.

Laura W. Lamps
Andrew M. Bellizzi
Wendy L. Frankel
Scott R. Owens
Rhonda K. Yantiss

1

Introduction to Diagnosis and Reporting of Gastrointestinal Tract Neoplasia

ANDREW M. BELLIZZI

INTRODUCTION

This chapter introduces key terminology used throughout this book, including neoplasia, dysplasia, and the benign–malignant dichotomy. General criteria for grading non-neuroendocrine carcinomas, neuroendocrine neoplasms, lymphomas, gastrointestinal stromal tumors (GISTs), and sarcomas are discussed, as are broad issues pertaining to staging. The importance of synoptic reporting of cancer resection specimens is emphasized. Prognostic and predictive markers are distinguished, and several key examples are presented. The concepts of screening and surveillance are reviewed, again with several key examples. The chapter concludes with a general approach to the diagnosis and reporting of biopsy and resection specimens.

KEY TERMINOLOGY

Neoplasia

The term neoplasia is derived from Greek and literally means new growth, creation, or formation. Mid-twentieth century Australian pathologist Rupert Allan Willis's definition of neoplasia is often cited, stating that, "A neoplasm is an abnormal mass of tissue, the growth of which exceeds and is uncoordinated with that of the normal tissues and persists in the same excessive manner after cessation of the stimuli which evoked the change." This definition emphasizes the proliferative and autonomous nature of tumors. Neoplasms need not form "masses of tissue," however.

For example, the precursor lesions of inflammation-associated adenocarcinomas are typically flat, and tubular adenomas initially arise in a single crypt.

Clonality and the Benign/Malignant Dichotomy

The idea that all the neoplastic cells in a tumor are the progeny of a single mutated cell is referred to as **clonality**. Although clonality implies neoplasia, it does not equate with malignancy, as benign neoplasms are also clonal. Recent investigations have further emphasized that neoplasms, particularly malignant ones, typically have unstable genomes in addition to being clonal.

Malignancy is characterized by invasive growth and the capacity for metastasis. For epithelial tumors in the tubal gut, the relationship between the anatomic extent of invasion and metastatic risk varies with anatomic site. For example, invasion into the lamina propria in the esophagus, stomach, and small intestine denotes metastatic risk (albeit low). In the colon, invasive neoplasms confined to the mucosa (sometimes termed intramucosal carcinoma) do not metastasize. Conversely, benign tumors typically do not recur after complete excision and do not metastasize.

As suggested by the example of intramucosal carcinoma of the colon above, the benign–malignant dichotomy and the terms associated with this concept are insufficient to describe the spectrum of all tumor behavior. Some neoplasms are locally destructive, yet nonmetastasizing; this phenotype has been described as "intermediate." Examples include verrucous carcinoma of the esophagus or anus and desmoid fibromatosis. For other tumors, the assessment of risk of metastasis, and thus the assessment of whether or not a tumor can be expected to behave in a benign or a malignant fashion, cannot be predicted on histologic appearance alone and attention to other clinico-pathologic parameters is needed. For example, parameters of risk stratification for GIST include anatomic location, tumor size, and mitotic rate, with the risk of metastasis or tumor-related death for various combinations of these three parameters ranging from 0% (essentially benign) to 90% (a high expectation of malignant behavior).

Risk Factors for Neoplasia

There are four basic contexts in which neoplasms arise. Many neoplasms arise in a **background of inflammation**. Carcinomas of the esophagus and stomach are particularly apt to arise in inflammatory backgrounds. Barrett-esophagus-associated adenocarcinomas and chronic-gastritis-associated intestinal-type adenocarcinomas are believed to arise through an inflammation→ metaplasia→dysplasia→carcinoma sequence, and gastric adenocarcinomas are etiologically linked to *Helicobacter pylori* gastritis. A large subset (~65%) of gastric neuroendocrine tumors (NETs) arise in a background of autoimmune atrophic gastritis, and extranodal marginal zone lymphomas of the stomach and small intestine (mucosa-associated lymphoid tissue [MALT] lymphomas) are also etiologically linked to *Helicobacter pylori* and *Campylobacter jejuni* infection, respectively. In the small intestine, patients with celiac disease are at increased risk for adenocarcinoma and lymphoma, including enteropathy-associated T-cell lymphoma. Patients with idiopathic inflammatory bowel disease (IBD) are at increased risk for developing colorectal cancer, and this risk is modulated by factors including disease duration, anatomic extent of disease, histologic inflammatory activity, family colon cancer history, and the presence of concomitant primary sclerosing cholangitis. Across the spectrum of inflammation-associated neoplasms, effective treatment of the underlying inflammatory disease is typically associated with improved outcomes and decreased risk of neoplasia. For example, *Helicobacter pylori* eradication has been shown to decrease disease recurrence in early gastric cancer and, in many gastric MALT lymphomas, leads to disease regression. Furthermore, a declining risk of IBD-associated colon cancer in contemporary series has been also attributed, at least in part, to improved medical management of colitis.

Epithelial, lymphoid, and even mesenchymal neoplasms may also arise in association with **oncogenic viruses**. The most common implicated viruses include human papillomavirus (HPV), the major cause of anal intraepithelial neoplasia (AIN) and anal squamous cell carcinoma; Epstein–Barr virus (EBV), which is associated with numerous neoplasms including most cases of gastric carcinoma with lymphoid stroma (also known as lymphoepithelioma-like carcinoma or medullary carcinoma), many types of lymphoma, and smooth muscle tumors in immunosuppressed individuals; and human herpesvirus 8 (HHV8; also known as Kaposi-sarcoma-associated herpesvirus), which drives primary effusion lymphoma, multicentric Castleman disease, and Kaposi sarcoma. Patients with a primary or secondary immunodeficiency, the latter including stem cell or solid organ transplantation, HIV infection, and in some instances, merely advanced age, are at increased risk for this class of tumors. Immunohistochemistry, in situ hybridization, or molecular methods for detection of virus, or surrogate markers (eg, p16 in HPV-driven tumors), may be useful diagnostic adjuncts in this group of tumors.

Neoplasms may also arise in the setting of a **genetic predisposition to cancer**. Hereditary cancer predisposition syndromes are due to highly penetrant germline mutations and share the following features:

1. They are generally autosomal dominant.
2. The tumors occur in relatively young persons (compared to sporadic tumors).
3. The tumors occur at a defined set of anatomic sites.
4. The tumors are often multiple (synchronous or metachronous).

In addition, these tumors, their associated precursors, or other syndromic "marker lesions" often have characteristic clinical and/or histologic features, such as the morphologic features that are seen in Lynch-syndrome-associated colorectal adenocarcinoma.

Most of the tumors that arise in hereditary cancer syndromes are carcinomas, but NETs, GISTs, other mesenchymal tumors, and lymphomas occur in select settings. For example, multiple duodenal gastrinomas and enterochromaffin-like (ECL)-cell gastric NETs may be seen in patients with multiple endocrine neoplasia type I (MEN1), and rarely, patients with neurofibromatosis type I (NF1) manifest periampullary somatostatin-producing NETs. GISTs are seen in patients with NF1, Carney–Stratakis syndrome (due to germline succinate dehydrogenase subunit mutations), and in rare patients with germline mutations in *KIT* or *PDGFRA*. Among other mesenchymal tumors, desmoid fibromatosis is seen in 10% to 30% of patients with familial adenomatous polyposis (FAP), and diffuse-type ganglioneuromatosis is essentially an NF1 or MEN2B-defining lesion. Lymphomas often develop in the very rare patients who inherit two defective copies of a given DNA mismatch repair gene (ie, constitutional Lynch syndrome).

The recognition of a hereditary cancer syndrome may affect the management of a presenting tumor, trigger syndrome-specific surveillance, inform the decision to undergo various prophylactic resections, and, perhaps most importantly, permit the identification of other at-risk family members. The approach to the recognition, diagnosis, and reporting of HCPSs involving the gastrointestinal (GI) tract will be presented in more detail in Chapter 6.

While hereditary cancer syndromes account for a small percentage of GI malignancies, more commonly, cancers aggregate in families without an obvious Mendelian inheritance pattern. For example, 20% to 30% of colon cancers arise in this setting. These tumors have been referred to as "familial" (rather than hereditary). This phenomenon is believed to reflect shared environment and/or inheritance of (possibly multiple) low-penetrant susceptibility alleles. Patients with a non-Mendelian family history are at increased cancer risk, a fact that is taken into account in screening guidelines.

The majority of neoplasms, including carcinomas, neuroendocrine neoplasms, lymphomas, and mesenchymal tumors appear to arise **sporadically**, that is, outside of any of the predisposing contexts described in the preceding paragraphs.

Dysplasia

Dysplasia is defined as an unequivocal neoplastic alteration of the epithelium, frequently within the confines of a basement membrane in the tubal gut. Dysplastic epithelium is often a precursor to the development of malignancy. The distinction of reactive atypia from dysplasia, especially in the context of an inflammatory background, is perhaps one of the most difficult exercises in neoplastic GI pathology.

Applying the concept of clonality in the distinction between dysplastic and reactive changes is a useful and powerful concept. The histologic correlate of clonality is the abrupt transition from a non-neoplastic background to dysplasia (Figure 1.1A). Stated another way, dysplasia "stops and starts;" in contrast, reactive atypia usually blends imperceptibly into adjacent areas that are non-neoplastic (Figure 1.1B). Immunohistochemical stains are sometimes useful to highlight an area of abrupt transition when one is concerned about dysplasia/clonality. Examples include p53 in Barrett esophagus (Figures 1.2A–B), chronic gastritis, and IBD; MLH1 in serrated polyps (Figure 1.2C); and SMAD4 in the pancreatobiliary tree (Figure 1.2D). These immunohistochemical applications will be discussed in greater detail in Chapter 13.

Some pathologists use the terms "atypia" and "dysplasia" interchangeably. Epithelial atypia simply refers to cytologic and/or architectural features that deviate from normal. Because dysplasia is, by definition, neoplastic, while the meaning of atypia is less specific, the two terms are not synonymous. Use of the term "atypia" on the diagnostic line, even if qualified as reactive, is therefore discouraged.

Grading of Dysplasia

From an historical standpoint, the Inflammatory Bowel Disease-Dysplasia Morphology Study Group (IBD-DMSG) undertook the key early effort of developing a standardized nomenclature and classification for dysplasia in IBD. "Dysplasia in inflammatory bowel disease: a standardized classification with provisional clinical applications," published by Riddell and colleagues in *Human Pathology*

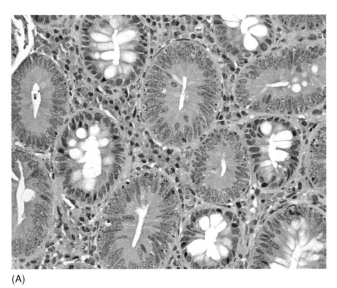

(A)

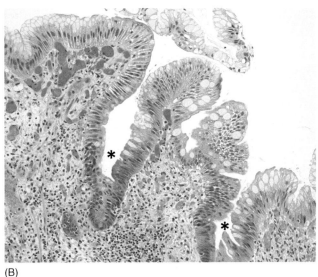

(B)

FIGURE 1.1 Adenomatous crypts with nuclear elongation and slight stratification as well as striking epithelial apoptosis are sharply demarcated from background, non-neoplastic crypts with small, basally located nuclei and preservation of goblet cells. An abrupt transition is characteristic of a dysplastic process (A). In this biopsy of Barrett mucosa, the greatest degree of atypia is seen in the crypt bases (*), with gradual diminution of nuclear size and progressive accumulation of cytoplasm as cells approach the surface, in keeping with a reactive process (B). Note also the lack of an abrupt transition between the reactive epithelium and the adjacent mucosa.

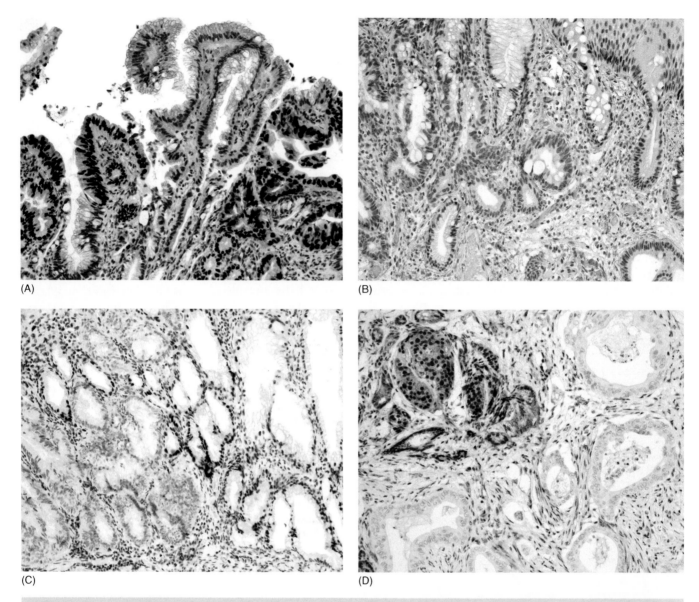

FIGURE 1.2 A p53 immunostain in an esophageal biopsy demonstrates abrupt transitions between foci of diffuse, strong staining in the nuclei of Barrett mucosa with high-grade dysplasia (likely due to *TP53* missense mutation) and focal weak or negative staining in the background Barrett epithelium without dysplasia (A). A p53 immunostain demonstrates the abrupt transition between foci of completely absent staining in dysplastic Barrett epithelium (likely due to *TP53* deletion or truncating mutation) and moderately intense (wild-type pattern) staining in non-dysplastic Barrett mucosa and adjacent squamous epithelium (B). Clonal loss of MLH1 expression corresponding to the acquisition of cytologic dysplasia in a background of sessile serrated polyp (C). Clonal loss of SMAD4 expression in a pancreatic ductal adenocarcinoma, compared to intact expression in stroma and adjacent non-neoplastic islets and ductules (D).

in 1983, remains a seminal reference work in GI pathology. This classification forms the foundation of dysplasia assessment in Western GI pathology, and has been adopted for columnar lesions throughout the tubal gut.

Whereas previously dysplasia was graded as mild, moderate, or severe, the IBD-DMSG introduced the categories "negative for dysplasia," "indefinite for dysplasia," and "positive for dysplasia." The "positive for dysplasia" group is subdivided into "low-grade dysplasia (LGD)" and "high-grade dysplasia (HGD)". Due to their work and the

recognition of the limits of interobserver reproducibility, the "mild, moderate, severe" classification scheme has been largely discarded and is no longer appropriate for grading dysplasia in the tubal gut. Grading of dysplasia will be discussed in more detail in the organ-specific chapters that follow.

By including "indefinite for dysplasia," the group formally recognized diagnostic uncertainty in the form of lesions that could not be readily classified as negative or positive. In clinical practice, when a lesion is worrisome

TABLE 1.1   Key Features of the Inflammatory Bowel Disease-Dysplasia Morphology Study Group Classification of Dysplasia

Defined dysplasia as "unequivocally neoplastic epithelium"
As a consequence, the term "atypia" could no longer be used synonymously with dysplasia
Established the category of indefinite for dysplasia
Established the categories of low-grade dysplasia and high-grade dysplasia and made provisional clinical recommendations based on these diagnoses
Recommended seeking a second opinion in diagnostically challenging cases
Contained an interobserver variability study
Provided an atlas of 84 images
Stated that low-grade dysplasia could directly give rise to adenocarcinoma

for dysplasia but is very focal, there is significant background inflammation, or the transition between the lesion and adjacent non-neoplastic mucosa is not well-visualized, the term "indefinite for dysplasia" is appropriate.

Another key goal of the group was to create a classification scheme that was clinically actionable. The group made provisional clinical recommendations based on their classification that, for dysplasia in IBD, have largely stood the test of time. Recommendations included short interval follow-up for diagnoses of LGD or indefinite for dysplasia, and consideration of colectomy for HGD. The results of the interobserver variability component of the group's work highlighted the importance of seeking a second opinion in diagnostically challenging cases, which is emphasized today in multidisciplinary medical position statements/practice guidelines regarding the management of Barrett esophagus and IBD. The contributions of the IBD-DMSG are summarized in Table 1.1.

Dysplasia detected at an index examination (or within 1 year) is referred to as "prevalent," while that detected in the context of surveillance is "incident." The natural history of prevalent dysplasia appears more aggressive than incident dysplasia.

Alternative Classifications

Western pathologists generally use a modified IBD-DMSG definition of dysplasia that defines it as a "*pre-invasive* unequivocal neoplastic epithelial proliferation." When used as such, dysplasia is a carcinoma precursor. The third edition of the *WHO Classification of Tumours of the Digestive System* (*WHO GI Blue Book*) introduced the generally synonymous term "intraepithelial neoplasia," and an alternative international consensus classification known as the Vienna system refers to "non-invasive neoplasia." For practical purposes, this textbook will refer to "dysplasia" throughout, except in the anus, where intraepithelial neoplasia (anal intraepithelial neoplasia [AIN]) has gained more widespread usage.

Carcinoma In Situ and Intramucosal Carcinoma

Historically, carcinoma in situ (CIS) generally refers to a tumor that is "cytologically malignant" but has yet to breach the basement membrane. As such, it has no metastatic potential, and is essentially equivalent to dysplasia. Theoretically, CIS is considered "more advanced" than HGD, but the distinction between these entities is not reproducible. Some authors have also used CIS to refer to tumors without metastatic potential, regardless of whether or not they are confined to the basement membrane (this broader definition encompasses colonic tumors that have invaded into but not beyond the mucosa). Again, given the lack of reproducibility in distinguishing HGD and CIS, compounded by the ambiguity of meaning, use of the term "carcinoma in situ" in reporting specimens from the tubal gut is strongly discouraged.

In intramucosal carcinoma (IMC), tumor cells have breached the basement membrane to invade into, but not beyond, the mucosa. This includes tumors that have invaded into the lamina propria and those that have invaded into, but not through, the muscularis mucosae. In the esophagus and stomach, IMC is associated with a small but definite risk of lymph node metastasis (4% or less) and is staged as T1a (as are small intestinal adenocarcinomas). In contrast, in the colon, IMC is not associated with lymph node metastasis and, thus, is staged as Tis (as are appendiceal tumors). Because the distinction of IMC from HGD in the colon is not as biologically meaningful as it is in the upper GI tract, some pathologists avoid this term and do not diagnose IMC in the colon.

Similar to the grading of dysplasia, the diagnosis of IMC is subject to significant interobserver variability. Cases in which single cells or small groups of cells are present in the lamina propria are readily recognized as IMC (Figure 1.3A), as are those characterized by large expanses of anastomosing glands (Figure 1.3B) or sheets of cells. Since IMC is defined by tumor cells having breached the basement membrane, and pathologists do not directly visualize that breach, the degree of architectural perturbation that is required to distinguish a small focus of IMC from HGD is not well defined (Figure 1.4). Two groups have published criteria for a category intermediate between HGD and IMC, referred to as "high-grade dysplasia with marked glandular architectural distortion, cannot exclude intramucosal carcinoma" and "high-grade dysplasia with features 'suspicious' for invasive carcinoma." These concepts will be discussed further in Chapter 7.

As with the distinction of dysplasia from reactive changes, the concept of clonality is again applicable to grading dysplasia and distinguishing HGD from early carcinoma; the notion of "neoplastic progression" is additionally useful. As one considers the diagnosis of HGD, it is useful if one can identify a specific area that is cytologically and/ or architecturally distinct from the background LGD (ie, a

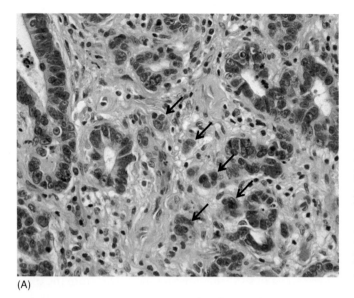
(A)

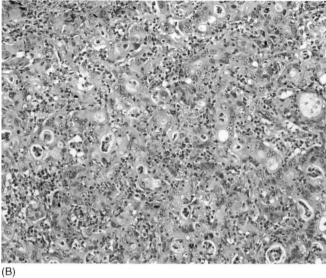
(B)

FIGURE 1.3 Intramucosal carcinoma is readily diagnosed when single cells or small groups of cells (arrows) are visualized in the lamina propria (A) or in the setting of an expansive anastomosing gland pattern (the so-called never-ending gland pattern) (B). These examples are from Barrett esophagus-associated neoplasms.

clonal area that has progressed) (Figure 1.5). This assumes, of course, confidence in the underlying diagnosis of dysplasia, and one may not always have the luxury of a background of LGD (although it is nearly always present in an adenomatous colon polyp with HGD). A similar approach may be used when one is considering a diagnosis of IMC in a background of HGD in the setting of Barrett esophagus.

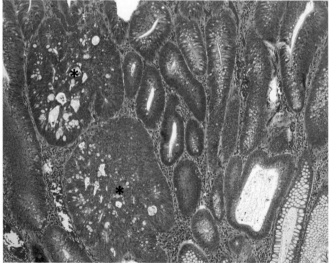

FIGURE 1.5 The right half of this mucosal biopsy specimen shows low-grade dysplasia. The discrete foci of more complex, cribriformed architecture (*) on the left are characteristic of a higher-grade lesion.

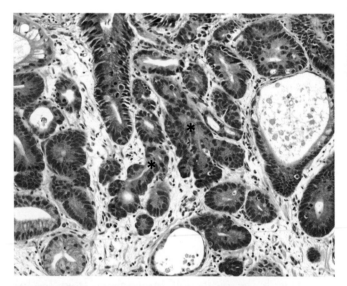

FIGURE 1.4 This focus of dysplastic Barrett epithelium shows at least high-grade dysplasia, and some would consider the degree of gland branching and budding (*) compatible with intramucosal carcinoma. The dilated glands with intraluminal debris also suggest a more advanced lesion.

Discrepancies Between Western and Eastern Neoplasia Assessment

The histologic features of LGD and HGD presented here and in subsequent chapters, and the concept that invasion defines carcinoma, represent distinctly Western viewpoints. It has long been recognized that many lesions classified as LGD or HGD by Western pathologists are diagnosed as early carcinomas by Japanese pathologists.

While Western pathologists seek "objective" evidence of invasion to secure a diagnosis of carcinoma, Japanese pathologists place greater weight on nuclear and architectural features, and, actually arrive at a diagnosis of carcinoma independent of the presence of invasion. These very different approaches to diagnosis profoundly affect the comparability of the incidence and survival rates for early carcinoma in Western and Japanese series (this applies mainly to gastric cancer, since Barrett-associated neoplasia is rare in Japan and colonic IMC lacks the capacity to metastasize). This textbook will reflect the Western viewpoint throughout because it is the one we have learned, the one we apply in our practices, and the one upon which Western clinical guidelines are based.

Submucosally Invasive Carcinoma

Once tumors invade beyond the muscularis mucosae, they initially encounter the submucosa, and are thus submucosally invasive. As the submucosa is frequently not well-represented in endoscopic mucosal biopsy material, this diagnosis can be challenging. In cases where the boundary between the mucosa and submucosa is not readily apparent, there are two histologic clues that suggest a diagnosis of submucosal invasion. First, the presence of desmoplastic (ie, cellular, fibroblastic, often blue-tinged) stroma strongly correlates with the presence of submucosal invasion (Figures 1.6A–B). Second, one can search for the close approximation of neoplastic epithelium to thick-walled, muscular submucosal blood vessels. These vessels are readily apparent in endoscopic mucosal resections (Figure 1.7A) and can usually be identified in well-oriented polypectomy specimens of larger, pedunculated

lesions (Figure 1.7B). A desmin immunostain can also help define the boundaries of the muscularis mucosae (as well as the muscularis propria), which is especially useful in cases where the microanatomy is obscured by fibrosis or inflammation (Figure 1.8A–B). This is less helpful in cases that are tangentially embedded.

GRADING AND STAGING OF GASTROINTESTINAL MALIGNANCIES

Tumor Grading

Tumor grading has traditionally represented an assessment of how well (or poorly) a given tumor resembles the normal tissue type it recapitulates (ie, differentiation). This assessment is inherently qualitative. For some tumor types, grading has incorporated more objective, reproducible features (eg, mitotic rate). Grade is prognostically significant and in many instances influences clinical management. For example, in pT3 N0 colon cancer, patients with poorly differentiated/high-grade tumors may be offered adjuvant chemotherapy, and patients with resected high-risk GISTs generally receive adjuvant tyrosine kinase inhibitor therapy. In addition, chemotherapy regimens are entirely different for low-grade versus high-grade lymphomas and well-differentiated NETs versus neuroendocrine carcinomas (NECs). Table 1.2 compares the grading of the major categories of tumor in the tubal gut.

For non-neuroendocrine carcinomas of the tubal gut, mainly adenocarcinomas and squamous cell carcinomas, there is no uniformly agreed upon, extensively clinically validated grading system as there is in breast (Nottingham

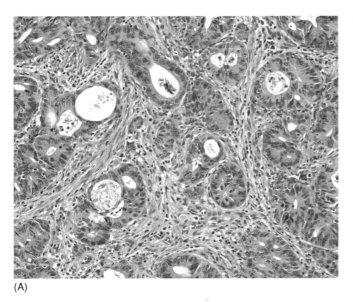

(A)

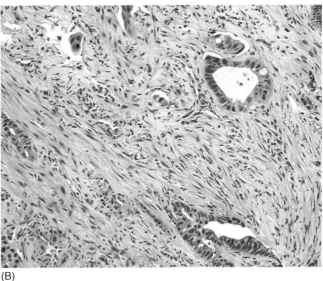

(B)

FIGURE 1.6 Stromal desmoplasia is an indicator of submucosal invasion. These are two examples of desmoplastic stroma, one more cellular (A) and the other more fibrotic (B).

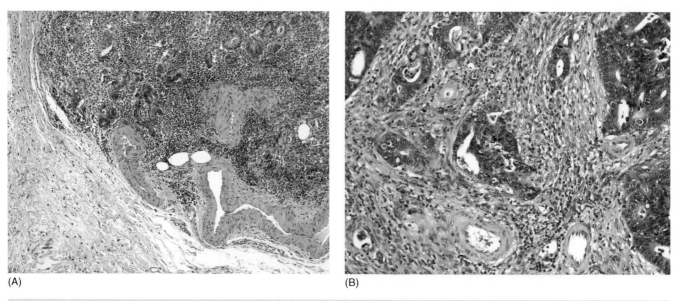

FIGURE 1.7 Barrett esophagus-associated adenocarcinoma (A) and adenocarcinoma arising in an adenomatous polyp (B) each infiltrate up to and around thick-walled muscular blood vessels, suggesting a diagnosis of submucosal invasion. Stromal desmoplasia is also seen in (B).

grade), kidney (Fuhrman grade), or prostate (Gleason grade). For adenocarcinomas of the colon and rectum, the WHO suggests that tumors may be graded based on the extent of gland formation, although this only applies to "adenocarcinoma, NOS" (ie, adenocarcinoma with no special morphologic features). Throughout the tubal gut, grading may be two-, three-, or four-tiered, with two-tiered grading (high-grade versus low-grade) increasingly advocated based on greater reproducibility and clinical utility.

Tumor grading will be discussed in greater detail in the organ-specific chapters.

The grading system for neuroendocrine neoplasms is entirely different from that used for non-neuroendocrine tumors. In the World Health Organization (WHO) 2010 Classification, gastroenteropancreatic neuroendocrine epithelial neoplasms are graded based on mitotic rate and Ki-67 proliferation index. In this system, morphologically well-differentiated neuroendocrine neoplasms are referred

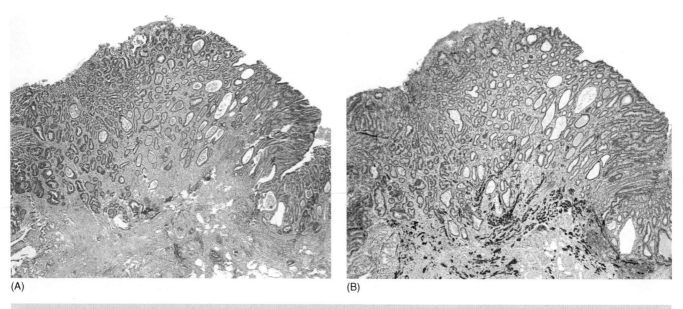

FIGURE 1.8 While this Barrett esophagus-associated adenocarcinoma was suspicious for invasion into the superficial submucosa (A), a desmin immunostain clarified that, at its deepest point, the tumor is confined by strands of muscularis mucosae (B).

TABLE 1.2   Tumor Grading in the Tubal Gut

Epithelial Neoplasms, Non-Neuroendocrine

Grade (Four-Tiered)	Grade (Two-Tiered)	% Gland Formation: Adenocarcinomas	Qualitative Features: Squamous Cell Carcinoma
Well-differentiated	Low-grade	>95%	Prominent keratinization with squamous pearl formation
Moderately differentiated	Low-grade	50%–95%	Less frequent keratinization; squamous pearls generally absent
Poorly differentiated	High-grade	>0%–49%	Predominance of basal-like cells; few, if any, keratinized cells
Undifferentiated	High-grade	Not applicable	Not applicable

Neuroendocrine Epithelial Neoplasms

Qualitative Grade (Two-Tiered)	WHO 2010 Grade (Three-Tiered)	Mitotic Rate		Proliferation Index (Ki-67 Labeling)
Well-differentiated	G1	<2 per 10 HPF	and/or	≤2%
	G2	2–20 per 10 HPF		3%–20%
Poorly differentiated	G3	>20 per 10 HPF		>20%

Lymphomas: Grade is Based on Tumor Type

Grade (Two-Tiered)   Representative Tumor Types
Low-grade   Extranodal marginal zone lymphoma of mucosa-associated lymphoid tissue (MALT lymphoma), mantle
                            cell lymphoma, follicular lymphoma
High-grade   Diffuse large B-cell lymphoma, Burkitt lymphoma

Gastrointestinal Stromal Tumor

Grade (Two-Tiered)   Mitotic Rate
Low-grade (G1)   ≤5 per 5 mm^2
High-grade (G2)   >5 per 5 mm^2

Sarcoma: Fédération Nationale des Centre de Lutte Contre le Cancer (FNCLCC) System

Grade (Three-Tiered)	Total Score	Tumor Differentiation	Mitotic Count	Tumor Necrosis
Grade 1	2 or 3	1: Closely resembles normal tissue	1: 0–9 per 10 HPF	0: None
Grade 2	4 or 5	2: Histologic typing certain	2: 10–19 per 10 HPF	1: <50%
Grade 3	6, 7, or 8	3: Embryonal and undifferentiated sarcomas, synovial sarcoma, sarcomas of uncertain type	3: >19 per 10 HPF	2: ≥50%

to as "neuroendocrine tumors (NETs)," while poorly differentiated examples (small cell and large cell) are termed "neuroendocrine carcinomas (NECs)." NETs with a low mitotic rate (less than 2 per 10 high-power fields [HPFs]) and proliferation index (2% or less) are considered G1, while those with a mitotic rate between 2 and 20 per 10 HPF and/or a proliferation index of 3% to 20% are G2. NECs (G3 in this classification) demonstrate more than 20 mitotic figures per 10 HPF and/or a proliferation index greater than 20%. This classification supplants the WHO 2000 Classification, in which well-differentiated tumors were "graded" based on the absence (well-differentiated endocrine tumor) or presence (well-differentiated endocrine carcinoma) of metastases and/or gross local invasion,

with the former category further stratified based on the following parameters: size, angioinvasion, perineural invasion (PNI), mitotic count, and Ki-67 proliferation index. Of note, the current mitotic threshold for G3/NEC (greater than 20 per 10 HPF) is greater than in the 2000 system (greater than 10 per 10 HPF). Rarely, morphologically well-differentiated tumors demonstrate a mitotic rate and/or proliferation index in the G3 range; these behave somewhat better than typical, poorly differentiated G3 tumors.

Tumor type largely defines the grade (low vs. high grade) in lymphoma. Follicular lymphoma (FL) can be further graded based on the number of centroblasts in neoplastic follicles per HPF, based on an assessment of at least 10 HPFs. In the *2008 WHO Classification of Tumours of Haematopoietic and Lymphoid Tissues*, the separation of grade 1 from grade 2 FL is discouraged, as this is not a clinically meaningful distinction. The presence of diffuse architecture distinguishes diffuse large B-cell lymphoma (DLBCL) from FL, grade 3. Grading of GI lymphomas will be further discussed in Chapter 4.

GISTs are graded based on mitotic rate. Low-grade/G1 tumors demonstrate 5 or fewer mitotic figures per 5 mm^2, while high-grade/G2 tumors contain 5 or more mitotic figures per 5 mm^2. Grade, tumor size, and anatomic location are combined to determine the overall "risk assessment" in GIST (none, very low risk, low risk, intermediate risk, high risk, overtly malignant/metastatic), which correlates with the likelihood of metastasis or tumor-related death. Of special note, mitotic rates in GIST were historically described in relation to 50 HPFs. It was recently discovered that the microscopes used to count mitotic figures in the initial clinical studies that form the evidence basis of the risk assessment had much smaller field areas than most modern microscopes. For many modern microscopes, 5 mm^2 is equal to approximately 20 high-power (40×) fields. Grading of mesenchymal tumors will be discussed in more detail in Chapter 5.

For sarcomas, the American Joint Committee on Cancer (AJCC), the College of American Pathologists (CAP), and the WHO each advocate use of the Fédération Nationale de Centre de Lutte Contre le Cancer (FNCLCC) grading system. Tumors are assessed for differentiation, mitotic rate, and tumor necrosis. Each of these three parameters is given a score, and the overall grade is assigned based on the sum of the scores. FNCLCC grade correlates with metastatic risk and overall survival, while adequacy of excision is a better predictor of local recurrence.

Tumor Staging

Historically, tumor stage has represented the anatomic extent of disease. It is typically expressed in the form of the tumor, node, metastasis (TNM) classification. Aside from tumor type, stage is the single most important determinant of an individual patient's therapy and prognosis. Accurate staging is also critical to the conduct of clinical trials and facilitates the comparison of cancer outcomes on large scales (eg, regionally, nationally, and internationally). The TNM Committee of the Union for International Cancer Control (UICC) and the AJCC work together to define T, N, and M stage categories and stage groups (also known as anatomic stage/prognostic groups) for each anatomic site. For a given site, any combination of T, N, and M can be expressed as an overall stage group (I through IV), with combinations of similar prognosis assigned to the same stage group (eg, T4a N1 M0 and T1 N2b M0 colon cancers are each considered stage IIIB disease).

The UICC/AJCC Classification is periodically revised (most recently at 6–8-year intervals), increasingly based on large, population-based clinical datasets. The AJCC first published a staging manual in 1977; the *AJCC Cancer Staging Manual* is now in its seventh edition (*AJCC 7*). This classification went into effect on January 1, 2010. It includes, for the first time, TNM staging for GISTs and NETs. Appendiceal carcinomas, classified with colorectal tumors in the sixth edition, are now separately classified. For every site in the tubal gut (except the anal canal), various T, N, and M categories were redefined or subclassified and various stage groupings were reassigned. For pathologists, the most significant change to their routine practices was perhaps the creation of the N1c category in colon cancer, defined as the presence of "tumor deposit(s) in the subserosa, mesentery, or nonperitonealized pericolic or perirectal tissues without regional nodal metastasis" (discussed further in Chapter 11).

In the past, stage groupings at a given site in the tubal gut were determined exclusively by TNM. In *AJCC 7* this is no longer the case. The so-called nonanatomic factors, including tumor type, location within an organ, grade, and mitotic rate, affect staging at some sites (summarized in Table 1.3). Additional nonanatomic factors, including molecular-based ones, will have increasing influence on stage groupings going forward. For the foreseeable future, however, anatomic factors will continue to form the core of tumor staging, as they permit comparisons of stage data over time and because they are applicable to the majority of patients worldwide who may not have access to advanced medical technologies.

Clinical Versus Pathologic Staging

Clinical staging is performed at disease presentation, before definitive treatment, and takes into account data obtained by any combination of history and physical examination, diagnostic imaging, endoscopy, biopsy (of the primary tumor and/or a regional lymph node), and surgical exploration without resection. If a biopsy is performed, the pathologist's role in clinical staging is to confirm the presence of tumor, rather than to define its anatomic extent, the latter of which is based on nonpathologic information (eg, imaging results). Clinical staging provides an estimate of prognosis and, most importantly, determines the initial treatment course.

The pathologic stage is based mainly on histologic examination of a surgically resected specimen. This provides more precise prognostic information and informs the need for additional treatment (eg, adjuvant chemotherapy or radiation). The value of synoptic reporting as a tool to ensure completeness of reporting of pathologic stage and other clinically significant parameters will be discussed in the section on synoptic reporting.

TABLE 1.3 "Nonanatomic Factors" Influencing AJCC/UICC Tubal Gut Stage Groupings

Anatomic Site (or Tumor Type)	Factor	Notes
Esophagus	Tumor type	Separate stage groupings for squamous cell carcinoma (SCC) and adenocarcinoma (AdCa)
	Tumor location (ie, upper, middle, lower)	Applies to SCC
	Grade (ie, 1, 2, 3)	Applies to SCC and AdCa
Appendix	Grade (ie, 1, 2, 3)	Low-grade appendiceal mucinous neoplasm with extra-appendiceal spread is considered G1; separate stage groupings for G1 vs. G2/3 tumors with intraperitoneal metastasis beyond the right lower quadrant
Gastrointestinal stromal tumor (GIST)	Mitotic rate (ie, ≤5 per 5 mm^2 vs. >5 per 5 mm^2)	
	Tumor location (ie, stomach/omentum vs. small intestine/esophagus/colorectum/ mesentery/peritoneum)	Separate stage groupings for gastric/omental GISTs vs. nongastric/nonomental GISTs based on increased aggressiveness of the latter
Neuroendocrine tumor (NET)	Tumor location	Separate stage groupings for appendiceal NETs vs. all other tubal gut NETs
Stomach, small intestine, colon, and rectum	None	Stage groupings based purely on TNM

Staging After Neoadjuvant Therapy

Neoadjuvant therapy refers to the use of chemotherapy and radiation, either singly or in combination, *prior* to surgical resection. Adjuvant therapy refers to chemotherapy and/or radiation administered after the definitive surgical procedure. In the *adjuvant* setting, radiation is generally applied to improve local control, while chemotherapy is used to achieve a systemic effect. Chemotherapy may also sensitize the tumor to the effects of radiation. In the *neoadjuvant* setting, combined chemoradiotherapy aims to downstage tumors and treats occult metastatic disease. In some patients it converts locally advanced, unresectable tumors to resectable ones, and it may improve the resectability of "borderline-resectable" tumors. In patients who are marginal surgical candidates (eg, due to comorbid conditions), a period of neoadjuvant therapy may provide the opportunity for metastasis to declare itself, sparing these patients surgery from which they would not derive benefit.

Neoadjuvant chemoradiotherapy is the standard of care for clinical stage T3/4 rectal cancer, in which it has been proven in clinical trials to significantly decrease the risk of local recurrence (compared to adjuvant therapy). It is also generally applied in patients with clinical nodal disease. Neoadjuvant chemoradiotherapy is also the evolving standard of care for patients with clinical stage T2 or greater esophageal/gastroesophageal junction/proximal gastric cancers. Its application in distal gastric cancers is more variable. In addition, neoadjuvant imatinib therapy may be used in locally advanced and/or high-risk GISTs.

Pathologic staging after neoadjuvant therapy is designated by the prefix "y" (ie, ypTNM). The use of this symbol is a vital component of accurate staging. For example, the prognosis of a patient with pT2 N0 disease may be very different than that of a patient with ypT2 N0 disease, who may have had clinically positive lymph nodes at presentation. Furthermore, for the purpose of research, these stages are not comparable. The ypTNM stage is based on the extent of viable tumor. Evidence of regressed tumor in the form of fibrosis, calcifications, and acellular mucin pools does not affect stage. Significant tumor regression in the face of neoadjuvant therapy may be associated with improved prognosis. Assessment of treatment effect after neoadjuvant therapy is a CAP required data element for carcinomas of the esophagus, stomach, pancreas, colorectum, and anal canal; assessment in GIST is optional, with a recommendation to report the percentage of viable tumor. There are several published regression grading systems, including three-, four-, and five-tiered examples. The *CAP Cancer Protocols* include a four-tiered example (see Table 1.4). This is discussed in more detail in Chapter 11.

TABLE 1.4 Tumor Regression Grading in Neoadjuvant Treated Tumors (Four-Tiered)

Grade	Histologic Description
0 (complete response)	No residual viable tumor
1 (moderate response)	Single cells or small groups of tumor cells
2 (minimal response)	Residual tumor outgrown by fibrosis
3 (poor response)	Little or no tumor kill; extensive residual tumor

SYNOPTIC VERSUS NARRATIVE REPORTING

For cancer resections, synoptic reporting (also known as checklist-based, template-driven, and pro forma reporting) has largely supplanted traditional narrative (ie, free-text) reporting. Multiple published studies have shown that synoptic reporting improves the completeness (and thus the prognostic and therapeutic relevance) of cancer reporting. A 1991 CAP Q-Probes Quality Improvement Study, based on data from 15,940 reports of resected primary colorectal cancers from 532 laboratories, related the completeness of reporting for 11 gross and microscopic parameters to: (a) use of a cancer checklist; (b) use of a microscopic description; (c) teaching institution status; (d) whether the institution had a pathology residency; and (e) bed size. The use of a cancer checklist was the single most important predictor of completeness of reporting, statistically significant for 8 of 11 parameters. Interestingly, at that time, only 12.5% of the 532 laboratories surveyed employed synoptic reporting.

More contemporary data demonstrating the significance of the adoption of synoptic reporting in an individual laboratory are presented in Table 1.5. Messenger and colleagues found synoptic reporting to significantly increase the completeness of reporting for 7 of 10 data elements in a series of 498 rectal cancer resections. Several of these increases are quite dramatic and affect parameters that are highly clinically actionable, such as lymphovascular invasion, perineural invasion, and tumor deposits. They also showed that while narrative reports from GI pathologists were more complete for the data elements lymphovascular invasion and extramural venous invasion, after the adoption of synoptic reporting, reports from non-GI and GI pathologists were equally complete. Furthermore, detection rates for lymphovascular invasion, perineural invasion, and extramural venous invasion dramatically increased (tripled to quadrupled) with the advent of synoptic reporting, presumably because pathologists prompted by checklist items performed more diligent searches for these features.

Synoptic reporting also increases the clarity of reporting, and thus the effectiveness of communication, between the pathologist and the treating clinicians. Sheldon Markel and Samuel Hirsch, credited with coining the term "synoptic reporting," expressed frustration over the disconnect between their perception of carefully crafted "conventional paragraphic" reports and occasional dissatisfaction with these reports by their clinicians, stating, "To our chagrin, surgeons and other clinicians frequently questioned why certain information, which was actually in the body or our reports, was not." Synoptic reports also facilitate data mining and reporting to cancer registries.

Not surprisingly, the quality of oncology reporting is of interest to laboratory accrediting bodies. The *CAP Laboratory Accreditation Program Anatomic Pathology Checklist* includes the Phase II requirement that "All data elements required in applicable *CAP Cancer Protocols* are included in the surgical pathology report." (Phase II deficiencies on inspection require a written response *and* documentation demonstrating compliance.) Furthermore, the required data elements must relate to the current edition of the protocols, with an 8-month grace period. The American College of Surgeons Commission on Cancer (CoC), which accredits cancer programs, similarly mandates the inclusion of *CAP Cancer Protocol* required data elements in surgical pathology reports. While neither the CAP nor the CoC dictates the specific use of the *CAP Cancer Protocols*, but rather that reports contain the required data elements from those protocols, *AJCC 7* specifically recommends the use of *CAP Cancer Protocols* for pathology reporting.

The *CAP Cancer Protocols* were originally developed in 1989 and are frequently updated by the CAP Cancer Committee and CAP Cancer Protocol Review Panels. At the time of writing this chapter, all the protocols relevant to the

TABLE 1.5   Effect of Report Format on Reporting of Data Elements

Parameter	Report Format		*P* Value
	Narrative (n = 183), % Complete	Synoptic (n = 315), % Complete	
Tumor size	99	99	NS
TNM stage	24	96	<0.001
Tumor type	99	99	NS
Tumor grade	92	98	0.004
Circumferential/radial margin (CRM) status	100	100	NS
Distance to CRM	86	97	<0.001
Lymphovascular invasion	39	98	<0.001
Extramural venous invasion	41	97	<0.001
Perineural invasion	14	94	<0.001
Regional deposits	13	83	<0.001

Source: Messenger DE, McLeod RS, Kirsch R. What impact has the introduction of a synoptic report for rectal cancer had on reporting outcomes for specialist gastrointestinal and nongastrointestinal pathologists? *Arch Pathol Lab Med*. 2011 Nov;135(11):1471–1475.

TABLE 1.6   College of American Pathologists Required Data Elements for Carcinomas and Neuroendocrine Tumors of the Tubal Gut, Regardless of Anatomic Site

Specimen (ie, organs received)
Procedure
Tumor site
Tumor size
Histologic type
Histologic grade
Microscopic tumor extension
Margin status
Distance to closest margin, if uninvolved
Treatment effect*
Lymphovascular invasion**
Number of regional lymph nodes examined and involved***
Pathologic staging (pTNM)

*not mentioned in appendix checklist
**not required for anal canal
***applies to resections

tubal gut had been updated within the prior 4 months. The protocols contain both "required" and "not required" data elements, the latter denoted by a "+." The required data elements are considered essential for cancer care and have a strong evidence base. A summary of required data elements common to all the checklists germane to this textbook is presented in Table 1.6. At each anatomic site, there may be additionally required data elements (eg, perineural invasion in colon cancer, mitotic rate per 10 HPF in NETs, risk assessment in GIST), which will be further discussed in subsequent chapters. Nonrequired elements have less data to support them or are less routinely used in patient care (eg, histologic features suggestive of microsatellite instability [MSI] in colon cancer, tumor necrosis in NET, treatment effect in GIST).

Further information about synoptic reporting is available in the following document:

www.cap.org/apps/docs/committees/cancer/cancer_protocols/synoptic_report_definition_and_examples.pdf. Finally, the *CAP Cancer Protocols* are accessible online in PDF and Word format at the CAP website through the "Reference Resources and Publications" tab.

PROGNOSTIC AND PREDICTIVE MARKERS

Prognostic Markers

A prognostic marker provides information that allows one to make a probabilistic statement about a patient's anticipated disease course. Although we typically think of these in the setting of overt malignancies (eg, tumor grade, microscopic tumor extension, presence or absence of lymphovascular invasion), the presence of Barrett esophagus, the extent of a patient's chronic colitis, the absence or presence and grade of flat dysplasia, and the number and size of neoplastic colon polyps can all be considered prognostic markers. Many prognostic markers are directly clinically

actionable (eg, influence decision to place a patient into surveillance and determine surveillance intensity; inform decision to give adjuvant chemotherapy), emphasizing the importance of accuracy of assessment and completeness of reporting. This textbook will specifically highlight issues related to the pathologic assessment of the most clinically significant prognostic markers.

Predictive Markers

Predictive markers provide information about whether a given patient will (or will not) respond to a specific therapy. Estrogen receptor and HER2 status in breast cancer represent the most well-known examples. At present, there are four main clinical applications of predictive markers in the GI tract:

1. HER2 testing to select patients for anti-HER2 therapy in advanced esophageal, gastroesophageal, and gastric adenocarcinoma;
2. *KRAS* mutation testing (and in some instances, assessment of related molecular markers) to determine the appropriateness of anti-EGFR (epidermal growth factor receptor) therapy in metastatic colorectal cancer;
3. DNA mismatch repair function testing (ie, mismatch repair protein immunohistochemistry and/or MSI testing) in colorectal cancer to inform the decision regarding adjuvant chemotherapy in stage II disease;
4. *KIT* and *PDGFRA* mutation analysis in GIST to predict response to specific tyrosine kinase inhibitors.

Predictive marker assays are generally held to a "higher standard," in terms of clinical validation and reporting than are purely diagnostic markers. These four sets of markers will be discussed further in the relevant organ-specific chapters, as well as Chapters 13 and 14.

SCREENING AND SURVEILLANCE

Screening

Screening refers to an effort to identify early, treatable disease in asymptomatic individuals. In the setting of neoplasia, the goal is to identify lesions at risk for neoplastic progression or early, treatable cancers. Screening may be undertaken in "average-risk" individuals or targeted to specific at-risk groups, based on factors such as the disease burden in the population and a precursor lesion's risk for neoplastic progression. These data, along with the availability of good screening tests and the cost of a screening program to the population, are considered in the construction of clinical guidelines.

As an example, the lifetime risk of developing colon cancer is 5% to 6%, with more than 90% of new diagnoses and cancer deaths occurring in patients over age 50. Cancer arises in neoplastic polyps, with a fairly long interval between a polyp becoming macroscopically evident and progression to cancer. Several reasonably sensitive tests exist to identify polyps or early cancers (eg, flexible sigmoidoscopy, colonoscopy, and/or fecal occult blood test), and polypectomy or treatment of early cancers has been proven to lead to decreased mortality from colon cancer. In this setting, the United States Preventative Services Task Force, the American Cancer Society (ACS), the American College of Radiology (ACR), and the United States Multi-Society Task Force (USMSTF; a collaboration between the American College of Gastroenterology, the American Society for Gastrointestinal Endoscopy [ASGE], and the American Gastroenterological Association [AGA]) each recommend colorectal cancer screening in average-risk individuals beginning at age 50. Screening recommendations are modifiable based on the presence of additional risk factors. In patients with colon cancer or adenomatous polyps diagnosed in a first-degree relative 60 years or older or with colorectal cancer diagnosed in two second-degree relatives, an ACS/USMSTF/ACR guideline recommends that screening commence at age 40.

In contrast, the lifetime risk of developing esophageal adenocarcinoma is only 0.5%. Cancer arises in Barrett esophagus, which is found in 1% to 2% of the general population and up to 10% of patients with chronic gastroesophageal reflux disease (GERD) (by comparison, 30% of average-risk patients 50 years or older will have polyps at an index colonoscopy). The risk of progression from Barrett esophagus to adenocarcinoma is reportedly 0.25%

or less per year. Barrett esophagus is not as amenable to eradication as are neoplastic colon polyps, and endoscopic ablative techniques are associated with a significant risk of stricture. Up to half of the patients presenting with esophageal adenocarcinoma do not report a history of GERD symptoms. Fifty to sixty percent of patients present with locally advanced or metastatic disease, and even in patients with localized disease, the 5-year survival is less than 40% (though substantially better in patients with T1 and especially T1a disease). Thus, in the general population, the costs associated with screening for esophageal adenocarcinoma clearly outweigh the benefits. In a 2011 medical position statement, the AGA recommended screening for Barrett esophagus specifically in patients with multiple risk factors associated with esophageal adenocarcinoma (age 50 years and above, male, Caucasian, chronic GERD, hiatal hernia, elevated body mass index, and intra-abdominal distribution of body fat), in whom the benefits of screening would appear to outweigh the costs. Table 1.7 summarizes GI conditions in which screening may be considered, the means of screening, the lesion the screening test aims to detect, and relevant expert guidelines.

Surveillance

Surveillance refers to testing in patients with "at-risk" lesions with the goal of identifying more advanced lesions or

TABLE 1.7   Screening for Neoplasia in the Tubal Gut

Underlying Condition	Procedure	Target Lesion	Comment(s)	Reference*
Gastroesophageal reflux disease (GERD)	Upper endoscopy	Barrett esophagus, prevalent dysplasia	In patients with multiple risk factors for esophageal adenocarcinoma (ie, age ≥ 50, male, White, chronic GERD, hiatal hernia, elevated body mass index, intra-abdominal distribution of body fat) Screening not recommended in general population with GERD	AGA 2011
Pernicious anemia (autoimmune atrophic gastritis)		Intestinal metaplasia, prevalent dysplasia, neuroendocrine proliferations	Insufficient data to support routine surveillance after single endoscopy	ASGE 2006
Long-standing idiopathic inflammatory bowel disease	Colonoscopy	Colitis, prevalent dysplasia	To determine if disease extent warrants surveillance	AGA 2010
Primary sclerosing cholangitis				
Age ≥ 50 years in patients with average colon cancer risk	Multiple options including flexible sigmoidoscopy, colonoscopy, double contrast barium enema, computed tomography colonography, fecal occult blood test, fecal immunochemical test, or stool DNA test	Adenoma and sessile serrated polyp, early colon cancer	Positive screening tests are followed up with colonoscopy	ACS/ USMSTF/ ACR 2008
Age 40 years in patients with a family history of colon cancer/polyps (defined here as colon cancer or adenomas in a first-degree relative ≥ age 60 or two second-degree relatives with colon cancer)				

*references available in the Screening and Surveillance section of the references

early, treatable cancers. It is the presence of a baseline "at-risk" lesion that distinguishes surveillance from screening. The "at-risk" lesion may represent an inflammatory condition, neoplasm, known germline mutation, or even a family history highly suspicious for a family cancer syndrome. Patients with a positive screening test are typically entered into surveillance. (A positive fecal occult blood test is an exception; it is followed up with colonoscopy, and patients may be entered into surveillance based on the results of this second test.) For example, if a patient with chronic GERD and the multiple risk factors for esophageal adenocarcinoma discussed previously undergoes screening endoscopy, the detection of Barrett esophagus (the "at-risk" lesion) would dictate patient placement into endoscopic surveillance. Patients in whom the "at-risk" lesion is genetic are generally placed directly into surveillance, without first undergoing screening. For example, in a patient with a known germline mutation in a DNA mismatch repair gene (ie, Lynch syndrome), surveillance colonoscopy, at an interval of 1 to 2 years, should commence at age 20 to 25, or 10 years earlier than the youngest colon cancer in the immediate family. Another characteristic of surveillance is that the intensity (ie, the surveillance interval and, in some instances, the number of biopsies) is adjusted based on biopsy results. For example, for the patient with chronic GERD and Barrett esophagus discussed previously, the finding of no dysplasia on biopsy might dictate a surveillance interval of 3 to 5 years with four-quadrant biopsies taken every 2 cm of metaplasia (as recommended in a recent AGA guideline), while follow-up in 6 to 12 months with biopsies every 1 cm would be recommended, given a biopsy finding of LGD.

Major indications for GI surveillance are listed in Table 1.8. The ones most frequently encountered include Barrett esophagus, extensive IBD, and precancerous colon polyps.

GENERAL APPROACH TO THE BIOPSY SPECIMEN

When faced with a biopsy specimen, the pathologist should seek the answers to a series of questions. Patient age, gender, and the clinical indication for the biopsy inform the further evaluation of the specimen.

First, is the tissue normal or abnormal? If the tissue is apparently normal, does that make clinical sense, and if not, would step sections be helpful? Step sections should be considered in many situations, particularly if the endoscopist saw a lesion or abnormality, yet the initial biopsy sections are normal.

If the tissue is abnormal, is the lesion inflammatory or neoplastic? The answer to this question is not always obvious. As discussed previously, neoplasms are clonal. As a consequence of this, pre-invasive epithelial neoplasms (dysplasias) are characterized by abrupt transitions from the non-neoplastic background. Epithelial lesions worrisome for dysplasia but for which the diagnosis cannot be made with certainty may be interpreted as "indefinite for dysplasia." The distinction of lymphoma from a reactive inflammatory process may require the demonstration of immunoglobulin heavy chain or T-cell receptor gene rearrangements or evidence of an aberrant immunophenotype.

If neoplastic, what is the tumor type? Primary considerations include epithelial (generally columnar or squamous), neuroendocrine, hematolymphoid, mesenchymal, melanocytic, mesothelial, and germ cell.

If the histogenesis is uncertain, could immunohistochemistry be helpful? For especially poorly differentiated tumors, broad spectrum keratins, LCA/CD45, and S100 are a useful start. Even if the broad tumor type is fairly certain (eg, lymphoma), immunohistochemistry may be useful to secure a more specific diagnosis (eg, demonstration of CD20 and cyclin D1 expression to support a diagnosis of mantle cell lymphoma).

If epithelial, is the lesion pre-invasive or invasive? Pre-invasive neoplasms are confined to the basement membrane. Single cells or small groups of cells, a never-ending gland pattern, and sheets of cells suggest invasion.

If pre-invasive, what is the grade of dysplasia? Two-tiered grading is recommended (low-grade or high-grade).

If invasive, what is the microscopic tumor extension? For columnar lesions, stromal desmoplasia and the juxtaposition of glands and thick-walled muscular blood vessels suggest a tumor is at least submucosally invasive.

Are there any other potentially clinically actionable histologic parameters that should be sought out? Tumor type and microscopic tumor extension are the key parameters. Additional features are important in select settings. For example, in polypectomy specimens of pedunculated adenomas in which an associated adenocarcinoma invades the stalk submucosa, tumor grade, LVI status, and margin status determine the adequacy of polypectomy versus the need for segmental colectomy.

Could the reporting of any additional histologic information be helpful to the clinician or to a pathologist interpreting a subsequent resection specimen from this patient? This is especially applicable to resections seen as intraoperative consultations. For example, a diagnosis of "invasive adenocarcinoma," though perhaps sufficient to drive neoadjuvant chemoradiotherapy and resection in esophageal carcinoma, is not as useful as one of "invasive adenocarcinoma, poorly differentiated, intestinal-type/tubular (or diffuse-type/poorly cohesive or mixed)," as signet ring cells, especially in small numbers, are notoriously difficult to interpret at a frozen section.

Finally, are any additional studies indicated on the biopsy material? For example, HER2 testing should be considered for esophageal/gastroesophageal/gastric adenocarcinomas; Ki-67 immunohistochemistry is necessary

TABLE 1.8   Surveillance for Neoplasms in the Tubal Gut

Condition	Qualifier	Surveillance Method	Surveillance Interval	Reference*
Barrett esophagus	No dysplasia	Upper endoscopy with random four-quadrant biopsies every 2 cm of Barrett length**	3–5 years	AGA 2011
	Indefinite for dysplasia	Not defined	Not defined	
	Low-grade dysplasia	Four-quadrant biopsies every 1 cm**	6–12 months	
	High-grade dysplasia	Four-quadrant biopsies every 1 cm**	3 months (strongly consider endoscopic eradication)	
History of caustic ingestion	Begin surveillance 15–20 years after ingestion	Upper endoscopy	1–3 years	ASGE 2006
Extensive inflammatory bowel disease (ie, left-sided, subtotal, or pan-ulcerative colitis; or Crohn's colitis involving at least one third of the colon)*** ****	No dysplasia	Colonoscopy with four-quadrant biopsy specimens approximately every 10 cm of colitic segment; 33 and 64 biopsy specimens detect dysplasia with 90% and 95% confidence, respectively; consider increased sampling (eg, every 5 cm) in rectosigmoid	1–3 years****	AGA 2010
	Indefinite for dysplasia		3–12 months	
	Polypoid low-grade dysplasia, adenoma-like		If entirely removed and no other flat dysplasia, regular or increased surveillance	
	Unifocal flat low-grade dysplasia		3–6 months (consider colectomy)	
	Multifocal flat low-grade dysplasia		3–6 months (consider colectomy)	
	Polypoid dysplasia, non-adenoma-like	Indication for colectomy		
	Flat high-grade dysplasia	Indication for colectomy		
Colon polyps at prior examination, otherwise average risk	Findings at baseline colonoscopy:	Colonoscopy with polypectomy		USMSTF 2012
	No polyps		10 years	
	Small (ie, <1 cm) rectosigmoid hyperplastic polyps		10 years	
	1–2 small tubular adenomas		5–10 years	
	3–10 tubular adenomas OR any adenoma ≥ 1 cm OR any adenoma with villous features OR any adenoma with high-grade dysplasia		3 years	
	>10 adenomas		<3 years	
	Sessile serrated polyp(s) <1 cm without cytologic dysplasia		5 years	
	Sessile serrated polyp(s) ≥1 cm OR with cytologic dysplasia OR Traditional serrated adenoma		3 years	
	Serrated polyposis syndrome		1 year	

(continued)

TABLE 1.8 Surveillance for Neoplasms in the Tubal Gut (*continued*)

Condition	Qualifier	Surveillance Method	Surveillance Interval	Reference*
Personal history of colon cancer	Patients should undergo removal of all polyps (perioperative clearing) within 6 months of surgery with curative intent	Colonoscopy with polypectomy	1 year from surgery or perioperative clearing; if negative, next examination at 3 years; if again negative, next at 5 years	ACS/ USMSTF/ ACR 2008
Strong family history*****	Colonoscopy beginning at 40 years or 10 years before the youngest case in the immediate family		5 years (or more frequent based on findings)	
Lynch syndrome	Colonoscopy beginning at 20–25 years or 10 years before the youngest case in the immediate family		1–2 years	

*references available in the Screening and Surveillance section of the references
**any mucosal abnormalities should be separately biopsied
***extent of disease is clarified at a screening endoscopy performed 8 years after onset of symptoms; patients with pancolitis and left-sided colitis are entered into surveillance within 1 to 2 years; patients with ulcerative proctitis, ulcerative proctosigmoiditis, and limited Crohn's colitis are not at increased risk of developing colon cancer and are managed as average risk (see table entry "Colon polyps")
****patients with primary sclerosing cholangitis should undergo screening colonoscopy at the time of that diagnosis, as patients may have long-standing subclinical IBD; for these patients entering surveillance, yearly colonoscopy (for no dysplasia) is recommended
*****defined here as colon cancer or adenomas in a first-degree relative [FDR] before age 60 or in 2 or more FDRs at any age

to accurately grade NETs; and mismatch repair protein immunohistochemistry should be considered for colorectal adenocarcinomas.

GENERAL APPROACH TO THE RESECTION SPECIMEN

Analogous to the approach to biopsy specimens described previously, evaluation should begin with patient age, gender, and the clinical indication for the procedure. Often, however, pathologists evaluating a resection specimen have access to the results of a diagnostic biopsy and all of the information that is included in that evaluation, which may make the evaluation of the resection specimen easier.

Given an established diagnosis, the first step in interpreting a resection specimen is to confirm that diagnosis. If available, review of prior diagnostic material is sometimes helpful. Once the diagnosis is confirmed, a systematic assessment of key histologic parameters, as represented by the required data elements of the appropriate synoptic reporting form, should be undertaken. As with biopsy specimens, additional immunohistochemical or molecular studies may be appropriate. For example, repeat HER2 testing may be considered on gastroesophageal adenocarcinomas as overexpression may be heterogeneous and, thus, not identified on a biopsy specimen. If a Ki-67 immunostain has been performed on the biopsy of a NET, repeat testing may again be useful, as the proliferation index may also be heterogeneous. MSI testing may be useful to confirm normal mismatch repair protein immunohistochemistry results,

as up to 5% of Lynch syndrome mutations abrogate protein function (resulting in MSI), while maintaining antigenicity (resulting in falsely normal immunohistochemistry results).

SELECTED REFERENCES

Key Terminology

Hanahan D, Weinberg RA. The hallmarks of cancer. *Cell*. 2000;100(1): 57–70. Epub 2000/01/27.

Hanahan D, Weinberg RA. Hallmarks of cancer: the next generation. *Cell*. 2011;144(5):646–674. Epub 2011/03/08.

Riddell RH, Goldman H, Ransohoff DF, et al. Dysplasia in inflammatory bowel disease: standardized classification with provisional clinical applications. *Hum Pathol*. 1983;14(11):931–968.

Schlemper RJ, Itabashi M, Kato Y, et al. Differences in diagnostic criteria for gastric carcinoma between Japanese and western pathologists. *Lancet*. 1997;349(9067):1725–1729.

Schlemper RJ, Kato Y, Stolte M. Review of histological classifications of gastrointestinal epithelial neoplasia: differences in diagnosis of early carcinomas between Japanese and Western pathologists. *J Gastroenterol*. 2001;36(7):445–456.

Willis RA. *The Spread of Tumours in the Human Body*. 2nd ed. London: Butterworth & Co; 1952.

Grading and Staging of Gastrointestinal Malignancies

Brierley JD, Greene FL, Sobin LH, Wittekind C. The "y" symbol: an important classification tool for neoadjuvant cancer treatment. *Cancer*. 2006;106(11):2526–2527.

Chang F, Deere H, Mahadeva U, George S. Histopathologic examination and reporting of esophageal carcinomas following preoperative neoadjuvant therapy: practical guidelines and current issues. *Am J Clin Pathol*. 2008;129(2):252–262.

College of American Pathologists. *Cancer Protocols and Checklists.* www.cap.org/cancerprotocols

Edge SB, Byrd DR, Compton CC, Fritz AG, Greene FL, Trotti A, eds. *AJCC Cancer Staging Manual.* 7th ed. New York, NY: Springer; 2010.

Fletcher CDM, Bridge JA, Hogendoorn PCW, Mertens F, eds. *WHO Classification of Tumours of Soft Tissue and Bone.* 4th ed. Lyon: IARC; 2013.

Markel SF, Hirsch SD. Synoptic surgical pathology reporting. *Hum Pathol.* 1991;22(8):807–810.

Messenger DE, McLeod RS, Kirsch R. What impact has the introduction of a synoptic report for rectal cancer had on reporting outcomes for specialist gastrointestinal and nongastrointestinal pathologists? *Arch Pathol Lab Med.* 2011;135(11):1471–1475.

Miettinen M, Lasota J. Gastrointestinal stromal tumors: pathology and prognosis at different sites. *Semin Diagn Pathol.* 2006;23(2):70–83.

Rindi G, Kloppel G, Alhman H, et al. TNM staging of foregut (neuro) endocrine tumors: a consensus proposal including a grading system. *Virchows Archiv.* 2006;449(4):395–401.

Ryan R, Gibbons D, Hyland JM, et al. Pathological response following long-course neoadjuvant chemoradiotherapy for locally advanced rectal cancer. *Histopathology.* 2005;47(2):141–146.

Swerdlow SH, Campo E, Harris NL, et al, eds. *WHO Classification of Tumours of Haematopoietic and Lymphoid Tissues.* 4th ed. Lyon: IARC; 2008.

Synoptic Versus Narrative Reporting

World Health Organization Classification of Tumours. *WHO Classification of Tumours of the Digestive System.* 4th ed. Bosman FT, Carneiro F, Hruban RH, Theise ND, eds. Lyon: IARC; 2010.

Zarbo RJ. Interinstitutional assessment of colorectal carcinoma surgical pathology report adequacy. A College of American Pathologists Q-Probes study of practice patterns from 532 laboratories and 15,940 reports. *Arch Pathol Lab Med.* 1992;116(11):1113–1119.

Prognostic and Predictive Markers

Bellizzi AM. Contributions of molecular analysis to the diagnosis and treatment of gastrointestinal neoplasms. *Semin Diagn Pathol.* 2013;30(4):329–361.

Screening and Surveillance

Farraye FA, Odze RD, Eaden J, et al. AGA medical position statement on the diagnosis and management of colorectal neoplasia in inflammatory bowel disease. *Gastroenterology.* 2010;138(2):738–745.

Farraye FA, Odze RD, Eaden J, Itzkowitz SH. AGA technical review on the diagnosis and management of colorectal neoplasia in inflammatory bowel disease. *Gastroenterology.* 2010;138(2):746–774, 74 e1–e4; quiz e12–e13.

Hirota WK, Zuckerman MJ, Adler DG, et al. ASGE guideline: the role of endoscopy in the surveillance of premalignant conditions of the upper GI tract. *Gastrointest Endosc.* 2006;63(4):570–580.

Levin B, Lieberman DA, McFarland B, et al. Screening and surveillance for the early detection of colorectal cancer and adenomatous polyps, 2008: *a joint guideline* from the American Cancer Society, the US Multi-Society Task Force on Colorectal Cancer, and the American College of Radiology. *Gastroenterology.* 2008;134(5):1570–1595.

Lieberman DA, Rex DK, Winawer SJ, Giardiello FM, Johnson DA, Levin TR. Guidelines for colonoscopy surveillance after screening and polypectomy: a consensus update by the US Multi-Society Task Force on Colorectal Cancer. *Gastroenterology.* 2012;143(3):844–857.

Spechler SJ, Sharma P, Souza RF, Inadomi JM, Shaheen NJ. American Gastroenterological Association medical position statement on the management of Barrett's esophagus. *Gastroenterology.* 2011;140(3):1084–1091.

2

Approach to Epithelial Neoplasms of the Gastrointestinal Tract

WEI CHEN AND WENDY L. FRANKEL

INTRODUCTION

The epithelial lining of the gastrointestinal (GI) tract provides an extremely large interface between the outside environment and the luminal surfaces of the GI tract (approximately 2,000,000 cm^2). Given the amount of epithelium required to create this interface, it is not surprising that the majority of gastrointestinal neoplasms are epithelial in origin.

EPIDEMIOLOGY

According to 2013 cancer statistics from the American Cancer Society, the five most common digestive system cancers in the United States, by decreasing incidence, are colorectal (49.2%), pancreatic (15.6%), liver/intrahepatic bile duct (13.9%), gastric (7.4%), and esophageal (6.2%). These account for 35.2%, 26.6%, 15.0%, 7.6%, and 10.5% of GI cancer-related deaths, respectively. The male to female ratios for these cancers are 1.1:1 (colorectal), 1:1 (pancreatic), 2.9:1 (liver/intrahepatic bile duct), 1.6:1 (gastric), and 4.1:1 (esophageal). Overall, colorectal cancer is the third most common malignant neoplasm worldwide, and the second leading cause of cancer deaths in the United States.

SUBTYPES OF EPITHELIAL NEOPLASMS

Epithelial neoplasms of the GI tract are broadly classified as adenocarcinomas, squamous cell carcinomas, neuroendocrine tumors (NETs), and mixtures of those cell types. Adenocarcinomas arise from the columnar epithelia of the GI tract, and this type of carcinoma is the most common epithelial neoplasm in the stomach and colon. There is well-documented evidence of a dysplasia/adenoma–carcinoma development sequence in both the colon and stomach as well. Histologic variants include tubular, papillary, mucinous, cribriform comedo-type, medullary, micropapillary, hepatoid, serrated, and signet ring cell carcinoma. When compared to glandular adenocarcinomas, signet ring cells are poorly cohesive, show a diffuse infiltrative growth pattern, and generally carry a worse prognosis. A more extensive discussion of specific histologic variants can be found in Chapters 7–11.

Squamous cell carcinoma most commonly arises in the parts of the GI tract lined by squamous mucosa, that is, the upper to middle esophagus and anus. Worldwide, squamous cell carcinoma is still the predominant carcinoma in the esophagus, whereas adenocarcinoma has surpassed squamous cell carcinoma in the esophagus in Western countries in recent years. Anal squamous cell carcinoma is associated with human papillomavirus (HPV) infection and immunosuppression; in contrast, HPV is detected in only a small number of esophageal squamous cell carcinomas, and its role in esophageal carcinogenesis is unclear.

Neuroendocrine cells are present throughout the GI tract, which is considered to be the largest endocrine organ of the human body. Given the distribution of neuroendocrine cells in the gut, it is not surprising that neuroendocrine tumors (NETs) occur throughout the tubular GI tract. An estimated 8,000 people in the United States are diagnosed with an NET arising in the GI tract each year.

Appendiceal NETs are the most common neoplasms of the appendix, and NETs also surpassed adenocarcinomas as the most common small bowel tumor reported to the National Cancer Data Base in the year 2000. In contrast, adenocarcinoma and squamous cell carcinomas are still the dominant primary malignant neoplasms in other parts of the GI tract, as discussed previously.

Malignant mixed epithelial neoplasms are those that are composed of more than one distinct histologic type. They are less common overall than pure adenocarcinomas in the GI tract. There are several different types of mixed neoplasms, and some types are more common in certain locations within the GI tract than others. Some of the most common examples of mixed tumors of the luminal GI tract are discussed briefly in the following paragraphs.

Mixed Carcinoma of the Stomach

This tumor is a mixture of discrete cohesive glandular (tubular and/or papillary) elements, as well as signet ring cell or poorly cohesive cellular components (Figure 2.1). The presence of any percentage of the latter is associated with a poor prognosis.

Adenosquamous Carcinoma

Adenosquamous carcinoma is a mixture of neoplastic glandular and neoplastic squamous elements (Figure 2.2A–B). The presence of benign metaplastic squamoid foci within an adenocarcinoma does not fulfill the criteria for adenosquamous carcinoma. In contrast to the ampulla and pancreas, no specific percentages of squamous differentiation are required in the tubular GI tract for this diagnosis to be made (WHO 2010 classification). Adenosquamous carcinomas are rare, but can be found throughout the GI tract, with esophagus and colorectum the most common sites.

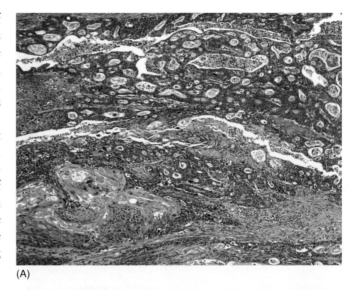

(A)

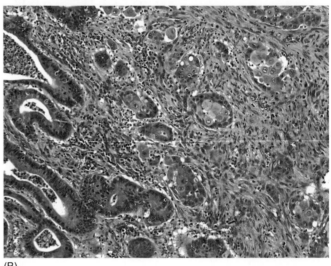

(B)

FIGURE 2.2 This adenosquamous carcinoma of the small bowel contains both a neoplastic glandular component and a neoplastic squamous component (A–B).

Mixed Adenoneuroendocrine Carcinoma (MANEC)

These tumors are a mixture of neoplastic glandular (exocrine) and neuroendocrine components (Figure 2.3A–C), and diagnosis requires at least 30% of each component present in the tumor. Common sites in the GI tract include stomach, ampullary/periampullary region, and appendix (see also Chapter 3).

DETERMINATION OF MALIGNANCY

Making a definite diagnosis of malignancy (versus one of a benign lesion or dysplasia) can be challenging, particularly

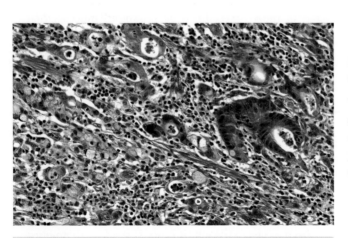

FIGURE 2.1 This mixed adenocarcinoma of the stomach contains a cohesive well-developed glandular component admixed with dyscohesive signet ring cells.

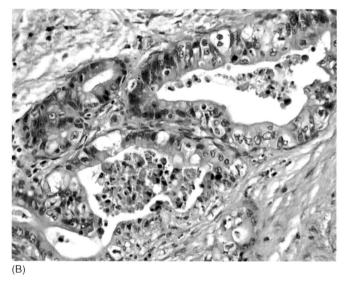

(A)

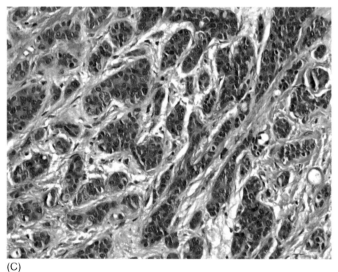

(B)

(C)

FIGURE 2.3 Mixed adenoneuroendocrine carcinoma (MANEC) of the colon showing a mixture of neoplastic glandular (A, left) and neuroendocrine components (A, right). High power views of the glandular (B) and neuroendocrine (C) components.

TABLE 2.1 Histologic Features Useful in Distinguishing Benign and Malignant Epithelial Lesions in the GI Tract

	Benign	Malignant
Architecture		
Preserved	+	−
Regular borders	+	−
Fused/cribriform glands	−	+/−
Cytology		
Nuclear atypia	−/+	++
Loss of polarity	−	+
Mitotic figures	−/+	+
Stroma		
Desmoplasia	−	+
Hemorrhage	−/+	−
Glands associated with lamina propria	+	−
Immunohistochemistry		
Ki-67	−/+	++
P53	−/+	++

on small biopsies. Numerous pitfalls and differential diagnoses are encountered, many of which vary with the exact location of the lesion within the GI tract. Table 2.1 summarizes some histologic features that can be useful in differentiating benign from malignant lesions. In general, benign lesions are circumscribed with regular borders, and show preserved architecture without desmoplastic stromal reactions. Malignant lesions, in contrast, often have irregular, poorly circumscribed borders with an associated desmoplastic reaction. Cytologically, benign lesions retain cellular polarity and lack prominent cytologic atypia, whereas malignant lesions demonstrate more significant atypia and often loss of nuclear polarity. Mitotic figures are typically more frequent in malignant neoplasms, although some inflammatory conditions may contain significantly increased mitoses and significant cytologic atypia. A background of inflammation may be very helpful in diagnosing a reactive lesion, although an inflammatory background can certainly be seen in malignant conditions as well.

Potential pitfalls exist when a small biopsy sample contains atypical reactive cells at the edge of an ulcer, but the ulcer or ischemic area is not clearly present in the biopsy. In difficult cases, immunohistochemical stains for Ki-67 and p53 may be helpful in distinguishing benign from malignant. Malignant lesions usually show a high Ki-67 proliferative labeling index and strong p53 staining, whereas benign lesions generally show negative to weak staining (Figure 2.4A–D).

PRIMARY VERSUS METASTATIC EPITHELIAL MALIGNANCY

One of the most important issues when evaluating epithelial malignancies of the GI tract is whether or not a tumor is primary or metastatic. Secondary tumors of the

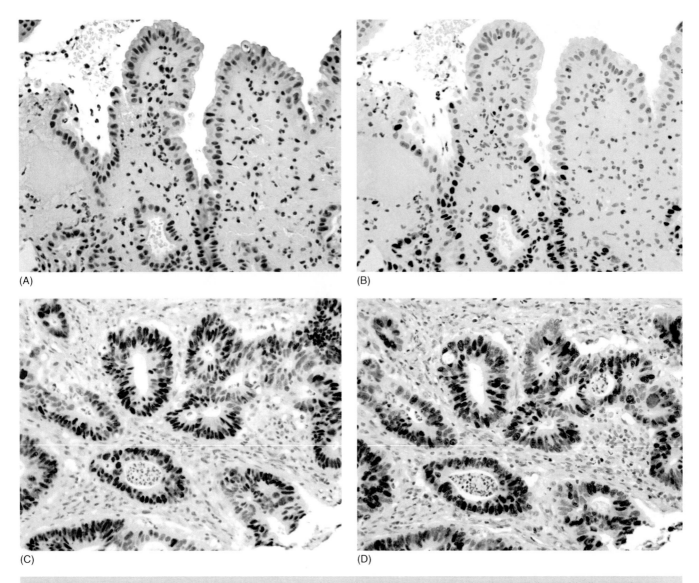

FIGURE 2.4 Ki-67 and p53 immunostains can be helpful in distinguishing between benign reactive epithelium and a malignancy. Reactive gastric epithelium is negative for p53 (A), and shows only focal positivity for Ki-67 (B) at the base of proliferating gastric pits. Malignant epithelial cells from a gastric adenocarcinoma are diffusely positive for both p53 (C) and Ki-67 (D).

GI tract are not uncommon, particularly in the small bowel, where metastatic disease occurs more frequently than primary malignancies. The most common metastatic tumors to the GI tract overall are malignant melanoma, lung adenocarcinoma, and breast cancer. The most common metastatic malignancies to the GI tract by site are listed in Table 2.2, and features useful in distinguishing primary from metastatic tumors in the GI tract are listed in Table 2.3. Knowledge of the clinical, radiographic, and endoscopic findings is crucial, as are morphologic features of the tumor, and the presence of multiple lesions favors a metastasis rather than a primary tumor. When the primary tumor is available for review, comparing it

TABLE 2.2 Most Common Metastatic Malignancies to the GI Tract by Site

Site of GI Tract	Most Common Subsite	Most Common Metastatic Tumors
Esophagus	Middle third	Breast, lung, melanoma
Stomach	Upper two thirds	Breast (two thirds are lobular carcinoma), melanoma, lung, esophagus, pancreas
Small intestine	Any site	Melanoma, breast, ovary, lung, pancreas
Colon and rectum	Any site	Breast, lung, ovary, kidney, pancreas

TABLE 2.3 Clinical and Pathologic Features Useful in Distinguishing Primary From Metastatic Epithelial Tumors

Features	Primary	Metastatic
Age	Younger	Older
History	No previous malignancy	Previous malignancy
Radiology	Single tumor	Multiple tumors
Endoscopy	Mucosal lesion	Submucosal lesion or lesion pushing into lumen
Gross	Mucosa-based rather than serosa-based	Serosa-based rather than mucosa-based
Microscopic	In situ precursor (dysplasia) in adjacent mucosa	No in situ precursor or undermines mucosa

with the metastatic lesion may be all that is required to make a diagnosis, but immunohistochemistry may also be helpful in some cases to make the distinction between primary and metastatic carcinomas. In metastatic lesions, tumors often undermine, rather than arise from, the mucosa (Figure 2.5A), or the tumor may be present only in the serosa or within the muscular wall. However, in some cases the metastatic tumor cells are intimately admixed with benign mucosal glands (Figure 2.5B). The identification of an in situ lesion is generally helpful in determining that a neoplasm is primary, but there are pitfalls. Metastatic tumors to the GI tract can involve the mucosal surface and superficial glands (Figure 2.5C), and thus mimic carcinoma in situ or a dysplastic mucosal lesion. In the small bowel, tumor growth along the

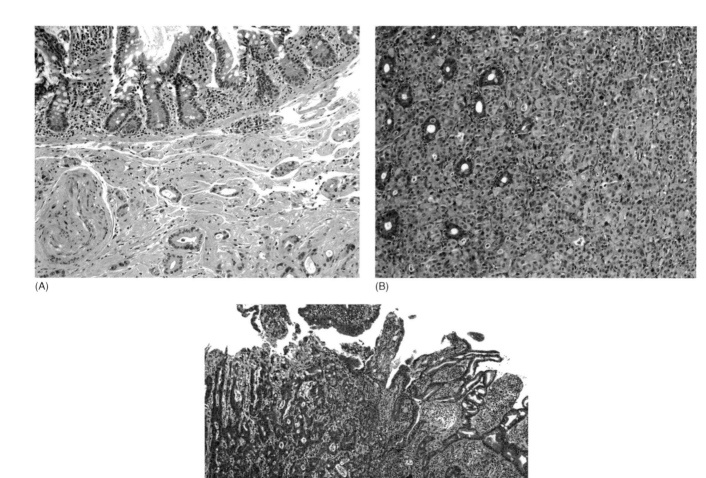

(A)

(B)

(C)

FIGURE 2.5 This metastatic colonic adenocarcinoma undermines the small bowel mucosa. This is a typical growth pattern for a metastasis to the GI tract (A). Metastatic poorly differentiated gastric adenocarcinoma infiltrates between benign rectal glands (B). Metastatic adenocarcinoma involving the mucosa and surface epithelium of the small bowel mimics carcinoma in situ (C).

basement membrane and the presence of an apparent adenoma cannot be assumed to be definite evidence of a primary neoplasm for similar reasons.

DIAGNOSTIC PITFALLS

There are many benign and/or non-neoplastic epithelial lesions in the GI tract that mimic malignant tumors both radiographically, endoscopically, and histologically. Some can be seen throughout the GI tract, while others are more common in certain anatomic locations. Some common diagnostic pitfalls in the differential diagnosis of GI epithelial neoplasms and their diagnostic clues are listed in Table 2.4 and discussed here.

Endometriosis/Endosalpingiosis

Endometriosis and endosalpingiosis frequently involve the GI tract, and these diagnoses should always be considered in the differential diagnosis of a glandular lesion in a woman of reproductive age. The rectum (73%), sigmoid colon (20%), and ileum (7%) are the three most commonly involved sites. Endometriosis may present clinically as a mass, stricture, or perforation, and thus suggest malignancy. The glands of endometriosis and endosalpingiosis may also mimic malignancy histologically, as they may infiltrate anywhere from serosa to mucosa.

The detection of endometrial or tubal-type glands, stroma, and hemosiderin on routine slide preparations is usually sufficient for diagnosis, but immunostains may be helpful in differentiating the glands of endometriosis from those of gastrointestinal origin. Typically, glands arising from the GI tract are cytokeratin (CK)20 and CDX2 positive, and in general PAX8 and CK7 will mark glands of Müllerian origin. When endometriosis involves the intestinal mucosal surface, the diagnosis may be particularly challenging, as the endometrial glands may contain mucin-depleted cells with enlarged nuclei on or near the luminal surface, mimicking dysplasia (Figure 2.6A–B). However, there is usually hypercellular endometrial stroma underlying the glands, and the endometrial glands may have cilia (tubal metaplasia). When endometriosis involves the colonic wall, the irregularly shaped glands lined by hyperchromatic cells may mimic an invasive colonic adenocarcinoma. The recognition of endometrial stroma is important, in contrast to the desmoplastic stroma typically seen in adenocarcinoma. Endometrial stroma is usually composed of densely packed small cells (Figure 2.6C) but can also contain large pink decidualized cells. Occasionally, the endometrial stroma may be inconspicuous. Endometriosis tends to be circumscribed, often shows mural concentric smooth muscle hyperplasia and hypertrophy, and frequently contains hemorrhage and hemosiderin deposition (Figure 2.6D). Rarely, the ectopic endometrial glands may give rise to endometrioid adenocarcinoma or Müllerian adenosarcoma. Immunohistochemically, these tumors stain similarly to endometriosis.

Ectopic Pancreas

Ectopic pancreatic tissue may present as a mucosal polyp or a submucosal mass lesion on endoscopy, and is most frequently located in the stomach or duodenum, especially within a few centimeters of either side of the gastroduodenal junction. Less often, ectopic pancreatic tissue is seen in the jejunum, ileum, or colon. Ectopic pancreas is composed of variable proportions of pancreatic acinar tissue, ducts, and islets, arranged in a rounded or lobular configuration. Histologically, it can mimic adenocarcinoma in the submucosa (particularly on the frozen section), especially if only ducts are present (Figure 2.7A–B). The lobulated architecture and lack of cytologic atypia are very useful findings in supporting a diagnosis of ectopic pancreas. Knowing the location of the endoscopic biopsy is also helpful for the correct diagnosis. The minor papilla in the duodenum can show the same histologic appearance as heterotopic pancreas, with surface intestinal epithelium undermined by submucosal pancreatic tissue. Most diseases of the pancreas, including pancreatic intraepithelial neoplasia and carcinoma, have been rarely reported arising from ectopic pancreas.

TABLE 2.4 Common Diagnostic Pitfalls in the Diagnosis of GI Epithelial Neoplasms

Pitfall	Mimic	Clue	Site
Endometriosis/endosalpingiosis	Adenocarcinoma	Endometrial or tubal-type glands, stroma, hemorrhage	Anywhere (most common in rectum and sigmoid colon)
Ectopic pancreas	Adenocarcinoma	Lobular arrangement, no atypia, islets	Anywhere (most common in stomach and duodenum)
Prolapse change/misplaced epithelium	Adenocarcinoma in a polyp	Fibromuscular stroma, hemorrhage, lack cytologic atypia	Rectum, sigmoid colon, stomach
Pseudo-signet ring cells (xanthoma, crushed gastric glands, ischemia)	Signet ring cell carcinoma	Lack atypia, background	Stomach, colon

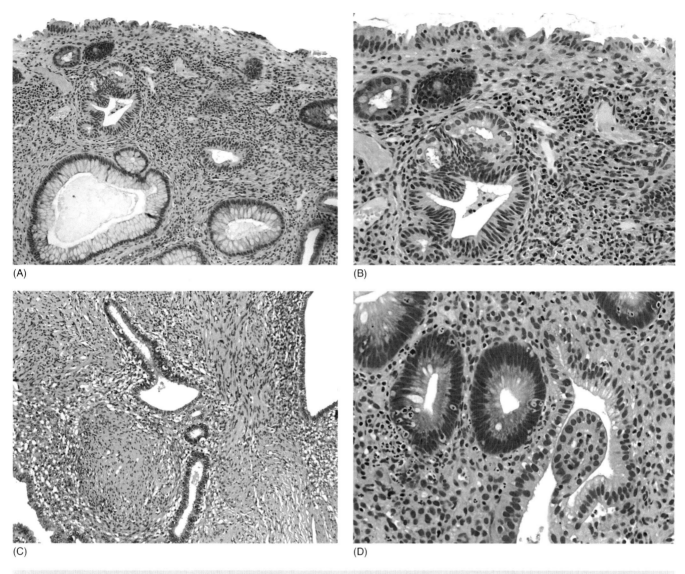

(A)

(B)

(C)

(D)

FIGURE 2.6   Endometriosis can be a major pitfall in the diagnosis of epithelial neoplasia. This example of endometriosis near the mucosal surface shows mucin-depleted cells with enlarged nuclei that mimic dysplastic crypts (A–B), but there is surrounding endometrial-type stroma. Endometrial stroma is composed of densely packed small cells, and should be distinguished from true desmoplasia (C). Endometrial stroma may be inconspicuous in some cases, but hemosiderin deposition can also be a clue to the diagnosis (D).

Prolapse Change or Misplaced Epithelium

The solitary rectal ulcer syndrome, colitis cystica profunda, and other forms of mucosal prolapse are a related spectrum of disorders in which benign, often dilated glands may herniate into the submucosa, often due to excessive straining during defecation. These misplaced benign glands in the submucosa may mimic adenocarcinoma, although the misplaced epithelium typically shows no dysplasia and is associated with a surrounding rim of lamina propria. There are often neighboring diamond-shaped, focally dilated, distorted crypts located between hypertrophic disorganized fibromuscular fibers that extend upwards, perpendicular to the muscularis mucosae (Figure 2.8A–B). Gastritis cystica profunda is a

similar condition found in the stomach, in which cystic gastric glands are misplaced into the submucosa due to chronic inflammation, ischemia, or surgery. Other scenarios in which mucosal entrapment can mimic invasive adenocarcinoma include misplaced epithelium in small intestinal Peutz–Jeghers polyps, adenomatous polyps of the left colon, and hyperplastic polyps of the sigmoid colon and rectum. Misplaced glands in adenomas can be particularly problematic due to the dysplasia inherently present in adenomatous epithelium (Figure 2.8C–D). Key findings that can help distinguish these glands from invasive adenocarcinoma include similar degrees of atypia in the misplaced and surface adenomatous glands, lack of desmoplastic stroma, and surrounding hemorrhage and hemosiderin deposition.

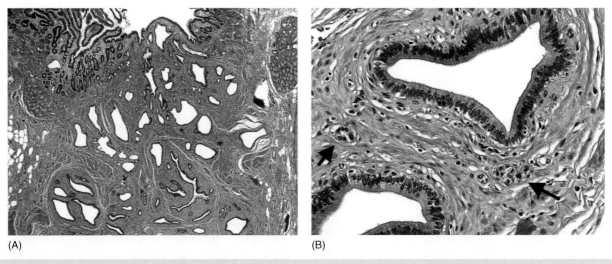

FIGURE 2.7 Ectopic pancreas composed primarily of dilated pancreatic ducts in the submucosa can closely mimic invasive adenocarcinoma (A). Note the lobular configuration of the glands. This high power image shows small islets associated with the pancreatic ducts (B, arrows).

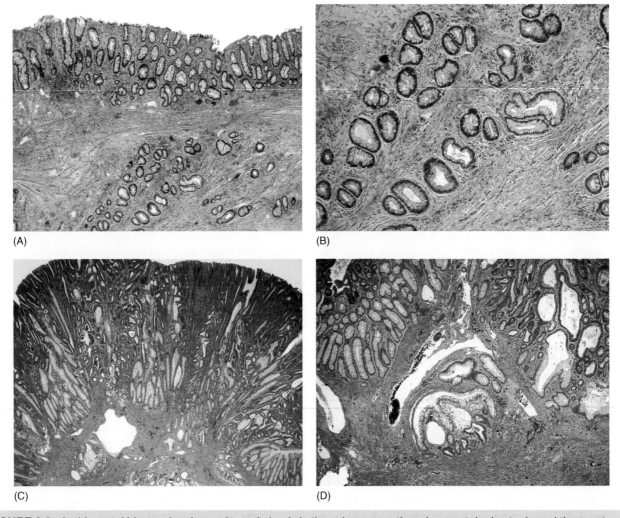

FIGURE 2.8 In this rectal biopsy showing prolapsed glands in the submucosa, there is no cytologic atypia and the crypts are surrounded by hypertrophic and disorganized fibromuscular fibers (A–B). In this tubulovillous adenoma with submucosal epithelial displacement, the downwardly displaced epithelium shows continuity with the surface epithelium (C). At higher power, the misplaced glands show the same degree of atypia as the surface adenomatous glands (D). Note also the lack of desmoplastic stroma.

Approximately 10% of Peutz–Jeghers polyps contain misplaced epithelium, which may herniate into the submucosa, muscularis propria, or subserosa with frequent associated mucin-containing cysts. Demonstration of continuity of the misplaced epithelium with the overlying mucosa, surrounding associated lamina propria, associated chronic inflammation and hemorrhage, lack of cytologic atypia, and lack of desmoplastic response are helpful in correctly diagnosing such cases as misplaced epithelium rather than true invasive adenocarcinoma (see also Chapter 6).

Signet Ring Cells and Pseudo-Signet Ring Cells

Signet ring cells are malignant epithelial cells found in adenocarcinoma, and are the hallmark of signet ring cell adenocarcinomas. However, several types of benign reactive cells can mimic neoplastic signet ring cells (pseudo-signet ring cells), most commonly of epithelial or histiocytic origin.

Malignant signet ring cells contain a large cytoplasmic vacuole that displaces the crescent-shaped nucleus to the periphery of the cell (Figure 2.9A). In reactive processes such as mucosal ulceration or ischemia, degenerated or sloughed mucin-containing epithelial cells may mimic malignant signet ring cells (pseudo-signet ring cells). Pseudo-signet ring cells are usually limited to the mucosa or luminal fibrinopurulent debris, although they are occasionally seen in the lamina propria. They should lack cytologic atypia and an associated desmoplastic stromal response. Common diseases associated with benign epithelial signet ring cells are pseudomembranous colitis (Figure 2.9B–C), ischemia, ulcerative colitis, gastritis, and cystic fibrosis, among others. Pseudo-signet ring cells can also be seen in ulcerated adenomas and Peutz–Jeghers polyps. In difficult cases, immunostains for E-cadherin, p53, and Ki-67 may be used; benign epithelial pseudo-signet ring cells are usually positive for E-cadherin, and negative for the latter two stains (Figure 2.9D–I). However, reactive processes may occasionally stain with proliferation markers.

Benign histiocytic cells residing in the GI tract may engulf mucin, lipid, or other materials and also simulate malignant signet ring cells. Examples include normal muciphages in the rectum (Figure 2.9J), xanthoma cells anywhere in the GI tract (Figure 2.9K), and other foamy histiocytes. Immunostains for histiocyte markers such as CD68 and CK are positive and negative in histiocytes respectively, with malignant signet ring cells showing the opposite staining pattern.

DIFFERENTIAL DIAGNOSIS OF EPITHELIAL NEOPLASMS

Most epithelial neoplasms have an epithelioid morphology; however, many neoplasms in the GI tract with epithelioid features are not, in fact, epithelial in origin. For example, 20% to 25% of gastric gastrointestinal stromal tumors (GIST) are epithelioid (Figure 2.10A), with many cases showing a mixed spindle and epithelioid histology. Many sarcomas also contain focal areas of epithelioid morphology that mimic carcinomas. Conversely, sarcomatoid carcinomas can be confused with sarcomas, and may lack CK positivity. Metastatic melanoma (Figure 2.10B) frequently has well developed epithelioid features as well. In such cases, a previous history of a cutaneous pigmented lesion, less cohesive tumor cells with cytoplasmic pigment and prominent nucleoli, and positive melanoma markers are all helpful. Malignant mesotheliomas (Figure 2.10C) can be composed of large epithelioid cells arranged in nests or pseudoglands, and are well-known mimics of adenocarcinomas. Lymphomas of the GI tract (Figure 2.10D), in particular large B cell lymphomas, can appear epithelioid but are usually dyscohesive, and a previous history of lymphoma may be an important clue.

Table 2.5 summarizes the initial, "first-line" immunochemical markers that aid in distinguishing between the major categories of tumors, including epithelial tumors (carcinomas and NETs), sarcoma, melanoma, and lymphoma. Table 2.6 summarizes immunohistochemical markers that are commonly used in the diagnosis of epithelial neoplasms, as well as their most frequent uses. The utility of immunohistochemistry in the diagnosis of neoplasms of the GI tract will be discussed in more detail in Chapter 13.

GENERAL APPROACH TO THE DIAGNOSIS OF EPITHELIAL NEOPLASMS

The general approach to the diagnosis of any epithelial neoplasm in the GI tract begins with a review of the patient's history, including age, gender, and previous malignancies or lesions such as adenomas or hamartomatous polyps. Radiologic and endoscopic findings can be very important as well.

Figure 2.11 illustrates a basic algorithmic approach to epithelial lesions of the GI tract. Initially, neoplastic lesions should be differentiated from a reactive or inflammatory process, an ectopic lesion (eg, ectopic pancreas), or a hamartomatous lesion (such as Peutz–Jeghers or juvenile polyps). The morphologic features, together with history, site, and background histologic findings are very helpful in this initial determination. Once an epithelial neoplasm is confirmed, attention should be focused on whether it is benign or malignant. Malignant neoplasms in the GI tract can be primary, but the possibility of metastatic disease should be always considered (see section on primary versus metastatic epithelial malignancy). If a primary tumor is diagnosed in a resection specimen, it must then be graded and staged (see Chapters 7–12 for more details). If the tumor

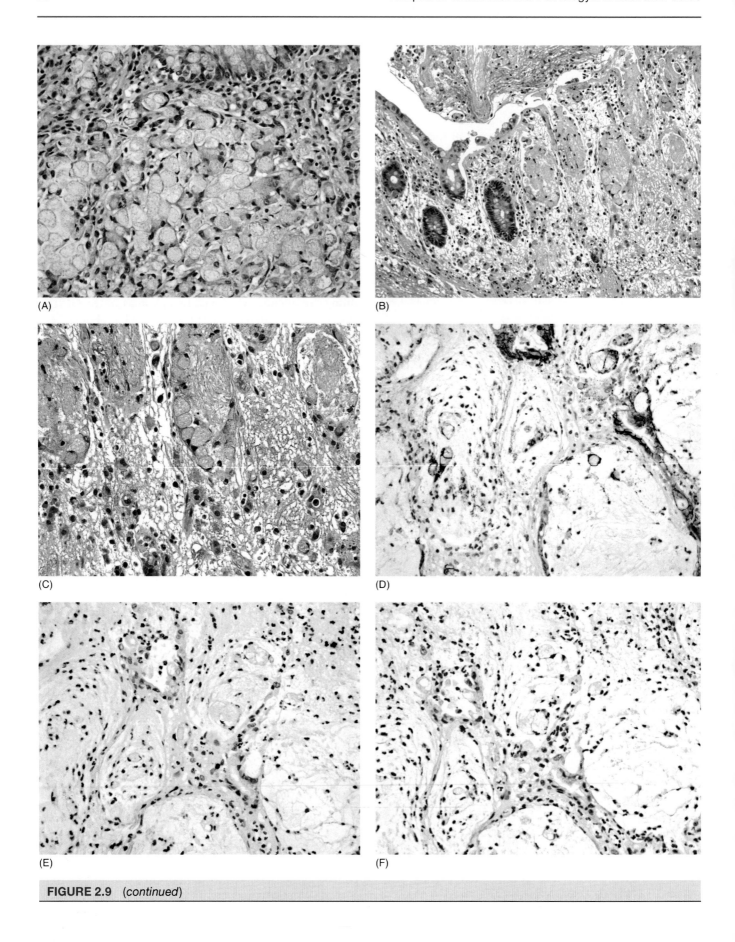

(A)

(B)

(C)

(D)

(E)

(F)

FIGURE 2.9   (*continued*)

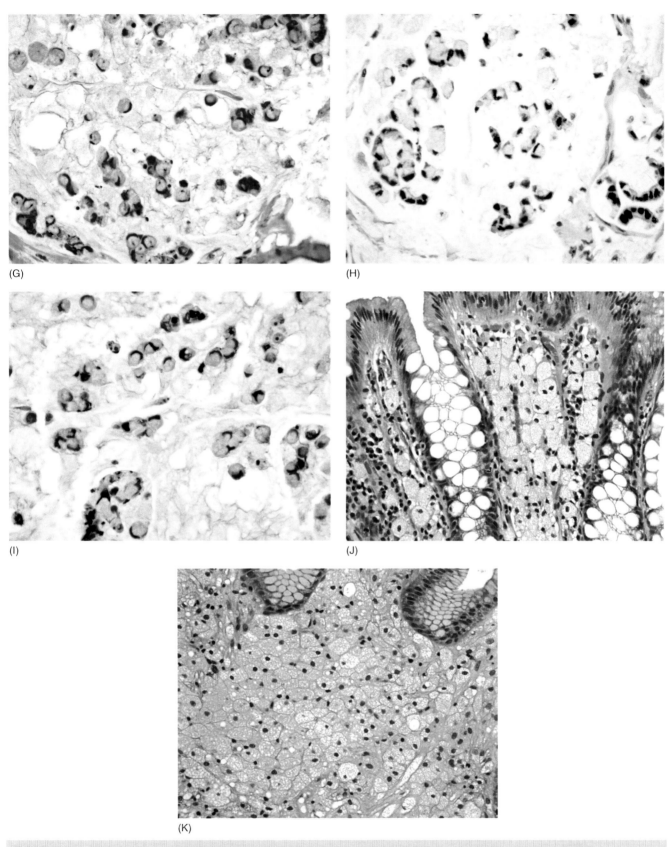

FIGURE 2.9   Signet ring cells within a colonic adenocarcinoma, showing infiltrative atypical cells with signet-shaped nuclei that are displaced by cytoplasmic vacuoles (A). Degenerating mucin-containing epithelial cells in pseudomembranous colitis mimicking signet ring cells (B–C). Epithelial pseudo-signet ring cells in a case of ischemic colitis are positive for E-cadherin (D), but negative for Ki-67 (E) and p53 (F). In contrast, neoplastic signet ring cells are negative for E-cadherin (G), and positive for Ki-67 (H) and p53 (I). Benign foamy macrophages including muciphages (J) and xanthoma cells (K) resemble signet ring cells, but have round, bland-appearing nuclei.

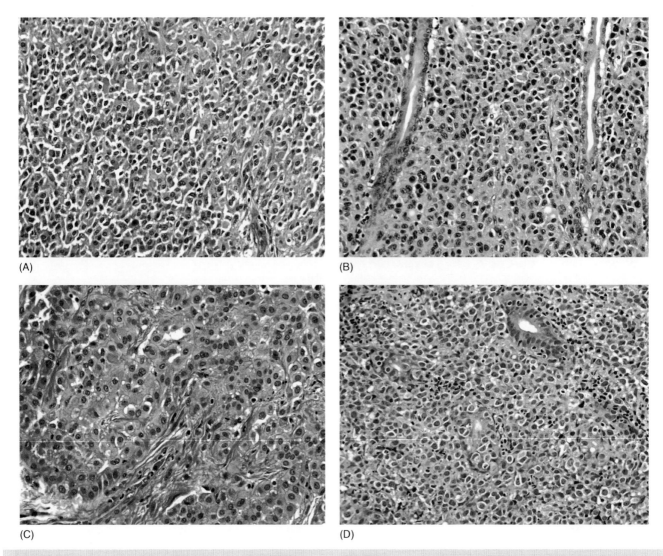

FIGURE 2.10 Common epithelioid neoplasms that involve the GI tract, but are not epithelial in origin, include epithelioid gastrointestinal stromal tumor (GIST) (A), metastatic melanoma (B), malignant mesothelioma (C), and diffuse large B cell lymphoma (D).

TABLE 2.5 Basic Panel of Immunohistochemical Stains Useful in the Differential Diagnosis of Epithelioid Neoplasms

	Carcinoma	NET	Sarcoma	Melanoma	Lymphoma
CKAE1/3*	+	+	–	–	–
CK5/6	+ (SCCA)	–	–	–	–
Chromogranin	–	+	–	–	–
Synaptophysin	–	+	–	–	–
S100	–	–/+	+ (Neural)	+	–
Vimentin	–/+	–/+	+	+	+/–
HMB-45	–	–	–	+	–
Melan A	–	–	–/+	+	–
KIT/DOG1	–	–	+ (GIST)	–	–
CD31	–	–	+ (Vascular)	–	–
SMA	–	–	+ (Muscle)	–	–
CD45	–	–	–	–	+

Abbreviations: CK, cytokeratin; GIST, gastrointestinal stromal tumor; NET, neuroendocrine tumor; SCCA, squamous cell carcinoma.

*Other useful cytokeratins include high and low molecular weight cytokeratin cocktails, CAM 5.2, CK7, CK19, and CK20 depending on the site of origin.

TABLE 2.6   Immunohistochemical Markers Useful in the Diagnosis of Gastrointestinal Epithelial Neoplasms

Epithelial Marker	Common Uses	Most Common GI Site
CK AE1/3	First-line marker	Broad spectrum (squamous and nonsquamous)
CK CAM 5.2/Low Molecular Weight CK (LMWK)	First-line marker	Broad spectrum (nonsquamous), complementary to CKAE1/3 for detecting CK18+ carcinomas, such as hepatocellular carcinoma
EMA	Second-line marker	Broad spectrum (glandular epithelia)
High Molecular Weight CK (HMWK; K903, 34βE12)	Second-line marker	Broad spectrum, predominantly in squamous epithelia and in basal cells
CK7	Site of origin	Stomach, biliary
CK19	Site of origin	Bile duct
CK20	Site of origin	Colorectal
CDX2	Site of origin	Intestinal
SATB2	Site of origin	Intestinal
CK5/6	Squamous cell, mesothelium	Esophagus, anorectal, mesothelium
p63	Squamous cell	Esophagus, anorectal

Abbreviation: CK, cytokeratin;

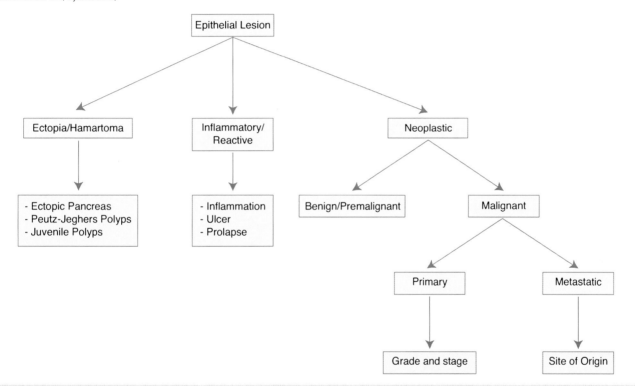

FIGURE 2.11   General algorithmic approach to evaluating epithelial neoplasms of the GI tract.

is metastatic, the site of origin should be addressed to the extent that it is possible, using clinical findings, morphology, and immunohistochemical panels.

More detailed diagnostic descriptions of individual epithelial tumors are in the organ-specific chapters that follow, but the following paragraphs summarize a basic approach to the initial evaluation of hematoxylin and eosin (H&E) stained sections of epithelial neoplasms. An important initial step in tumor diagnosis is the assignment of a general morphologic pattern (Figure 2.12) to the lesion. Once the pattern is identified, a differential diagnosis is generated, which can then be further

investigated with immunohistochemistry and other ancillary testing as necessary. For each pattern, there are specific epithelial tumors that are most likely to fall into that category, as well as nonepithelial tumors that must be considered in the differential diagnosis. The final diagnosis should, of course, correlate the results of immunohistochemical panels with the clinical and morphologic findings, and basing a diagnosis on the interpretation of a single immunostain should be avoided. The ability to make a diagnosis may be further limited, in many cases, by the size of the tissue sample, crush or cautery artifact, and necrosis.

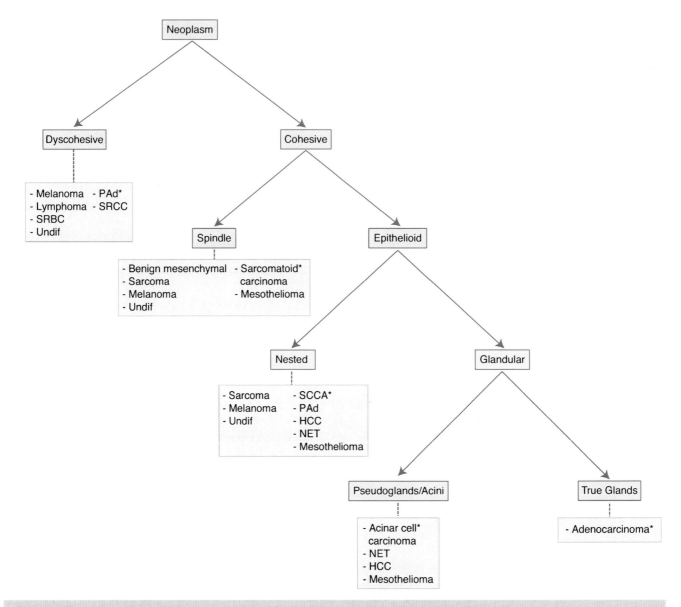

FIGURE 2.12 Algorithmic approach to general morphologic patterns in epithelioid neoplasms.

*Indicates epithelial tumors

Abbreviations: HCC, hepatocellular carcinoma; NET, neuroendocrine tumor; PAd, poorly differentiated adenocarcinoma; SCCA, squamous cell carcinoma; SRBC, small round blue cell tumor; SRCC, signet ring cell carcinoma; Undif, undifferentiated tumor.

Many epithelial neoplasms may be divided as to their cohesiveness, whether they have predominantly epithelioid or spindled patterns, and whether they are composed of nests, glands, signet ring cells, etc.

Dyscohesive Tumors

The most classic dyscohesive epithelial tumor is signet ring cell adenocarcinoma. However, many poorly differentiated carcinomas can be dyscohesive as well. The differential diagnosis for dyscohesive tumors is broad, and includes epithelial as well as nonepithelial neoplasms such as melanoma, lymphoma, small round blue cell tumors (such as Ewing sarcoma/primitive neuroectodermal tumor

and desmoplastic small round cell tumor), and undifferentiated neoplasms. Tumors that are actually cohesive may appear to be dyscohesive due to artifacts (such as that introduced during needle biopsy or fine needle aspiration) or necrosis. Prior to ordering immunohistochemical stains, useful morphologic features include brown pigment and cherry red nucleoli in melanomas, keratinization in squamous cell carcinomas, and mucin production in adenocarcinomas. Mucicarmine or periodic acid–Schiff (PAS) with diastase histochemical stains may be useful for detecting mucin, but are frequently negative or only show very focal positivity in poorly differentiated adenocarcinomas. Immunohistochemical stains that are most useful for dyscohesive tumors include a broad spectrum CK such as

AE1/3 for carcinomas, leukocyte common antigen (CD45) for lymphomas, and S100 for melanoma. Other markers may be useful if a sarcoma is in the differential diagnosis, and these are discussed later in Chapters 5 and 13 as well as in the organ-specific chapters. Additional stains may be necessary depending on the findings from this initial panel, and in the case of limited material, cutting several unstained slides on the front end may avoid wasting tissue in the block if it has to be refaced.

Cohesive Tumors

Cohesive tumors may be categorized further into a number of morphologic patterns, including spindle cell and epithelioid patterns, and epithelioid lesions can be further subdivided into nested, glandular, and pseudoglandular/acinar patterns. Some tumors show combinations of these patterns.

Although spindled tumors are most often mesenchymal in origin, carcinomas and malignant mesothelioma can also have spindle cell features. One of the most common spindled carcinomas of the GI tract is sarcomatoid carcinoma, which is most often seen in the esophagus and pancreas. Immunohistochemical stains can be very useful in distinguishing these tumors, and panels should consist of CK (both a broad spectrum keratin and a low molecular keratin such as CAM 5.2 may be useful), smooth muscle actin, KIT, S100 (for neural and melanocytic lesions), and CD31 (for vascular lesions). It is important to note that sarcomatoid carcinomas may not express CK at all in some cases. In addition, sarcomatoid malignant mesothelioma and some sarcomas can express CKs, leading to possible confusion with carcinoma. Additional immunohistochemical stains useful in this differential will be further discussed in the next two paragraphs and in Chapter 13.

Cohesive epithelial tumors that are nested and lack gland formation include squamous cell carcinoma, NETs, poorly differentiated adenocarcinoma, malignant mesothelioma, and hepatocellular carcinomas. Immunohistochemical stains useful in differentiating between poorly differentiated adenocarcinoma and squamous cell carcinoma include CK5/6, p63, and p40 for squamous cell carcinoma, and MOC31, BerEp4, and mucicarmine for adenocarcinoma. Many benign and malignant nonepithelial lesions also can feature a cohesive nested morphologic pattern, including granular cell tumors, paragangliomas, epithelioid sarcoma, angiosarcoma, malignant peripheral nerve sheath tumor, and GISTs. Melanomas frequently show a nested epithelioid pattern as well.

The initial immunohistochemical panel for the differential diagnosis of a cohesive epithelioid tumor with a nested pattern may include CK AE1/3, a neuroendocrine marker (synaptophysin, chromogranin, or CD56), SMA, KIT, S100, and CD31. Beware of weak CK AE1/3

staining in angiosarcomas and some other epithelioid sarcomas. Depending on the site, mesothelioma may also be worthy of consideration when there are positive epithelial markers. CK5/6, WT-1, and calretinin positivity favors mesothelioma, while MOC31, BerEp4, and pCEA favor adenocarcinoma. One pitfall of using CK AE1/3 alone to screen for carcinomas is that some carcinomas (eg, hepatocellular carcinoma) may be weak or negative. However, adding CAM5.2 to a panel may complement CK AE1/3 by detecting CK18, an additional low molecular weight keratin that is not present in the AE1/3 cocktail.

Cohesive glandular tumors can be divided into those composed of true glands and those that are pseudoglandular or acinar. True glandular tumors are adenocarcinomas, in which the glandular epithelium is lined by a basement membrane, forms a central lumen (true gland), and characteristically has intracytoplasmic mucin. In contrast, pseudoglandular/acinar tumors are composed of nests of tumor cells that are arranged around a small lumen (acinus), central necrosis, or centrally dilated space that mimics a lumen; this pattern lacks intracytoplasmic mucin. Examples of acinar/pseudoglandular epithelial neoplasms in the digestive tract include malignant mesothelioma, NETs, hepatocellular carcinoma, pancreatic solid pseudopapillary tumor, and acinar cell carcinoma. Immunohistochemical stains for CKs and neuroendocrine markers are most helpful in this setting. If malignant mesothelioma is in the differential diagnosis, the immunohistochemical stains discussed in the preceding paragraphs should be considered.

ILLUSTRATIVE EXAMPLES

The following three cases are presented to illustrate how to integrate the above algorithms in the workup of an epithelial lesion in the GI tract.

Case 1

A 32-year-old woman with a history of chronic abdominal pain and no previous history of malignancy presented with diarrhea and rectal bleeding. She was found to have a submucosal rectal mass at colonoscopy. Biopsy of the rectal mass (Figure 2.13A) showed a few glands in the submucosa of colon, and thus corresponds to the category of "epithelial lesion" in the Figure 2.11 algorithm. The next step is to determine whether the lesion is inflammatory/reactive, ectopic/hamartomatous (or another benign lesion), or neoplastic (which, given the presence of submucosal glands in this case, would be worrisome for invasive adenocarcinoma). Histologic evaluation using features previously described in the section determination of malignancy and in Table 2.1 shows that the

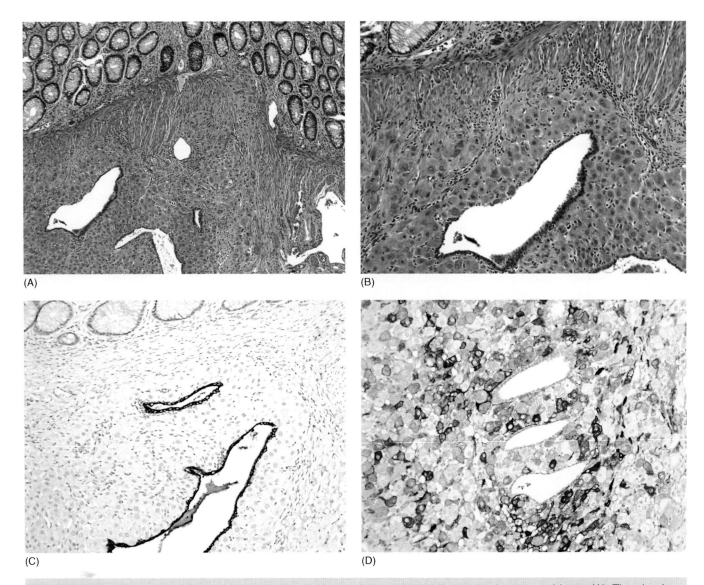

FIGURE 2.13 A submucosal glandular proliferation with prominent eosinophilic stroma is seen on biopsy (A). The glands are composed of cuboidal epithelium with scant cytoplasm and small, regular nuclei. The surrounding stroma is composed of large eosinophilic cells (B). CK7 expression confirms that the glands are not colonic in origin (C). CD10 expression is seen in the decidualized stroma (D).

lesion is somewhat circumscribed. A higher power view (Figure 2.13B) demonstrates benign appearing glands, with intact cellular polarity. No nuclear atypia, mitoses, or desmoplastic stromal reaction is noted. The lack of prominent inflammatory cells, mucosal ulcers, or history of trauma or surgery makes an inflammatory/reactive lesion less likely. In addition, large epithelioid cells with abundant pink cytoplasm surround the glands, reminiscent of decidualized endometrial stroma.

Immunostains revealed that the glandular cells are positive for CK7 (Figure 2.13C) and the stroma is positive for CD10, consistent with decidualized endometrial stroma (Figure 2.13D). The morphologic features on H&E, together with the immunohistochemical findings, are diagnostic of endometriosis. In difficult cases, additional

immunohistochemical markers may be employed. In endometriosis, for example, glands express PAX8 and CK7 and are negative for CK20 and CDX2, whereas colonic adenoma or adenocarcinoma typically shows the opposite staining pattern. In addition, estrogen receptor (ER) immunostain can also be helpful to highlight glands and stroma in endometriosis.

Case 2

A 67-year-old man with no known past medical history presented with nausea, vomiting, and constipation. He was found to have a complex pelvic mass with partial small bowel obstruction on CT scan. Small bowel biopsy (Figure 2.14A) shows a neoplasm involving the mucosa and submucosa of the small bowel. The distinction between benign and malignant in this case is fairly straightforward, since the tumor is poorly circumscribed with an invasive growth pattern and a desmoplastic stromal reaction, and thus one would begin with the "neoplastic" category in the Figure 2.11 algorithm. The definite site of origin is not discernible from this biopsy, however; thus the next step in the algorithm is to assess whether the malignant tumor is a primary tumor of the small bowel or a metastasis. Morphologic features that favor a metastatic tumor in this case include the lack of an associated in situ lesion and the fact that the majority of the tumor is present beneath the mucosa (see also Table 2.3).

As mentioned previously, the site of origin (primary vs. metastatic) is often an issue in glandular neoplasms in the GI tract, depending on the clinical findings, morphologic features (eg, the presence of an in situ precursor lesion), and site of the tumor. When necessary, the most frequently employed immunohistochemical stain panels to determine the site of origin include CK7, CK20, CDX2, and SATB2 to confirm the GI tract origin. No site of origin is characterized by an entirely distinct immunophenotype, and there is significant immunophenotypic overlap. Additional discussion on immunohistochemical stains and the site of origin will be presented in Chapters 7–13.

At this point, the Figure 2.12 algorithm is useful to elucidate the cell origin of the tumor. At the first branch point, the tumor is determined to be cohesive, and the cells are epithelioid and arranged in nests (Figure 2.14B).

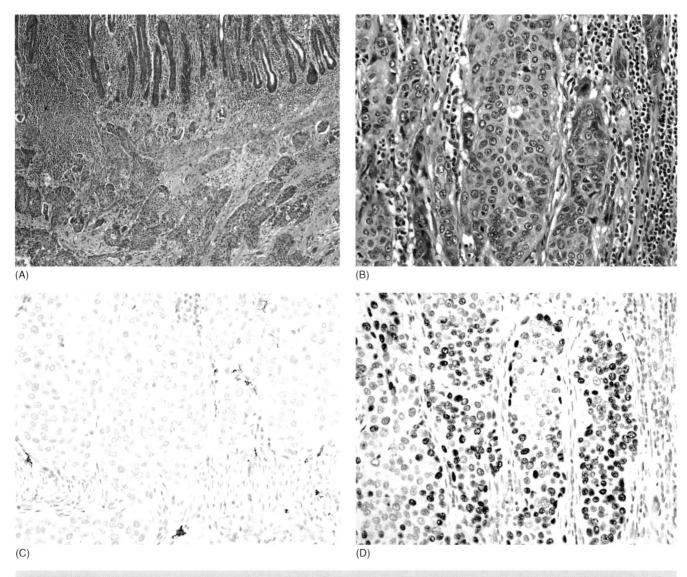

(A)

(B)

(C)

(D)

FIGURE 2.14 An epithelioid neoplasm in the small bowel, consisting of a predominantly submucosal proliferation of cells arranged in nests (A). Higher power view showing nests of epithelioid cells with small nucleoli (B). Synaptophysin expression is negative in the tumor (C). p63 immunostaining supports the diagnosis of metastatic urothelial carcinoma to the small bowel (D).

The primary differential diagnoses for a tumor with nests of bland epithelioid cells without prominent nucleoli in the small bowel are a metastatic carcinoma or an NET.

Selected immunohistochemical stains show that the tumor is positive for CKs AE1/3, CK7, and CK20 and negative for synaptophysin (Figure 2.14C), chromogranin, and CDX2. Expression of both CK7 and CK20 is frequently seen in metastatic urothelial carcinoma, but is also common in the peridiaphragmatic GI organs including pancreas, biliary tree, and stomach. As metastatic carcinomas are far more common than primary ones in the small bowel, and the immunophenotype suggested urothelial carcinoma as a diagnostic consideration, a p63 stain was performed and the positive staining (Figure 2.14D) supported the diagnosis. Further clinical and radiographic workup revealed urothelial carcinoma of the bladder.

Case 3

A 72-year-old man with weight loss and lethargy was found to have a mass in his right colon at colonoscopy. Upon resection, the tumor consisted of plump spindle cells with marked pleomorphism, arranged in a fascicular pattern (Figure 2.15A). The degree of cellular pleomorphism and nuclear atypia in this tumor excludes benign lesions, and thus using the Figure 2.12 algorithm, this tumor would be classified as cohesive and spindled. The main entities under consideration include sarcoma, melanoma, sarcomatoid carcinoma, and sarcomatoid malignant mesothelioma. Immunohistochemical stains showed that the tumor cells were positive for CK AE1/3 (Figure 2.15B) and vimentin (Figure 2.15C), and negative for DOG1, KIT, CD31, SMA, and S100. The coexpression

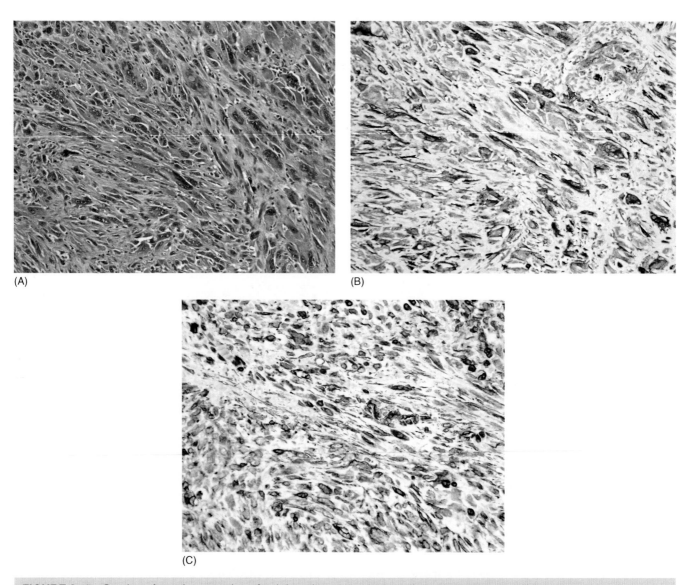

(A)

(B)

(C)

FIGURE 2.15 Sections from the resection of a right colon mass show malignant spindle cells with marked nuclear pleomorphism (A). The tumor cells were positive with CK AE1/3 (B) and vimentin (C), supporting the diagnosis of a sarcomatoid carcinoma.

of CK AE1/3 and vimentin suggests that the tumor is a carcinoma with sarcomatous differentiation (ie, sarcomatoid carcinoma). Further examination of the tumor identified a small area of poorly formed glands, further supporting the diagnosis.

The preceding three cases illustrate that using an algorithmic approach when evaluating epithelial and epithelioid lesions of the GI tract is helpful in establishing a differential diagnosis that can be evaluated systematically, thus helping to avoid pitfalls. This algorithmic approach, together with the selective use of immunostains, is a helpful general approach to a great majority of tumors that are encountered in the daily practice of GI pathology.

SELECTED REFERENCES

Epidemiology

Siegel R, Naishadham D, Jemal A. Cancer statistics. *CA Cancer J Clin.* 2013;63:11–30.

Subtypes of Epithelial Neoplasms

Bilimoria KY, Bentrem DJ, Wayne JD, et al. Small bowel cancer in the United States: changes in epidemiology, treatment, and survival over the last 20 years. *Ann Surg.* 2009;249:63–71.

Bosman F, Carneiro F, Hruban R, et al. eds. *World Health Organization Classification of Tumours of the digestive system.* 4th ed. Lyon, France:IARC Press;2010.

Deschamps L, Couvelard A. Endocrine tumors of the appendix: a pathologic review. *Arch Pathol Lab Med.* 2010;134:871–875.

Schlemper RJ, Riddell RH, Kato Y, et al. The Vienna classification of gastrointestinal epithelial neoplasia. *Gut.* 2000;47:251–255.

Yong F, Xudong N, Lijie T. Human papillomavirus types 16 and 18 in esophagus squamous cell carcinoma: a meta-analysis. *Ann Epidemiol.* 2013;23:726–734.

Primary Versus Metastatic Malignancy

Disibio G, French SW. Metastatic patterns of cancers: results from a large autopsy study. *Arch Pathol Lab Med.* 2008;132:931–939.

Estrella JS, Wu TT, Rashid A, Abraham SC. Mucosal colonization by metastatic carcinoma in the gastrointestinal tract: a potential mimic of primary neoplasia. *Am J Surg Pathol.* 2011;35:563–572.

Telerman A, Gerard B, van den Hevle B, Bleiberg H. Gastrointestinal metastases from extra-abdominal tumors. *Endoscopy.* 1985;17:99–101.

Diagnostic Pitfalls

De Petris G, Leung ST. Pseudoneoplasms of the gastrointestinal tract. *Arch Pathol Lab Med.* 2010;134:378–392.

Detlefsen S, Fagerberg CR, Ousager LB, et al. Histiocytic disorders of the gastrointestinal tract. *Hum Pathol.* 2013;44:683–696.

Distler M, Rückert F, Aust D, et al. Pancreatic heterotopia of the duodenum: anatomic anomaly or clinical challenge? *J Gastrointest Surg.* 2011;15:631–636.

Greene FL. Epithelial misplacement in adenomatous polyps of the colon and rectum. *Cancer.* 1974;33:206–217.

Huang CC, Frankel WL, Doukides T, et al. Prolapse-related changes are a confounding factor in misdiagnosis of sessile serrated adenomas in the rectum. *Hum Pathol.* 2013;44:480–486.

Jiang W, Roma AA, Lai K, et al. Endometriosis involving the mucosa of the intestinal tract: a clinicopathologic study of 15 cases. *Mod Pathol.* 2013;26(9):1270–1278.

Muto T, Bussey HJR, Morson BC. Pseudocarcinomatous invasion in adenomatous polyps of the colon and rectum. *J Clin Pathol.* 1973;26:25–31.

Petersen VC, Sheehan AL, Bryan RL, et al. Misplacement of dysplastic epithelium in Peutz-Jeghers Polyps: the ultimate diagnostic pitfall? *Am J Surg Pathol.* 2000;24:34–39.

Differential Diagnosis of Epithelial Neoplasms

Adair C, Ro JY, Sahin AA, et al. Malignant melanomas metastatic to gastrointestinal tract: A clinico-pathologic study. *Int J Surg Pathol.* 1994;2:3–9.

Agaimy A, Wünsch PH. Epithelioid and sarcomatoid malignant pleural mesothelioma in endoscopic gastric biopsies: a diagnostic pitfall. *Pathol Res Pract.* 2006;202:617–622.

Allison KH, Yoder BJ, Bronner MP, Goldblum JR, Rubin BP. Angiosarcoma involving the gastrointestinal tract: a series of primary and metastatic cases. *Am J Surg Pathol.* 2004;28:298–307.

Bellizzi AM. Immunohistochemical in gastroenterohepatopancreatobiliary epithelial neoplasia: Practical application, pitfalls, and emerging markers. *Surg Pathol Clin.* 2013;6:567–609.

Filippa DA, Lieberman PH, Wiengrad DN, et al. Primary lymphomas of the gastrointestinal tract: Analysis of prognostic factors with emphasis on histologic type. *Am J Surg Pathol.* 1983;7:363–372.

Guarino M, Tricomi P, Giordano F, Cristofori E. Sarcomatoid carcinomas: pathological and histopathogenetic considerations. *Pathology.* 1996;28:298–305.

Iezzoni JC, Mills SE. Sarcomatoid carcinomas (carcinosarcomas) of the gastrointestinal tract: A review. *Semin Diagn Pathol.* 1993;10:176–187.

Kende AI, Carr NJ, Sobin LH. Expression of cytokeratins 7 and 20 in carcinomas of the gastrointestinal tract. *Histopathology.* 2003;42:137–140.

Miettinen M, Lasota J. Histopathology of gastrointestinal stromal tumor. *J Surg Oncol.* 2011;104:865–873.

Ordóñez NG. Broad-spectrum immunohistochemical epithelial markers: a review. *Human Pathology.* 2013;44:1195–1215.

3

Approach to Neuroendocrine Neoplasms

ANDREW M. BELLIZZI

INTRODUCTION

The term "neuroendocrine epithelial neoplasms" (NENs) encompasses both well-differentiated tumors, historically referred to as carcinoid tumors, and poorly differentiated ones (small cell and large cell neuroendocrine carcinomas). These neoplasms have been variously referred to as endocrine (eg, in the 2000 WHO Classification) and neuroendocrine. The current World Health Organization (WHO) Classification refers to them as neuroendocrine, which emphasizes their dual nature. Many of these tumors' products are distinctly neural. For example, the same serotonin produced by midgut neuroendocrine tumors (NETs) is also a monoamine neurotransmitter, while the general neuroendocrine marker synaptophysin, a component of synaptic vesicles, is highly expressed by gray matter neuronal processes.

NENs can be characterized by three general features:

- Expression of the general neuroendocrine markers chromogranin A and/or synaptophysin.
- Production of peptide hormones and/or biogenic amines.
- Elaboration of the intermediate filament keratin.

Neuroendocrine neoplasms that do not make keratins (eg, pheochromocytoma/paraganglioma) and endocrine epithelial neoplasms lacking hybrid "neural" characteristics (eg, thyroid follicular neoplasms, gonadal sex cord stromal tumors) lie beyond this definition, though the thyroid (medullary thyroid carcinoma) and gonads (carcinoid and small cell carcinoma-pulmonary type) can certainly harbor primary neoplasms showing dual neuroendocrine nature. Of these three overlapping tumor types (neuroendocrine/epithelial, neuroendocrine/nonepithelial, and strictly endocrine/epithelial), primary tumors in the gastrointestinal (GI) tract are of the former.

HISTORICAL PERSPECTIVE

The term *karzinoide* (translated as carcinoid; literally "carcinoma-like") was introduced by the German pathologist Siegfried Oberndorfer in his 1907 seminal description of six patients with multifocal ileal tumors that histologically resembled carcinoma, but were unique in that they were unusually small, well-circumscribed, and associated with a benign clinical course. Although their function remained elusive, Rudolf Peter Heidenhain had identified neuroendocrine cells in the stomach, based on their histochemical reaction with chromium salts (the basis of the term enterochromaffin [EC] cell), 39 years earlier. A year before that, Theodor Langhans had provided the first histologic description of a carcinoid tumor. Neuroendocrine cells in the pancreas and intestine were subsequently described by Paul Langerhans (1869) and Nikolai Kulchitsky (1897), respectively. In 1914 Andre Gosset and Pierre Masson made the link between carcinoid tumors and EC cells, demonstrating that each reacted similarly with silver salts (the basis of the term argentaffin), and further speculating that these tumors and cells were neuroendocrine in nature. In 1929 Oberndorfer published a series of 36 additional carcinoid tumors of the small intestine and appendix and acknowledged that some of these tumors were, in fact, malignant.

In 1931 A.J. Scholte coined the term *carcinoid syndrome* to describe the edema, sweating, flushing, and diarrhea in a patient found at autopsy to have a 1 cm ileal carcinoid tumor; the patient died of heart failure and was also found to have a thickened tricuspid valve and right atrial subendocardial fibrosis. Serotonin (5-hydroxytryptamine) was isolated and characterized by Maurice Rapport in 1948. Five years later, Vittorio Erspamer demonstrated that EC cells produced serotonin, and

39

Fred Lembeck isolated serotonin from an ileal carcinoid. Andrew Schally and Roger Guillemin are credited with the codiscovery of somatostatin, for which in part they received (along with Rosalyn Yalow) the 1977 Nobel Prize in Physiology or Medicine. In 1979 Wilfried Bauer synthesized the somatostatin analogue octreotide, which has become a mainstay in the treatment of NETs. Jean-Claude Reubi, S.W. Lamberts, E.P. Krenning, and colleagues demonstrated high-level expression of somatostatin receptors in a subset of NENs, and in 1989 published the first study of the use of radiolabeled octreotide in the imaging of endocrine tumors (ie, somatostatin receptor scintigraphy) (Figure 3.1). The late 1990s saw the first trials of radiolabeled octreotide as a therapeutic agent (ie, peptide receptor radionuclide therapy). More recently (2011), positive clinical trials in pancreatic NETs have introduced mTOR inhibitors and sunitinib into the therapeutic armamentarium. At present, high-throughput DNA sequencing holds promise to unlock the molecular genetic basis of this class of tumors, which will hopefully suggest new avenues for directed biologic therapy.

Based on histologic, histochemical, and clinical observations, E.D. Williams and M. Sandler (1963) proposed that carcinoids, rather than representing a single monolithic entity, could be logically divided into foregut-, midgut-, and hindgut-derived types. In 1971 Jun Soga and Kenji Tazawa introduced a histologic-pattern-based classification that correlates with the site of origin and biology. The WHO first published a histologic classification of endocrine tumors in 1980, which was substantially updated in 2000. This textbook makes use of the 2010 WHO Classification of gastroenteropancreatic (GEP) NENs, introduced in the fourth edition of the *WHO GI Blue Book*. These classifications will be discussed in more detail in the section on classification.

HORMONE PRODUCTION IN NEUROENDOCRINE NEOPLASMS

Although a myriad of immunostains for hormones are commercially available, these are generally of limited clinical utility outside of the context of neuropathologic examination of pituitary adenomas (eg, prolactin, adrenocorticotropic hormone [ACTH], growth hormone). Immunohistochemical demonstration of hormones in an NEN does not equate with functionality, which is instead defined by the presence of a characteristic clinical syndrome attributable to hormone production by the tumor (eg, Whipple's triad with insulinoma; glucagonoma syndrome; diabetes mellitus, steatorrhea, gallstones, and hypochlorhydria with somatostatinomas; Zollinger–Ellison syndrome (ZES); Verner–Morrison syndrome, carcinoid syndrome, and Cushing syndrome). There are occasional situations in which hormone

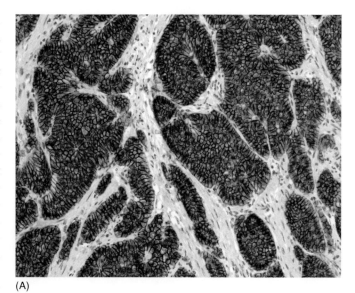

(A)

4 HR   IN-111 OCTREOTIDE

(B)

FIGURE 3.1 Neuroendocrine neoplasms, in particular well-differentiated tumors, tend to express high levels of somatostatin receptors, as illustrated by this immunohistochemical stain for somatostatin receptor type 2A in an ileal tumor (A). This expression is the basis of somatostatin receptor scintigraphy, as demonstrated by this OctreoScan showing extensive hepatic uptake in multiple foci (B).

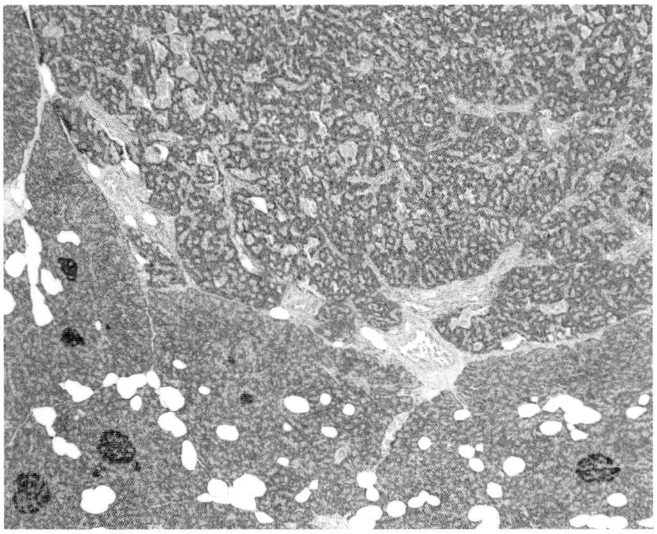

FIGURE 3.2 This patient presented with Whipple's triad and was found to have an insulinoma, as demonstrated by the diffuse, strong staining in the tumor and adjacent islets (insulin immunoperoxidase stain). The patient subsequently was diagnosed with a bronchopulmonary neuroendocrine tumor that did not express insulin, and thus likely represented a new primary.

immunohistochemistry (IHC) may be useful, however. Combined expression of insulin, glucagon, and somatostatin favors islet hyperplasia over a pancreatic NET, which is more likely to express a dominant hormone. In patients with a functional syndrome and multiple tumors (eg, as often occurs in combined multiple endocrine neoplasia type 1 Zollinger-Ellison syndrome), hormone IHC may be useful in identifying which tumor is responsible for the syndrome. Finally, in a patient with a tumor known to express a dominant hormone presenting with a new tumor, hormone IHC can be useful in distinguishing a metastasis from a separate primary (Figure 3.2).

GENERAL FEATURES OF WELL-DIFFERENTIATED NEUROENDOCRINE TUMORS

Well-differentiated NENs (formerly known as carcinoid tumors in the tubular gut or islet cell tumors in the pancreas) are referred to as NETs in the contemporary WHO (2010) Classification. They are characterized by a variety of growth patterns, including nested, trabecular, gyriform, glandular, tubuloacinar, pseudorosette-forming, solid, and mixed, which are collectively referred to as "organoid" (Figure 3.3A). The nuclear chromatin is typically granular, often referred to as "salt and pepper," and nucleoli are generally inconspicuous, although there is variation from case to case depending on the quality of the histologic

preparation (Figure 3.3B). Cytoplasm is moderate to abundant and may be granular (or less commonly microvesicular, vacuolated, or containing "rhabdoid" inclusions). The neuroendocrine nature of these neoplasms is usually evident on hematoxylin and eosin (H&E) staining, but can be confirmed with IHC for general neuroendocrine markers (Figure 3.3C). Synaptophysin and chromogranin A are favored over CD56 and neuron-specific enolase (NSE), due to lack of specificity of the latter. The biology of NETs varies widely, ranging from entirely benign, to indolent and generally nonprogressive, to metastatic with long-term survival, to metastatic and rapidly fatal. Improved prognostication is an area of ongoing research. To this end, the past several years have seen the introduction of a new grading system for NETs based on mitotic rate and Ki-67 proliferation index, and the American Joint Committee on Cancer (AJCC) has published, for the first time, an NET staging system (Figure 3.3D).

GENERAL FEATURES OF NEUROENDOCRINE CARCINOMAS

Poorly differentiated NENs are referred to as neuroendocrine carcinomas (NECs) in the WHO 2010 Classification. NEC encompasses small cell and large cell neuroendocrine carcinomas (as well as mixed small and large cell carcinomas). Small cell neuroendocrine carcinoma (SCNEC) typically demonstrates a diffuse growth pattern, although it may show some evidence of organoid architecture (eg, peripheral palisading of nuclei or rosette formation) (Figure 3.4A). Tumor cells are "small" (up to three times the diameter of a resting lymphocyte) with scant cytoplasm, finely (or sometimes coarsely) granular chromatin, inconspicuous to absent nucleoli, and a tendency for nuclear molding (Figure 3.4B). Mitotic activity and necrosis are conspicuous. Encrustation of vessels by basophilic material representing tumor DNA may be seen in up to a third of cases (referred to as the Azzopardi effect). SCNEC is often an "H&E diagnosis," though the diagnosis can be supported with IHC for general neuroendocrine markers. In addition, tumors may show dot-like expression of broad-spectrum keratins, and TTF-1 is frequently expressed, regardless of the site of origin (Figures 3.4C–D).

Compared to SCNEC, large cell neuroendocrine carcinoma (LCNEC) is more likely to demonstrate a "neuroendocrine" or organoid growth pattern and is characterized by larger cell size, more voluminous cytoplasm, variable nuclear chromatin, and, typically, prominent nucleoli (Figure 3.5A–B). It is similarly mitotically active and prone to extensive necrosis. Because of substantial morphologic overlap with non-neuroendocrine large cell undifferentiated carcinoma, the diagnosis formally requires demonstration of a neuroendocrine immunophenotype (Figure 3.5C–D). LCNEC stains similarly to

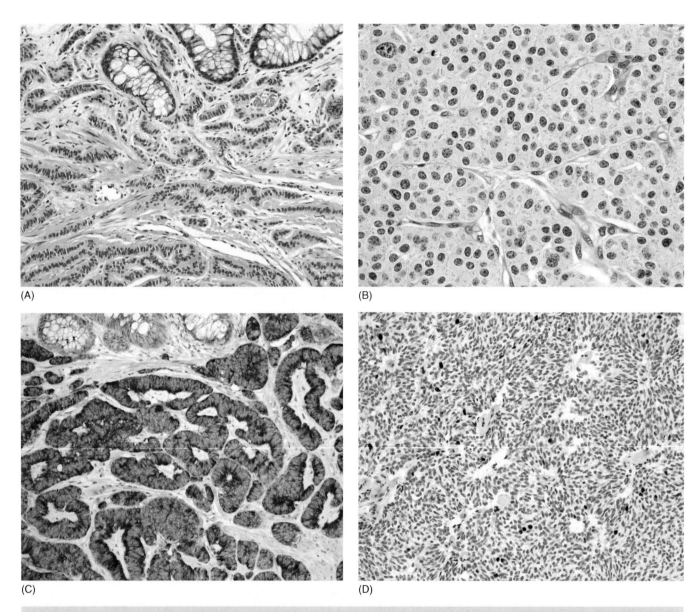

FIGURE 3.3 The trabecular pattern seen in this rectal NET exemplifies organoid architecture (A). NETs typically have a "salt-and-pepper" nuclear chromatin pattern and inconspicuous nucleoli. Note also the occasional large nucleus at the upper left, as well as an adjacent mitotic figure (B). NETs express general neuroendocrine markers, as illustrated by this synaptophysin IHC stain (C). In the WHO 2010 system, neuroendocrine tumors are graded based on mitotic rate and Ki-67 proliferation index. This appendiceal tumor has a low proliferation index at 3.2% (D).

SCNEC, though it is less likely to express TTF-1. Some tumors demonstrate mixed small cell and large cell morphology and in others, tumor cells are neither small nor large. In this latter group, the designation "neuroendocrine carcinoma with 'intermediate cell' morphology" may be used. Regardless of morphologic subtype or site of origin, NECs are highly aggressive tumors.

EPIDEMIOLOGY

NETs are uncommon but not rare, and their incidence is rising, due at least in part to increased recognition and

reporting. Based on data from Surveillance, Epidemiology, and End Results (SEER) registries, the annual age-adjusted incidence has increased from 1.09/100,000 in 1973 to 5.25/100,000 in 2004. By comparison, the age-adjusted incidence of colon cancer for 2007 to 2011 was 43.7/100,000. Although these lesions are relatively uncommon, because NETs are generally indolent, they are fairly prevalent. Based again on SEER data, Yao and colleagues estimated the 29-year-limited duration prevalence of NETs at 103,312 (35/100,000). This number refers to the number of people alive on a given date diagnosed with an NET anytime in the preceding 29 years. This far exceeds the 29-year-limited duration prevalence of gastric cancer

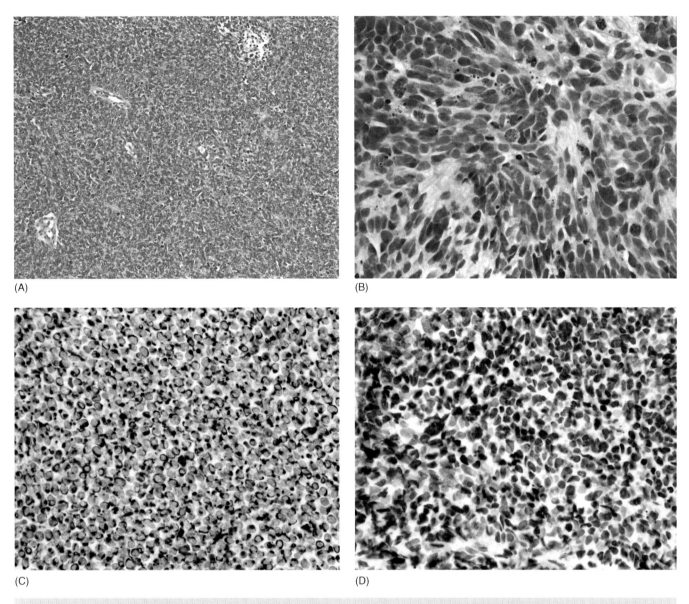

(A)

(B)

(C)

(D)

FIGURE 3.4 Small cell NECs are composed of small oval- to spindle-shaped cells with a very high nucleus: cytoplasm (N:C) ratio and a diffuse growth pattern; tumor necrosis is evident at the upper right (A). Tumor cells have fine chromatin, inconspicuous nucleoli, and demonstrate nuclear molding (B). Dot-like keratin expression may be seen (C). TTF-1 expression is usually seen in lung primaries but is also frequently seen in extrapulmonary visceral NECs (D).

(66K), pancreatic cancer (32K), and esophageal cancer (29K). Two thirds to three quarters of NETs arise in the gastro-entero-pancreatic system, although the single most frequently involved organ is the lung (25%–33%). In the GI tract, tumors present in the following organs in order of decreasing frequency: rectum, jejunoileum, pancreas, stomach, duodenum, and appendix. Because the SEER registries only capture "malignant" cases, rectal and appendiceal tumors, in particular, are likely underrepresented.

The male to female ratio is 1.1:1, although it varies from site to site (eg, 1.4:1 in both jejunoileum and pancreas; 0.9:1 in lung, stomach, and appendix). The median age at presentation is 63 for both men and women, although patients with rectal tumors (median age 56), which tend to be incidentally detected at screening colonoscopy, and appendiceal tumors (median age 47), which tend to be incidentally detected in association with acute appendicitis, are identified significantly earlier. Overall, 40% of disease is localized, 19% is regional, and 21% is distantly metastatic at presentation. Again, localized disease may be underreported to SEER, and practitioners at cancer centers will encounter more metastatic disease. The site of origin is strongly correlated with biologic potential in NETs. For example, while only 5% of rectal tumors are associated with distant metastasis at presentation and the median survival is 240 months, those figures for pancreatic tumors

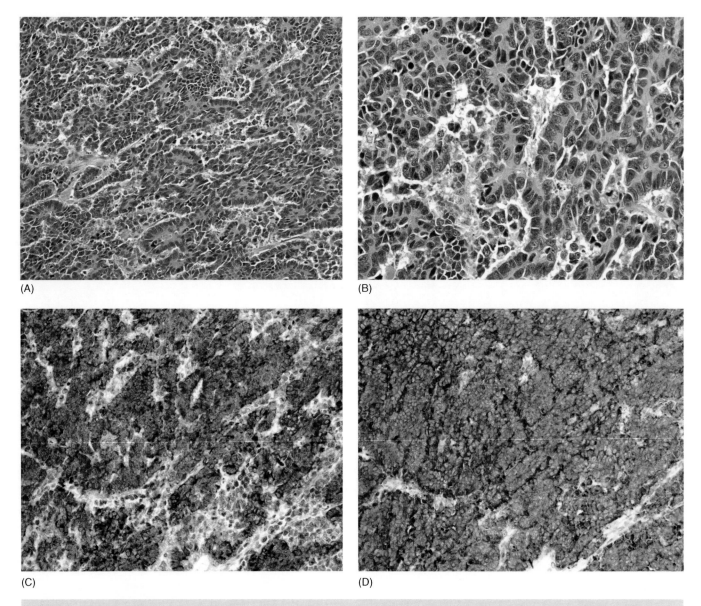

FIGURE 3.5 Compared to small cell NEC, large cell tumors are more likely to demonstrate organoid architecture (A). Tumor cells are larger with moderate amounts of cytoplasm and readily identifiable nucleoli (B). Convincing expression of at least one general neuroendocrine marker is required for the diagnosis, as illustrated here by chromogranin A (C) and synaptophysin (D) IHC.

are 64% and 42 months. Additional details regarding relative frequency, percentage of patients presenting with distant metastasis, and median survival for NETs stratified by the site of origin are provided in Table 3.1.

Extrapulmonary NECs are uncommon, with the annual incidence of Merkel cell carcinoma estimated at 1,600 and visceral extrapulmonary NEC at 1,000. Up to a quarter of extrapulmonary visceral NECs arise in the GI tract. Twenty-five percent to fifty percent of GI primaries arise in association with a non-neuroendocrine component, and an associated squamous or columnar dysplasia may be identified, regardless of the presence of a non-neuroendocrine carcinoma (Figure 3.6A–B). The prognosis

for patients with extensive-stage extrapulmonary visceral NEC is similar to that for lung (median survival for limited-stage and extensive-stage disease of 16–24 months and 6–12 months, respectively), while median survival may be slightly better for limited-stage disease (up to 43 months).

CLASSIFICATION OF NEUROENDOCRINE NEOPLASMS

Williams and Sandler Classification

Carcinoid tumors were originally described in the small intestine, though it was subsequently discovered that

TABLE 3.1   Site of Origin and Outcome in 35,825 Neuroendocrine Tumors From the Surveillance, Epidemiology, and End Results Registry (1973–2004)

Site of origin	Frequency (%)*	Distant Metastasis (%)	Median Survival (Months)
Foregut			
Lung	27	28	193
Thymus	0.4	31	77
Stomach	6.0	15	124
Duodenum	3.8	9	99
Pancreas	6.4	64	42
Liver	0.8	28	23
Midgut			
Jejunum/Ileum	13	30	88
Appendix	3.0	12	NR
Cecum	3.2	44	83
Colon	4.0	32	121
Hindgut			
Rectum	17	5	240
Other/Unknown Primary	15	NA	NS

Source: Yao JC, et al. One hundred years after "carcinoid": epidemiology of and prognostic factors in neuroendocrine tumors in 35,825 cases in the United States. *J Clin Oncol.* 2008;26(18):3063–3072.

Note: *data in this column based on years 2000–2004; NA, not applicable; NR, not reached; NS, not stated.

similar tumors arose in the lung and throughout the tubal gut. E.D. Williams and M. Sandler (1963), based on histologic, biochemical, and clinical observations, suggested that these tumors could be classified based on embryologic origin: foregut, midgut, or hindgut. Typical jejunoileal tumors, with nested architecture, a positive argentaffin reaction, high serotonin content, and a propensity to give rise to the carcinoid syndrome are of midgut origin. Foregut tumors include pulmonary, gastric, duodenal, and pancreatic primaries. These are more likely to show trabecular or mixed growth patterns, a negative argentaffin reaction, low serotonin content, and, with the exception of lung primaries, are unlikely to give rise to carcinoid syndrome. Hindgut tumors are nearly all rectal in origin. They tend to demonstrate trabecular growth, produce a negative argentaffin reaction, have low serotonin content, and do not result in carcinoid syndrome.

Soga and Tazawa Classification

J. Soga and K. Tazawa (1971) proposed that carcinoid tumors could be classified based on their predominant histologic patterns (see Table 3.2 and Figure 3.7A–E). They found that these histologic patterns correlated with the site of origin, and thus, their classification scheme supplements that of Williams and Sandler. Midgut tumors nearly always had a predominant nested growth pattern (type A), and were occasionally mixed, in which the secondary growth pattern was apt to be pseudoglandular (type C). The most frequent predominant pattern in foregut-derived tumors was trabecular or ribbon-like (type B), though half of the tumors showed mixed patterns. They reported a predominance of mixed patterns in hindgut tumors, though in subsequent reports, and in our experience, rectal NETs typically demonstrate an anastomosing trabecular pattern.

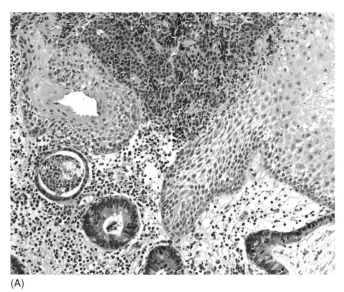

(A)

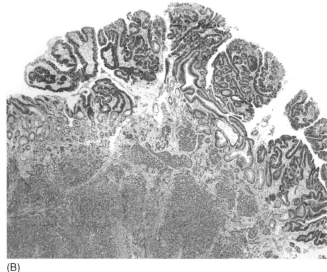

(B)

FIGURE 3.6   Small cell NEC arising in association with Barrett esophagus with low-grade dysplasia (A). "Intermediate cell" NEC arising in association with a gastric adenoma (B).

TABLE 3.2 Soga and Tazawa Classification

Type	Description	Comment(s)
A	Nested	Typical of midgut tumors
B	Trabecular	Typical of rectal tumors
C	Pseudoglandular	Characteristic of periampullary somatostatin-producing tumors; also common as a secondary pattern in midgut tumors
D	Diffuse	Prognostically adverse
Mixed	Any combination of the above-mentioned four patterns	Common outside of the midgut and rectum

WHO 2010 CLASSIFICATION OF GASTROENTEROPANCREATIC NEUROENDOCRINE EPITHELIAL NEOPLASMS

As discussed in the preceding paragraphs, in the 2010 WHO Classification of gastro-entero-pancreatic neuroendocrine neoplasms, well-differentiated neoplasms are classified as "neuroendocrine tumors," while poorly differentiated examples are referred to as "neuroendocrine carcinomas." NETs are further stratified into G1 and G2 based on mitotic rate and/or Ki-67 proliferation index. NECs are by definition G3 (see Table 3.3). Up to 40% of NETs that appear G1 by mitotic count are found to be G2 based on Ki-67 IHC, while up to a third of tumors that are G2 by mitotic count have proliferation indices greater than 20%, upgrading them to G3 (see Table 3.4). This data highlights the importance of performing Ki-67 IHC in all morphologically well-differentiated NENs, even those found to be G2 by mitotic count. For these grade-discrepant cases, the WHO recommends assigning the higher grade. This classification scheme also contains the category "mixed adenoneuroendocrine carcinoma" (MANEC), defined as a mixed tumor with at least 30% of each component. Most MANECs consist of NEC with a coexistent component of adenocarcinoma (Figure 3.8A–E). The WHO specifically states that adenocarcinomas in which scattered neuroendocrine cells are identified immunohistochemically (reported in up to 40% of cases) are not considered to be MANECs.

The 2010 WHO Classification supplants the WHO 2000 Classification, in which well-differentiated tumors were classified as well-differentiated endocrine tumor (WDET) or well-differentiated endocrine carcinoma (WDEC) based on the absence or presence of gross local invasion or metastasis. WDETs were further stratified into "benign behavior" or "uncertain behavior" based on a combination of angioinvasion, perineural invasion, local anatomic extent, size, mitotic count, and Ki-67

proliferation index, with the criteria differing slightly from site to site. While we have observed strong support and use of the 2010 classification, the WHO 2000 Classification was not widely embraced by U.S. pathologists, and has been criticized for several reasons including complexity, inclusion of features typically used to assign stage (local anatomic extent, gross local invasion, metastasis), and lack of comfort with the "benign behavior" category. This final criticism has been supported by the recognition that, on occasion, even small NETs may metastasize (see the following discussion of jejunoileal tumors). Of note, the gastro-entero-pancreatic neuroendocrine neoplasia classification is entirely different from the *2004 WHO Classification of Tumours of the Lung, Pleura, Thymus, and Heart.*

FEATURES OF NEUROENDOCRINE TUMORS BY ANATOMIC SITE

Esophagus

Esophageal NETs are rare, representing 0.06% (n = 6) of 13,175 "carcinoid" tumors reported to SEER registries from 1973 to 1999. They have been described arising de novo or in association with an invasive adenocarcinoma.

Stomach

Gastric NETs arise in three distinctive clinical settings, with implications for prognosis and management (summarized in Table 3.5). Type I tumors, representing 70% to 80%, arise in autoimmune atrophic gastritis. Type II tumors (5%–10%) arise in combined MEN1–ZES. Type III tumors (20%–25%) arise sporadically. Type I and II tumors are found in the gastric body, are typically confined to the mucosa or submucosa, and have a tendency to be multifocal (Figure 3.9A–B). They are composed of enterochromaffin-like (ECL) cells (ie, histamine-producing) and are driven by hypergastrinemia. Patients with small type I and II tumors may be managed with endoscopic removal and surveillance, while patients with type II tumors additionally benefit from removal of the gastrinoma, in which case their NET(s) may spontaneously regress. Hypergastrinemia-driven tumors, especially type I, are indolent. In a series of 193 gastric NETs, there were no tumor-related deaths in 152 type I tumors and 1 (8%) in 12 type II tumors.

Type III tumors are nearly always solitary and may arise anywhere in the stomach. They, too, are generally composed of ECL-cells, although approximately 25% are composed of alternative cell types (eg, gastrin, somatostatin, or serotonin-producing). Type III tumors are inherently aggressive. They tend to invade the muscularis propria or beyond and demonstrate frequent lymphovascular

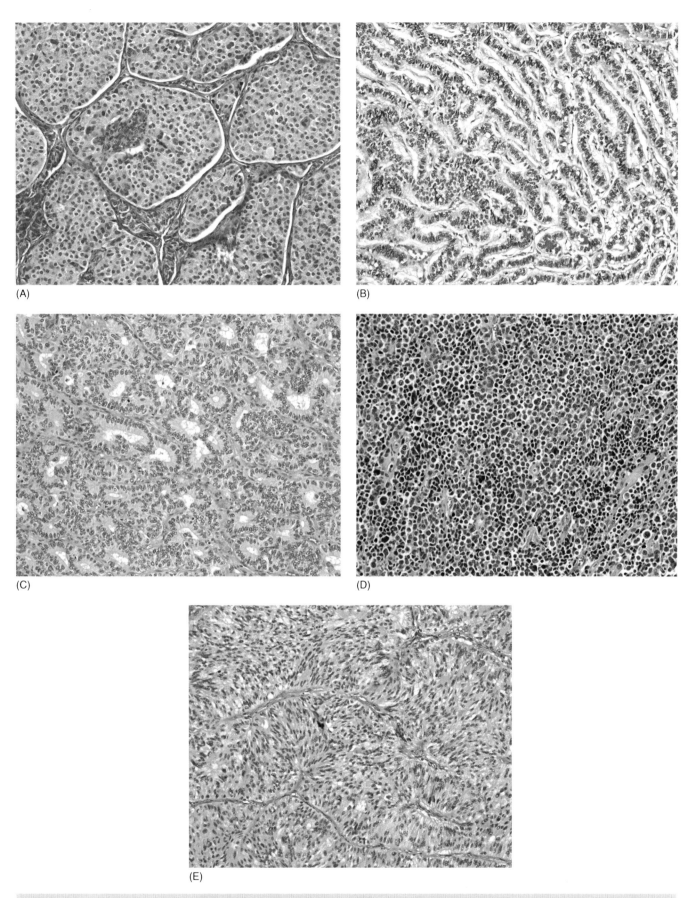

FIGURE 3.7   These pancreatic NENs illustrate the types of tumors within the Soga and Tazawa classification: Type A, nested (A); type B, trabecular (B); type C, pseudoglandular (C); and type D, diffuse (D). This tumor has mixed types A and C, as well as spindle cell morphology (E). All of these tumors except for "D" are well-differentiated.

TABLE 3.3 Grading of Gastroenteropancreatic Neuroendocrine Epithelial Neoplasms—Comparison of World Health Organization 2010 and 2000 Systems

WHO 2010

Category	Defined by
Neuroendocrine tumor (NET) G1	• Well-differentiated histology • <2 mitotic figures per 10 high-power fields (HPFs) and/or • Ki-67 proliferation index ≤2%
Neuroendocrine tumor (NET) G2	• Well-differentiated histology • 2–20 mitotic figures per 10 HPF and/or • Ki-67 proliferation index 3%–20%
Neuroendocrine carcinoma (NEC) G3	• Poorly differentiated histology • >20 mitotic figures per 10 HPF and/or • Ki-67 proliferation index >20%
Mixed adenoneuroendocrine carcinoma (MANEC)	• Mixed tumor with at least 30% of each component

WHO 2000

Category	Defined by
Well-differentiated endocrine tumor (WDET)*	• Well-differentiated histology • No gross local invasion or metastasis
Well-differentiated endocrine carcinoma (WDEC)	• Well-differentiated histology • Gross local invasion and/or metastasis
Poorly differentiated endocrine carcinoma (PDEC)/small cell carcinoma	• Poorly differentiated histology
Mixed exocrine–endocrine carcinoma (MEEC)	• Mixed tumor with endocrine component comprising at least 1/3

Note: *WDETs were further divided into "benign behavior" and "uncertain behavior" based on features including angioinvasion, perineural invasion, local anatomic extent, size, mitotic count, and Ki-67 proliferation index with criteria differing slightly based on primary site; for example, for pancreas "benign behavior" = nonangioinvasive, <2 cm, ≤2 mitotic figures and ≤2% Ki-67 positive cells per 10 HPF and "uncertain behavior" = 1 or more of the following: ≥2 cm, >2 mitotic figures per 10 HPF, >2% Ki-67 positive cells per 10 HPF, and angioinvasive.

TABLE 3.4 Grade Discordance in Neuroendocrine Tumors Based on Mitotic Rate Versus Ki-67 Proliferation Index

Mitotic Figures per 10 HPF	Ki-67 Proliferation Index ≤ 2%	Ki-67 Proliferation Index 2%–20%	Ki-67 Proliferation Index > 20%
<2 (n = 41)	25 (61%)	16 (39%)	None
2–20 (n = 13)	None	9 (69%)	4 (31%)

Source: Rege TA, King EE, Barletta JA, Bellizzi AM. Ki-67 proliferation index in pancreatic endocrine tumors: comparison with mitotic count, interobserver variability, and impact on grading. *Mod Pathol.* 2011;24(1S):372A.

invasion (Figure 3.9C–D). They are managed with gastrectomy and regional lymph node dissection. In the series of 193 tumors mentioned in the preceding paragraph, 7 (26%) of 27 type III tumors resulted in tumor-related deaths.

In the stomach, intramucosal tumors greater than 500 μm and submucosally invasive tumors are classified as NETs, while lesions measuring 150 to 500 μm are termed neuroendocrine dysplasias, and those less than 150 μm classified as hyperplasias. The distinction of these seems arbitrary, and lesions as small as 200 μm have been shown to be neoplastic based on molecular studies.

Duodenum

While the vast majority of duodenal NETs (90% or above) arise sporadically, they may also arise in association with MEN1 or neurofibromatosis type 1 (NF1). The biology of sporadic duodenal tumors appears to be somewhat less aggressive than sporadic gastric tumors. Tumors tend to be small and superficial, and those less than 1 to 2 cm may be managed endoscopically, while larger tumors or those with evident lymph node metastases require surgical resection. Duodenal NETs demonstrate the entire range of organoid architectural patterns, and tumors are often "mixed." Peptide hormones can be detected in

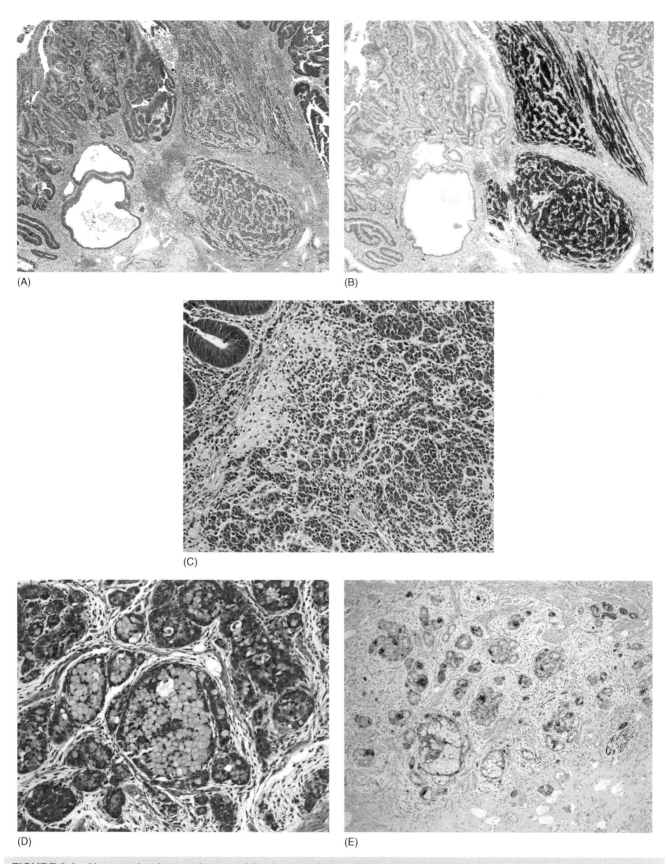

FIGURE 3.8   Neuroendocrine carcinoma arising in association with a rectal adenoma/adenocarcinoma (A). The neuroendocrine component expresses synaptophysin diffusely and strongly (B). Higher power view demonstrating the juxtaposition of an adenoma (top left) with the neuroendocrine carcinoma (C). This right colon cancer arose in association with a tubulovillous adenoma (D). Synaptophysin is expressed by more than 30% of tumor cells (E).

TABLE 3.5   Clinicopathologic Types of Gastric Neuroendocrine Tumors

Type	Disease Association	Relative Frequency	Focality	Biology
I	Autoimmune atrophic gastritis	70%–80% of gastric NETs	Multifocal	Indolent
II	Combined MEN1–ZES	5%–10%	Multifocal	Intermediate
III	None (sporadic)	20%–25%	Unifocal	Aggressive

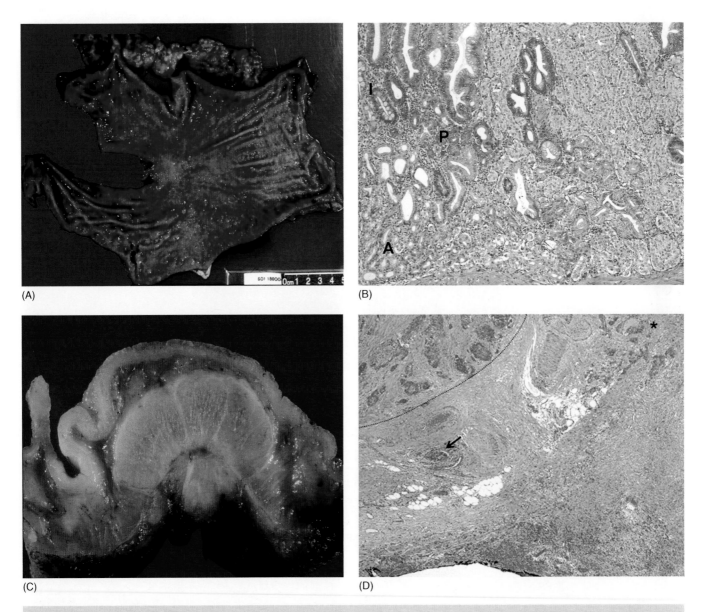

FIGURE 3.9 This patient underwent gastrectomy for approximately 50 neuroendocrine tumors arising in the context of autoimmune atrophic gastritis (type I). Note the nodularity, erythema, and decreased rugae in the gastric body (A). A representative section of the NEN from this patient also shows adjacent pancreatic acinar (P), intestinal (I), and antral/pyloric (A) metaplasia (B). Gross photograph of a transmurally invasive gastric tumor arising sporadically (type III) (C). The tumor has invaded beyond the muscularis propria into the subserosa (dashed line highlights this boundary); perineural (*) and lymphovascular invasion (arrow) are evident (D).

more than 95%, including serotonin (40%), somatostatin (50%), and gastrin (60%), but expression is only very rarely associated with a functional syndrome, and thus peptide-hormone IHC is not routinely recommended. Twenty to sixty percent of MEN1 patients are found to have multiple duodenal gastrinomas, which are typically quite small (up to 0.5 cm) and difficult to identify, even in a resection specimen. As discussed in the preceding section, these may be associated with ECL-cell tumors in the stomach. Patients with MEN1 may also manifest multiple gastrin and/or somatostatin-expressing neuroendocrine hyperplasias (see previous definition) and small NETs in the duodenum, and multiple glucagon/pancreatic polypeptide-expressing neuroendocrine hyperplasias and microadenomas in the pancreas. Again, the distinction between these terms seems arbitrary, as lesions as small as 200 μm have been shown to be neoplastic based on loss of heterozygosity for MEN1.

One percent of NF1 patients manifest somatostatin-producing tumors. These characteristically demonstrate type C histology and psammomatous calcifications, and are present at the ampulla (Figure 3.10A–B). Similar tumors are also seen sporadically, and thus, although the so-called "psammomatous somatostatinoma" should prompt consideration of NF1, it is not an NF1-defining lesion.

One final distinctive tumor in this area is worthy of mention. Gangliocytic paraganglioma demonstrates triphasic histology with neuroendocrine, spindle cell (Schwann cells and axons), and ganglion cell components, present in variable proportions (Figure 3.11). The ganglion cells may be singly dispersed or form clusters. In the largest published series of 51 cases, 49 occurred in the duodenum and all behaved in a benign fashion. Tumors may rarely metastasize to regional lymph nodes, and even more rarely to distant sites, but even in these settings, the clinical course may be indolent. This entity is discussed in greater detail in Chapters 5 and 9.

Jejunum and Ileum

Jejunoileal NETs are among the most aggressive, with a median survival of 88 months. In the Armed Forces Institute of Pathology (AFIP) series of jejunoileal tumors, the proportion of patients presenting with localized, regional, and distant metastatic disease was approximately equal. Seventy-seven percent of 159 tumors invaded beyond the muscularis propria, and small tumors were frequently metastatic. For example, 17% of submucosal tumors involved regional lymph nodes (without distant metastasis), while 25% were associated with distant metastasis; 21% of tumors less than 1 cm involved regional lymph nodes (without distant metastasis), as did 29% of tumors 1 to 2 cm; 29% of 1 to 2 cm tumors were associated with distant metastasis.

The ratio of ileal to jejunal tumors is 6.5:1. Rarely, morphologically and biologically similar tumors are detected in a Meckel's diverticulum. Twenty-five percent of jejunoileal NETs are multiple (Figure 3.12A). Whereas multiple NETs in the pancreas suggest a hereditary cancer predisposition syndrome (especially MEN1), the same

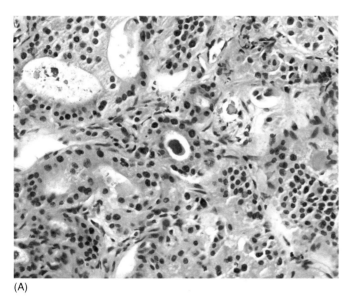
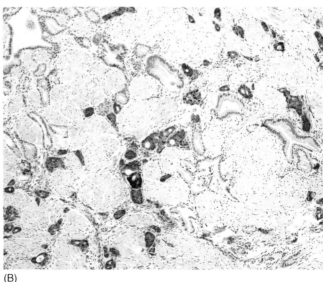

(A)   (B)

FIGURE 3.10 Somatostatin-expressing NETs may arise sporadically or in association with neurofibromatosis type I. They typically arise around the ampulla, demonstrate type C growth, and have intraluminal calcifications; given this growth pattern, it may be mistaken for adenocarcinoma (A). Somatostatin expression is demonstrated by immunohistochemistry (B).

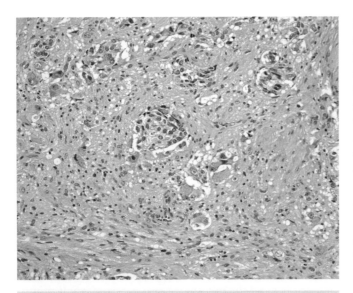

FIGURE 3.11 Gangliocytic paragangliomas have triphasic histology with neuroendocrine, spindle cell, and ganglion cell components. This tumor type typically arises in a periampullary location.

does not hold true at this anatomic site. Jejunoileal NETs are not associated with a known cancer syndrome, though up to 5% of patients have a first-degree relative with the same tumor type. The presence of multifocal disease may be prognostically adverse, though in the AFIP series this did not remain significant in a multivariate analysis.

Greater than 90% of these tumors demonstrate the type A (nested) growth pattern histologically, sometimes mixed with type C (pseudoglandular) (Figure 3.12B). The cytoplasm is typically replete with eosinophilic granules containing serotonin, which is immunohistochemically detectable in approximately 90% of tumors (Figure 3.12C). Tumors with high serotonin content reduce silver salts to metallic silver (the basis of the argentaffin reaction), which was used in the pre-IHC era to support a diagnosis of carcinoid tumor. Serotonin is responsible for the "carcinoid syndrome," which is only seen in 5% of patients with jejunoileal NETs in the AFIP series (in the setting of large volume hepatic disease). More frequently, patients present with obstruction, abdominal pain, or GI bleeding. Serotonin (and/or related peptides) induces fibroelastosis, and segments of small intestine containing transmural invasion by tumor are often "kinked," while mesenteric vessels frequently demonstrate elastosis, an underrecognized cause of intestinal ischemia in these patients (Figure 3.12D–E).

Appendix

Appendiceal NETs tend to involve the appendiceal tip, and often present incidentally at the time of appendectomy

for acute appendicitis (Figure 3.13A). According to SEER data, about one-third are not localized at the time of diagnosis. While most of these tumors pursue a benign clinical course, it is important for pathologists to recognize and report characteristics associated with increased aggressiveness, particularly tumor size greater than 2 cm. Moreover, the North American Neuroendocrine Tumor Society (NANETS) recommends right hemicolectomy in patients with an appendiceal NET found to exhibit one or more of the features listed in Table 3.6.

Most appendiceal NETs are composed of serotonin-producing EC cells, similar to jejunoileal tumors (Figure 3.13B). They typically have type A predominant or mixed architectural patterns. Ten to twenty percent of tumors are composed of L cells (glucagon-like peptide-1-producing); many of these have either tubular or tubular and trabecular architecture and have been referred to as "tubular carcinoids" (Figure 3.13C–D). Given their growth pattern and the fact that they often do not express chromogranin A (although they do express synaptophysin), tubular carcinoids may be mistaken for adenocarcinoma. Tubular carcinoids are typically minute and pursue a benign clinical course. Occasional appendiceal NETs show cytoplasmic microvesicular change and/or vacuolization (Figure 3.13E). These tumors are referred to as clear cell NETs, and this appears to represent a degenerative phenomenon in otherwise typical EC-cell tumors. Clear cell NETs express general neuroendocrine markers, but do not express mucins (Figure 3.13F).

Goblet cell carcinoid is an unusual tumor that is virtually restricted to the appendix. It demonstrates circumferential appendiceal involvement and appears to "drop off" the crypt bases, without an overlying in situ component (Figure 3.14A). Histologically, the tumor invades as small crypts composed of mixtures of relatively bland goblet, enteroendocrine, and Paneth cells, recapitulating the crypts of Lieberkühn (thus one of the alternative designations "crypt cell carcinoma") (Figure 3.14B). In the WHO 2010 Classification, goblet cell carcinoids and adenocarcinomas (including signet ring cell and poorly differentiated types) arising in goblet cell carcinoids are considered mixed adenoneuroendocrine tumors although their classification as such is not universally accepted. These tumors must be distinguished from appendiceal involvement by metastatic adenocarcinoma; the characteristic circumferential growth pattern and invasion as identifiable crypts suggest the diagnosis. These tumors are tumor, node, metastasis (TNM)-staged and are generally managed as adenocarcinomas.

Colorectum

The vast majority of colorectal NETs involve the rectum. In the AFIP series of 84 colonic tumors, 81 involved the rectum and 3 the distal sigmoid. Tumors are typically

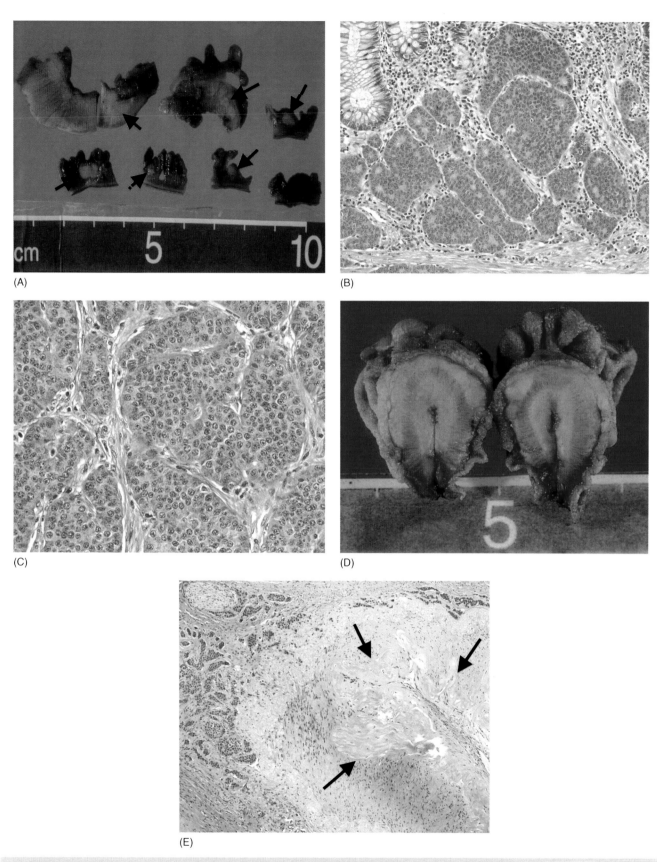

FIGURE 3.12 Twenty-five percent of jejunoileal tumors are multifocal (A) as shown in this resection specimen containing multiple white-tan nodules (arrows). Type A growth predominates in jejunoileal neuroendocrine tumors, but is sometimes mixed with type C, as in this example; note also the dense eosinophilic cytoplasmic granularity (B). Higher power of another tumor demonstrates cytoplasmic granularity (C). Transmurally invasive tumors tend to "kink" segments of intestine, leading to obstruction (D). Mesenteric vascular elastosis is common; note especially the marked adventitial elastosis (E, arrows).

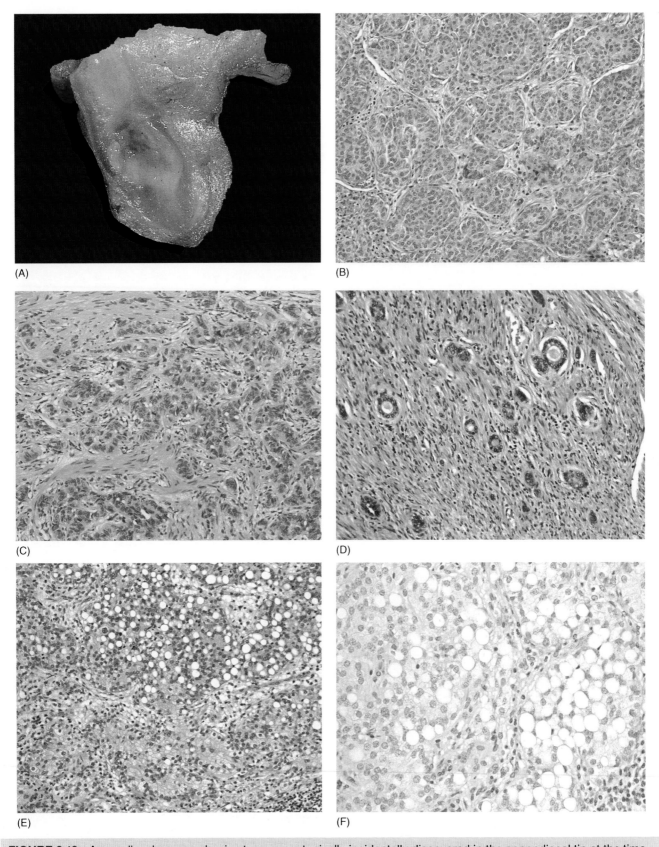

FIGURE 3.13 Appendiceal neuroendocrine tumors are typically incidentally discovered in the appendiceal tip at the time of appendectomy for acute appendicitis (A). Most tumors are composed of EC cells, similar to jejunoileal primaries (B). Occasional tumors are composed of L cells, which may demonstrate trabecular (C) or tubular architecture (D). Clear cell change may manifest as cytoplasmic vacuolization or microvesiculation (E). This appears to represent a degenerative change in otherwise typical EC-cell tumors. The clear cell change is due to cytoplasmic lipid accumulation, and mucin stains, like this alcian blue, are negative (F).

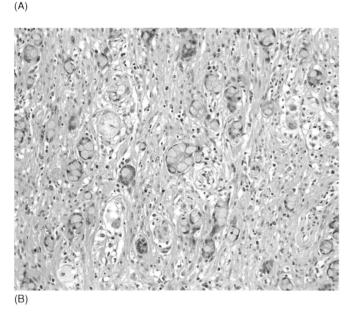

(A)

(B)

FIGURE 3.14 Goblet cell carcinoids invade circumferentially (A). They are composed of crypt-like structures with an admixture of bland goblet and enteroendocrine cells (B).

TABLE 3.6 NANETS Recommendations for Right Hemicolectomy in Appendiceal Neuroendocrine Tumors

Tumor size > 2 cm (or if size cannot be determined)
Tumor location in base of appendix
Positive margins on appendectomy
Lymphovascular invasion
Mesoappendiceal invasion
G2 (and goblet cell carcinoid)
Gross mesenteric nodal involvement

Source: Boudreaux JP, Klimstra DS, Hassan MM, Woltering EA, Jensen RT, Goldsmith SJ, Nutting C, Bushnell DL, Caplin ME, Yao JC; North American Neuroendocrine Tumor Society (NANETS). The NANETS consensus guideline for the diagnosis and management of neuroendocrine tumors: well-differentiated neuroendocrine tumors of the jejunum, ileum, appendix, and cecum. *Neuroendocrinology.* 2012;95(2):135–156.

incidentally discovered, small, and benign. In the SEER database of 4,701 tumors (1973–2004), the median size was 0.6 cm, and 4% and 2.4% of patients presented with regional and distant metastatic disease, respectively. Similarly, in the AFIP series, 3.6% of patients presented with lymph node metastases. Surgical series have identified size greater than 1 cm and lymphovascular invasion as features associated with aggressive behavior, and patients with these features may undergo resection with lymph node dissection. Histologically, rectal NETs typically demonstrate type B (trabecular) growth, are composed of L cells, and may fail to stain for chromogranin A (Figure 3.15A–B). Ninety percent express prostatic acid phosphatase, and as such, they may be mistaken for locally advanced prostate cancer in small, crushed biopsies.

CLINICAL SIGNIFICANCE OF RECOGNIZING NEUROENDOCRINE EPITHELIAL NEOPLASMS

The correct diagnosis of NET has prognostic and therapeutic significance, relative to the diagnosis of non-neuroendocrine tumors. For example, multiple small NETs arising in a background of autoimmune atrophic gastritis and small, solitary tumors in the duodenum or rectum may be managed endoscopically, whereas similarly sized adenocarcinomas at these anatomic locations might result in a resection. Patients with resected NETs metastatic to regional lymph nodes have not been shown to benefit from adjuvant chemotherapy, while such therapy is the norm in colorectal adenocarcinoma. In patients presenting with extensive hepatic metastases, a diagnosis of non-neuroendocrine carcinoma is considered incurable disease, and patients receive palliative chemotherapy. In NET, patients with less than "diffuse, multifocal liver metastases" may be offered surgery with curative intent. Complete resection (R0/R1) is associated with a 5-year survival of 60% to 80%, double that of patients whose liver metastases are not resected. Although it is recognized that this benefit may in part reflect a selection bias, it is clinically significant nonetheless. Patients in whom hepatic disease is unresectable may still be candidates for tumor ablation, especially in the face of a functional syndrome. The associated primary tumors, especially jejuno-ileal ones, may also be resected to prevent complications including obstruction and ischemia.

NECs often present with distant metastases, in which case the chemotherapy (a platinum-based agent and etoposide) is the same regardless of the site of origin. Patients with extrapulmonary visceral NECs with locoregional disease may undergo resection and then receive adjuvant chemotherapy.

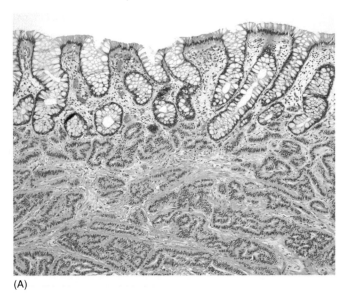

(A)

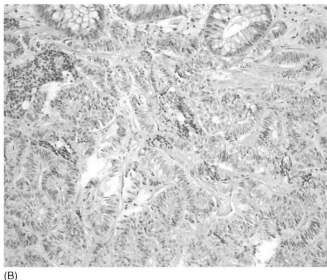

(B)

FIGURE 3.15 Rectal neuroendocrine tumors frequently exhibit an anastomosing trabecular architecture (A). Chromogranin A is negative in up to half, similar to other L-cell tumors (B).

DIFFERENTIAL DIAGNOSIS

The primary entities in the differential diagnosis of well-differentiated NETs include non-neuroendocrine carcinomas, neuroendocrine hyperplasias, and NECs. Periampullary somatostatin-expressing tumors, appendiceal tubular carcinoids, and other tumors exhibiting type B or C histology may be mistaken for adenocarcinoma. Tumors with nested growth may be mistaken for squamous cell carcinoma or solid adenocarcinoma, and clear cell NETs may be mistaken for "foamy gland" adenocarcinoma. Furthermore, NETs may produce luminal or stromal mucin, a potential source of diagnostic confusion (Figure 3.16A). Rectal NETs usually express prostatic acid phosphatase and may be mistaken for prostatic adenocarcinoma. In all these instances, neuroendocrine chromatin may be evident, although its "obviousness" varies from case to case. NETs are also characterized by relative monomorphism, which is often punctuated by scattered large cells (so-called "endocrine atypia"), while non-NECs tend to exhibit greater pleomorphism (Figure 3.16B). In the liver, tumors composed of large, polygonal cells may be mistaken for hepatocellular carcinoma as well. When a tumor diagnosis is in question, pathologists should consider NET and have a low threshold for ordering IHC for general neuroendocrine markers.

Adrenal cortical carcinomas may also be mistaken for NETs. These tumors are often cytologically diverse, with wildly pleomorphic areas alternating with deceptively bland ones (Figure 3.16C). At least half of these tumors express synaptophysin, and this in large part leads to the diagnostic confusion (Figure 3.16D). They do not express

chromogranin, however, nor epithelial membrane antigen (EMA). IHC for broad-spectrum keratins is often weak and patchy. If a diagnosis of adrenal cortical carcinoma is suspected, more specific immunostains including melan-A (clone A103), inhibin, and steroidogenic factor 1 may be helpful (Figure 3.16E).

Glomus tumors, especially in the stomach, may be mistaken for NETs, especially since they often express synaptophysin (albeit weakly) (Figure 3.16F–G). Tumors are often multinodular and/or plexiform, and tend to grow within blood vessel walls (subendothelially). Tumor cells are round with moderate amounts of eosinophilic to clear cytoplasm. Demonstration of strong smooth muscle actin expression is useful in securing the diagnosis (Figure 3.16H).

Neuroendocrine tumors may be mistaken for NECs as well. This may be a particular problem in small or crushed specimens (Figure 3.16I–J). In contrast to NETs, NECs have high nucleus: cytoplasm ratios and are highly proliferative, generally with readily observable mitotic activity and abundant karyorrhectic debris. Tumor necrosis is often prominent, although it tends to be "punctate" in G2 NETs, and is rarely observed in G1 tumors. Ki-67 IHC readily distinguishes NET from NEC and is strongly recommended if there is any concern about the diagnosis of NEC, especially in small, crushed biopsies (Figure 3.16 K–L).

The primary entities in the differential diagnosis of NECs also include non-neuroendocrine carcinomas, as well as other high-grade round cell tumors, and chronic inflammation. NECs should show characteristic cytomorphology and demonstrate diffuse expression of at least one general neuroendocrine marker. Significant pleomorphism, although it may be encountered focally in NEC, suggests the diagnosis of a non-neuroendocrine carcinoma.

Small cell neuroendocrine carcinoma is rarely mistaken for a non-neuroendocrine carcinoma. Basaloid squamous cell carcinoma can exhibit overlapping morphologic features on occasion, though, and thus it may be prudent to perform a limited immunohistochemical panel in many cases (eg, a general neuroendocrine marker such as synaptophysin, a broad-spectrum keratin, and possibly p63, TTF-1, and/or cytokeratin [CK]20). Large cell neuroendocrine carcinoma is rarer and thus less familiar, and generally does not demonstrate typical neuroendocrine

chromatin. Given its relative monomorphism and occasionally prominent nucleoli, cases may be mistaken for high-grade prostatic adenocarcinoma, and given its frequently nested architecture, squamous cell carcinoma and solid adenocarcinoma may also enter the differential. The previously mentioned panel of immunohistochemical stains is similarly useful in this situation, as well.

NECs must also be distinguished from other round cell tumors including lymphomas, melanomas, and some sarcomas. NECs should express broad-spectrum keratins, which may appear perinuclear or dot-like, as well as general neuroendocrine markers. CD45 is helpful in

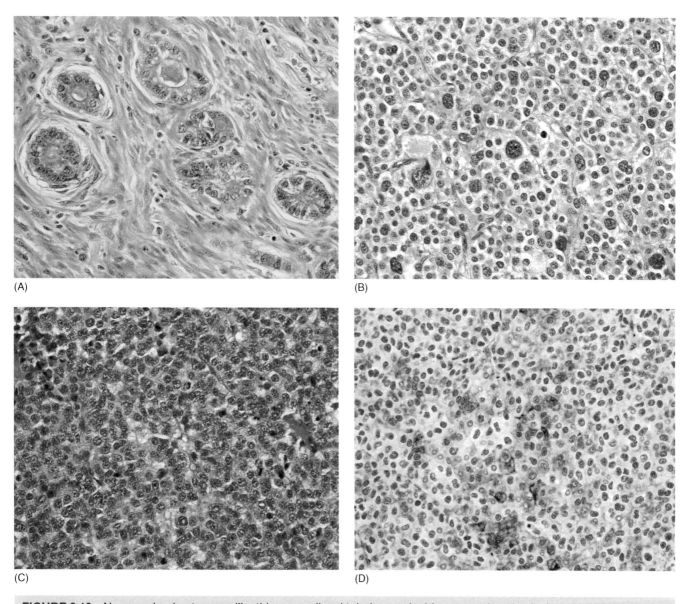

(A)

(B)

(C)

(D)

FIGURE 3.16 Neuroendocrine tumors, like this appendiceal tubular carcinoid, may produce luminal or stromal mucin, though intracytoplasmic mucin is uncommon (A, mucicarmine). Scattered larger nuclei are common in well-differentiated NETs, and do not affect grading (B). A core biopsy of this adrenal cortical carcinoma demonstrates monomorphous, low-grade cytomorphology and granular chromatin, initially diagnosed as an NET (C). Synaptophysin expression is seen in about half of adrenal cortical carcinomas (D). (*continued*)

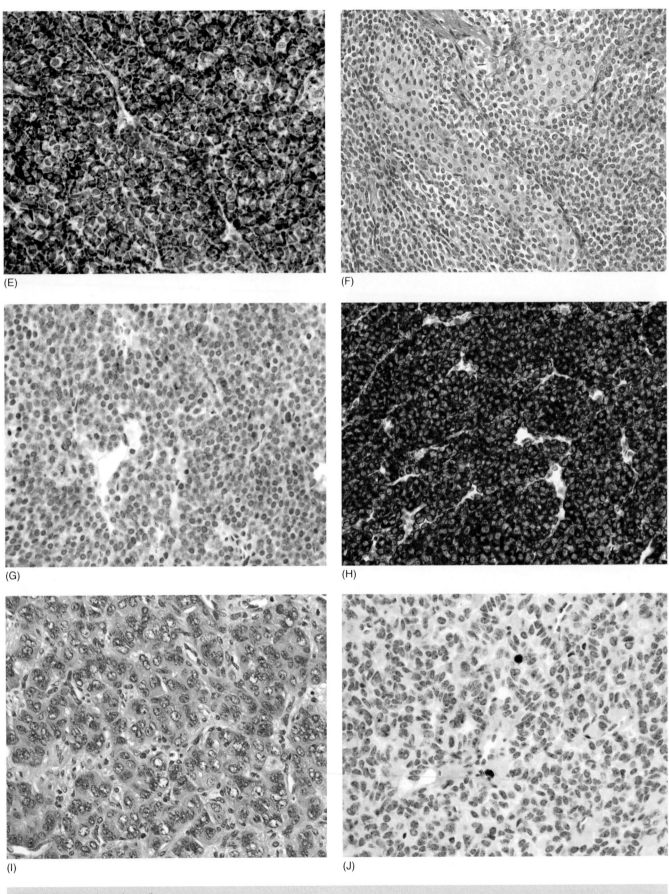

(E)

(F)

(G)

(H)

(I)

(J)

FIGURE 3.16   (*continued*)

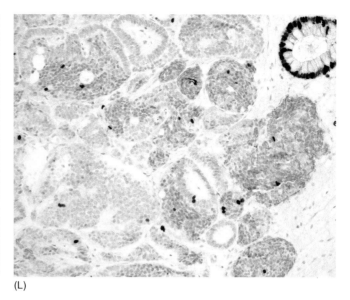

(K)   (L)

FIGURE 3.16 *(continued)* Negative chromogranin A and positive melan-A immunostains suggest the correct diagnosis (E, melan-A IHC). This gastric glomus tumor was also initially diagnosed as a neuroendocrine tumor (F). Weak staining for synaptophysin in glomus tumors may lead to diagnostic confusion as well (G). Glomus tumors consistently demonstrate strong staining with antibodies to smooth muscle actin (H). This pancreatic neuroendocrine tumor, with vesicular rather than granular chromatin, was initially diagnosed as a poorly differentiated neuroendocrine carcinoma based on morphology (I). Mitotic figures were rare, and the Ki-67 proliferation index was 1.4%, confirming the diagnosis of NET (J, Ki-67 IHC). This rectal neuroendocrine tumor was concerning for NEC because the crushed foci on the right were worrisome for small cell carcinoma (K). A Ki-67 proliferation index of 3.9% confirms the diagnosis of a G2 neuroendocrine tumor (L, Ki-67 IHC).

excluding lymphoma, and S100 for excluding melanoma. Among sarcomas, desmoplastic small round cell tumor (dot-like immunopositivity for desmin, NSE, and nuclear WT-1 with antibodies to the carboxy but not the amino terminus), Ewing sarcoma (diffuse, strong membranous CD99), rhabdomyosarcoma (desmin, myogenin, MyoD1 positivity), and poorly differentiated synovial sarcoma (TLE1) are often differential considerations. In crushed small biopsies, IHC for broad-spectrum keratins (and/ or general neuroendocrine markers) and CD45 may be used to distinguish NEC from chronic inflammation (Figure 3.17A–B).

True MANECs of the tubal gut are rare, and combined adenocarcinoma–NEC is the most commonly encountered. In these cases, the key is recognizing areas of typical small cell or large cell NEC in addition to areas of adenocarcinoma.

Not uncommonly, poorly differentiated carcinomas (usually adenocarcinomas) are mistakenly classified as MANECs, and a diagnosis is rendered such as "poorly differentiated (adeno)carcinoma with neuroendocrine features" or "poorly differentiated (adeno)carcinoma with neuroendocrine differentiation." This situation often occurs in the setting of an especially high-grade, solid adenocarcinoma (Figure 3.18A) in which a diagnosis of NEC is contemplated (eg, a medullary-type microsatellite unstable tumor that has lost expression of CK20 and/or

CDX2) and thus IHC for general neuroendocrine markers is performed (Figure 3.18B–C). As discussed previously, GI tract adenocarcinomas frequently (up to 40% of tumors) contain scattered neuroendocrine cells, but by definition 30% of cells must show neuroendocrine differentiation before a diagnosis of MANEC can be assigned. A diagnosis of "poorly differentiated (adeno)carcinoma with neuroendocrine features" is ambiguous, and strongly discouraged, because it is frustrating for clinicians who do not know whether to give chemotherapy for adenocarcinoma (eg, FOLFOX) or NEC (eg, cisplatin/etoposide).

NETs, especially in the stomach, ampulla, and pancreas, occasionally entrap benign glands or ductules (Figure 3.18D), mimicking a component of adenocarcinoma. In a true MANEC, the non-neuroendocrine component must be overtly cytologically malignant.

GENERAL APPROACH TO DIAGNOSIS AND REPORTING OF PRIMARY NEUROENDOCRINE TUMORS

To summarize, there are five key aspects to the diagnosis of an NET:

- Recognition of a histologic pattern suggestive of NET.
- Performance of supportive diagnostic IHC as needed.

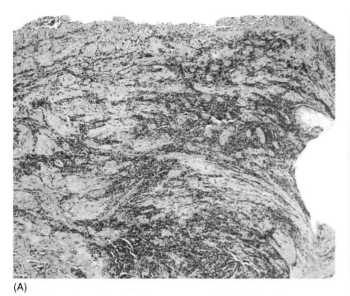

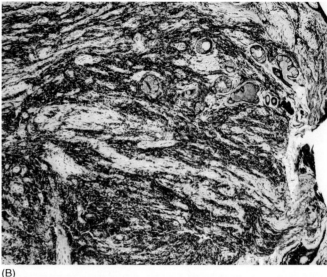

(A)   (B)

FIGURE 3.17   Crushed foci of small cell NEC in small biopsies must be distinguished from chronic inflammation (A). Pan-cytokeratin positivity confirms the diagnosis of carcinoma (B).

- Assessment of the mitotic index.
- Performance of Ki-67 IHC to assess proliferation index.
- Consideration of associated conditions.

As discussed previously in the section on morphology, NETs characteristically demonstrate one or more "organoid" architectural patterns. Chromatin is typically "salt and pepper" and nucleoli are generally inconspicuous, but there is variation from case to case. Tumors appear to arise "de novo," without an associated precursor lesion, with the exception of type I and II gastric NETs that arise in the context of neuroendocrine hyperplasia, and very rare tubal gut NETs that appear to arise in association with a columnar dysplasia (eg, tubular adenoma) (Figure 3.19).

As noted previously in the "General Features" sections, the most useful supportive diagnostic immunostains include the general neuroendocrine markers chromogranin A and synaptophysin. In a recent consensus conference of NET experts, however, 53% agreed that "routine immunohistochemical staining is not necessary to diagnose histologically typical examples of well-differentiated NETs (carcinoid tumors) of the ileum, appendix, and stomach or certain pancreatic endocrine tumors." If general neuroendocrine markers are performed, it is often useful to do two markers in tandem. As discussed previously in the section on hormone expression, IHC for peptide hormones is only appropriate in very select circumstances.

Once a diagnosis of NET is rendered, the mitotic count and proliferation index should be assessed. Mitotic counts are expressed per 10 high-power fields (HPFs). The *AJCC Cancer Staging Manual* recommends evaluating at

least 40 fields and the *WHO GI Blue Book* recommends examining at least 50 fields in areas of greatest mitotic activity. It is useful to scan at low power looking for any mitotic activity, and to begin the count in a field containing a mitotic figure. Mucosal biopsies (and core biopsies of metastatic lesions) rarely contain the requisite number of fields, and in these instances it is helpful to report precisely what was observed (eg, 1 mitotic figure in 7 HPF).

Ki-67 IHC is essential for correct WHO 2010 NET grading, and some authorities perform Ki-67 staining on both biopsies and resections of primary NETs. The proliferation index is generally quantified in one of three ways:

- Estimation by regular light microscopy.
- Manual counting of a digitally captured image.
- Automated image analysis.

Many experienced pathologists estimate ("eyeball") proliferation indices with confidence, though this takes some practice. For example, many cases clearly have a proliferation index of less than 2%, while others are clearly greater than 5% or greater than 20%. For cases in the 2% to 5% range and those around 20%, it is useful to formally count at least 500 tumor cells (generally 500–1,000) in the areas of highest labeling (so-called "hot spots"). Of note, the *AJCC Cancer Staging Manual* recommends counting 2,000, and the *WHO GI Blue Book* 500–2,000, nuclei. A 400× HPF generally includes at least 500 tumor nuclei. It can be very helpful to take a digital photomicrograph, which can then be printed out and the nuclei "checked off" as they are counted (Figure 3.20). It may be easier to count the positive nuclei on the computer monitor, especially if the printout is in black and

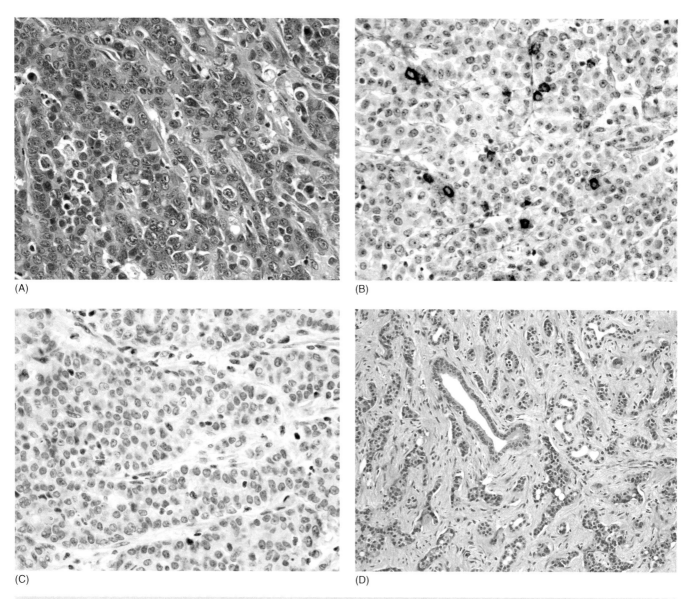

(A)

(B)

(C)

(D)

FIGURE 3.18 This poorly differentiated adenocarcinoma (A, note the scattered small droplets of intracytoplasmic mucin) was initially interpreted as a "poorly differentiated adenocarcinoma with neuroendocrine differentiation," based in part on this chromogranin A immunostain showing occasional positive cells (B). PMS2 immunostain from the same case demonstrates absent expression in tumor cells with intact internal control staining (C); the tumor was also MLH1 deficient, while MSH2 and MSH6 were intact. Tumors with deficient DNA mismatch repair function, particularly those with solid growth patterns or that lack typical markers of GI differentiation, are especially apt to be overinterpreted as showing "neuroendocrine differentiation." Neuroendocrine tumors entrapping benign non-neoplastic glands or ducts are occasionally misinterpreted as mixed adenoneuroendocrine carcinomas (D).

white. Results are expressed in percentage. One may also state either the numerator and denominator, and/or state that the proliferation index was "formally quantified." Although seemingly complicated, this entire process takes about 5 minutes. The utility of automated image analysis has been limited by the cost (exceeding 100K) and thus availability of image analyzers. Counting nontumor cells (eg, tumor infiltrating lymphocytes are often Ki-67 positive) is a source of error. Free online image analysis

programs such as ImmunoRatio have recently become available as well (153.1.200.58:8080/immunoratio).

Pertinent associated conditions should also be reported. In gastric NETs, these include autoimmune atrophic gastritis and MEN1–ZES. The presence of a corpus-restricted chronic gastritis with pyloric, intestinal, and pancreatic acinar metaplasia and ECL-cell hyperplasia is typical of autoimmune gastritis. Patients with ZES demonstrate giant rugal folds with parietal cell hypertrophy

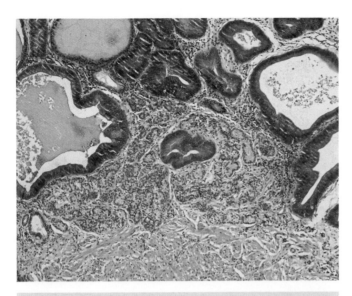

FIGURE 3.19 Compared to neuroendocrine carcinomas, well differentiated neuroendocrine tumors only rarely arise in association with a columnar dysplasia. This gastric tumor is present in a background of polypoid low-grade intestinal type dysplasia.

and hyperplasia and ECL-cell hyperplasia. The presence of multiple duodenal or pancreatic NETs suggests the diagnosis of MEN1. A periampullary, type C, somatostatin-expressing NET raises the differential of NF1. In resection

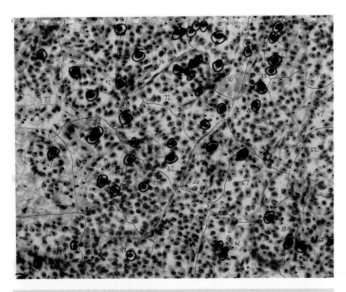

FIGURE 3.20 To manually count a Ki-67 immunolabeled slide, a photomicrograph of a proliferation index "hot spot" is taken. The brown staining nuclei are counted (53), as are the total neuroendocrine tumor nuclei (1363), to arrive at a proliferation index of 3.9%. The photomicrograph has been segmented to facilitate counting (courtesy of Frank A. Mitros, MD).

specimens of jejunoileal tumors, mesenteric vessels should be examined for vascular elastosis.

A report on the biopsy of a primary NET should include the tumor type, tumor size, and WHO 2010 grade, followed by the mitotic rate, the Ki-67 proliferation index, the presence or absence of nonischemic tumor necrosis, and any associated conditions. For resection specimens, a synoptic reporting form is recommended (see Table 3.7).

APPROACH TO METASTATIC NEUROENDOCRINE TUMORS OF UNKNOWN ORIGIN

The same five key aspects discussed in the prior section regarding primary NETs apply to the diagnosis and reporting of metastatic NETs. Although some consider Ki-67 IHC to be optional in this setting, particularly in resected metastases, there is evidence that the proliferation index in metastases predicts progression-free survival. There is one additional critical element in the metastatic setting, which is determination of the site of origin. Ten to twenty percent of all NETs present as metastases of unknown origin, even after investigations including computed tomography, magnetic resonance imaging, positron emission tomography, and upper and lower endoscopy. OctreoScan (somatostatin receptor scintigraphy) is able to localize the primary in up to 40% of these, but is limited by a range of detection of around 2 cm. In patients who are surgically explored, many occult primaries are of jejunoileal origin, followed by pancreas. Occult primaries average about 1.5 cm (recall that the frequencies of regional and distant disease for jejunoileal tumors this size in the AFIP series were each 33%).

Determination of the site of origin is both prognostically and therapeutically significant. In the SEER dataset, the median survival for patients with distant disease from jejunoileal and pancreatic NETs was 56 and 24 months, respectively. While somatostatin analogues are the mainstay of medical antiproliferative therapy in metastatic jejunoileal tumors, there are several additional options including alkylating agents, mTOR inhibitors, and tyrosine kinase inhibitors in pancreatic NETs.

IHC can be useful in assigning the primary site in metastatic NETs of unknown origin. Around 90% of jejunoileal metastases express CDX2, which is typically diffuse and strong (Figure 3.21). Although up to 15% of pancreatic NETs also express CDX2, in one recent study these tumors always coexpressed the transcription factors PAX6 and/or islet 1. Many laboratories have found that polyclonal PAX8 antibodies, which cross-react with PAX4 and PAX6, are fairly sensitive and specific for pancreatic primaries. Prostatic acid phosphatase, expressed in most rectal NETs, is also detected in at least 40% of jejunoileal

TABLE 3.7 Sample Gastroenteropancreatic Neuroendocrine Neoplasm Synoptic Report Format

Tumor Diagnosis ([well-differentiated] neuroendocrine tumor; [poorly differentiated] neuroendocrine carcinoma):

Tumor Site (eg, terminal ileum, pancreas, etc.):

Tumor Size (cm):

Tumor Focality (unifocal, multifocal):

Mitotic Rate (assess 50 HPF in most mitotically active areas; report average per 10 HPF):

Proliferation Index (% Ki-67 labeled nuclei in areas of highest labeling; assess 500–2,000 cells):

Grade (WHO 2010):
___ G1: mitotic rate <2 per 10 HPF AND proliferation index ≤2%
___ G2: mitotic rate 2–20 per 10 HPF OR proliferation index 3%–20%
___ G3: mitotic count >20 per 10 HPF OR proliferation index >20% (vast majority of G3 tumors are morphologically poorly differentiated)

Nonischemic Tumor Necrosis (present, absent):

Extent of Invasion (eg, for tubal gut, depth of invasion into/through gut wall; for pancreas, invasion into peripancreatic soft tissue, duodenum, ampulla, or extrapancreatic common bile duct):

Resection Margins (mucosal, mesenteric, radial, as appropriate; positive, negative):

Distance to Closest Margin (specify which margin):

Lymphovascular Invasion (present, absent):

Perineural Invasion (present, absent):

Associated Diseases (eg, atrophic gastritis; MEN1; mesenteric vascular elastosis, functional syndrome):

Regional Lymph Nodes (positive/total):

Pathologic Staging (pTNM) (the following apply to WDNET; PDNEC staged according to site-specific TNM guidelines for carcinoma):

TNM Descriptors (required only if applicable):
___ m (multiple)
___ r (recurrent)
___ y (posttreatment)

Stomach Primary Tumor (T):
___ TX: Primary tumor cannot be assessed
___ T0:   No evidence of primary tumor
___ Tis: Carcinoma in situ/dysplasia (tumor size less than 0.5 mm, confined to mucosa)
___ T1:   Tumor invades lamina propria or submucosa and size 1 cm or less
___ T2:   Tumor invades muscularis propria or more than 1 cm in size
___ T3:   Tumor invades subserosa
___ T4:   Tumor invades visceral peritoneum or other organs/structures

Duodenum/Ampulla/Jejunum/Ileum Primary Tumor (T):
___ TX: Primary tumor cannot be assessed
___ T0:   No evidence of primary tumor
___ T1:   Tumor invades lamina propria or submucosa and size 1 cm or less (small intestine); tumor 1 cm or less (ampulla)
___ T2:   Tumor invades muscularis propria or size >1 cm (small intestine); size > 1 cm (ampulla)
___ T3:   Tumor invades subserosa (jejunum, ileum); or pancreas or retroperitoneum (duodenum, ampulla); or nonperitonealized tissues (any)
___ T4:   Tumor invades visceral peritoneum or other organs/structures

Pancreas Primary Tumor (T):
___ TX: Primary tumor cannot be assessed
___ T0:   No evidence of primary tumor

(continued)

TABLE 3.7   Sample Gastroenteropancreatic Neuroendocrine Neoplasm Synoptic Report Format (*continued*)

___ T1:   Tumor limited to the pancreas, size 2 cm or less
___ T2:   Tumor limited to the pancreas, size >2 cm
___ T3:   Tumor extends beyond the pancreas but without involvement of the celiac axis or the superior mesenteric artery
___ T4:   Tumor involves the celiac axis or the superior mesenteric artery

Appendix Primary Tumor (T):
___ TX: Primary tumor cannot be assessed
___ T0:   No evidence of primary tumor
___ T1a: Tumor size 1 cm or less
___ T1b: Tumor size >1 cm but ≤2 cm
___ T2:   Tumor size >2 cm but ≤4 cm or extension to the cecum
___ T3:   Tumor size >4 cm or extension to the ileum
___ T4:   Tumor invades other organs/structures

Colon/Rectum Primary Tumor (T):
___ TX: Primary tumor cannot be assessed
___ T0:   No evidence of primary tumor
___ T1a: Tumor invades lamina propria or submucosa and size 1 cm or less
___ T1b: Tumor invades lamina propria or submucosa and size 1–2 cm
___ T2:   Tumor invades muscularis propria or size more than 2 cm
___ T3:   Tumor invades subserosa or nonperitonealized pericolorectal tissues
___ T4:   Tumor invades visceral peritoneum or other organs/structures

Regional Lymph Nodes (N):
___ NX: Regional lymph nodes cannot be assessed
___ N0:   No regional lymph node metastasis
___ N1:   Regional lymph node metastasis

Distant Metastasis (M):
___ M1:   Distant metastasis

Note: MX and M0 no longer exist as pathologic M stage designations.
The pathologic stage based on available pathologic material is: __pT__N__M__
The optimal tissue block for molecular studies on tumor is:
The optimal tissue block for molecular studies on nontumor is:
Abbreviations: WDNET, well-differentiated neuroendocrine tumor; PDNEC, poorly differentiated neuroendocrine carcinoma.

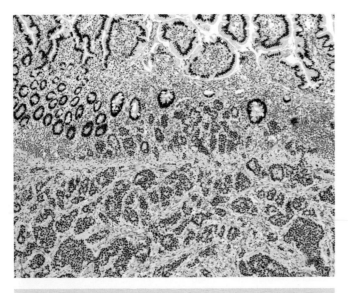

FIGURE 3.21   Ninety percent of tumors of midgut origin, like this ileal primary, express CDX2, while only 15% of pancreatic tumors do. Pancreatic tumors may express PR, PAX6, and/or islet 1, while midgut tumors do not.

primaries. For laboratories that do not have PAX6, islet 1, or polyclonal PAX8 antibodies, progesterone receptor is a good substitute, as it is detected in two thirds of pancreatic tumors. TTF-1 is specific, though fairly insensitive (30%–40%) for bronchopulmonary primaries. The immunophenotype of NETs by site of origin is summarized in Table 3.8.

Morphology is complementary to the results of IHC. Metastases from occult ileal and pancreatic primaries are most likely; most ileal tumors will demonstrate type A histology and contain eosinophilic cytoplasmic granules, while pancreatic tumors can show any growth pattern.

GENERAL APPROACH TO DIAGNOSIS AND REPORTING OF NEUROENDOCRINE CARCINOMAS

Of the five key aspects discussed in the preceding section on general approach to neuroendocrine tumors, the first two are also germane to the diagnosis of an NEC:

TABLE 3.8 Immunophenotype of Neuroendocrine Tumors by Site of Origin

| Marker | Site | | | |
	Lung	Jejunoileum	Pancreas	Rectum
TTF-1	30%–40%	<1%	<1%	<1%
CDX2	<5%	>90%	15%	20%–30%
Polyclonal PAX8/ monoclonal PAX6	5%	<1%	60%–70%	60%
Islet 1	<10%	<5%	70%–90%	85%
PR	5%	5%	60%–70%	20%
PrAP	<1%	40%–60%	5%	90%

recognition of a suggestive histologic pattern and performance of supportive diagnostic IHC. Ki-67 IHC is generally not needed, as tumors are by definition G3. Small cell neuroendocrine carcinomas generally demonstrate a diffuse growth pattern, with "small" cell size, little cytoplasm, finely granular chromatin, inconspicuous to absent nucleoli, and prominent nuclear molding. Large cell neuroendocrine carcinoma may show organoid architecture, "large" cell size with more abundant cytoplasm, variable chromatin, and prominent nucleoli. In the GI tract, SCNEC is more common in the esophagus and anus, while LCNEC predominates elsewhere. Twenty-five to fifty percent of GI NECs arise in association with a non-neuroendocrine carcinoma.

Depending on the morphology, immunostains may be important for tumor diagnosis. NECs should express at least one general neuroendocrine marker, preferably diffusely and strongly, as well as broad-spectrum keratins (eg, CAM5.2). In occasional instances in which synaptophysin and chromogranin A are negative, TTF-1 or dot-like keratin expression may serve as surrogate "neuroendocrine markers." Extrapulmonary visceral NECs also express TTF-1 in 40% to 50% of cases; CK20 is rarely expressed, and when it is, it is often focal. Aside from these two markers, in contrast to NETs, IHC is not useful in assigning the site of origin in NECs. In fact, NECs frequently express multiple transcription factors irrespective of the site of origin, a phenomenon that has been referred to as "transcription factor infidelity" (Figure 3.22). According to the *AJCC Cancer Staging Manual*, NECs are staged identically to non-neuroendocrine carcinomas, and organ-specific synoptic reports for carcinomas of the same site may be utilized.

SPECIFIC ILLUSTRATIVE EXAMPLES

Case 1

A 66-year-old man with a history of gastroesophageal reflux disease (GERD) symptoms, including dysphagia, was referred for upper endoscopy. The endoscopist

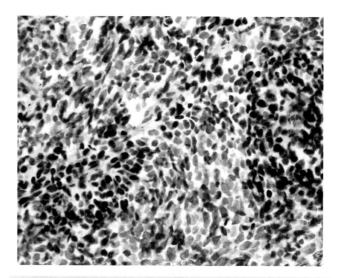

FIGURE 3.22 NECs tend to express multiple transcription factors irrespective of site of origin, like p63 in this metastasis from a lung primary.

noted "gastritis" in the body of the stomach and a normal antrum. Five random biopsies, encompassing proximal and distal stomach, were taken (Figures 3.23A–C), showing features suggestive of autoimmune gastritis. A special stain for *Helicobacter* was negative. One biopsy fragment contained a 0.17 cm NET (Figure 3.23D) that also expressed chromogranin A and had a low Ki-67 proliferation index of 1% (Figure 3.23E).

The patient was found to have antiparietal and intrinsic factor antibodies and a serum gastrin of 896 pg/mL (reference range 0–100). The patient was taken off his proton pump inhibitor, so as not to further exacerbate the hypergastrinemia driving the ECL-cell proliferation.

Endoscopy was repeated at 6 months, with topographic mapping of the stomach. Another NET was detected in a random biopsy from the proximal greater curvature (Figure 3.23F); tumor was no longer present on the slide prepared for Ki-67 staining. In addition, random biopsies from the lesser curve demonstrated high-grade

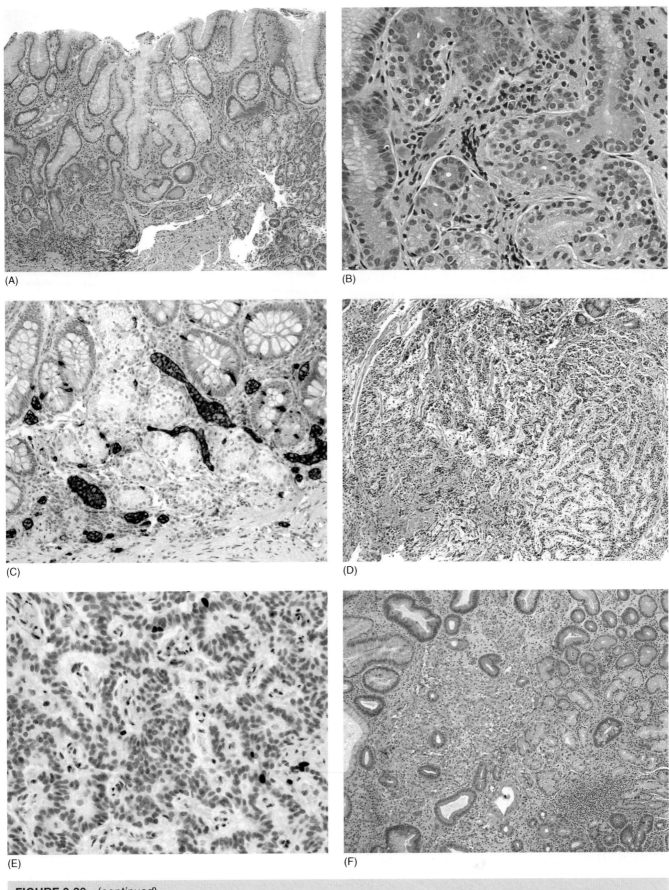

FIGURE 3.23   (*continued*)

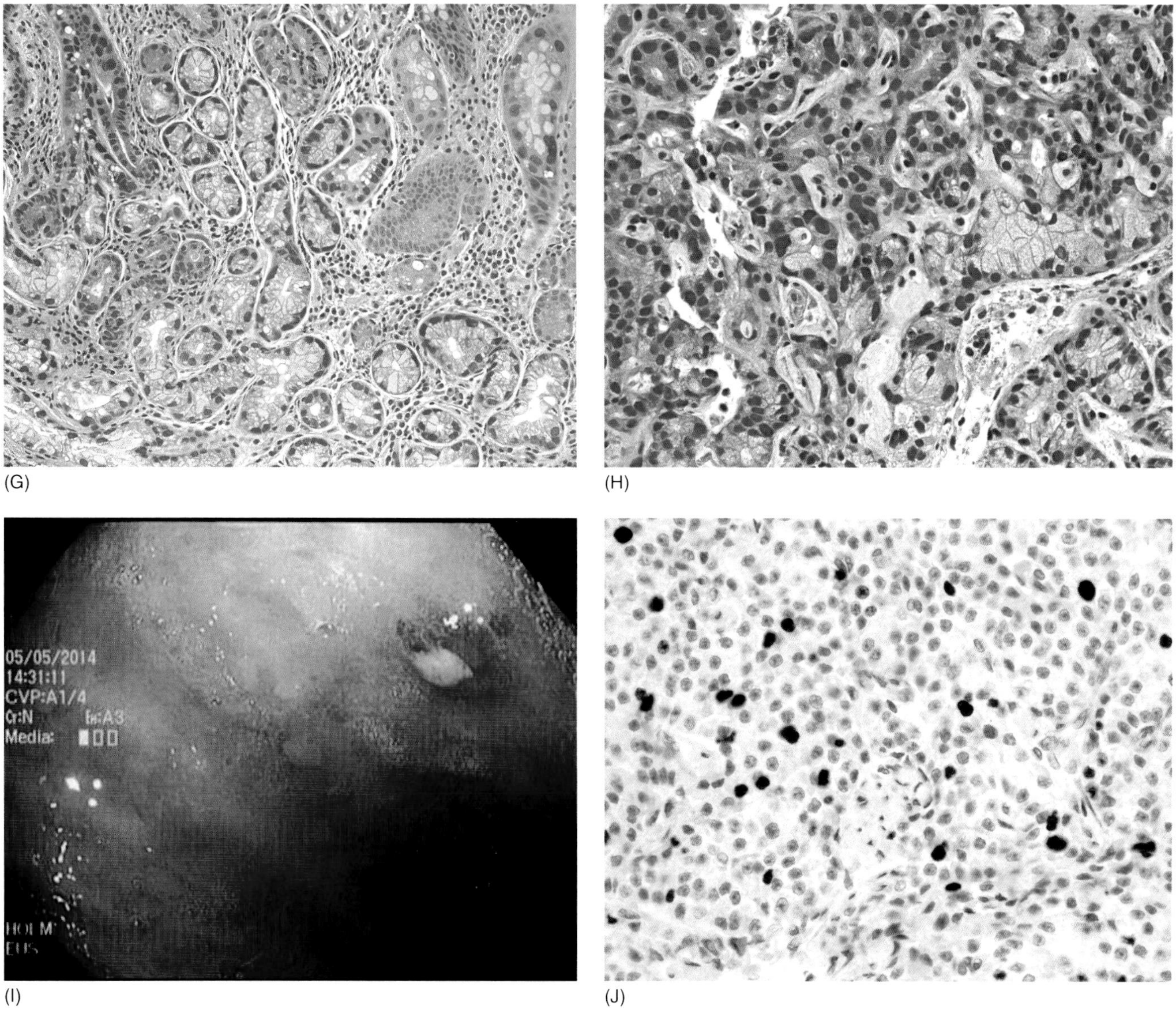

(G)

(H)

(I)

(J)

FIGURE 3.23 Fragments of gastric corpus demonstrate chronic gastritis with pancreatic acinar, intestinal, and antral/pyloric metaplasia, as well as a suggestion of neuroendocrine hyperplasia (A). Neuroendocrine hyperplasia seen at higher power (B) and confirmed by chromogranin A immunostain highlighting micronodular hyperplasia (C). A 0.17 cm NET was also present, composed of cords of cells (D). The lesion had a low Ki-67 proliferation index of 1% (E). The second endoscopy showed a second NET in a random biopsy from the proximal greater curvature (F). Random biopsies from the lesser curve also demonstrated high-grade glandular dysplasia (G), as well as a focus suspicious for intramucosal adenocarcinoma (H). A third small NET was detected at subsequent endoscopy (I), with a proliferation index of 7% (J).

glandular dysplasia (Figure 3.23G), as well as a focus suspicious for intramucosal adenocarcinoma (Figure 3.23H).

Endoscopy was repeated 1 week later, this time with endoscopic ultrasound. A small nodule was detected along the lesser curvature (Figure 3.23I), and an endoscopic mucosal resection was performed, revealing another NET. A Ki-67 immunostain demonstrated a proliferation index of 7% (Figure 3.23J). The ultrasound portion of the examination failed to detect foci of invasion or lymphadenopathy. The patient was referred to surgery for consideration of gastrectomy.

This case highlights some of the clinical and pathologic aspects of type I gastric NETs, as well as a relatively uncommon associated condition, the latter of which is driving clinical management. The initial biopsy series demonstrated autoimmune atrophic gastritis, and this diagnosis was supported by the subsequent laboratory studies. Around 10% of patients with autoimmune atrophic gastritis develop NETs. Tumors tend to be small, superficial, and relatively innocuous, as seen on this case. Proliferation indices are usually low. The higher proliferation index in the final NET is unusual and may denote a more aggressive clinical course. Patients with small type I gastric NETs can often be managed with endoscopic removal and surveillance. In this case, the initial diagnosis of an NET arising in autoimmune gastritis led to endoscopic follow-up at 6 months. High-grade glandular dysplasia (at least) was detected on random biopsies. According to the American Society for Gastrointestinal Endoscopy guidelines, gastrectomy or endoscopic resection is recommended in the face of a diagnosis of high-grade dysplasia. Given that the glandular dysplasia is endoscopically inapparent, the former is a strong consideration. Gastric cancer develops in 1% to 3% of patients with autoimmune atrophic gastritis.

Case 2

A 64-year-old man with a history of coronary artery disease and diverticular disease presented with a few months of left lower quadrant pain and diarrhea. A CT of the abdomen and pelvis was ordered to evaluate for probable diverticulitis. It instead demonstrated multiple lesions throughout the liver, measuring up to 8.5 cm. An ultrasound-guided liver biopsy was performed (Figure 3.24A–C), and a diagnosis of metastatic well-differentiated NET, WHO 2010 grade 2 was rendered. An OctreoScan demonstrated uptake in multiple liver lesions but failed to localize the primary (Figure 3.24D). Based on the morphology and CDX2 expression, a jejunoileal origin was strongly favored.

The patient underwent surgical exploration and 16 nodules, ranging in size from 0.2 to 1 cm, were palpated

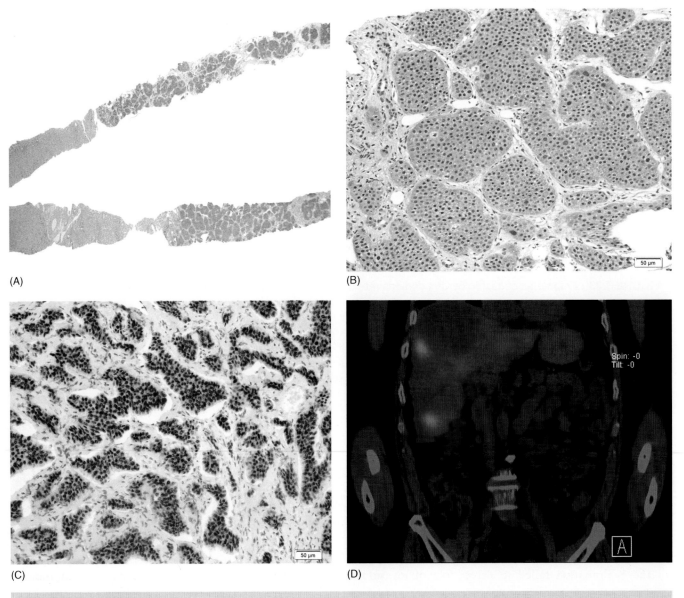

(A) (B) (C) (D)

FIGURE 3.24 *(continued)*

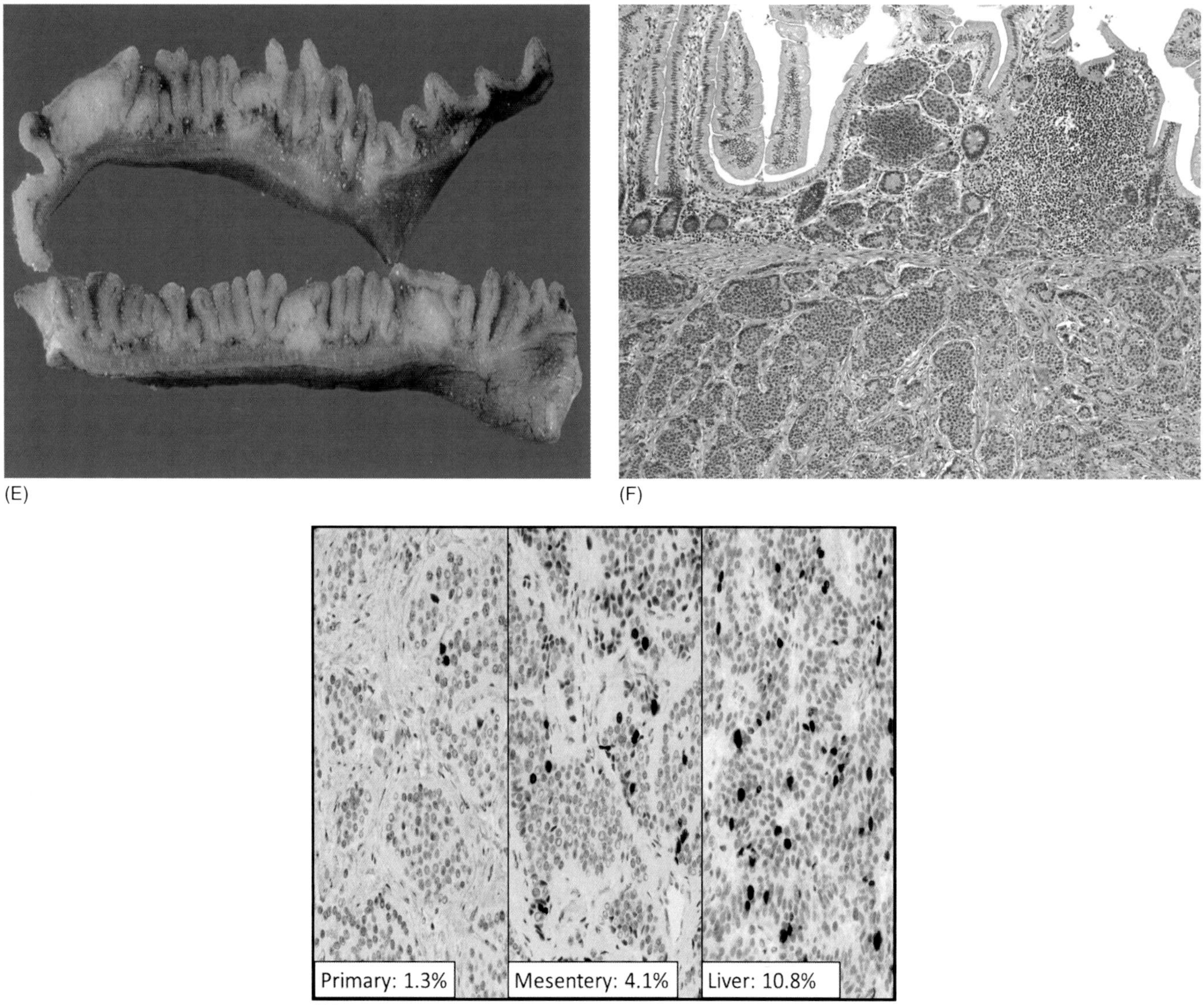

(E)

(F)

Primary: 1.3%   Mesentery: 4.1%   Liver: 10.8%

(G)

FIGURE 3.24   A low-power view shows nests of cells within fibrous stroma (A). The tumor is composed of nests of uniform cells with scattered larger nuclei (B). There is prominent eosinophilic cytoplasmic granularity. The tumor expressed CDX2 consistent with gastrointestinal origin (C). OctreoScan shows uptake in multiple liver lesions but did not localize the primary (D). The ileal resection showed 16 tumors along a 50 cm segment of ileum (E). Typical features of a midgut NET were seen (F). Proliferation indices were 1.3% in the primary tumor, 4.1% in the mesenteric lesion, and 10.8% in the liver metastasis (G).

along a 50 cm length of ileum, which was excised (Figure 3.24E). Multiple liver metastases were resected and ablated also, though several small liver metastases were left behind. Histology showed features of a typical midgut NET (Figure 3.24F), also involving lymph nodes and liver; the tumor was staged as pT2 N1 M1. Ki-67 immunohistochemistry was performed on a representative primary tumor, a mesenteric deposit, and a liver metastasis, demonstrating proliferation indices of 1.3%, 4.1%, and 10.8%, respectively (Figure 3.24G). The patient was started on long-acting octreotide.

This case highlights the typical presentation of a metastatic NET of initially occult origin, clues to

detecting the site of origin, the characteristically aggressive biology of jejunoileal NETs, and caveats as regards the determination of proliferation index in NETs. The histology in the liver core biopsy is classic for a midgut NET (nested growth pattern; eosinophilic cytoplasmic granularity). Once the neuroendocrine nature of this neoplasm is recognized on the liver biopsy, a reasonable IHC panel might include chromogranin A and synaptophysin (to confirm neuroendocrine nature); Ki-67 (to assess proliferation index); and CDX2, PR (or PAX6 or Islet 1 or polyclonal PAX8), and TTF-1 (to suggest the site of origin). Given the classic histology in this case, one could make an argument for limiting the "site of origin"

IHC to CDX2. CK7 and CK20 are less useful markers for assigning the site of origin in NETs due to variability in staining.

Up to 20% of NETs present as metastases of occult origin. The most likely primary sites are jejunoileum, followed by pancreas. An OctreoScan failed to highlight the primary tumors in this patient, which is not unexpected given their small size.

Historically, NETs of this size would have been considered benign, but as illustrated in the AFIP series and in this case, even small jejunoileal tumors are frequently metastatic. Twenty-five percent of jejunoileal NETs are multifocal, which may be associated with a more adverse prognosis.

The Ki-67 proliferation index in the initial liver biopsy in this case was originally estimated ("eye-balled") as 1%. Although there were areas in the tumor in which the proliferation index was that low, it was not uniform throughout, as is typical. Manual counting of a digitally captured image subsequently demonstrated a proliferation index in the WHO 2010 G2 range. Ki-67 IHC was repeated on the resection specimen (primary tumor, regional disease, distantly metastatic disease). Since the tumor was already G2 on the biopsy, an argument could be made that repeating these studies on the resection was not necessary. However, a proliferation index of 10.8% on a resected metastasis (versus 3% on a biopsied metastasis) was of interest to the clinician. A reasonable approach is to repeat Ki-67 IHC on at least one primary tumor and one metastatic tumor in resected specimens.

Case 3

A 73-year-old man presented to the Emergency Department with 4 weeks of headaches and 10 days of progressively unsteady gait. A head CT demonstrated right frontal (3 × 3 cm) and left cerebellar (5 × 4 cm) cystic lesions. The patient was admitted, and a follow-up MRI with contrast revealed that these lesions were ring-enhancing (Figure 3.25A). Neurosurgery was consulted, and a posterior fossa craniotomy with tumor debulking was planned. In the meantime, CT of the chest, abdomen, and pelvis demonstrated a 9 cm long segment of midesophageal thickening with associated necrotic mediastinal adenopathy, multiple liver lesions, and nodular thickening of bilateral adrenal glands, suspicious for metastatic disease. A specimen from the cranial debulking showed abundant high-grade tumor with extensive necrosis, admixed with fragments of cerebellum (Figure 3.25B–F). Given the CT findings and the results of IHC, an initial diagnosis of metastatic esophageal adenocarcinoma was favored.

Another pathologist noted that in addition to lacking glands, papillae, or mucin, the tumor cells were fairly monomorphous, and areas of trabecular architecture were seen (Figure 3.25G). Basophilic material encrusting thin-walled blood vessels was identified in necrotic areas (Figures 3.25H–I). Diffuse, strong staining for chromogranin A and synaptophysin (Figures 3.25J–K) supported a diagnosis of LCNEC, presumably from the esophagus. Upon further questioning, the patient related a 2-month history of dysphagia and 40-pound weight loss. The

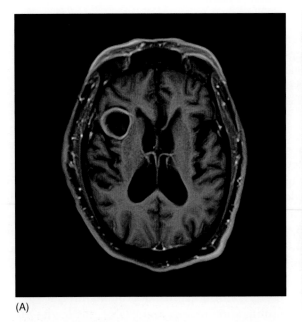

(A)

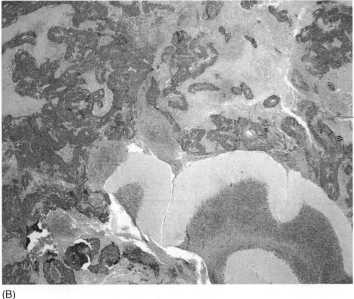

(B)

FIGURE 3.25 MRI with contrast showed ring-enhancing cranial lesions (A). The cranial debulking showed a high grade neoplasm with extensive necrosis, admixed with fragments of cerebellum (B). (*continued*)

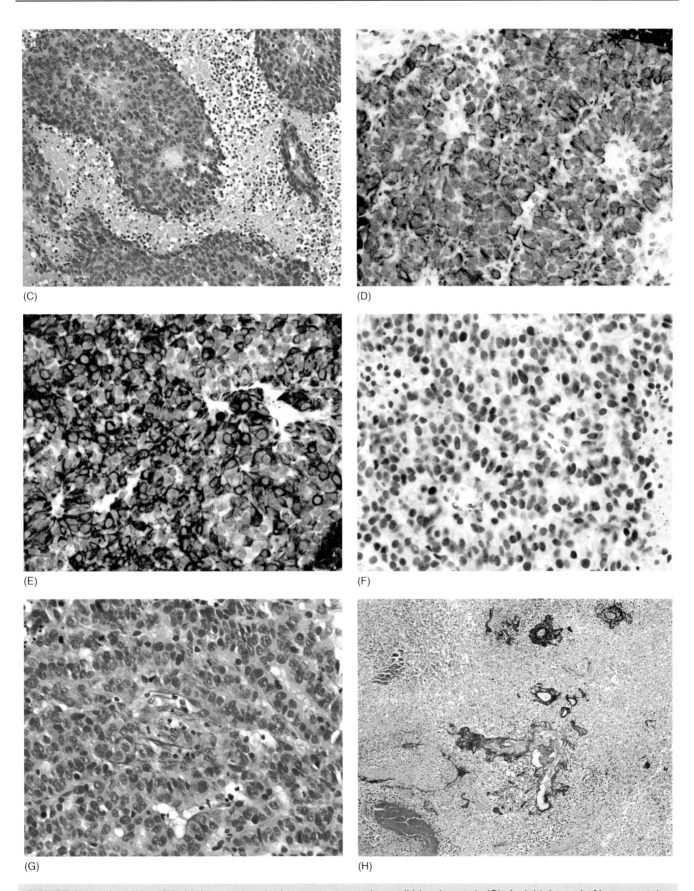

FIGURE 3.25 (*continued*) At higher power, viable tumor surrounds small blood vessels (C). An initial panel of immunostains showed that the tumor expresses CK7 (D), CK20 (E), and CDX2 (F), but not TTF-1 or prostate-specific antigen (PSA). The tumor cells were noted to be fairly monomorphous, and areas of trabecular architecture were seen (G). (*continued*)

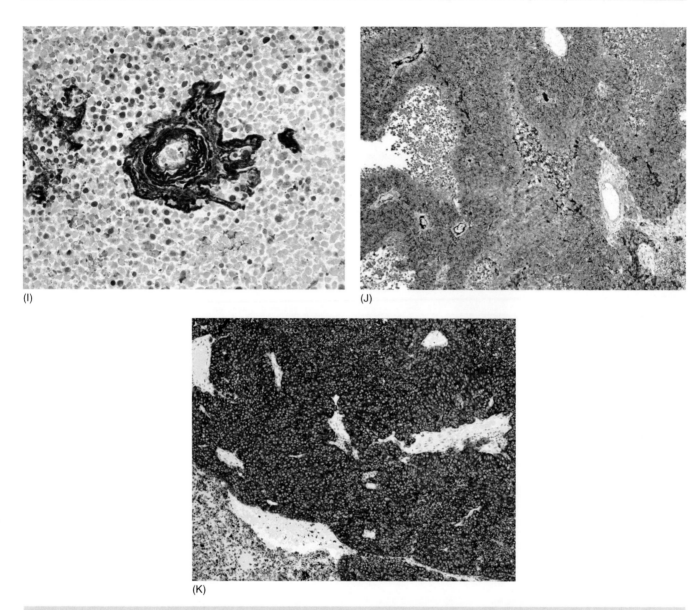

(I)

(J)

(K)

FIGURE 3.25 (*continued*) Basophilic material encrusts thin-walled blood vessels (Azzopardi effect), and there is extensive necrosis (H–I). The tumor cells diffusely and strongly expressed chromogranin A (J) and synaptophysin (K), supporting a diagnosis of LCNEC.

patient underwent a course of whole brain irradiation, but given his declining performance status chemotherapy was deferred, and he was placed in hospice.

This case highlights the difficulty in recognizing LCNECs. A diagnosis of solid esophageal adenocarcinoma was strongly entertained, which seemed to be corroborated by the results of initial immunostains (positivity for CK7/CK20/CDX2). Careful attention to the H&E revealed cellular monomorphism, organoid architecture, and Azzopardi effect, and the morphologic impression was then confirmed by the results of chromogranin A and synaptophysin IHC. Although CDX2 is expressed in this case, IHC is generally not useful in assigning the site of origin

in NECs, because they typically express multiple transcription factors regardless of primary site. The tumor followed a typical aggressive clinical course.

SELECTED REFERENCES

Historical Perspectives

Banck MS, Kanwar R, Kulkarni AA, et al. The genomic landscape of small intestine neuroendocrine tumors. *J Clin Invest.* 2013;123(6):2502–2508.

Bauer W, Briner U, Doepfner W, et al. SMS 201-995: a very potent and selective octapeptide analogue of somatostatin with prolonged action. *Life Sci.* 1982;31(11):1133–1140

Erspamer V, Asero B. Identification of enteramine, the specific hormone of the enterochromaffin cell system, as 5-hydroxytryptamine. *Nature.* 1952;169(4306):800–801.

Francis JM, Kiezun A, Ramos AH, et al. Somatic mutation of CDKN1B in small intestine neuroendocrine tumors. *Nat Genet.* 2013;45(12):1483–1486.

Krenning EP, Bakker WH, Breeman WA, et al. Localisation of endocrine-related tumours with radioiodinated analogue of somatostatin. *Lancet.* 1989;1(8632):242–244.

Lembeck F. 5-hydroxytryptamine in a carcinoid tumour. *Nature.* 1953;172:910–911.

Modlin IM, Shapiro MD, Kidd M, Eick G. Siegfried Oberndorfer and the evolution of carcinoid disease. *Arch Surg.* 2007;142(2):187–197.

Raju TN. The Nobel chronicles. 1977: Roger Charles Louis Guillemin (b 1924); Andrew Victor Schally (b 1926); Rosalyn S Yalow (b 1921). *Lancet.* 1999;354(9188):1481.

Raymond E, Dahan L, Raoul JL, et al. Sunitinib malate for the treatment of pancreatic neuroendocrine tumors. *N Engl J Med.* 2011;364(6):501–513.

Smith MC, Liu J, Chen T, et al. OctreoTher: ongoing early clinical development of a somatostatin-receptor-targeted radionuclide antineoplastic therapy. *Digestion.* 2000;62 Suppl 1:69–72.

Yao JC, Shah MH, Ito T, et al. Everolimus for advanced pancreatic neuroendocrine tumors. *N Engl J Med.* 2011;364(6):514–523.

Epidemiology

Brennan SM, Gregory DL, Stillie A, Herschtal A, Mac Manus M, Ball DL. Should extrapulmonary small cell cancer be managed like small cell lung cancer? *Cancer.* 2010;116(4):888–895.

Yao JC, Hassan M, Phan A, et al. One hundred years after "carcinoid": epidemiology of and prognostic factors for neuroendocrine tumors in 35,825 cases in the United States. *J Clin Oncol.* 2008;26(18):3063–3072.

Classifications

Foley EF, Gaffey MJ, Frierson HF, Jr. The frequency and clinical significance of neuroendocrine cells within stage III adenocarcinomas of the colon. *Arch Pathol Lab Med.* 1998;122(10):912–914.

Rege TA, King EE, Barletta JA, Bellizzi AM. Ki-67 proliferation index in pancreatic endocrine tumors: comparison with mitotic count, interobserver variability, and impact on grading. *Mod Pathol.* 2011;24(1S):372A.

Rindi G, Arnold R, Bosman FT, et al. Nomenclature and classification of neuroendocrine neoplams of the digestive system. In: Bosman FT, Carneiro F, Hruban RH, Theise ND, eds. *World Health Organization Classification of Tumours: WHO Classification of Tumours of the Digestive System.* 4th ed. Lyon: IARC; 2010: 13–14.

Smith DM, Jr., Haggitt RC. The prevalence and prognostic significance of argyrophil cells in colorectal carcinomas. *Am J Surg Pathol.* 1984;8(2):123–128.

Soga J, Tazawa K. Pathologic analysis of carcinoids. Histologic reevaluation of 62 cases. *Cancer.* 1971;28(4):990–998.

Solcia E, Kloppel G, Sobin LH, eds. *Histological Typing of Endocrine Tumours.* 2nd ed. New York, NY: Springer-Verlag; 2000.

Travis WD. The concept of pulmonary neuroendocrine tumours. In: Travis WD, Brambilla E, Muller-Hermelink HK, Harris CC, eds. *World Health Organization Classification of Tumours: Pathology and Genetics of Tumours of the Lung, Pleura, Thymus and Heart.* 3rd ed. Lyon: IARC Press; 2004:19–20.

Williams ED, Sandler M. The classification of carcinoid tumours. *Lancet.* 1963;1(7275):238–239.

Clinicopathologic Features of Neuroendocrine Tumors by Anatomic Site

Esophagus

Hoang MP, Hobbs CM, Sobin LH, Albores-Saavedra J. Carcinoid tumor of the esophagus: a clinicopathologic study of four cases. *Am J Surg Pathol.* 2002;26(4):517–522.

Modlin IM, Lye KD, Kidd M. A 5-decade analysis of 13,715 carcinoid tumors. *Cancer.* 2003;97(4):934–959.

Soga J. Esophageal endocrinomas, an extremely rare tumor: a statistical comparative evaluation of 28 ordinary carcinoids and 72 atypical variants. *J Exp Clin Cancer Res.* 1998;17(1):47–57.

Stomach

Bordi C, Yu JY, Baggi MT, et al. Gastric carcinoids and their precursor lesions. A histologic and immunohistochemical study of 23 cases. *Cancer.* 1991;67(3):663–672.

Bordi C. Gastric carcinoids: an immunohistochemical and clinicopathologic study of 104 patients. *Cancer.* 1995;75(1):129–130.

La Rosa S, Inzani F, Vanoli A, et al. Histologic characterization and improved prognostic evaluation of 209 gastric neuroendocrine neoplasms. *Hum Pathol.* 2011;42(10):1373–1384.

Rindi G, Bordi C, Rappel S, La Rosa S, Stolte M, Solcia E. Gastric carcinoids and neuroendocrine carcinomas: pathogenesis, pathology, and behavior. *World J Surg.* 1996;20(2):168–72.

Thomas RM, Baybick JH, Elsayed AM, Sobin LH. Gastric carcinoids. An immunohistochemical and clinicopathologic study of 104 patients. *Cancer.* 1994;73(8):2053–2058.

Duodenum

Anlauf M, Garbrecht N, Bauersfeld J, et al. Hereditary neuroendocrine tumors of the gastroenteropancreatic system. *Virchows Arch.* 2007;451 Suppl 1:S29–S38.

Burke AP, Federspiel BH, Sobin LH, Shekitka KM, Helwig EB. Carcinoids of the duodenum. A histologic and immunohistochemical study of 65 tumors. *Am J Surg Pathol.* 1989;13(10):828–837.

Burke AP, Helwig EB. Gangliocytic paraganglioma. *Am J Clin Pathol.* 1989;92(1):1–9.

Burke AP, Sobin LH, Federspiel BH, Shekitka KM, Helwig EB. Carcinoid tumors of the duodenum. A clinicopathologic study of 99 cases. *Arch Pathol Lab Med.* 1990;114(7):700–704.

Burke AP, Sobin LH, Shekitka KM, Federspiel BH, Helwig EB. Somatostatin-producing duodenal carcinoids in patients with von Recklinghausen's neurofibromatosis. A predilection for black patients. *Cancer.* 1990;65(7):1591–1595.

Mullen JT, Wang H, Yao JC, et al. Carcinoid tumors of the duodenum. *Surgery.* 2005;138(6):971–977; discussion 7–8.

Jejunoileum

Anthony PP, Drury RA. Elastic vascular sclerosis of mesenteric blood vessels in argentaffin carcinoma. *J Clin Pathol.* 1970;23(2):110–118.

Burke AP, Thomas RM, Elsayed AM, Sobin LH. Carcinoids of the jejunum and ileum: an immunohistochemical and clinicopathologic study of 167 cases. *Cancer.* 1997;79(6):1086–1093.

Lorenzen AW, O'Dorisio TM, Howe JR. Neuroendocrine tumors arising in Meckel's diverticula: frequency of advanced disease warrants aggressive management. *J Gastrointestinal Surg.* 2013;17(6):1084–1091.

Soga J. Carcinoids of the small intestine: a statistical evaluation of 1102 cases collected from the literature. *J Exp Clin Cancer Res.* 1997;16(4):353–363.

Appendix

Boudreaux JP, Klimstra DS, Hassan MM, et al. The NANETS consensus guideline for the diagnosis and management of neuroendocrine tumors: well-differentiated neuroendocrine tumors of the jejunum, ileum, appendix, and cecum. *Pancreas.* 2010;39(6):753–766.

Burke AP, Sobin LH, Federspiel BH, Shekitka KM, Helwig EB. Goblet cell carcinoids and related tumors of the vermiform appendix. *Am J Clin Pathol.* 1990;94(1):27–35.

Burke AP, Sobin LH, Federspiel BH, Shekitka KM. Appendiceal carcinoids: correlation of histology and immunohistochemistry. *Mod Pathol.* 1989;2(6):630–637.

Glasser CM, Bhagavan BS. Carcinoid tumors of the appendix. *Arch Pathol Lab Med.* 1980;104(5):272–275.

Isaacson P. Crypt cell carcinoma of the appendix (so-called adenocarcinoid tumor). *Am J Surg Pathol.* 1981;5(3):213–224.

Pape UF, Perren A, Niederle B, et al. ENETS Consensus Guidelines for the management of patients with neuroendocrine neoplasms from the jejuno-ileum and the appendix including goblet cell carcinomas. *Neuroendocrinology.* 2012;95(2):135–156.

Sandor A, Modlin IM. A retrospective analysis of 1570 appendiceal carcinoids. *Am J Gastroenterol.* 1998;93(3):422–428.

Tang LH, Shia J, Soslow RA, et al. Pathologic classification and clinical behavior of the spectrum of goblet cell carcinoid tumors of the appendix. *Am J Surg Pathol.* 2008;32(10):1429–1443.

Colorectum

Federspiel BH, Burke AP, Sobin LH, Shekitka KM. Rectal and colonic carcinoids. A clinicopathologic study of 84 cases. *Cancer.* 1990;65(1):135–140.

Landry CS, Brock G, Scoggins CR, McMasters KM, Martin RC, 2nd. A proposed staging system for rectal carcinoid tumors based on an analysis of 4701 patients. *Surgery.* 2008;144(3):460–466.

Park CH, Cheon JH, Kim JO, et al. Criteria for decision making after endoscopic resection of well-differentiated rectal carcinoids with regard to potential lymphatic spread. *Endoscopy.* 2011;43(9):790–795.

Shields CJ, Tiret E, Winter DC. Carcinoid tumors of the rectum: a multi-institutional international collaboration. *Ann Surg.* 2010;252(5):750–755.

Clinical Significance of Recognizing Neuroendocrine Epithelial Neoplasms

Elias D, Lasser P, Ducreux M, et al. Liver resection (and associated extrahepatic resections) for metastatic well-differentiated endocrine tumors: a 15-year single center prospective study. *Surgery.* 2003;133(4):375–382.

Pavel M, Baudin E, Couvelard A, et al. ENETS Consensus Guidelines for the management of patients with liver and other distant metastases from neuroendocrine neoplasms of foregut, midgut, hindgut, and unknown primary. *Neuroendocrinology.* 2012;95(2):157–176.

Salazar R, Wiedenmann B, Rindi G, Ruszniewski P. ENETS 2011 Consensus Guidelines for the Management of Patients with Digestive Neuroendocrine Tumors: an update. *Neuroendocrinology.* 2012;95(2):71–73.

Sarmiento JM, Heywood G, Rubin J, Ilstrup DM, Nagorney DM, Que FG. Surgical treatment of neuroendocrine metastases to the liver: a plea for resection to increase survival. *J Am Coll Surg.* 2003;197(1):29–37.

Strosberg JR, Coppola D, Klimstra DS, et al. The NANETS consensus guidelines for the diagnosis and management of poorly differentiated (high-grade) extrapulmonary neuroendocrine carcinomas. *Pancreas.* 2010;39(6):799–800.

Approach to Diagnosis and Reporting of Primary Neuroendocrine Tumors

Adsay V. Ki67 labeling index in neuroendocrine tumors of the gastrointestinal and pancreatobiliary tract: to count or not to count is not the question, but rather how to count. *Am J Surg Pathol.* 2012;36(12):1743–1746.

College of American Pathologists. *Cancer Protocols and Checklists.* www.cap.org/cancerprotocols

Klimstra DS, Modlin IR, Adsay NV, et al. Pathology reporting of neuroendocrine tumors: application of the Delphic consensus process to the development of a minimum pathology data set. *Am J Surg Pathol.* 2010;34(3):300–313.

Neuroendocrine Tumors. In: Edge SB, Byrd DR, Compton CC, Fritz AG, Greene FL, Trotti A, eds. *AJCC Cancer Staging Manual.* 7th ed. New York, NY: Springer; 2010:181–189.

Tang LH, Gonen M, Hedvat C, Modlin IM, Klimstra DS. Objective quantification of the Ki67 proliferative index in neuroendocrine tumors of the gastroenteropancreatic system: a comparison of digital image analysis with manual methods. *Am J Surg Pathol.* 2012;36(12):1761–1770.

Approach to Diagnosis and Reporting

Bellizzi AM. Assigning site of origin in metastatic neuroendocrine neoplasms: a clinically significant application of diagnostic immunohistochemistry. *Adv Anatomic Pathol.* 2013;20(5):285–314.

Dhall D, Mertens R, Bresee C, et al. Ki-67 proliferative index predicts progression-free survival of patients with well-differentiated ileal neuroendocrine tumors. *Hum Pathol.* 2012;43(4):489–495.

Kirshbom PM, Kherani AR, Onaitis MW, Feldman JM, Tyler DS. Carcinoids of unknown origin: comparative analysis with foregut, midgut, and hindgut carcinoids. *Surgery.* 1998;124(6):1063–1070.

Savelli G, Lucignani G, Seregni E, et al. Feasibility of somatostatin receptor scintigraphy in the detection of occult primary gastro-entero-pancreatic (GEP) neuroendocrine tumours. *Nucl Med Commun.* 2004;25(5):445–449.

Wang SC, Parekh JR, Zuraek MB, et al. Identification of unknown primary tumors in patients with neuroendocrine liver metastases. *Arch Surg.* 2010;145(3):276–280.

4

General Approach to Lymphomas of the Gastrointestinal Tract

SCOTT R. OWENS

INTRODUCTION

The gastrointestinal (GI) tract is the most common extranodal site of involvement by lymphoma. Any pathologist who regularly encounters GI specimens is likely to come across cases that either contain overt lymphoma, or findings suspicious for lymphoma, with some frequency. Thus, it is important to have a coherent and pragmatic approach to evaluation and diagnosis when confronted with such specimens. The "front-line" pathologist may be able to make a definite diagnosis in many cases by using such an approach and, for rarer or more equivocal entities, can at least initiate the diagnostic process and facilitate further testing. This chapter outlines a pragmatic approach to the workup of lymphomas in the GI tract, beginning with a review of the basics of lymphoid populations and the general principles related to lymphoid tissue in the GI tract, followed by a brief overview of specific lymphomas encountered in this organ system. A paraffin-embedded tissue-based approach, using immunohistochemistry for diagnosis, is emphasized, as this is routinely available to most pathologists. In addition, this discussion will focus on mature B and T lymphocytes, as the vast majority of hematolymphoid neoplasms encountered in the GI tract involve mature lymphoid subtypes. Individual lymphomas will be explored in greater detail in Chapters 8, 9, and 11.

BASICS OF LYMPHOID ANTIGENS

B and T lymphocytes normally express a variety of antigens on their surfaces and/or in the cytoplasm, many of

which are part of the "cluster of differentiation" (CD) system. For some time, these antigen expression patterns have been used to identify normal subpopulations of lymphocytes in the GI tract and elsewhere, and to demonstrate aberrant expression of antigen(s) associated with various hematolymphoid neoplasms.

B Lymphocytes

The pattern of antigen expression by normal B lymphocytes depends somewhat on their level of maturity (or degree of *differentiation*), as well as their associated location in lymphoid tissues. Normal B cells typically express the pan-B cell antigens CD20 and CD79a. CD19 is also expressed by all B cells, but is not usually the target of tissue-based immunohistochemistry. Normal B cells also express the transcription factor PAX-5 in their nuclei, as well as surface immunoglobulins. Immunoglobulin (Ig) expression reaches its fullest form in plasma cells (derived from B cells), and these immunoglobulins consist of a variety of heavy chain types (IgM, IgG, IgA, IgD, and IgE) that are associated with either kappa or lambda light chain expression. The normal pattern of expression of these light chains results in about two-thirds of cells expressing kappa light chain, and the other one-third lambda light chain. Demonstration of exclusive kappa or lambda light chain expression by plasma cells or B lymphocytes (the latter usually accomplished by flow cytometry) is a convenient method to establish the clonality of a lymphoid population. Other antigens expressed by subpopulations of B cells can give rise to subtypes of B cell lymphoma, meaning that patterns of antigen expression are useful in diagnosing these lymphomas. For instance, CD10 and BCL-6 are expressed by follicle center B lymphocytes as well as follicular lymphoma (FL), and plasma cells express CD38 and CD138, as do neoplasms with plasmacytic differentiation. Aberrant expression of antigens not normally expressed by B cells can also be helpful in lymphoma diagnosis. Expression of the T cell marker CD5 is characteristic of certain B cell lymphomas, and expression of BCL-2 characterizes the majority of B cell lymphomas regardless of type, but is diagnostically useful in selected situations.

T Lymphocytes

Like B lymphocytes, T cells have a normal antigen expression pattern that varies with their maturity and function. The pan-T cell markers, expressed by all mature T lymphocytes, are CD2, CD3, CD5, and CD7. Depending on their function, T cells may also express either CD4 (generally, the helper T cell phenotype) or CD8 (the cytotoxic phenotype). Analogous to surface Ig expression, T cells express surface receptors (T cell receptors [TCRs]) that are most often composed of alpha and beta chains (α/β). Receptors composed of gamma and delta (α/β) chains are less common, and there is no definitive marker of clonality in T cells analogous to the light chains in B lymphocytes. Of the four types of TCR chains, only the beta chain has routinely available antibodies for immunohistochemistry. Natural killer (NK) cells express a mixture of T cell antigens (CD2, CD7 and, occasionally, CD5), with other antigens including CD16, CD56, CD57, and CD94. They do not express TCR chains or surface CD3. One important caveat is that CD56, like CD138 on plasma cells, is not a specific marker and can be found in a variety of malignancies including carcinomas and neuroendocrine tumors.

Just as aberrant gain of expression by lymphocytes (eg, CD5 in B cells) can characterize lymphoid neoplasms, aberrant loss of normal markers can also be helpful. Thus, Ig light-chain-negative plasma cells are aberrant by definition, as are B cells lacking the pan-B cell antigens previously described in the "B Lymphocytes" section. Similarly, T cells lacking one or more of the pan-T cell antigens should raise the suspicion of a T cell lymphoma, as should cells expressing both CD4 and CD8 ("double positive"), or neither of these antigens ("double negative"). An important caveat associated with this principle is that reactive T cells in intense inflammatory reactions may have diminished expression of CD7 and occasionally of CD5.

Finally, normally organized lymphoid tissues have a characteristic expression of antigens reflecting the composition and organization of a mixture of T and B cells. This pattern is best illustrated in normal lymph nodes, but analogous patterns of expression can be found in the GI tract, particularly those areas with well-organized lymphoid populations such as Peyer's patches commonly seen in the distal ileum (Figure 4.1). B cells are organized into follicles and/

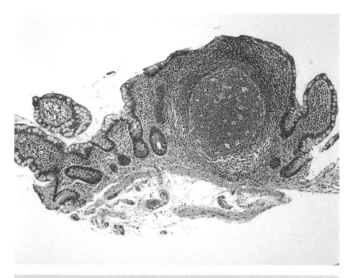

FIGURE 4.1 Peyer's patch in the terminal ileum. The terminal ileum contains a variable lymphoid population, typically most prominent in younger patients. The lymphocytes are a mixture of B cells, organized into follicular structures with surrounding mantle, and surrounding T cells, recapitulating the structures of lymph node cortex. In this example, note the mild distortion of mucosal architecture by the large lymphoid follicle, complete with polarized germinal center. The surface epithelium overlying the follicle and the epithelium of the surrounding crypts contain infiltrating lymphocytes, a normal finding in this situation.

or germinal centers (Figure 4.2A), which are surrounded by mantle and marginal zones (also composed of B lymphocytes), while T cells fill the interfollicular areas (Figure 4.2B). In addition to the B and T cell populations, the follicular structures contain a meshwork of follicular dendritic cells, which express CD21 and CD23 (Figure 4.2C).

UNIQUE FEATURES OF GASTROINTESTINAL LYMPHOID TISSUE

The diagnosis of lymphomas in the GI tract has some unique aspects and challenges. First, many lymphoid processes in the GI tract are sampled, at least initially, by a small biopsy obtained endoscopically. For this reason, the pathologist is quite dependent on the endoscopic description of the process or lesion during the assessment of a putatively atypical lymphoid population. As an example, an "atypical lymphoid infiltrate" in a gastric biopsy may become much more ominous when associated with the endoscopic description of a mass or large ulcer. The often limited nature of a biopsy sample can also make it difficult to fully assess the architectural features and extent of a lymphoid infiltrate that would be easier to diagnose if more tissue were sampled. This also means that obtaining

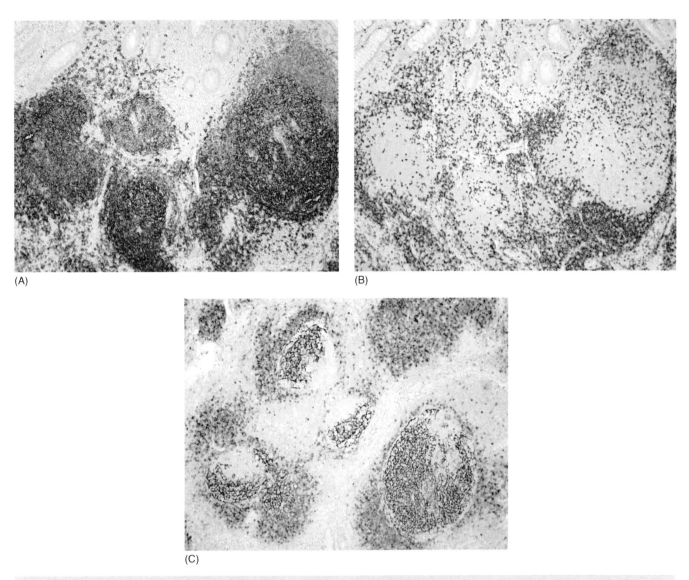

(A)

(B)

(C)

FIGURE 4.2 Immunostaining pattern of reactive follicles/germinal centers. In this example, an intensely reactive lymphoid infiltrate in an appendix is composed of both primary follicles and germinal centers with surrounding mantle zones, all of which are positive for CD20 (A). Surrounding these structures are normal T cells, positive for CD3 (B). Finally, a CD23 stain (C) highlights the meshwork of follicular dendritic cells in the germinal centers, as well as some activated B cells in the mantle zones around the germinal centers.

tissue for ancillary studies often used to diagnose lymphoma, such as flow cytometry and molecular diagnostics may be very difficult, such that optimizing an immunohistochemical approach to diagnosis is often the most helpful tactic. One must also, however, take care in the application of immunohistochemistry to the investigation of a lymphoid population in the GI tract; the combination of a comprehensive "lymphoma panel" of immunostains may, in fact, provide too much information, which increases the complexity of the assessment. This may be a particular problem in the context of a very small sample where the architecture and arrangement of the cells is already difficult to gauge.

The GI tract also has normal lymphoid populations that vary depending on the site, and GI lymphoid tissue can easily expand, or new foci can develop, in response to a variety of stimuli. The lymphoid tissue in the GI tract can be divided into so-called "native" mucosa-associated lymphoid tissue (MALT) and "acquired" MALT. Native MALT is epitomized by Peyer's patches of the distal ileum, which are well-developed lymphoid follicles with germinal centers that are most prominent in young patients. These can sometimes create a nodular endoscopic appearance in the terminal ileum, or may be perceived as small, sessile "polyps," prompting a biopsy during endoscopic examination. When exuberant, this normal lymphoid tissue can mildly alter the mucosal architecture, and some of the lymphocytes can encroach on the overlying mucosa or on the underlying muscularis mucosae. Either of these features can be misinterpreted as an ominous sign, potentially leading to the attribution of the descriptor "atypical." Similar lymphoid aggregates can be seen in and around the appendix, and a protrusion or eversion of appendiceal tissue into the cecum can be interpreted as a "mass" that, when sampled by biopsy, contains a sea of lymphocytes that may raise the specter of lymphoma as well. Individual lymphoid aggregates can occur anywhere in the GI tract, and are sampled frequently as tiny polyps, particularly as endoscope technology improves and makes smaller and smaller mucosal "abnormalities" visible.

If native MALT creates problems of interpretation, acquired MALT can present even more of a challenge. The paradigm of acquired lymphoid tissue in the GI tract is that associated with *Helicobacter pylori* infection in the stomach. This infection classically results in a dense, band-like lymphoplasmacytic infiltrate in the superficial gastric mucosa (Figure 4.3B) that is frequently accompanied by well-formed lymphoid follicles in the deeper mucosa, complete with germinal centers and surrounding mantle and marginal zones (Figure 4.3A). Other inflammatory conditions can initiate the development of or markedly expand existing lymphoid tissue within the GI tract and, because the underlying inflammatory condition can put the patient at risk of developing both epithelial and lymphoid neoplasia, the problem with acquired MALT often involves a

decision about when the line from "reactive" to "neoplastic" has been crossed. It is particularly important, therefore, to understand and correlate the clinical presentation and endoscopic appearance with the histologic findings when investigating an infiltrate of acquired lymphoid tissue, in order to avoid an overdiagnosis of lymphoma. In addition, some low-grade lymphomas arising in a background of inflammation and acquired MALT may be treated by very conservative therapy aimed at eradication of the inciting entity (ie, *H. pylori*), and this adds another layer of complexity to the issue, particularly when it comes to follow-up biopsies to assess disease progression and/or response.

GENERAL PRINCIPLES OF GASTROINTESTINAL LYMPHOMA DIAGNOSIS

As noted in the Introduction, the GI tract is, overall, the most common extranodal site of involvement by lymphomas, accounting for 4% to 20% of all non-Hodgkin lymphomas (depending on what literature is cited). In addition, hematolymphoid neoplasms tend to hover in a "no-man's land" between the subdisciplines of gastrointestinal pathology and hematopathology. Gastrointestinal pathologists may fear that they are missing subtleties of lymphoma diagnosis, while hematopathologists worry that they may miss an important feature of the precursor process or another entity coexisting with the lymphoma. As a result, such cases are often traded back and forth

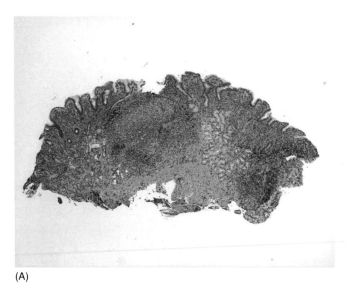

(A)

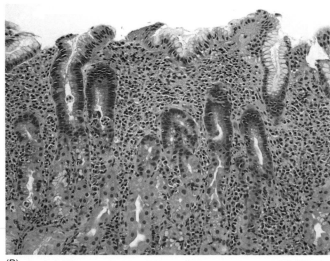

(B)

FIGURE 4.3 This low-power view of *H. pylori* gastritis highlights the typical, band-like superficial lymphoplasmacytic infiltrate involving the foveolar/pit compartment of the mucosa (A). This is punctuated by deeper lymphoid aggregates, including a well-formed germinal center in this case that spans almost the entire depth of the mucosa. Higher magnification reveals the prominent plasma cell component of the lamina propria inflammation, in this case involving gastric oxyntic mucosa (B). In addition, the chronic inflammation is accompanied by neutrophils infiltrating the epithelium of the deep pits and the transition between foveolar and gland epithelium (the so-called "mucous neck" region). Photomicrographs courtesy of H. D. Appelman, MD.

between experts in both fields before a diagnosis is settled upon. Thankfully, however, common entities remain common in the GI tract as elsewhere.

The most frequent lymphomas involving the GI tract are B cell lymphomas, as is the case everywhere in the body. Most lymphomas of the GI tract involve the stomach and the small intestine, followed by the colon. Lymphomas involving the esophagus and the solid GI organs (liver and pancreas) are very rare.

As noted earlier, correlation with the clinical impression and, particularly, the endoscopic appearance associated with a lymphoid population sampled by biopsy is crucial to an effective diagnostic approach. Atypical populations associated with a large destructive mass or malignant-appearing ulcer may be fairly easy to evaluate, whereas those coming from endoscopically normal (or very subtly abnormal) mucosa can pose a significant challenge. This challenge applies to both the clinical and the pathology side of the equation. If an outright diagnosis of lymphoma is made on a biopsy taken from endoscopically normal mucosa, it can be nearly impossible for the endoscopist to return to the same site to monitor or resample the disease process. By the same token, very compelling histologic evidence of malignancy in the context of only a subtle macroscopic abnormality (or a nebulous and randomly sampled finding such as "gastritis" or "erythema") should prompt consideration of rebiopsy or more extensive sampling for additional evidence of disease.

COMMON LYMPHOMAS AFFECTING THE GASTROINTESTINAL TRACT

While individual lymphomas are discussed and illustrated in much more detail in Chapters 8, 9, and 11, several of the most commonly encountered entities are briefly reviewed here, followed by a general, pragmatic overview to lymphoma diagnosis and a handful of specific illustrative scenarios that raise points of importance and potential pitfalls in GI lymphoma diagnosis. Table 4.1 summarizes the antigen expression patterns of the lymphomas discussed here.

Diffuse Large B Cell Lymphoma

Diffuse large B cell lymphoma (DLBCL) is the most common lymphoma affecting the GI tract. This lymphoma is, by definition, composed of diffuse sheets of intermediate-to-large B lymphocytes that typically have a high proliferative rate, vesicular nuclei, and scant cytoplasm. The neoplastic lymphocytes are dyscohesive, and obliterate the underlying tissue architecture as they infiltrate. A helpful clue to cell size is to compare the nuclei of the neoplastic lymphocytes to those of residual endothelial cells, which are a good internal measure of "large." DLBCL may arise de novo, or may evolve from a pre-existing low-grade lymphoma, which may still be found lurking in the background if not completely replaced by the large cell process.

Immunohistochemically, DLBCL is characterized by positivity for pan-B cell markers such as CD20 and PAX-5. This type of lymphoma also commonly expresses BCL-2, and may exhibit staining by the markers of follicle center cell differentiation, BCL-6 and CD10, depending on the specific subtype. It is negative for T cell markers such as CD3 (although about 10% may stain with CD5), and for cyclin-D1. DLBCL is a clinically aggressive lymphoma that often presents as a large, destructive mass. As with many other aggressive hematolymphoid neoplasms, however, it is potentially curable with appropriate chemotherapy, most often with a combination of cyclophosphamide, vincristine, doxorubicin, and dexamethasone (CHOP), and possibly with the addition of anti-CD20 immunotherapy such as rituximab.

MALT Lymphoma

The correct term for "MALT" lymphoma is actually "extranodal marginal zone lymphoma of mucosa-associated

TABLE 4.1   Antigen Expression Patterns of Various GI Lymphomas

Lymphoma	CD2	CD3	CD4	CD5	CD7	CD8	CD10	CD20	CD43	CD56	CD79a	BCL-2	BCL-6	Cyclin-D1	PAX-5
DLBCL	NH	NH	NH	−/+	NH	NH	+/−	+	+/−	−	+	+	+/−	−	+
MALT	NH	NH	NH	−	NH	NH	−	+	−/+	−	+	+	−	−	+
FL	NH	NH	NH	−	NH	NH	+	+	−	−	+	+	+	−	+
MCL	NH	NH	NH	+	NH	NH	−	+	+	−	+	+	−	+	+
BL	NH	NH	NH	−	NH	NH	+	+	−	−	+	−	+	−	+
EATL	+	+	−	−	+	−/+	NH	NH	+	−	NH	NH	NH	NH	NH
EATL-II	+	+	−	−	+	+/−	NH	NH	+	+	NH	NH	NH	NH	NH
ENKTL	+	−	−	−	−	−	NH	NH	+	+	NH	NH	NH	NH	NH

Abbreviations: BL, Burkitt lymphoma; DLBCL, diffuse large B cell lymphoma; EATL, enteropathy-associated T cell lymphoma; EATL-II, "type II" EATL; ENKTL, extranodal NK/T cell lymphoma, nasal type; FL, follicular lymphoma; MALT, mucosa-associated lymphoid tissue; MCL, mantle cell lymphoma; NH, not helpful.

lymphoid tissue." MALT lymphoma can occur throughout the GI tract, but is common in the stomach, where it is almost invariably associated with underlying *H. pylori* gastritis. As such, gastric MALT lymphomas are derived from *acquired* MALT that develops in response to immunogenic bacteria, a process that is enhanced when the organism is a strain harboring the *CagA* gene. This lymphoma is composed predominantly of small-to-intermediate-sized B cells, many with a morphology recapitulating that of centrocytes in the normal lymphoid follicle. In addition, a variable proportion of the neoplastic cells have ample cytoplasm with indented nuclei, imparting a "monocytoid" appearance. Scattered large, "centroblast-like" cells are also common, but this should not be the predominant cell type as this appearance would be best classified as DLBCL. Some cases have plasmacytic differentiation and, occasionally, MALT lymphomas are composed almost exclusively of plasma cells. Classically, the lymphoma cells expand the mucosa and destroy the normal mucosal structures, creating what are commonly referred to as "lymphoepithelial lesions." Macroscopically, MALT lymphomas may cause expansion of the mucosal folds, or produce ulcers. Unfortunately, this type of lymphoma has no specific immunophenotype, but the neoplastic B cells mark with CD20 and usually outnumber associated T cells (unlike reactive lymphoid infiltrates, in which T cells typically predominate). Around 30% to 50% of cases are reported to aberrantly coexpress CD43 on the neoplastic B cells, which can be a helpful feature when present. Finally, cases with plasmacytic differentiation contain abnormal plasma cells that will express only kappa or lambda light chain (also known as light chain restriction), a convenient marker of clonality when available. The association of gastric MALT lymphoma with *H. pylori* gastritis means that treatment of the underlying inflammatory condition can actually cure the lymphoma as well in most cases. Similarly, MALT lymphomas in other sites respond to eradication/resolution of the inciting inflammatory process, as typified by the mounting evidence of an association between *Campylobacter* infection and certain types of intestinal MALT lymphoma, which also respond to antibiotic therapy.

Follicular Lymphoma

The GI tract is often involved secondarily by follicular lymphoma that arises primarily in the retroperitoneal lymph nodes or elsewhere. Follicular lymphoma, as its name suggests, is a lymphoma of cells that recapitulate the follicle center B cells of a germinal center, and it is graded based on the proportion of small centrocyte-like cells (which often have grooved or "cleaved" nuclei) to large centroblast-like cells. Along with other B cell markers like CD20, the neoplastic B cells in FL express BCL-6 and CD10, which are markers of follicle center differentiation. The pattern of the

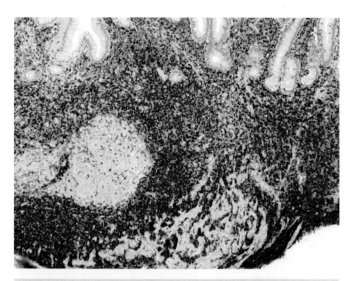

FIGURE 4.4 BCL-2 negativity in a reactive germinal center. Immunohistochemistry for BCL-2 staining can cause confusion in the workup of lymphoma in the GI tract and elsewhere. Many normal hematolymphoid cells, including T cells, plasma cells, and mantle zone B cells, express BCL-2. In addition, many B cell lymphomas are BCL-2 positive. Thus, the best use of this immunostain is in the distinction between reactive, non-neoplastic germinal centers like the one in the left of this photomicrograph, which are negative, and the neoplastic follicular structures of follicular lymphoma, which are usually positive for BCL-2 (see Chapter 9 for additional details and images).

lymphoma is nodular, with neoplastic "follicles" that also contain follicular dendritic cells, which can be highlighted with a CD21 or CD23 immunostain. FL is the one lymphoma where a BCL-2 immunostain can be crucial, as the cells in the neoplastic follicles express this antigen in most cases of FL. This helps separate true FL from reactive follicular hyperplasia (Figure 4.4). The common expression of BCL-2 by a very large number of other types of B cell lymphoma means that not everything that is BCL-2 positive is FL, a point that commonly causes confusion. FL is a relatively indolent lymphoma, but it commonly involves the bone marrow and can be difficult to cure. A relatively recently described entity, dubbed "primary intestinal FL," is usually found in the second part of the duodenum and is, by definition, isolated to the GI tract. This form of the disease, which has an identical immunophenotype to conventional FL, is reported to be very indolent, and some patients have long-term survival even without treatment.

Mantle Cell Lymphoma

Mantle cell lymphoma (MCL) has classically been associated with diffuse involvement of the GI tract that produces the appearance of numerous polypoid projections of the mucosa that can mimic inherited polyposis syndromes.

This so-called "lymphomatous polyposis" is regarded by some as synonymous with GI involvement by MCL, but this appearance has occasionally been reported in other types of lymphoma. MCL has a deceptively low-grade morphology, composed of small lymphocytes that often have angulated nuclei, which can infiltrate diffusely or have a nodular pattern. Most confusing is the "mantle zone" pattern, in which the neoplastic mantle cells are arranged around reactive germinal centers, because this appearance can be easily overlooked as malignant and misdiagnosed as a reactive process. Despite its bland morphology, MCL is quite aggressive and has a median survival of only 3 to 5 years (although it is not believed to transform to DLBCL, unlike the other lymphomas described thus far). MCL has a distinctive immunophenotype, aberrantly expressing the pan-T cell marker CD5 as well as typical B cell markers like CD20. In addition, almost all cases express nuclear cyclin-D1, which usually confirms the diagnosis and distinguishes MCL from GI involvement by chronic lymphocytic leukemia/small lymphocytic lymphoma (CLL/SLL), another B cell lymphoma that expresses CD5.

Burkitt Lymphoma

An aggressive B cell lymphoma, gastrointestinal Burkitt lymphoma (BL) is classically associated with large masses involving the ileocecal region, but it can occur anywhere in the GI tract. BL has several forms, including the endemic type, associated with Epstein–Barr virus (EBV) infection in certain parts of the world, and the sporadic type, found throughout the world. BL has an extraordinarily high proliferative rate, with nearly 100% of cells marking with the proliferation marker Ki-67 (Mib-1) in a typical case. This is also reflected in the easy identification of mitotic figures. BL has a characteristic low-magnification appearance referred to as "starry sky," because of the numerous tingible-body macrophages admixed with the lymphoma cells. BL is composed of monotonous, medium-sized neoplastic cells with inconspicuous nucleoli, which mark with CD20, CD10, and BCL-6, although they are almost always BCL-2 negative. Rearrangements in the *MYC* gene are characteristic as well. BL is an aggressive but potentially curable lymphoma, with an 80% to 90% survival rate when aggressively treated. In the past, lymphomas that did not fit precisely the immunophenotype and/or morphology of BL, but which had a similar high proliferative rate, were termed "atypical BL," although this terminology has recently fallen out of favor. Exactly how to handle such lymphomas remains controversial, but at least some have been found to harbor two or more abnormalities or rearrangements in the *MYC*, *BCL2*, and/or *BCL6* genes, and have been dubbed "double-hit" lymphomas. Currently, these reside in the nebulous and awkwardly named category of "B cell lymphoma, unclassifiable, with features intermediate between diffuse large

B cell lymphoma and Burkitt lymphoma" in the most recent (2008) WHO classification. This diagnosis may have implications for response to therapy, as there is some evidence that such lymphomas may not respond well to conventional DLBCL-type chemotherapy.

T Cell Lymphomas

While B cell lymphoma is by far the most common type of lymphoma involving the GI tract, there are two T cell lymphomas that merit mention in this brief introduction. First, enteropathy-associated T cell lymphoma (EATL) is, as the name suggests, usually related to an underlying gluten-sensitive enteropathy (celiac disease). EATL may arise in previously diagnosed celiac disease, or it may be the presenting event in undiagnosed patients, sometimes resulting in perforation of the small intestine (often the jejunum) by a large, destructive lymphomatous mass. EATL may also be preceded by a phase of celiac disease that is refractory to a gluten-free diet. As currently classified by the WHO, EATL comes in two forms, one referred to simply as "EATL" and the other as "Type II EATL." The Type II form comprises the minority of cases (up to 20%) and is composed of rather monotonous small- and medium-sized lymphocytes that usually express CD8 and CD56, along with the pan-T cell marker CD3. This form is less often associated with underlying celiac disease. The cells in the "conventional" form of the disease tend to be more pleomorphic and are most often CD8 and CD56 negative, while also being CD3 positive. The neoplastic T cells in this form also lose expression of CD5. EATL is an aggressive lymphoma, with poor overall survival. The association with an underlying malabsorption syndrome likely contributes to the poor prognosis.

Another T cell lymphoma that can involve the GI tract, and which can be confused with EATL, is extra-nodal NK/T cell lymphoma (ENKTL), nasal type. While its name indicates the most frequent site of involvement, which is in and around the nose (where it was previously termed "lethal midline granuloma," among other names), the GI tract is actually the most common extranasal site of involvement by this relatively rare entity. It tends to occur in adults, and has a predilection for Asian patients and native populations from Central America. Like EATL, this is a clinically aggressive disease. It is composed of neoplastic T cells that express CD2 and CD56, but which lack most other pan-T cell markers. The cells lack surface CD3, but contain cytoplasmic CD3ε, which may be identified by immunostains on paraffin-embedded tissue depending on the antibody specificity. In addition, the cells of ENKTL are essentially always positive for EBV by in situ hybridization (EBV-encoded ribonucleic acid [EBER] probe). They have a characteristic tendency to infiltrate the tissue with an angiocentric pattern that results in destruction of blood vessel walls, which also sets this entity apart from EATL.

GENERAL APPROACH TO LYMPHOMA DIAGNOSIS IN THE GASTROINTESTINAL TRACT

Approaches to evaluating GI specimens in which lymphoma is being considered vary greatly, particularly when dealing with small endoscopic tissue biopsies. While there is no absolutely correct or incorrect way to approach these diseases, a pragmatic diagnostic scheme that incorporates clinical, endoscopic, and morphologic features with ancillary testing (as needed) is outlined here.

First, as mentioned earlier, the endoscopic impression of the lesion or process that was biopsied is crucial, and should be sought actively if it is not immediately available when evaluating the biopsy. The endoscopist's viewpoint serves as the pathologist's "gross description" when dealing with small biopsies, and this information is invaluable to both parties. For the pathologist, it provides additional information regarding the extent and scope of the process, as a morphologically atypical lymphoid infiltrate takes on a more ominous tenor when associated with a large mass or ulcer. For the practitioner performing the endoscopic examination and clinical follow-up, the finding of a discrete lesion provides a landmark that can be targeted during subsequent examinations, either to obtain more tissue to reach a definite diagnosis, or to monitor the progress of potential therapy after the diagnosis is made. In addition, the pathologist must incorporate the background histologic features found in the biopsy, including whether there is an underlying inflammatory condition (eg, *H. pylori* infection) that may be contributing to the development of lymphoma, or evidence of underlying gluten-sensitive enteropathy in the case of EATL.

Once the pathologist determines that there is sufficient suspicion of lymphoma to warrant further diagnostic workup, he or she typically selects a battery of immunostains. While it can be tempting to try to be comprehensive and all-encompassing on the first pass, a tailored approach that takes into account the entities with the highest "pretest probability" is favored, as there is a significant risk of too much information when large immunostain panels are used at the outset. In addition, one does not want to cut entirely through the tissue in a small biopsy block when performing a large battery of immunostains, only to find out that different stains are needed, yet there is no tissue left in the block.

Specific staining patterns and approaches will be discussed in Chapters 8, 9, and 11, but a reasonable first-tier set of stains for most cases is CD3, CD20, and CD43. This panel allows the "balance" of T and B cells to be ascertained, and a predominance of small T cells with fewer B cells often points toward a reactive phenomenon. In addition, the architecture of the infiltrate can often be better seen when highlighted with immunostains, as B cell follicles are more easily recognizable. The addition

of CD43 is helpful in several ways. First, its expression should normally roughly parallel that of CD3, as it is normally expressed on T cells. It is also normally expressed by plasma cells, which are negative for CD20, so an infiltrate heavy in these plasma cells (such as *H. pylori* gastritis) may have increased CD43 staining. In addition, some B cell lymphomas aberrantly coexpress CD43, so definite staining in a B cell population is strong evidence for lymphoma. These CD43+ tumors include 30% to 50% of MALT lymphomas, as well as those B cell neoplasms that aberrantly coexpress CD5 (MCL and CLL/SLL). Finally, expression of *only* CD43 by a hematolymphoid infiltrate suggests that a myeloid neoplasm (such as GI involvement by acute myeloid leukemia) should be investigated.

BCL-2 immunohistochemistry is often included in initial "lymphoma panels," but this can create serious potential diagnostic pitfalls. There is a tendency to equate BCL-2 expression with FL, but this is not the case. Expression of this antigen is common with a variety of normal lymphoid cells, including cells of the normal mantle zone surrounding germinal centers, T cells, and plasma cells. In addition, most B cell lymphomas of any type express BCL-2. As suggested earlier, the best use of this stain is to differentiate between reactive follicular hyperplasia and follicular lymphoma, and a diagnosis of the latter should be restricted to a nodular/follicular pattern of B cells that express both a marker of follicular center cells (CD10 and/or BCL-6) and BCL-2 when it is used in this way. Additional evidence for follicular structures can be obtained by using a marker of follicular dendritic cells (CD21 and/or CD23).

The use of additional ancillary studies when evaluating putative GI lymphomas, particularly molecular diagnostic assays and flow cytometry, is somewhat controversial. The tissue typically obtained by endoscopic biopsy is scant enough that it is often most prudent to conserve it for a good look at the hematoxylin and eosin (H&E)-stained morphology combined with judicious immunohistochemistry, rather than attempting to subdivide it and send precious tissue (which may or may not contain tumor) to other labs. This is particularly true for flow cytometry, which is suboptimal for diagnosis of the most common type of GI lymphoma (DLBCL) due to poor cell survival during the disaggregation processes used to prepare tissue for flow cytometric analysis. Evaluation of GI biopsies by flow cytometry can also be affected by contamination by epithelial cells. There are a few situations where molecular studies can be quite helpful, but often after the actual diagnosis of lymphoma is made. Such situations will be addressed in Chapters 8, 9, and 11, but two worth mentioning are *H. pylori*-related MALT lymphoma and aggressive large B cell lymphomas where the differential diagnosis includes DLBCL with a high proliferative rate and the so-called "double-hit" B cell lymphoma. Some cases of *H. pylori*-related MALT lymphoma harbor a specific translocation, t(11;18)(q21;q21), that is associated with poor or absent response to conservative therapy aimed at *H. pylori* eradication, so identification of this abnormality by molecular diagnosis may be helpful in avoiding a fruitless trial of conservative therapy. Some authors recommend performing this test immediately at the time of initial diagnosis, even though the vast majority (greater than 80%–90%) of gastric and duodenal MALT lymphomas will respond to antibiotic therapy (even when *H. pylori* is not identified in biopsies). As discussed earlier, "double-hit" B cell lymphomas harbor molecular abnormalities in two or all three of the genes *MYC*, *BCL2*, and *BCL6*, and this information can help to cement the diagnosis and differentiate these aggressive lymphomas from conventional DLBCL, as well as potentially affecting therapy.

As with flow cytometric analysis and other molecular studies, the question of whether or not to order B or T cell gene rearrangement testing is one that can create struggles when making decisions about tissue allocation, especially for small diagnostic biopsies. This is further complicated by the fact that reactive, non-neoplastic T cell populations and, to an extent, B cell populations as well, can harbor small clonal populations. When subjected to amplification, these can potentially lead to an overdiagnosis of lymphoma. Therefore, while gene rearrangement studies can sometimes "tip the balance" and provide evidence for neoplasm in difficult or equivocal cases, it may be a better use of precious tissue to ensure a good look at H&E morphology and carefully selected immunohistochemical results in making a diagnosis of lymphoma, particularly because accurate subclassification is often important.

SPECIFIC ILLUSTRATIVE EXAMPLES

To help illustrate the concepts outlined in this introductory chapter on a pragmatic approach to the diagnosis of GI lymphomas, two specific clinical scenarios are worth exploring in more depth.

Lymphoid Tissue in the Terminal Ileum and Right Colon

A common question often asked in consultation is, "How much lymphoid tissue is normal in the terminal ileum and right colon?" The somewhat tongue-in-cheek answer is, "It depends."

Prominent lymphoid tissue is the norm in the right lower quadrant, particularly in young patients, but not uncommonly in patients of any age. Peyer's patches in the terminal ileum, a form of "native MALT," can be quite prominent, and as mentioned in the Unique Features of Gastrointestinal Lymphoid Tissue section, may impart an endoscopic picture of mucosal "nodularity" or even

small polyps. Similar tissue can be seen in the right colon, and the normally abundant lymphoid tissue surrounding the appendiceal orifice can prompt a biopsy as well. Under the microscope, even normal lymphoid tissue in an expected location can have a worrisome appearance, depending on the plane of section, the interaction with the associated mucosal structures, and the architecture. Worrisome microscopic findings combined with certain clinical settings, such as a middle-aged or older patient in whom prominent lymphoid tissue is somewhat surprising, can result in an expensive diagnostic workup that is undertaken in a valiant effort to avoid missing a diagnosis.

In this situation, it is important to understand what can create an "atypical" appearance in the normal lymphoid population of the right lower quadrant, and to combine this with an understanding of just how prominent the lymphoid aggregates in this region can be. A few specific features are most often the cause of diagnostic problems. The first is the interaction of lymphoid tissue with the fibers of the muscularis mucosae. Some observers regard any admixture of lymphocytes with the muscularis mucosae as evidence of aggressive or "invasive" behavior. In reality, however, odd planes of section, mild mucosal prolapse changes, and other normal variants can cause groups of lymphocytes to seemingly mix with the smooth muscle fibers; thus this is not necessarily evidence of malignancy. Large lymphoid aggregates can also give an impression of mucosal "distortion," when normal crypts are pushed out of the way and villi seem shortened, and individual lymphocytes can infiltrate the epithelium of the adjacent crypts, mimicking lymphoepithelial lesions of the type seen especially in MALT lymphomas (Figure 4.5). Finally, and perhaps most confusing, is the primary follicle. While we expect to encounter germinal centers in Peyer's patches and other large lymphoid aggregates such as those associated with the appendix, a tangential section or a sample containing primary follicles that have not developed into germinal centers can present the pathologist with nodules of monotonous mantle cells, which normally express BCL-2 (Figure 4.6). This is another important scenario where BCL-2 positivity is not equivalent to FL.

Gastritis Versus MALT Lymphoma

A second source of many specialty consultations is the question of gastric MALT lymphoma, particularly the effort to understand exactly where severe *H. pylori* gastritis ends and early MALT lymphoma begins. Unfortunately, there is no easy answer to this question, but application of a pragmatic approach can ease the pain of trying to provide one. Several features of this low-grade lymphoma make it potentially challenging. First, it is quite common and it is usually relatively easily treated, so the index of suspicion tends to be high when any lymphoid tissue is found in

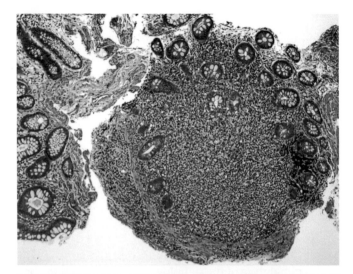

FIGURE 4.5 Effects of a benign Peyer's patch on mucosal structures. In addition to displacing the crypts and causing a localized blunting of overlying villi as illustrated in Figure 4.1, the lymphocytes of a normal Peyer's patch can both interdigitate with the fibers of the muscularis mucosae, seen at the bottom of this image, and infiltrate the epithelium of surrounding crypts. Neither of these features is diagnostic of a neoplastic process. When lymphocytes are found within the epithelium in a benign condition, the destructive infiltration characteristic of the "lymphoepithelial lesions" seen in MALT lymphoma is absent (see Chapter 8 for additional details and images).

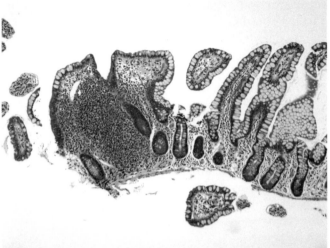

FIGURE 4.6 This ileal biopsy contains a lymphoid aggregate without an organized germinal center (Peyer's patch with primary lymphoid follicle). Otherwise, it has similar features to the Peyer's patch seen in Figure 4.1, with mild architectural disorganization and small lymphocytes infiltrating the adjacent surface and crypt epithelium. Characterizing this lymphoid population with immunostains would reveal a mixture of T cells and B cells, but the latter would also likely express BCL-2, because many of the B cells are mantle zone lymphocytes. This can cause confusion with lymphoid neoplasms, particularly follicular lymphoma (see also Chapter 9).

the gastric mucosa. The GI tract is the most common site for MALT lymphoma, and 85% of GI cases occur in the stomach in association with *H. pylori* gastritis. In addition, there are no specific immunohistochemical markers for MALT lymphoma, so the diagnosis relies heavily on the H&E morphology coupled with the balance of T and B lymphocytes identified by appropriate immunostains (and, on occasion, B cell gene rearrangement studies). Extensive plasmacytic differentiation can further confuse the issue, because a dense infiltrate of plasma cells can be regarded simply as part of the underlying gastritis and overlooked as a part of a neoplasm. Evidence of clonality using kappa and lambda light chain immunohistochemistry can easily solve this problem, and this should be kept in mind when evaluating a lymphoid infiltrate with plasmacytic features. Even when extensive plasmacytic differentiation is considered, there is another potential stumbling block; the use of a CD138 stain to highlight the plasma cells can lead to a different type of misdiagnosis, as many epithelial and mesenchymal neoplasms also express CD138.

As noted earlier, correlation with the endoscopic impression is important in the diagnosis of any lymphoma in the GI tract, but this is particularly true with regard to MALT lymphoma. Because of the overlap with severe *H. pylori* gastritis, atypical lymphoid infiltrates that raise the suspicion of MALT lymphoma are commonly found in biopsies that come from mucosa with rather nebulous endoscopic findings such as "gastritis" or "erythema." In this setting, one must be careful with an unequivocal diagnosis of lymphoma. It can be impossible, without a targetable endoscopic finding, for the patient to be easily monitored following diagnosis. Thus, in cases where the histologic suspicion is very high and the sample is considered too scant for a definite diagnosis, it may be best for the patient to undergo another examination that can better "map" the mucosa and obtain more tissue for diagnosis. When the suspicion is relatively low, the very high rate of MALT lymphoma response to conservative *H. pylori* eradication therapy means that treatment of the underlying disease is very likely to be sufficient in eradicating a possible lymphoma, in any case, and prudence may dictate simply treating the gastritis rather than wasting time and energy on wrestling with the diagnosis.

Even when accompanied by a finding of diffusely thickened gastric folds or a malignant-appearing ulcer, the diagnosis of MALT lymphoma, while easier to make, is not without potential pitfalls. In particular, earlier-than-optimal rebiopsy to assess response to therapy can do more harm than good, and can lead to confusion. While most MALT lymphomas are sensitive to eradication of the inciting *H. pylori* organisms, this process can take months to reach full histologic resolution. Cases taking greater than a year to resolve have even been reported. Thus, rebiopsy at 4 or 6 weeks may result in an appearance that is not appreciably different from the original diagnostic biopsy (although the success of *H. pylori* eradication may be assessed). Treatment of MALT lymphomas considered refractory to conservative therapy may be escalated to chemotherapy or other modalities, so it is important not to give the impression of refractoriness too early in the course of treatment. It is reasonable to diagnose "residual MALT lymphoma" and to comment on how the infiltrate compares to earlier biopsies (eg, "significantly improved from prior biopsy on [DATE]") to provide a record of continuing progress in resolution of the lymphoma.

Finally, the frequency of gastric MALT lymphoma may induce a tendency to regard almost any lymphoma in the stomach as this type of disease. It is important to consider the possibility of other types of lymphoma, in particular DLBCL, because these may not respond to *H. pylori* eradication therapy. Furthermore, DLBCL can evolve from MALT lymphoma, so recognition of a large cell component is very important, and will be discussed in greater detail in Chapter 8.

SELECTED REFERENCES

General

Burke JS. Lymphoproliferative disorders of the gastrointestinal tract: A review and pragmatic guide to diagnosis. *Arch Pathol Lab Med.* 2011;135:1283–1297.

Dickson BC, Serra S, Chetty R. Primary gastrointestinal tract lymphoma: diagnosis and management of common neoplasms. *Expert Rev Anticancer Ther.* 2008;6:1609–1628.

O'Malley DP, Goldstein NS, Banks PM. The recognition and classification of lymphoproliferative disorders of the gut. *Hum Pathol.* 2014;45:899–916.

Sagaert X, Tousseyn T, Yantiss RK. Gastrointestinal B-cell lymphomas: from understanding B-cell physiology to classification and molecular pathology. *World J Gastrointest Oncol.* 2012;4:238–249.

Smith LB, Owens SR. Gastrointestinal lymphomas: entities and mimics. *Arch Pathol Lab Med.* 2012;136:865–870.

B Cell Lymphomas

Harris NL, Swerdlow SH, Jaffe ES, et al. Follicular lymphoma. In: Swerdlow SH, Campo E, Harris NL, et al., eds. *WHO Classification of Tumours of Haematopoietic and Lymphoid Tissues.* Lyon, France: IARC Press; 2008:265–266.

Leoncini L, Raphael M, Stein H, et al. Burkitt lymphoma. In: Swerdlow SH, Campo E, Harris NL, et al., eds. *WHO Classification of Tumours of Haematopoietic and Lymphoid Tissues.* Lyon, France: IARC Press; 2008:262–264.

Owens SR. Large cell lymphoma. In: Greenson JK, Lamps LW, Montgomery EA, et al. *Diagnostic Pathology: Gastrointestinal.* Salt Lake City, UT: Amirsys, Inc. 2010:2.76–2.79.

Owens SR. MALT lymphoma. In: Greenson JK, Lamps LW, Montgomery EA, et al. *Diagnostic Pathology: Gastrointestinal.* Salt Lake City, UT: Amirsys, Inc. 2010:2.70–2.75.

Owens SR. Mantle cell lymphoma. In: Greenson JK, Lamps LW, Montgomery EA, et al. *Diagnostic Pathology: Gastrointestinal.* Salt Lake City, UT: Amirsys, Inc. 2010:2.80–2.83.

Psyrri A, Papageorgiou S, Economopoulos T. Primary extranodal lymphomas of stomach: clinical presentation, diagnostic pitfalls and management. *Ann Oncol.* 2008;19:1992–1999.

Zullo A, Hassan C, Ridola L, et al. Gastric MALT lymphoma: old and new insights. *Ann Gastroenterol.* 2014;27:27–33.

T Cell Lymphomas

Chan JKC, Quintanilla-Martinez L, Ferry JA, Peh S-C. Extranodal NK/T-cell lymphoma, nasal type. In: Swerdlow SH, Campo E, Harris NL, et al., eds. *WHO Classification of tumours of Haematopoietic and Lymphoid Tissues.* Lyon, France: IARC Press; 2008:285–288.

Ferreri AJ, Zinzani PL, Govi S, Pileri SA. Enteropathy-associated T-cell lymphoma. *Crit Rev Oncol Hematol.* 2011;79:84–90.

Isaacson PG, Chott A, Ott G, Stein H. Enteropathy-associated T-cell lymphoma. In: Swerdlow SH, Campo E, Harris NL, et al., eds. *WHO Classification of Tumours of Haematopoietic and Lymphoid Tissues.* Lyon, France: IARC Press; 2008:289–291.

5

Approach to Mesenchymal Neoplasms of the Gastrointestinal Tract

LAURA W. LAMPS AND MATTHEW R. LINDBERG

INTRODUCTION

Despite their overall rarity when compared to epithelial and other nonmesenchymal tumors, mesenchymal neoplasms are relatively common in the gastrointestinal (GI) tract. This large group of tumors encompasses a wide range of entities, including both conventional soft tissue entities (eg, lipoma, leiomyoma, and nerve sheath tumors) as well as entities that are almost entirely restricted to the GI tract (eg, gastrointestinal stromal tumor [GIST], plexiform fibromyxoma, Schwann cell hamartoma, and inflammatory fibroid polyp). GIST has the distinction of being the most common GI mesenchymal tumor overall, comprising 0.2% of all GI tumors.

Many pathologists are uncomfortable with the diagnosis of mesenchymal tumors, but GI mesenchymal neoplasms tend to pose less of a problem than their counterparts arising from soft tissue due to a more limited differential diagnosis. Histomorphologic evaluation, accompanied by basic clinical information (eg, site) and a small panel of immunohistochemical stains, is often sufficient to accurately classify a GI mesenchymal neoplasm. This chapter will discuss the basic approach to the evaluation of mesenchymal neoplasms, features of GISTs and their differential diagnosis, and current ancillary testing that is increasingly considered the standard of care from both a prognostic and a therapeutic standpoint.

GENERAL APPROACH TO SPECIMEN EVALUATION AND DIAGNOSIS

Clinical Evaluation

The importance of the location of a mesenchymal tumor within the GI tract cannot be overemphasized. Some mesenchymal tumors show a predilection for particular sites and are very uncommon in others. For example, the vast majority of mesenchymal neoplasms in the stomach are GISTs, whereas in the esophagus mesenchymal tumors are usually leiomyomas. Not uncommonly, a reasonable guess can be made as to the diagnosis before a histologic section is even seen, just by knowing the anatomic site. This information is summarized in Table 5.1.

Knowledge of the patient's clinical history may also provide useful information. For example, a solitary mural tumor arising in a patient with neurofibromatosis is usually a GIST (and not a malignant peripheral nerve sheath tumor), whereas multiple serosal or transmural nodules in the same demographic likely represent plexiform neurofibromas. In addition, the history of another malignancy (such as primary lung carcinoma or malignant melanoma) should always lead the pathologist to exclude a metastasis before investigating the possibility of a primary mesenchymal neoplasm.

TABLE 5.1 Distribution of Mesenchymal Tumors by Site in the Gastrointestinal Tract

Esophagus	Stomach	Small Bowel	Colon	Anus
Leiomyoma	GIST	GIST	GIST (particularly rectum)	Leiomyoma
Granular cell tumor	Schwannoma	Inflammatory fibroid polyp (particularly ileum)	Leiomyoma	GIST
Giant fibrovascular polyp	Inflammatory fibroid polyp (antrum)	Granular cell tumor (duodenum)	Granular cell tumor	Granular cell tumor
GIST	Glomus tumor		Perineurioma Ganglioneuroma Schwannoma	

Gross Evaluation

When approaching a gross specimen for evaluation of a mesenchymal neoplasm, it is particularly important to document the size of the tumor (this is particularly important for GISTs, as size is an important prognostic indicator). If possible, the specific anatomic layer (eg, submucosa, muscularis propria) of origin within the wall of the GI tract should be noted as well (see Table 5.2). If the tumor appears to be extraintestinal, such as from the mesentery or omentum, then its relationship to the GI tract and/or other organs in the resection specimen should be described. The presence of necrosis should be noted. Margins should be sampled, if applicable, and multiple sections of the tumor submitted (ideally one section per centimeter of the greatest tumor dimension). Consideration should also be given to reserving fresh tissue for molecular analysis or cytogenetic studies, although the majority of ancillary tests can be performed directly from the paraffin block.

Intraoperative Evaluation

Frozen section evaluation may be requested if the tumor type is in question at the time of surgery. For many mesenchymal tumors, the intraoperative diagnosis of "spindle cell neoplasm" is sufficient, with the caveat that a formal diagnosis must be deferred until multiple formalin-fixed hematoxylin and eosin (H&E) sections have been evaluated and any necessary ancillary diagnostic techniques have been incorporated. The differential diagnosis of epithelioid tumors on frozen section is, of course, more broad and challenging. If there is any chance that that tumor is an epithelioid mesenchymal neoplasm (mainly GIST), a preliminary diagnosis of "epithelioid neoplasm" with deferral to evaluation of permanent sections is warranted.

Histologic Evaluation

A reasonable histologic approach to GI tract mesenchymal tumors includes the following:

- Determination of growth pattern (circumscribed, infiltrative, polypoid, etc.).
- Evaluation of overall cellular morphology (spindled, epithelioid, or mixed).
- Assessment of the presence or absence of nuclear atypia/pleomorphism.
- Assessment for characteristic features that may be of diagnostic utility.

Growth Pattern

The differential diagnosis of a discrete mesenchymal polyp is often fairly limited and well-defined, whereas a submucosal or mural mass engenders a broader list of considerations,

TABLE 5.2 Classification of GI Mesenchymal Tumors by Location in the Wall of the GI Tract

Mucosa	Submucosa	Muscularis Propria	Serosa/Mesentery
Nerve sheath/neural tumors Perineurioma	Inflammatory fibroid polyp Nerve sheath tumors	GIST Schwannoma	Desmoid tumor Inflammatory myofibroblastic tumor
Leiomyoma of muscularis mucosae	Gangliocytic paraganglioma	Leiomyoma	Sclerosing mesenteritis
Kaposi's sarcoma	Lipoma	Glomus tumor	Extraintestinal GIST

Source: Adapted from Voltaggio L. and Montgomery EA: "Gastrointestinal spindle cell lesions: just like real estate, it's all about location." *Mod Pathol.* 2015;28 Suppl 1: S47-66.

including rarer entities. Some of the more common mesenchymal polyps include ganglioneuroma, leiomyoma, perineurioma, Schwann cell hamartoma, inflammatory fibroid polyp, and granular cell tumor, all of which are benign and generally of little clinical consequence. Entities such as GIST, schwannoma, mural leiomyoma/leiomyosarcoma, plexiform angiomyxoma, and glomus tumor are more likely to present clinically as masses, and not polyps. Importantly, as noted earlier, when dealing with a nonpolypoid subepithelial tumor, the anatomic layer of origin is important to note and often provides a useful clue to the diagnosis (see Table 5.2). For example, GIST arises in the muscularis propria, while schwannoma and inflammatory fibroid polyp arise in the submucosa. Inflammatory myofibroblastic tumor (IMFT) and desmoid tumor usually arise extrinsic to the GI tract (ie, mesentery) but may appear to arise in the serosa or the muscularis propria (if involved through local extension).

Overall Cellular Morphology

The differential diagnosis of a spindled mesenchymal neoplasm is quite broad, but most commonly includes GIST, schwannoma, leiomyoma/leiomyosarcoma, and inflammatory fibroid polyp. Knowing what portion of the GI tract is involved, as noted previously in the section on general approach to specimen evaluation and in Table 5.1, is often very helpful in narrowing down this list. Epithelioid neoplasms are generally more straightforward and almost always represent GISTs, provided that carcinoma and melanoma are fully excluded. Glomus tumor is also a noteworthy consideration. Tumors with a mixture of spindled and epithelioid cells are also usually GISTs. This information is summarized in Table 5.3.

Nuclear Atypia/Pleomorphism

Significant nuclear atypia/pleomorphism is generally uncommon in GI tract mesenchymal neoplasms. When faced with a pleomorphic submucosal or mural neoplasm, metastatic carcinoma and melanoma should always be promptly excluded first. Once this is done, leiomyosarcoma should be considered next, followed by entities such as GIST, symplastic leiomyoma, and other rare tumors. As a rule, nuclear pleomorphism in GIST is very uncommon, even in malignant cases. Two notable exceptions to this rule are pleomorphic epithelioid GIST, which may show prominent nuclear atypia (resembling carcinoma or melanoma) but almost no mitotic figures (Figure 5.1); and dedifferentiated GIST, which is defined as a classic KIT-positive spindled GIST containing an anaplastic KIT-negative component (Figure 5.2A–B).

Characteristic/Diagnostic Features

There are a few histologic findings or patterns that, if present, can help significantly narrow a broad differential diagnosis. Nuclear palisading in a GI tract mesenchymal tumor often indicates a GIST (Figure 5.3), despite its traditional association with neural neoplasms such as schwannoma. Peritumoral or intratumoral lymphoid aggregates (Figure 5.4) should suggest schwannoma, although they can be seen in other tumors as well. A multinodular or plexiform growth pattern suggests plexiform fibromyxoma, plexiform neurofibroma, or succinate dehydrogenase (SDH)-deficient GIST (Figure 5.5). Prominent myxoid stroma is a feature of many GISTs, but can also be seen in smooth muscle tumors, plexiform fibromyxoma, inflammatory fibroid polyp, IMFT, and desmoid

TABLE 5.3 Approach to Gastrointestinal Mesenchymal Neoplasms Based on Histologic Pattern

Spindle Cell	Epithelioid	Nested	Myxoid	Small Round Blue Cells	Pleomorphic
GIST	GIST	Gangliocytic Paraganglioma	GIST	DSRBCT	Leiomyosarcoma
Desmoid	PEComa	Clear-cell-sarcoma-like tumor of the GI tract	Inflammatory fibroid polyp	Round cell liposarcoma	MPNST
Schwannoma	Schwannoma		Plexiform fibromyxoma		GIST
Leiomyoma/ leiomyosarcoma	Epithelioid vascular tumors		Leiomyosarcoma		Liposarcoma
Inflammatory fibroid polyp	Glomus		IMFT		
Perineurioma	Granular cell tumor		Neurofibroma		
Neurofibroma	Rhabdoid tumor				
Inflammatory pseudotumors					
IMFT					
SFT					
Plexiform fibromyxoma					
Granular cell tumor					

Abbreviations: DSRBCT, desmoplastic small round blue cell tumor; IMFT, inflammatory myofibroblastic tumor; MPNST, malignant peripheral nerve sheath tumor; PEComa, perivascular epithelioid cell tumor; SFT, solitary fibrous tumor.

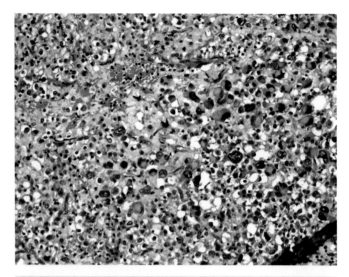

FIGURE 5.1 Pleomorphic GIST may show striking nuclear atypia, as seen here in a gastric tumor, but mitotic figures are scarce instead of not increased.

tumor. Large dilated/ectatic stromal vessels (ie, "staghorn" or hemangiopericytoma-like) may be seen in GIST, though not nearly as often or as prominently as in solitary fibrous tumor, which of course must be carefully excluded (Figure 5.6A–B). Tumor involvement of the mucosa is not typical of malignant GIST, and should lead to consideration of leiomyosarcoma, metastatic carcinoma/melanoma, and other malignancies (Figure 5.7).

Care must be taken when evaluating a GI tract mesenchymal tumor that has been sampled only by a small biopsy. Such biopsies are often only a minute portion of a much larger tumor, and therefore may not be representative, leading to misdiagnosis or undergrading. This is particularly problematic with GIST, as modern prognostication schemes require careful evaluation of numerous microscopic fields for the presence of mitotic figures. Accurate grading is often impossible on a small biopsy, particularly if only a few or no mitoses are present. Radiographic correlation may be helpful when evaluating needle biopsies of mesenchymal neoplasms, as they can provide information on size, relationship to anatomical structures, and the presence or absence of possible metastases.

Immunohistochemical Evaluation

Immunohistochemistry can be extremely helpful in the evaluation of GI tract mesenchymal tumors. The most commonly utilized antibodies include KIT, DOG1, S100 protein, smooth muscle actin (SMA), desmin, CD34, and broad-spectrum keratin. A summary of the basic immunohistochemical features and pitfalls in the evaluation of GI mesenchymal tumors is given in Table 5.4. It is extremely important to be aware of the sensitivity, specificity, and potential cross-reactivity of immunostains that are used in diagnosis and evaluation of mesenchymal tumors of the GI tract (or any other tumor), as well as staining artifacts.

KIT and DOG1

Diffuse KIT expression is characteristic of GIST (Figure 5.8A), and may be cytoplasmic or membranous (but not nuclear). It rarely shows a perinuclear dot-like pattern of expression (Figure 5.8B). DOG1 is nearly identical

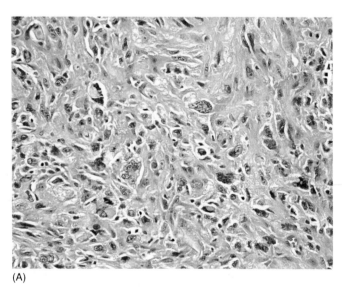

(A)

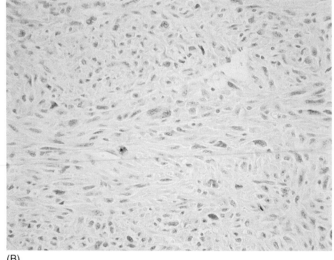

(B)

FIGURE 5.2 Dedifferentiated GIST is defined as a typical spindle cell GIST with characteristic immunostaining, which also contains an anaplastic component (A) that is either KIT negative or only weakly positive (B). Figures courtesy of Dr. Jason L. Hornick.

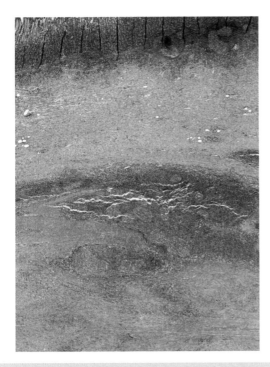

FIGURE 5.3 Despite the traditional association with schwannomas, GISTs frequently feature areas of nuclear palisading.

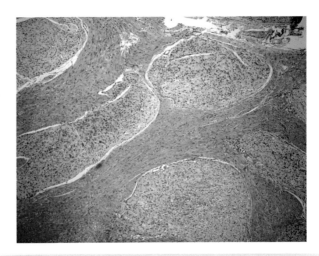

FIGURE 5.5 A multinodular or plexiform growth pattern, as seen here in a GIST, suggests either SDH-deficient GIST or plexiform fibromyxoma.

in sensitivity and specificity to KIT and may be used as an alternative. It may also be used in conjunction with KIT to increase sensitivity. Rare GISTs are KIT negative (usually those with epithelioid morphology), but DOG1 is often positive in these tumors. Exceptionally rare tumors are both KIT and DOG1 negative, and often require molecular analysis to make a diagnosis.

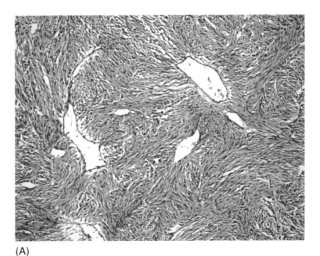

(A)

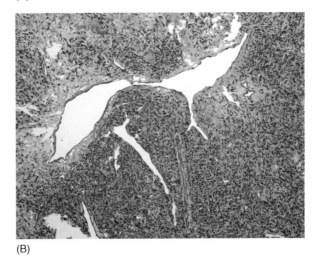

(B)

FIGURE 5.4 Peritumoral and/or intratumoral lymphoid aggregates are very common in gastrointestinal tract schwannomas, as seen here in this gastric tumor.

FIGURE 5.6 Although dilated or ectatic vessels (also known as "staghorn" or "hemangiopericytoma-like" vessels) may be seen in GIST (A), they are more often associated with solitary fibrous tumor (B). However, solitary fibrous tumor of the GI tract is very rare.

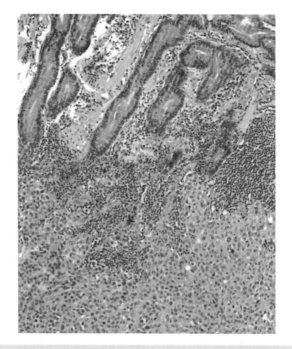

FIGURE 5.7 True mucosal invasion is not typical of GIST, and should lead to consideration of other entities such as malignant melanoma, as shown here.

Caveats

KIT is expressed by mast cells; thus it is important to differentiate KIT-positive mast cells from true tumor cells when intratumoral mast cells are prominent within a non-GIST mesenchymal tumor (Figure 5.9). One should always be reluctant to diagnose a GIST in the setting of scattered KIT-positive individual cells. KIT expression has been rarely reported in desmoid tumors, and DOG1 expression has been rarely reported in leiomyosarcomas and malignant peripheral nerve sheath tumors. KIT also stains a wide variety of nonmesenchymal tumors, including melanoma, Kaposi's sarcoma, plasma cell myeloma, urothelial carcinoma, chromophobe renal cell carcinoma, thymic carcinoma, and some breast carcinomas (Figure 5.10A–B). DOG1 positivity can also be seen in synovial sarcoma, gastric adenocarcinoma, acinic cell carcinoma of salivary gland, and rarely in malignant peripheral nerve sheath tumors.

S100 PROTEIN

Strong, diffuse nuclear and cytoplasmic expression is characteristic of schwannoma, Schwann cell hamartoma, granular cell tumor, and ganglioneuroma (Figure 5.11).

TABLE 5.4 Basic Panel of Immunostains Useful in the Diagnosis of Mesenchymal Tumors of the GI Tract

	GIST	**Leiomyoma**	**Leiomyosarcoma**	**Schwannoma**	**Desmoid**
KIT	95%	Negative	Negative	Negative	Rarely positive
DOG1	~90%	Negative	0.3%	Negative	Negative
CD34	70%	Negative	Negative	Negative	Negative
SMA	30%–40%	~100%	86%	Negative	Negative
Desmin	1%–2%	~100%	50%–80%	Negative	Negative
S100	1%–2%	Negative	Negative	100%	Negative
Cytokeratin	1%–2%	~20% (varies with keratin used)	20%–38%	Rare, focal	Negative

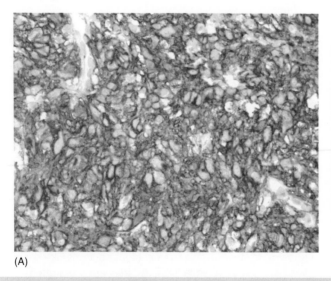

(A)

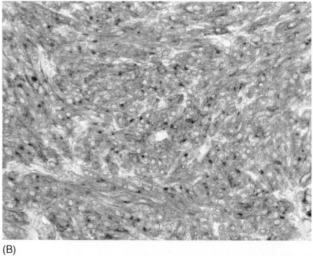

(B)

FIGURE 5.8 Diffuse cytoplasmic or membranous KIT expression is characteristic of GIST (A), but staining should not be nuclear. Rarely, KIT immunostaining produces a perinuclear dot-like pattern of expression (B).

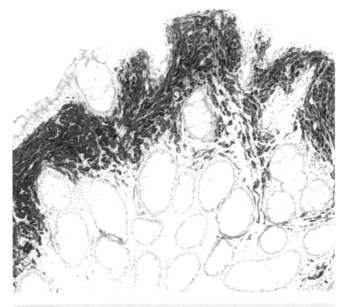

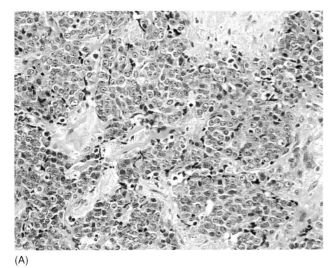

(A)

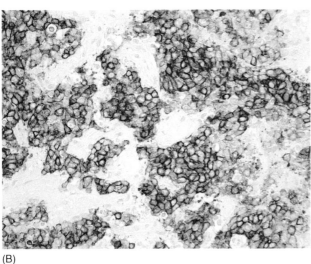

(B)

FIGURE 5.9   This KIT stain of a duodenal leiomyoma shows scattered intratumoral mast cells. KIT-positive mast cells should not be mistaken for staining of tumor cells.

FIGURE 5.10   This epithelioid thymic carcinoma (A) shows strong, diffuse cytoplasmic and membranous staining for KIT (B). Figures courtesy of Dr. Jason L. Hornick.

FIGURE 5.11   This gastric Schwann cell hamartoma shows strong, diffuse staining for S100.

Caveats

Scattered individual S100-positive cells within a tumor are likely dendritic-type cells. A proportion of GISTs that arise within the setting of neurofibromatosis also express S100 protein.

Smooth Muscle Actin

Diffuse cytoplasmic expression (Figure 5.12A) is most characteristic of smooth muscle neoplasms such as leiomyoma and leiomyosarcoma, but SMA positivity is also present in glomus tumors and PEComas. Expression can also be seen in plexiform fibromyxoma, IMFT, and desmoid, but it is usually more "wispy" and less impressive in these tumors (Figure 5.12B).

Caveats

In approximately 20% of cases, GIST can show focal to extensive SMA positivity (Figure 5.13). It may also be focally expressed in some gastric schwannomas.

Desmin

Strong, diffuse desmin expression is typical of smooth muscle neoplasms, particularly leiomyoma (Figure 5.14). Leiomyosarcoma is negative in approximately half of the cases. PEComa, desmoid, and IMFTs may also show patchy expression.

Caveats

Desmin may be expressed in rare cases of gastric schwannoma. In the GI tract, focal expression of desmin in the absence of SMA or similar antibodies is likely nonspecific.

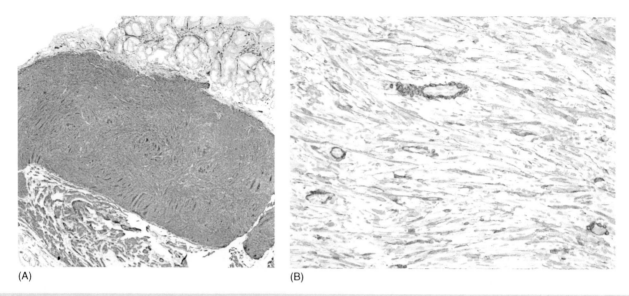

(A)   (B)

FIGURE 5.12   Diffuse cytoplasmic expression of smooth muscle actin is most characteristic of smooth muscle neoplasms, as seen here in a gastric leiomyoma of the muscularis mucosae (A). Wispy, weaker SMA expression can be seen in a variety of other tumors, including inflammatory myofibroblastic tumor (B, courtesy of Dr. Andrew Folpe).

CD34

CD34 expression is seen in a variety of tumors including GIST, solitary fibrous tumor, and inflammatory fibroid polyp, and therefore it is of limited utility in evaluating mesenchymal tumors of the GI tract.

Caveats

Many mesenchymal tumors, both intrinsic and extrinsic to the GI tract, express CD34. If it is used at all, it should be used as part of a panel rather than as a confirmatory stain on its own.

Keratin

In the evaluation of GI mesenchymal tumors, keratin is primarily used to exclude carcinoma. Diffuse cytoplasmic expression is typical of epithelial malignancies. Focal expression is nonspecific, but may also indicate carcinoma.

Caveats

Keratin may be focally expressed in gastric schwannomas. Some antibodies (such as cytokeratin [CK] AE1/AE3) may show patchy expression in smooth muscle tumors as well.

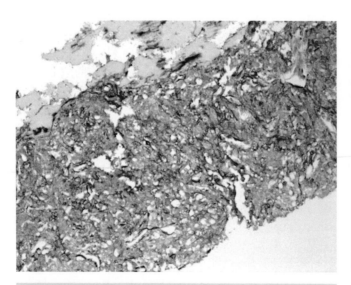

FIGURE 5.13   This needle biopsy of a small bowel GIST shows strong SMA positivity.

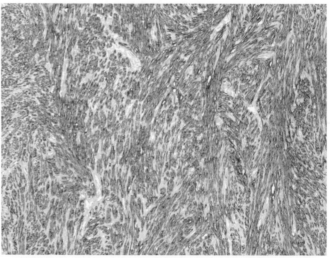

FIGURE 5.14   Strong, diffuse desmin expression is typical of smooth muscle tumors, particularly leiomyomas.

Other Markers

Nuclear β-catenin expression may be helpful in supporting the diagnosis of desmoid tumor (Figure 5.15). Melanocytic markers (HMB-45 and MART-1) are used mainly to evaluate for metastatic melanoma, but these markers are often coexpressed with SMA in PEComa (Figure 5.16). Focal MART-1 expression has also been reported in 30% to 40% of epithelioid GISTs.

Molecular Evaluation

Some mesenchymal tumors of the GI tract, particularly GISTs but not exclusively so, have well-elucidated

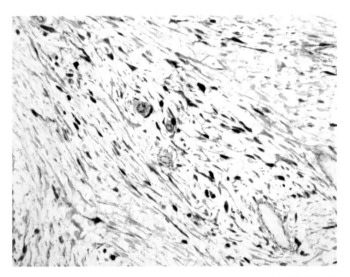

FIGURE 5.15 Nuclear β-catenin expression is helpful in supporting the diagnosis of desmoid tumors. Cytoplasmic expression is entirely nonspecific and is not diagnostically useful.

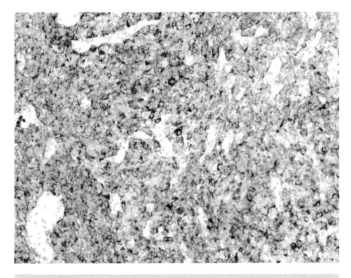

FIGURE 5.16 PEComas express HMB-45 (shown here, courtesy of Dr. Andrew Folpe) as well as SMA.

molecular characteristics. In addition, molecular and cytogenetic testing has become the standard of care in the diagnosis, prognosis, and therapeutic decision making in many GI mesenchymal tumors. A summary of molecular alterations and correlative tests is given in Table 5.5.

Diagnostic Pitfalls

The majority of diagnostic errors that occur when evaluating mesenchymal tumors of the GI tract are due to either failure to consider spindle cell lesions other than GIST in the differential diagnosis, or to incorrect interpretation of immunostains and lack of awareness of the spectrum of tumors that commonly used immunostains can mark (see section on immunohistochemical evaluation).

COMMON MESENCHYMAL TUMORS OF THE GI TRACT

Gastrointestinal Stromal Tumors

GISTs are the most common mesenchymal tumor of the GI tract. GISTs are believed to arise from the KIT-positive interstitial cells of Cajal, which are an innervated network of cells associated with Auerbach's plexus. These are known as "intestinal pacemaker cells," as they coordinate peristalsis. This chapter will provide a general overview and approach to these tumors, but additional discussion may be found in Chapters 8, 9, and 11.

GISTs present within a wide patient age range, with a peak in the fifth to seventh decades and an equal gender distribution. Symptoms depend on location and size of the tumor, and a significant proportion are incidental findings in imaging studies or procedures for unrelated conditions. The most common symptoms are nonspecific upper abdominal pain and GI bleeding. Other presenting signs and symptoms include bloating, early satiety, signs/symptoms of a mass, or obstruction in small bowel GIST.

Pathologic Features

GISTs are most common in the stomach (60% of tumors) followed by the small bowel (30%), esophagus, and colorectum (approximately 5% each). One percent or less of GIST arise in the omentum and mesentery, and are known as extraintestinal GIST (EGIST). Grossly, GISTs arise in the muscularis propria, and are usually somewhat centered in the wall of the tubular gut (Figure 5.17A–C). They vary widely in size, ranging from 1.0 mm to more than 40 cm, with a median size of 6 cm in the stomach, 4.5 cm in the duodenum, and 7.0 cm in the distal small bowel. Tumors may occasionally protrude into the lumen in a polypoid fashion (Figure 5.17D), and show overlying mucosal ulceration. The cut surface may show hemorrhage, calcification, or, less commonly, necrosis. GISTs

TABLE 5.5 Summary of Molecular Alternations in GI Mesenchymal Tumors

	GIST	IFP	IMFT	Desmoid	CSS
Affected gene	KIT PDGFRA SDH	PDGFRA (55%–70%)	ALK	APC (FAP cases) CTNNB1 (most sporadic cases)	EWSR1
Test	KIT IHC; SDH IHC; Mutational analysis	PDGFRA mutational testing (usually not necessary in this context)	IHC for ALK protein (results very variable) FISH	IHC for nuclear β-catenin	RT-PCR; FISH

Abbreviations: CSS, clear cell sarcoma; IFP, inflammatory fibroid polyp; IMFT, inflammatory myofibroblastic tumor; FAP, familial adenomatous polyposis.

are typically circumscribed, and although the overlying mucosa is often ulcerated, true invasion of the mucosa is rare, and is associated with a worse prognosis.

The majority (70%) of GISTs are spindle cell lesions (Figure 5.18A–B). Of the remaining 30%, 20% are epithelioid (Figure 5.18C–D), and 10% are mixed.

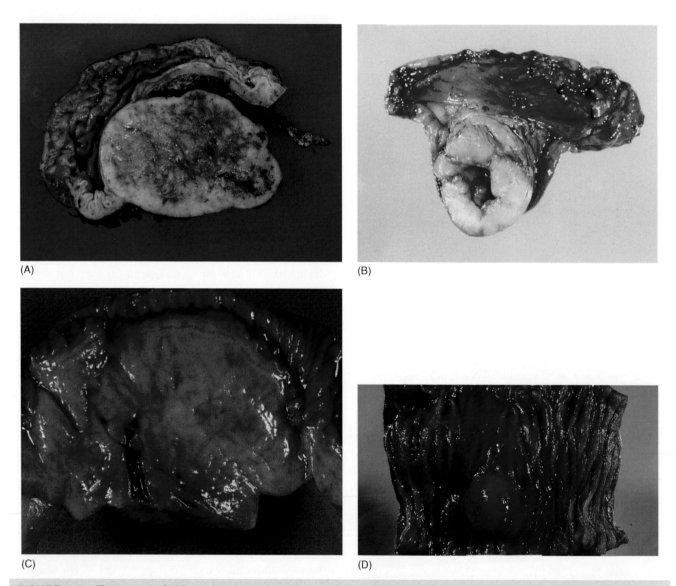

(A) (B) (C) (D)

FIGURE 5.17 This gastric GIST can be seen arising from the muscularis propria (A). The cut surface is hemorrhagic, and there are focal areas of necrosis. This partial gastrectomy specimen shows a GIST that is roughly centered in the bowel wall, beneath the mucosa (B). There is central cystic degeneration. This large small bowel GIST shows a firm, somewhat whorled cut surface (C). GISTs may protrude into the lumen in a polypoid fashion (D), and show overlying mucosal ulceration.

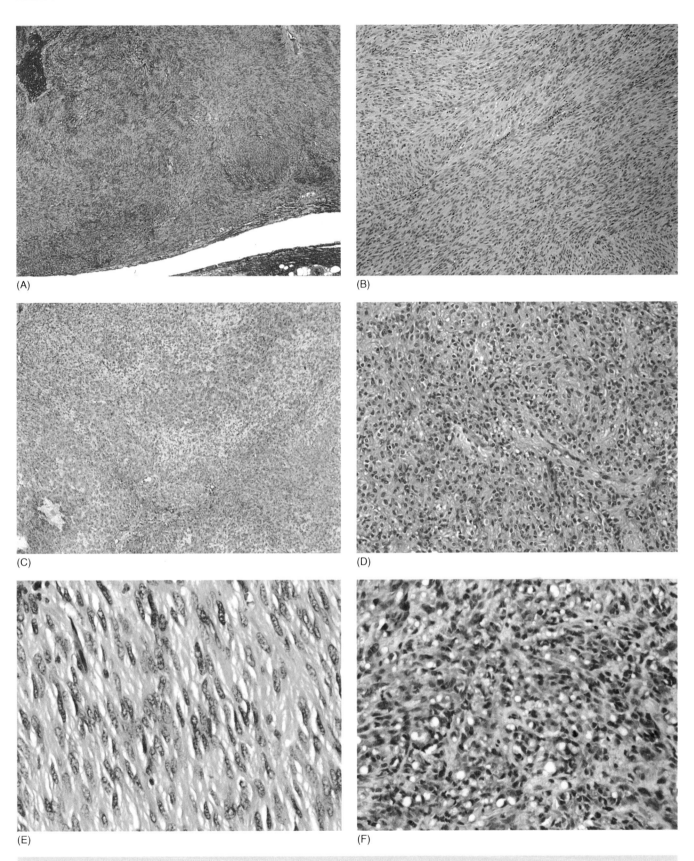

FIGURE 5.18 The majority of GISTs are spindled (A–B), and may also show nuclear palisading (A). Tumor cells are monomorphic, and lack nuclear pleomorphism (B). Approximately 20% of GISTs are epithelioid (C–D). In spindle cell tumors, nuclei are bland and elongated, with eosinophilic cytoplasm (E) and inconspicuous nucleoli. Some GISTs, especially in the stomach, have prominent perinuclear vacuoles (F). (*continued*)

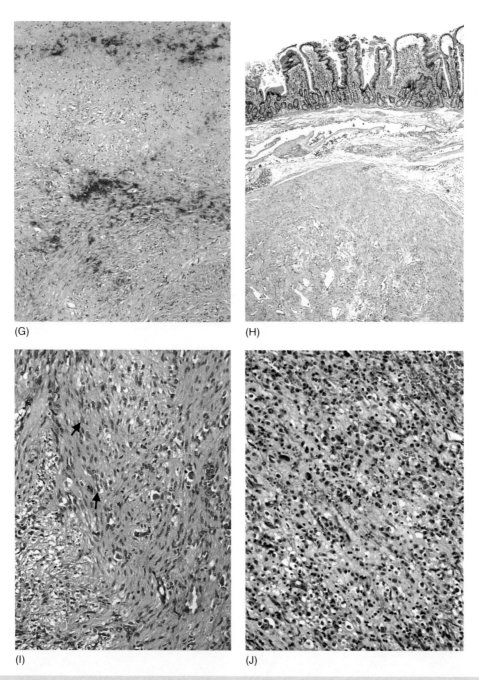

FIGURE 5.18 *(continued)* Stroma may be hyalinized or contain calcifications (G), and typically GISTs contain prominent vessels (H). Infrequently seen features include skeinoid fibers (arrows, I) and plasmacytoid cellular morphology (J).

Cellularity is quite variable. Nuclei are usually bland, elongated, and uniform, with pale eosinophilic cytoplasm (Figure 5.18E). Nucleoli are usually inconspicuous, and perinuclear vacuoles may be seen (Figure 5.18F). As noted in the section on nuclear atypia and pleomorphism, the majority of GISTs are monomorphic, and nuclear pleomorphism is rare even in malignant tumors. The appearance of the stroma is also variable, and it may be myxoid or hyalinized, with variably present calcifications (Figure 5.18G). GISTs are typically quite vascular (Figure 5.18H) and the vessels may be hyalinized.

Other features that may be infrequently seen in GISTs include skeinoid fibers (Figure 5.18I); nuclear palisading that mimics schwannoma (Figure 5.3); and plasmacytoid cellular morphology (Figure 5.18J). Nuclear palisading and cytoplasmic vacuolization are most often seen in gastric GIST, whereas skeinoid fibers are almost always found in small bowel GISTs.

The term "dedifferentiated GIST" refers to tumors with areas of morphologically typical GIST adjacent to areas of high-grade sarcoma (Figure 5.2). The sarcomatous component is typically KIT negative and more mitotically active than a typical GIST.

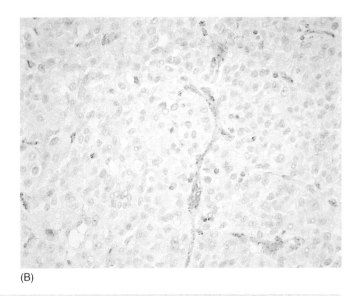

(A)   (B)

FIGURE 5.19 Succinate dehydrogenase (SDH) deficient GISTs have distinctive histology, featuring a multinodular or plexiform growth pattern (A). Virtually all of them demonstrate a loss of SDHB staining by immunohistochemistry (B). Figures courtesy of Dr. Jason L. Hornick.

A more recently described subtype of GIST is the SDH-deficient GIST (also known as pediatric GIST or type 2 GIST). These tumors often occur in female children (peak age of onset in the second decade) in the stomach or omentum. The distinctive histology features a multinodular or plexiform growth pattern (Figure 5.5 and Figure 5.19A–B), often with epithelioid or mixed cell types. These tumors are positive for KIT, but virtually all demonstrate a loss of SDHB staining by immunohistochemistry, and thus this stain is a good screening tool for this subtype of GIST. Only a minority of these tumors have an identifiable *SDH* mutation. Typical grading criteria are not applicable to this subtype (see the section on grading and risk stratification), and they are often imatinib resistant. Additionally, this subtype is more likely to metastasize to lymph nodes, although this finding does not appear to affect prognosis. These tumors are uncommon in adults, accounting for only 8% of gastric GISTs.

Immunohistochemistry

The most characteristic immunophenotypic feature of GIST is KIT immunoreactivity, which may be cytoplasmic, dot-like, or membranous (see Figure 5.8), or a mixture of these three patterns. Ninety-five percent of GISTs are KIT positive, and most (~99%) also mark with DOG1 and CD34. Approximately 5% of GISTs are KIT negative; the majority of these are epithelioid GISTs that have platelet derived growth factor receptor A (*PDGFRA*) mutations, and these typically arise in the stomach or are extraintestinal (see also Chapter 13).

A more recently described antibody that is very useful in the diagnosis of GIST is DOG1 or ANO-1. This is a very sensitive and specific marker that is present in the vast majority of GISTs (Figure 5.20). The majority of KIT-negative GISTs stain with DOG1, including 79% of PDGFRA-positive GISTs (as opposed to approximately 9% of PDGFRA-positive GISTs that stain with KIT). However, as the *Food and Drug Administration* (FDA)-approved therapies for GIST require the demonstration of KIT positivity, it is still necessary to confirm the diagnosis with KIT. Caveats regarding the use of KIT and DOG1 were discussed previously.

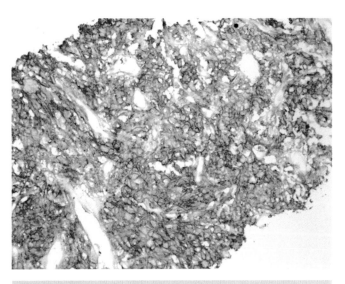

FIGURE 5.20 Diffuse DOG1 positivity is seen in this needle biopsy from a small bowel GIST.

Molecular Features

Approximately 80% of GISTs have *KIT* mutations. This gene encodes the *KIT* tyrosine kinase receptor, a membrane-associated member of the type III tyrosine kinase family that is involved in the proliferation of germ cells, mast cells, melanocytes, and the interstitial cells of Cajal. Oncogenic *KIT* mutations impair regulation of receptor activation or alter enzymatic function of tyrosine kinases.

Up to 20% of tumors contain wild-type *KIT*, however, and of these nearly 10% harbor mutations in *PDGFRA*, or platelet-derived growth factor A. This gene also encodes a type III tyrosine kinase receptor that is highly homologous to *KIT*. This subset of GISTs is more likely to occur in the stomach or proximal small bowel, or to be extraintestinal, and they are typically epithelioid with a myxoid stroma and occasional multinucleated or rhabdoid cells. They have a lower potential for malignant behavior as well. Immunohistochemistry for KIT in these tumors shows faint positive or negative staining (see case examples in the Specific Illustrative Examples section). Certain mutations (both *KIT* and *PDGFRA* mutations) may affect prognosis, and as a result molecular analysis of GISTs is increasingly regarded as the standard of care.

Some GISTs lack both *KIT* and *PDGFRA* mutations, and may be referred to as "wild-type" GIST. Some of these tumors harbor *BRAF V600E* mutations; these are KIT positive by immunohistochemistry. GISTs with *BRAF V600E* mutations are more commonly seen in the small bowel, and often show more aggressive behavior. Another subgroup of wild-type GIST shows mutations in subunits A, B, C, or D of *SDH*, which encodes succinate dehydrogenase. *SDH* mutations are mutually exclusive with other GIST mutations. Approximately 42% of wild-type GIST demonstrate loss of succinate dehydrogenase B (SDHB) expression by immunohistochemistry, and are known as SDH-deficient GIST (see also the previous discussion on

the morphology of SDH-deficient GIST). Wild-type GISTs are associated with tumors seen in the pediatric population, as well as those occurring in the setting of neurofibromatosis 1, Carney triad, and Carney–Stratakis syndrome.

Grading, Risk Stratification, and Prognosis

The most important parameters for grading and assessing behavior risk in GIST are size, anatomic location, and mitotic rate. These criteria should only be applied to primary, unifocal GIST that have not been treated with either neoadjuvant or adjuvant therapy.

There are multiple schemes for GIST risk stratification, including the National Institutes of Health (NIH) Consensus Criteria, the Armed Forces Institute of Pathology (AFIP) modification of the NIH criteria, and more recent modifications to the AFIP criteria known as the Joensuu criteria (see Table 5.6). Some authorities prefer the Joensuu criteria, as they are believed to be more accurate in identifying patients at high risk for developing recurrence or metastasis, and thus should receive adjuvant therapy. Mucosal invasion and rupture are associated with a high risk of disease progression, regardless of the site. Furthermore, if a GIST presents with metastases, this tumor should be regarded as malignant, and further evaluation is not necessary. EGISTs are evaluated according to the criteria for jejunum/ileum.

Conventional GISTs rarely metastasize to lymph nodes, but when metastases occur, they are more likely to be in the liver or within the abdomen. Metastases to lung, skin, and bone have been rarely described. Unlike conventional GISTs, SDH-deficient GISTs do have a tendency to metastasize to lymph nodes (approximately half of the cases), yet overall their behavior is indolent even in the context of lymph node metastases. Because of this unusual behavior, standard criteria for grading and risk stratification are probably not applicable to this subgroup of

TABLE 5.6   Risk Stratification of Primary GIST

Tumor Characteristics		Risk of Metastasis and/or Death From Disease			
Mitotic Index	Size	Stomach	Duodenum	Jejunum/Ileum	Colorectum
<5/HPF	<2 cm	Extremely low	Extremely low	Extremely low	Extremely low
	>2–< 5 cm	Very low (1.9%)	Low (8.3%)	Low (4.3%)	Low (8.5%)
	>5–< 10 cm	Low (3.6%)	Inadequate data	Intermediate (24%)	Inadequate data
	>10 cm	Intermediate (10%)	High (34%)	High (52%)	High (57%)
>5/HPF	< 2 cm	None but few cases	Inadequate data	High but few cases	High (57%)
	>2–< 5 cm	Intermediate (16%)	High (50%)	High (73%)	High (52%)
	>5–<10 cm	High (55%)	Inadequate data	High (85%)	Inadequate data
	>10 cm	High (86%)	High (86%)	High (90%)	High (71%)

Source: Adapted from Downs-Kelly E, Rubin BP, Goldblum JR. Mesenchymal Tumors of the Gastrointestinal Tract. In Odze RD, Goldblum JR, *Surgical Pathology of the GI Tract, Liver, Biliary Tract, and Pancreas.* Philadelphia: Elsevier, 2015; Fletcher CD, et al. Diagnosis of gastrointestinal stromal tumors: a consensus approach. *Hum Pathol.* 2002;33:459–465; Miettinen M et al. Gastrointestinal stromal tumors: pathology and prognosis at different sites. *Sem Diag Pathol.* 2006;23:70–83; Joensuu H. Risk stratification of patients diagnosed with gastrointestinal stromal tumor. *Hum Pathol.* 2008;39:1411–1419.

tumors, and it has been recommended that conventional criteria not be used in this specific context.

Therapy

The first-line therapy for GIST is complete resection. Because approximately 40% of GISTs recur or metastasize after complete resection, adjuvant therapy is common, and is based on targeting the mutant *KIT* or *PDGFRA* proteins. As previously mentioned in the section on molecular features, the type of mutation may predict response to therapy, and thus mutational analysis is strongly recommended for clinical management (see also Chapters 13 and 14).

Imatinib mesylate, or Gleevec, is a tyrosine kinase inhibitor that targets *KIT, PDGFRA, BCR-ABL,* and other mutations. It is the FDA-approved first-line therapy for *KIT*-positive GIST patients, and it is associated with therapeutic response rates up to 90%. Imatinib is occasionally used to treat primary, nonmetastatic disease if the tumor has a very high risk for malignant behavior. Tumors with exon 11 *KIT* mutations respond best to imatinib therapy, followed by those that are *KIT/PDGFRA* wild-type. GISTs with exon 9 *KIT* mutations may respond to a higher dose of imatinib or standard dosing with sunitinib.

Approximately 10% to 30% of GISTs show primary resistance, or progression of disease within 3 to 6 months of initiating therapy; tumors with primary resistance include those with wild-type *KIT, KIT* exon 9 mutations, and most common *PDGFRA* mutations. Some patients have what is known as delayed or secondary resistance, meaning that the tumors show partial response or stabilization of disease, only to progress 6 months or more after the initial response or disease stabilization. This typically happens within 2 years of initiation of therapy. Resistance may be generalized to the entire tumor or tumor burden, or limited to certain foci. Two of the most common mutations that confer resistance to imatinib are sensitive to the drug sunitinib, which has been approved for patients who have failed or cannot tolerate imatinib. Tumors deficient in SDH are often resistant to imatinib, but may show some response to therapy with sunitinib.

Pathologists may occasionally be asked to evaluate the percentage of viable GIST in a resection specimen. Treatment-associated changes include a decrease in cellularity, myxoid stroma, fibrosis, and necrosis, but islands of viable cells are usually present as well (Figure 5.21). Grading/ risk stratification criteria do not apply to treated GISTs.

Genetic Syndromes Involving GIST

Although the vast majority of GISTs are sporadic, there are a number of important genetic syndromes that involve GISTs, including Carney triad, Carney–Stratakis syndrome, neurofibromatosis type 1 (NF1), and familial GIST.

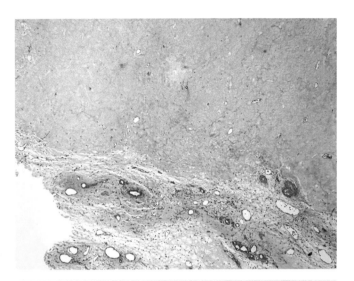

FIGURE 5.21 Treatment-associated changes in GISTs include fibrosis, decreased cellularity, and a myxoid stroma. No viable tumor cells are seen in this field, although they can usually be found on examination of multiple sections.

Patients with familial GISTs have germline mutations in either *KIT* or *PDGFRA* that are identical to sporadic mutations in the same sites. The pattern of inheritance is autosomal dominant, and there is approximately 100% penetrance. Patients often have multiple tumors, and may have associated hyperplasia of the interstitial cells of Cajal.

Up to 10% of patients with NF1 have GISTs as well; these tumors are often multiple and within the small bowel. NF1-associated GISTs lack *KIT* and *PDGFRA* mutations, and may contain skeinoid fibers histologically. Carney triad includes epithelioid gastric GIST, pulmonary chondroma, and paragangliomas; GISTs in this context are wild-type, and believed to be part of the spectrum of SDH-deficient GIST. Patients with Carney–Stratakis syndrome have epithelioid gastric GIST and paraganglioma. These patients have germline *SDH* subunit gene mutations and thus are also part of the spectrum of SDH-deficient GIST.

Differential Diagnosis

The most common entities in the differential diagnosis of GIST include smooth muscle tumors, schwannoma, and desmoid tumor. The immunophenotypic comparison of these neoplasms is summarized in Table 5.4, and it is important to note that a relatively small panel of antibodies can address the majority of entities in the differential diagnosis. Less common mesenchymal tumors that may enter into the differential diagnosis include inflammatory fibroid polyp, IMFT, neural tumors, glomus tumor, and PEComa. The differential diagnosis of GIST, including both common and uncommon entities, is discussed in more detail in the sections that follow.

Leiomyoma

Leiomyomas are the second most common mesenchymal tumor of the GI tract, and the most common mesenchymal tumor of the esophagus. The majority (approximately 80%) of these benign tumors present as polypoid lesions in the colon, and are often found incidentally at colonoscopy for some other indication. The second most common presentation is that of an intramural mass in the esophagus, most often at the gastroesophageal junction (Figure 5.22A–B). Multiple esophageal leiomyomas are referred to as "seedling" leiomyomas or, if large, leiomyomatosis. Leiomyomas may also present as mural masses in the stomach and small bowel, or in association with the anal sphincters.

Esophageal leiomyomas are most commonly seen in the fifth decade, and some studies report a male predominance. Rectal tumors are also most commonly encountered in the fifth to sixth decades. Leiomyomas may present incidentally, or with GI bleeding; esophageal lesions may be associated with a cough or dysphagia. Leiomyomas are very variable in size, ranging from a few millimeters to 20 cm in size. Esophageal tumors most often arise from the inner layer of the muscularis propria, but a significant minority arise from the muscularis mucosae. Colonic lesions tend to be smaller than esophageal leiomyomas, and arise from the muscularis mucosae. Grossly, these tumors are well-circumscribed, unencapsulated, and often lobulated, with a firm, white to tan, whorled, fibrous appearance on the cut section.

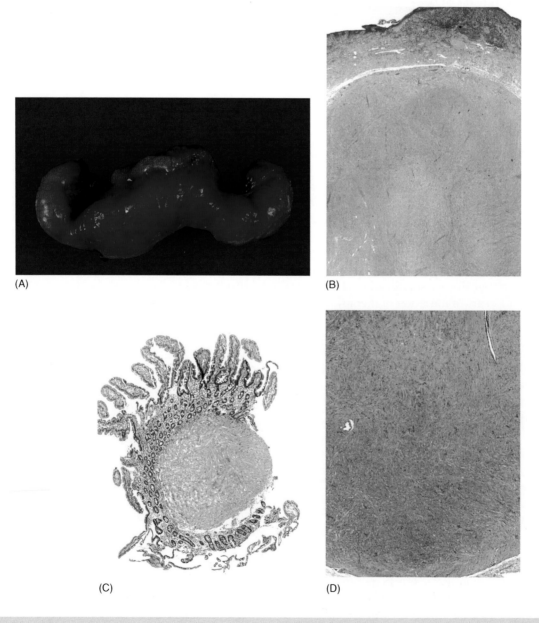

(A)

(B)

(C)

(D)

FIGURE 5.22 *(continued)*

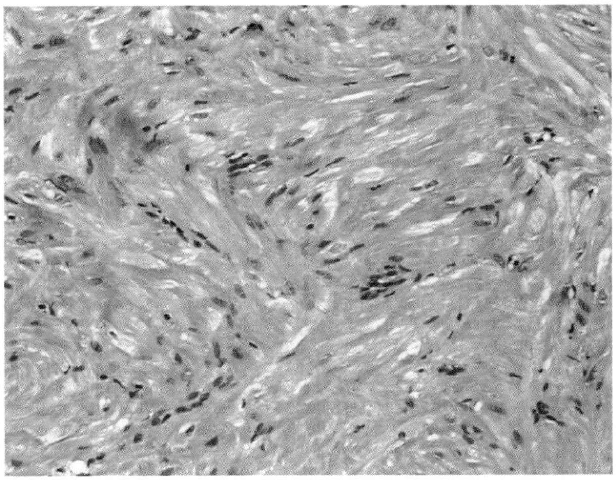

(E)

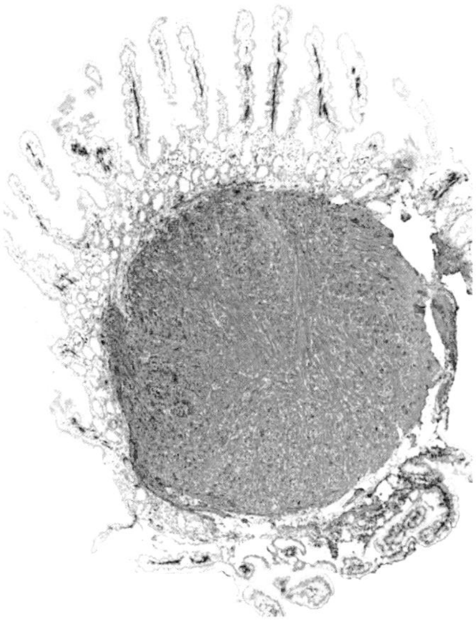

(F)

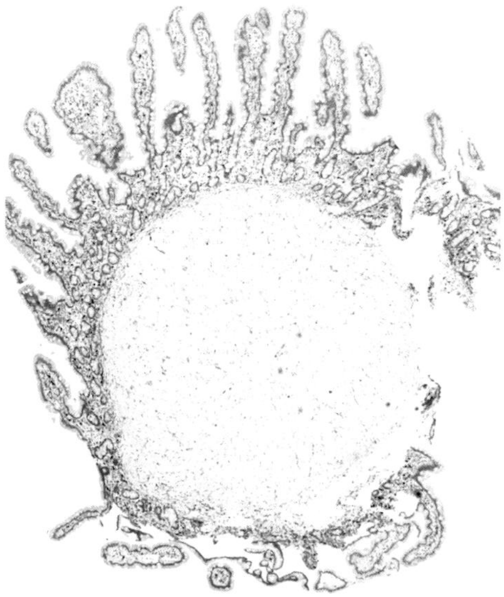

(G)

FIGURE 5.22   This gross photograph illustrates a large tubular leiomyoma with a small fragment of overlying normal mucosa (A). Leiomyomas of the esophagus are most often at the gastroesophageal (GE) junction, as seen here (B). This small, well-circumscribed duodenal leiomyoma arises from the muscularis mucosae (C). At low power, leiomyomas are composed of fascicles of spindle cells with eosinophilic cytoplasm and elongated, cigar-shaped nuclei (D–E). Leiomyomas are diffusely positive for desmin (F), but negative for KIT (G).

Histologically, leiomyomas feature fascicles of spindle cells with bright eosinophilic cytoplasm and elongated, cigar-shaped nuclei with tapering or blunt ends (Figure 5.22C–E). Cytologic atypia is rare, although degenerative atypia has been described, similar to symplastic leiomyomas in the uterus. Hyalinization and calcification may be present. Mitotic activity is low or absent, typically less than 1 mitosis/50 high-power field (HPF),

and necrosis should be absent. Epithelioid leiomyomas have not been described in the GI tract.

Leiomyomas show immunoreactivity for SMA, desmin, and caldesmon (Figure 5.22F–G). KIT, DOG1, and CD34 are characteristically negative, as is S100, although large intramural leiomyomas may rarely show KIT and/or DOG1 positivity. Mast cells within leiomyomas will, of course, stain with KIT.

Leiomyomatosis peritonealis disseminata is an unusual condition in which multiple tumors composed of smooth muscle arise beneath the peritoneum throughout the abdomen. This disease is seen almost exclusively in women of reproductive age, and many are on oral contraceptives or are pregnant, suggesting that estrogens may be a contributing factor. The histologic findings range from nodules or infiltrative foci of smooth muscle to a fibroblastic or myofibroblastic proliferation. Nuclear pleomorphism is minimal, and mitoses are rare. Many of these lesions regress after pregnancy or withdrawal of estrogens, and malignant degeneration is rare and somewhat debatable in the literature.

Schwannoma

Gastrointestinal schwannomas are most commonly found in the stomach, followed by the colorectum, esophagus, and small bowel. Patients are typically in the sixth or seventh decade, and gastric tumors are more common in women. Presenting symptoms are related to tumor location, and include dysphagia with esophageal tumors; dyspepsia, abdominal pain, and bleeding with gastric tumors; and bleeding or obstruction with intestinal lesions.

Schwannomas generally arise in the muscularis propria, but they may bulge into the lumen, with overlying mucosal ulceration (Figure 5.23A). Grossly, they are circumscribed, but unencapsulated, and measure from 1 cm to over 10 cm. The cut surface is homogeneous, firm, rubbery, and yellow gray to tan. Cystic change and hemorrhage are not usually seen. Colorectal lesions may present as polyps.

A notable feature in GI tract schwannomas (as opposed to those that occur in the soft tissues) is a dense lymphoplasmacytic cuff, often with germinal centers, present at the periphery of the tumor (Figures 5.4 and 5.23B). Numerous lymphocytes may also be seen admixed with tumor cells (Figure 5.23C). Schwannomas are moderately cellular, and are composed of spindle cells arranged in short bundles. Focal nuclear atypia is common (Figure 5.23D), but mitotic figures should be rare to absent, and atypical mitoses should not be seen. Unlike conventional soft tissue schwannomas, palisading is rare in the GI tract, as are foamy histiocytes. Epithelioid foci are very rare in GI tract schwannomas.

The variant known as microcystic or reticular schwannoma may occur in the GI tract, and may mimic mucinous adenocarcinoma. This variant of schwannoma also lacks the typical lymphoid cuff, and has a striking microcystic/reticular growth pattern (Figure 5.23E).

All GI tract schwannomas express S100 (Figure 5.23F), and generally lack immunoreactivity for KIT, DOG1, SMA, desmin, and other smooth muscle markers; however, rare tumors can show focal expression of keratin, SMA, or desmin. In addition, unlike their soft tissue counterparts, GI tract schwannomas do not express calretinin.

Given the S100 positivity, the differential diagnosis of schwannomas also includes melanoma (which should mark with other melanoma markers).

BENIGN NEURAL POLYPS

Granular Cell Tumor

Granular cell tumors, named for their abundant granular cytoplasm, are believed to be of neural (Schwannian) origin. The most common site in the GI tract is the esophagus, followed by the large bowel and perianal area. The vast majority of these lesions are benign, and they rarely recur even if inadequately excised. Tumors consist of polygonal or spindle cells with abundant granular eosinophilic cytoplasm, small uniform nuclei, and small nucleoli (Figure 5.24A–B). The spindled cell variant is most likely to cause confusion with GIST or other common spindle cell lesions of the GI tract (Figure 5.24C–D). Granular cell tumors are strongly and diffusely S100 positive (Figure 5.24E). Similar to their counterparts elsewhere, GI granular cell tumors may have overlying pseudoepitheliomatous hyperplasia or acanthosis, which may mimic squamous cell carcinoma (Figure 5.24A).

Ganglioneuroma/Ganglioneuromatosis

Ganglioneuromas (GNs) are composed of an admixture of Schwann cells, which are the predominant cell type, along with ganglion cells and nerve fibers (Figure 5.25A–C). There are three contexts in which these lesions are found in the GI tract. The sporadic, solitary GN is the most common; these are usually incidental findings on the left side of the colon, measuring less than 1.0 cm. Ganglioneuromas in the form of ganglioneuromatous polyposis are associated with Cowden syndrome and NF1, and diffuse ganglioneuromatosis is associated with MEN-2B and NF1. Unlike granular cell tumors, which form an expansile mass, ganglioneuromas entrap and surround the mucosal crypts. The Schwann cell component is S100 positive (Figure 5.25D), and the nerve fibers are neurofilament protein (NFP) positive.

Mucosal Schwann Cell Hamartoma

This is a recently described lesion that is distinct from other neural lesions in the GI tract, including neurofibroma and mucosal neuroma, which are associated with syndromes and rarely encountered sporadically. These usually incidental lesions are typically found in the rectosigmoid colon of middle-aged to older adults; there is a female predominance. They measure less than 5 mm, and consist of a proliferation of spindle-shaped, uniform Schwann cells with plump tapering nuclei and eosinophilic cytoplasm (Figure 5.26A–B). These lesions are purely composed of Schwann cells, with no ganglion cells or axons

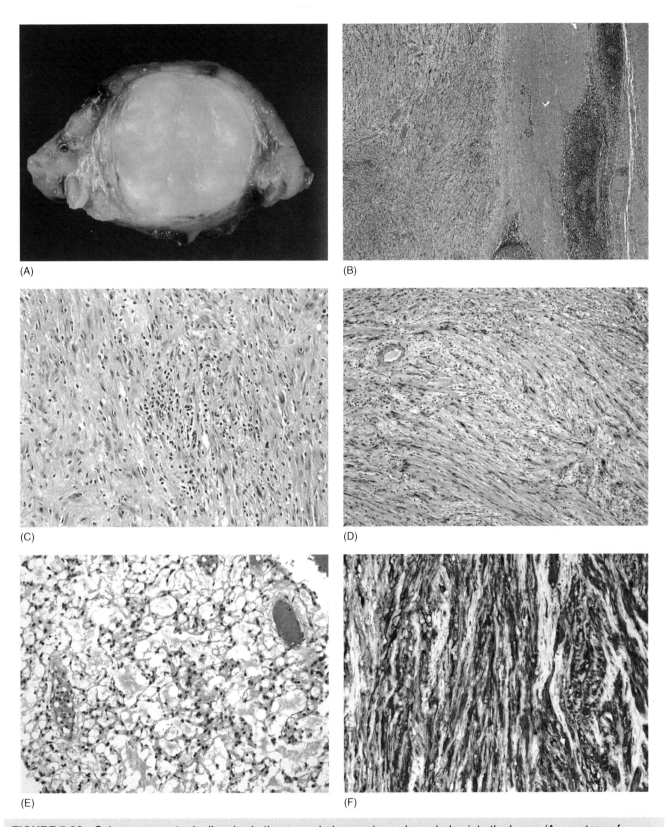

FIGURE 5.23 Schwannomas typically arise in the muscularis propria, and may bulge into the lumen (A, courtesy of Dr. Keisuke Goto). They are circumscribed but unencapsulated. The cut surface is yellow–tan, rubbery, and homogeneous. GI tract schwannomas have a dense peripheral lymphoplasmacytic cuff, often with lymphoid aggregates (B). Intratumoral lymphocytes are also common (C). Schwannomas are typically moderately cellular and are composed of bundles of spindle cells with focal nuclear atypia but no mitoses (D). Microcystic or reticular schwannomas may occur in the GI tract as well, and feature a striking microcystic or reticular growth pattern (E). They lack a lymphoid cuff, and may mimic mucinous adenocarcinoma. Schwannomas diffusely and strongly express S100 (F).

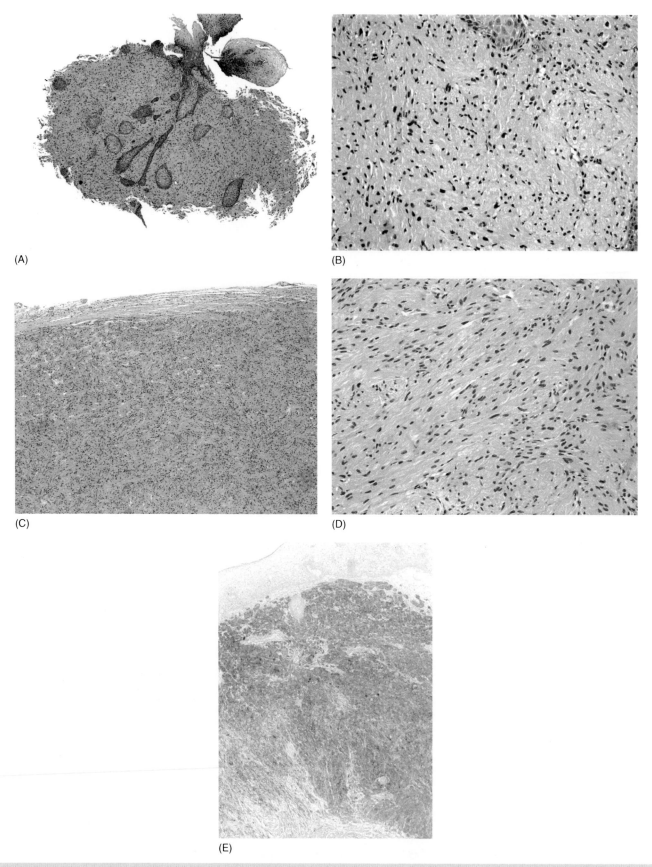

FIGURE 5.24 Granular cell tumors consist of polygonal or spindle cells with abundant granular eosinophilic cytoplasm. Associated pseudoepitheliomatous squamous hyperplasia is common (A). Tumor cells have small uniform nuclei, small nucleoli, and abundant granular eosinophilic cytoplasm (B). The spindled variant may cause confusion with GIST, but the abundant granular cytoplasm is usually still apparent (C–D). Granular cell tumors are strongly and diffusely S100 positive (E).

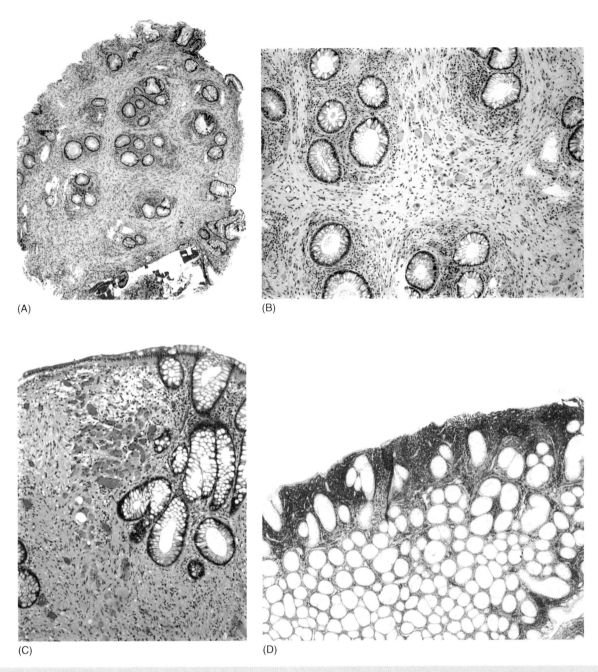

(A)

(B)

(C)

(D)

FIGURE 5.25 Ganglioneuromas consist of a proliferation of Schwann cells and ganglion cells that infiltrate between the crypts in the bowel mucosa (A–C). The Schwann cell component is strongly S100 positive (D).

(in contrast to ganglioneuroma). They are strongly S100 positive (Figure 5.11). Mucosal Schwann cell hamartomas are limited to the lamina propria, and often entrap crypts.

Perineurioma

Perineuriomas (also classified as benign fibroblastic polyps by some authors) are usually incidental findings in middle-aged adults undergoing colonoscopy for another reason. There is a female predominance. These are typically sessile polypoid lesions in the rectosigmoid colon, which endoscopically may be mistaken for a hyperplastic polyp or adenoma. These bland spindle cell lesions expand the lamina propria and entrap crypts (Figure 5.27A). They may have a lamellar or a whorled pattern, and consist of bland spindle cells with ovoid to tapering nuclei, fine fibrillary stroma, and no nuclear atypia or mitoses (Figure 5.27B). These lesions are positive for epithelial membrane antigen (EMA), although staining may be weak and extremely focal. They are

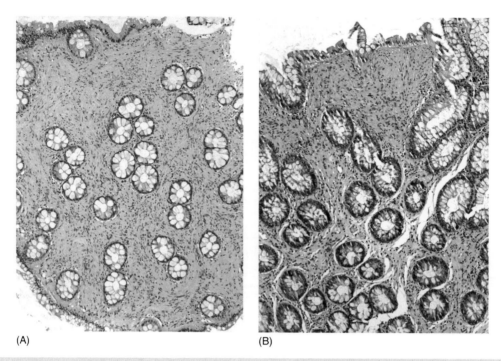

(A)   (B)

FIGURE 5.26 Schwann cell hamartomas consist of a proliferation of spindle-shaped, uniform Schwann cells with plump tapering nuclei and eosinophilic cytoplasm (A–B). No ganglion cells or axons are present, in contrast to ganglioneuromas. They often infiltrate between the crypts, and are strongly S100 positive.

negative for S100, and 40% to 90% express claudin-1 (Figure 5.27C). Of note, perineurioma-like proliferations frequently occur in association with both hyperplastic polyps and sessile serrated adenomas, although these areas may be focal (Figure 5.27D), and some authors have argued that these lesions represent a mixed stromal/epithelial polyp. Indeed, *BRAF* mutations are detected in the spindled and epithelial cell components of polyps with both elements.

A wide variety of neural tumors are associated with neurofibromatosis (NF1), including ganglioneuromatous polyposis, diffuse ganglioneuromatosis, neurofibromas (Figure 5.28A–B), diffuse neuromatosis, and gangliocytic paraganglioma. As previously mentioned in the section on genetic syndromes involving GISTs, NF1 patients also have an increased incidence of GIST.

Desmoid Tumor (Intra-Abdominal Desmoid Fibromatosis)

Intra-abdominal desmoid tumors primarily affect the mesentery or retroperitoneum, but when these lesions invade or encroach upon the bowel wall, they may mimic a primary GI mesenchymal neoplasm (particularly GIST). Tumors may occur in the abdomen or in the pelvis. Of note, 25% occur in the context of familial adenomatous polyposis/ Gardner syndrome. These tumors may present at any age, and there is no gender predilection. Patients can present in

a variety of ways, including a mass, abdominal pain, bleeding, or signs of obstruction or fistula formation.

Desmoid tumors are typically large at the time of resection, ranging from 4 to 25 cm. Grossly they are firm, infiltrative, poorly circumscribed tumors with a coarse, trabecular, gritty cut surface (Figure 5.29A). Histologically, these tumors are uniform and monotonous, consisting of long, sweeping, broad fascicles of slender spindle-shaped cells with elongated nuclei and eosinophilic cytoplasm (Figure 5.29B–D). Nuclei have fine chromatin and inconspicuous nucleoli. Mitotic activity is variable but usually low, and atypical mitoses should be absent. Vessels are typically prominent and may be ectatic or compressed between fascicles of tumor cells. Some tumors contain myxoid areas, dense (keloidal) hyalinization, fasciitis-like areas, or areas with a loose, storiform growth pattern.

Unlike some of the other entities in the differential diagnosis of GIST, these tumors arise in the mesentery and invade the bowel, rather than the reverse. However, they can be deeply infiltrative, extending all the way through the wall to the mucosa. Tumor cells express nuclear β-catenin (Figure 5.15) in most cases, and tumor cells are negative for DOG1, S100, desmin, and caldesmon. The vast majority of desmoid tumors are KIT negative, but positive staining has been reported very rarely.

Desmoid tumors lack the potential for metastasis, but have a high likelihood of local recurrence, and the clinical course is often unpredictable. Surgery is the mainstay of therapy.

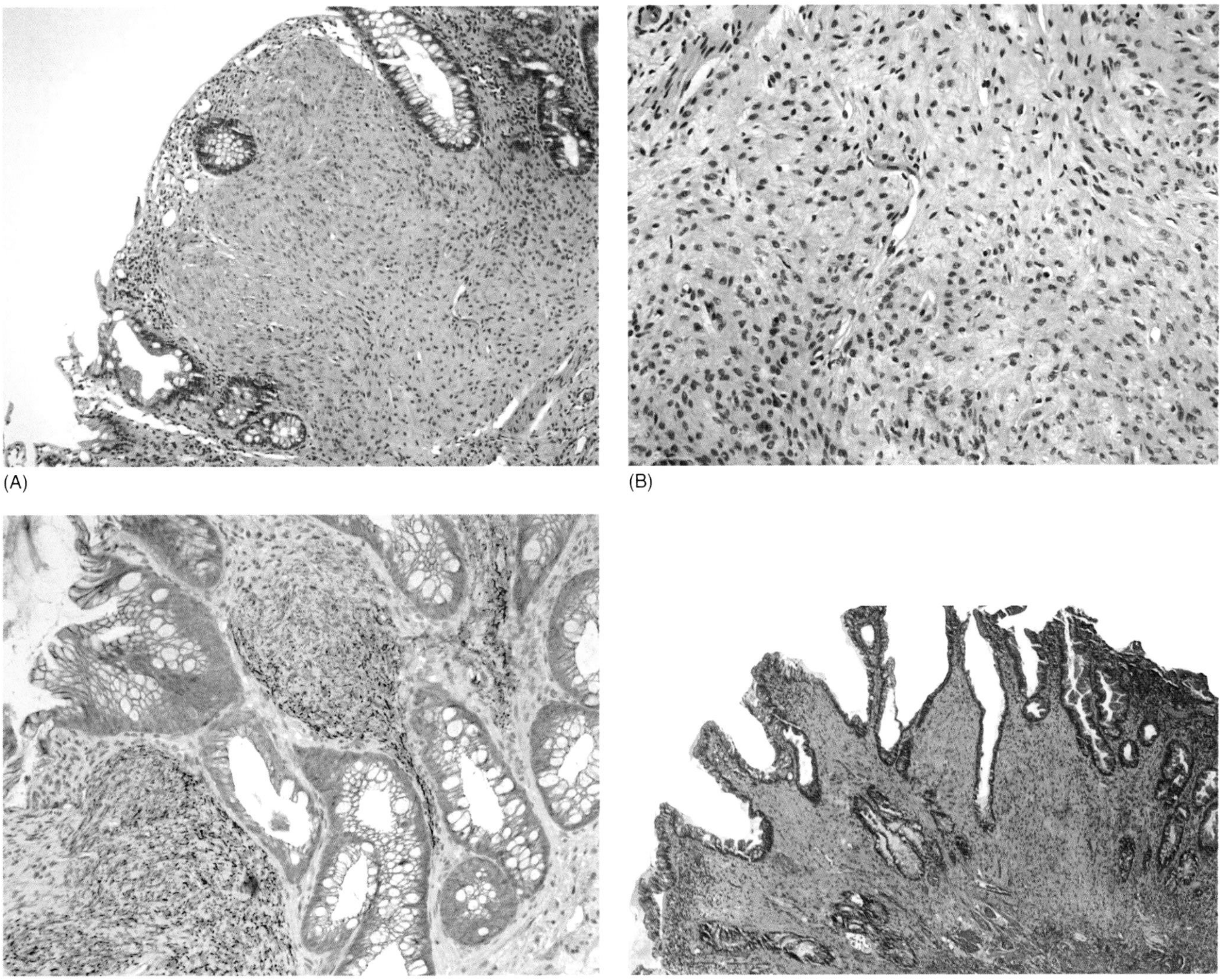

FIGURE 5.27   Perineuriomas are composed of a proliferation of bland spindle cells that expand the lamina propria and entrap crypts (A). The cells have ovoid to tapering nuclei, fine fibrillary stroma, and no nuclear atypia or mitoses (B). Many of these lesions stain with claudin-1 (C). Perineurioma-like proliferations frequently occur in association with both hyperplastic polyps and sessile serrated adenomas (D).

Sclerosing mesenteritis may also enter into the differential diagnosis of either GIST or desmoid tumor. This idiopathic disease, also known as mesenteric panniculitis, liposclerotic mesenteritis, mesenteric Weber–Christian disease, xanthogranulomatous mesenteritis, mesenteric lipogranuloma, systemic nodular panniculitis, inflammatory pseudotumor, or mesenteric lipodystrophy is a fibroinflammatory disorder that primarily affects the small bowel mesentery. It most often presents as a large, unifocal mass, although approximately 20% of patients have multiple lesions. These lesions consist of fibrous bands that infiltrate and encase fat lobules, with associated inflammation (predominantly mononuclear cells) and fat necrosis. The presence of inflammation and fat necrosis helps differentiate these from desmoid tumors, and nuclear

β-catenin staining is not seen in sclerosing mesenteritis. Of note, sclerosing mesenteritis has been rarely reported to express KIT.

LESS COMMON/RARE MESENCHYMAL TUMORS OF THE GI TRACT

Glomus Tumor

Glomus tumors are most commonly found in the skin and subcutis of the distal extremities, but they occasionally arise in the GI tract, most commonly in the antrum of the stomach. Patients are from a wide age range, and there is a female predominance in some series. Tumors may present

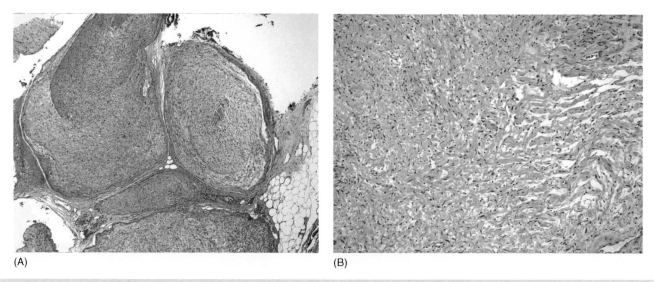

(A)   (B)

FIGURE 5.28   This patient with NF1 had multiple gastrointestinal plexiform neurofibromas, such as the colonic one shown here (A–B).

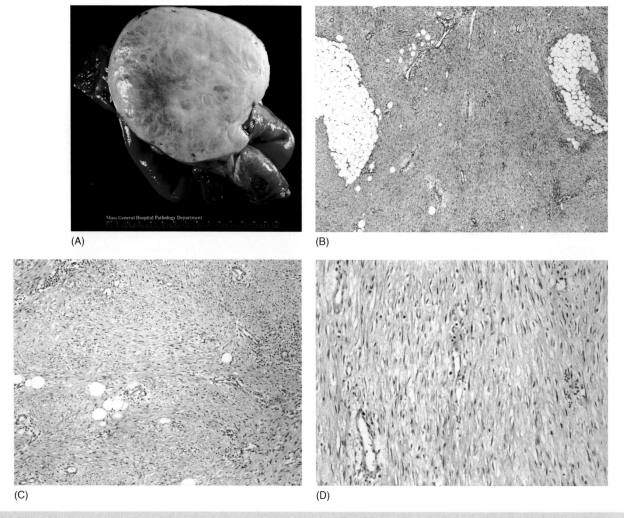

(A)   (B)

(C)   (D)

FIGURE 5.29   This desmoid tumor forms a large, homogeneous mass with a trabecular cut surface and adherent loops of bowel (A, courtesy of Dr. Petur Nielsen). These tumors contain a monotonous population of spindle cells arranged in long, sweeping, broad fascicles with prominent vessels (B). Cells are slender with elongated nuclei, fine chromatin, inconspicuous nucleoli, and eosinophilic cytoplasm (C–D).

with upper GI bleeding, abdominal pain, or as inciden-tal findings on evaluation for something unrelated. The majority of tumors are benign, but rare malignant glomus tumors have been reported.

Glomus tumors are typically 1 to 3 cm, arise in the muscularis propria, and feature cellular nodules or nests separated by bands of smooth muscle extending from the muscularis propria (Figure 5.30A–C). Prominent slit-like and dilated vessels are common, and the tumor cells show a subendothelial growth pattern within walls of blood vessels. The cells are uniform and rounded, with clear to eosinophilic cytoplasm and sharply defined cell borders. The nucleus appears "punched out" and round, and is well demarcated from the surrounding cytoplasm. There

is typically diffuse reactivity for SMA (Figure 5.30D), but KIT and DOG1 are negative, unlike GIST. Calponin and caldesmon are typically positive, but desmin is often nega-tive, in contrast to smooth muscle tumors. Some tumors are focally positive with CD34 and synaptophysin, but chromogranin and keratin should be negative. Pericellular membranous positivity is seen with laminin and collagen type IV.

Other vascular tumors occurring in the gut that may have spindle cell morphology include angiosarcoma and Kaposi's sarcoma. If the latter is suspected, HHV-8 and vas-cular markers are very helpful, but it is important to be aware that Kaposi's sarcoma will stain with KIT. Angiosarcoma occurs very rarely in the GI tract (see also Chapter 9).

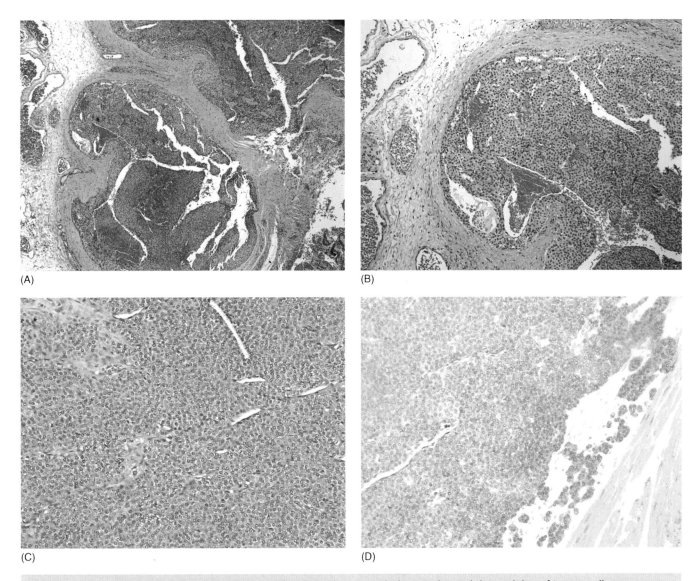

(A) (B) (C) (D)

FIGURE 5.30 This gastric glomus tumor is arising from the muscularis propria, and the nodules of tumor cells are surrounded by bands of smooth muscle. Prominent dilated and/or slit-like vessels are common (B). Tumor cells are uniform and round, with clear to eosinophilic cytoplasm (C, courtesy of Dr. Andrew Folpe). Reactivity for SMA is characteristic (D, courtesy of Dr. Andrew Folpe).

Inflammatory Fibroid Polyp

Inflammatory fibroid polyps are benign tumors that are most commonly found in the antrum of the stomach (see also Chapter 8) or the ileum (see also Chapter 9), and often present as a polyp. They present in a wide age range but are typically seen in adults from 60 to 80 years old, and may be associated with intussusception. These lesions arise from the submucosa, and the overlying mucosa is often ulcerated (Figure 5.31A). Tumors range in size from less than 0.5 cm to over 4.0 cm, with an average size of 1 to 2 cm. Histologically, they have ill-defined margins (Figure 5.31B), and consist of a bland proliferation of spindle cells and stellate cells with prominent admixed inflammatory cells, especially eosinophils (Figure 5.31C). Blood vessels are typically prominent, and may show surrounding "onion-skin" fibrosis (Figure 5.31D). If the surface is ulcerated, bizarre pleomorphic stromal cells can be seen, which should not be interpreted as a feature of malignancy. Occasionally, prominent multinucleated giant cells are present (Figure 5.31E). IFPs are positive for CD34 and variably positive for SMA; they are negative for KIT, desmin, and S100. The neoplastic nature of these lesions has been debated, but some IFPs have been found to have activating mutations in PDGFRA, so they in fact may be neoplastic. Giant fibrovascular polyps of the esophagus are histologically somewhat similar lesions, although they lack the eosinophilic component of IFP; these will be discussed in Chapter 7.

Inflammatory Myofibroblastic Tumor

IMFTs are most often seen in children and young adults. Historically, these have also been known as inflammatory pseudotumors of the GI tract, or plasma cell granulomas. They are considered lesions of intermediate risk, as they have a tendency to recur but rarely metastasize. Outside of the lung, the most common sites include abdomen (mesentery, omentum, and tubal gut), pelvis, and retroperitoneum. Patients typically present with abdominal pain and/or mass, and some have prominent systemic complaints including fever, weight loss, and malaise.

IMFTs are variably sized at presentation, with a mean of 8 to 10 cm, and are typically solitary and multinodular. Several patterns have been described, including spindle cell lesions with myxoid or hyalinized stroma, more storiform or fascicular growth patterns, and hypocellular sclerotic lesions. The spindle cells typically have ovoid to tapering nuclei and pale eosinophilic cytoplasm (Figures 5.32A–B). Approximately half contain ganglion-like cells (Figure 5.32C), and a prominent lymphoplasmacytic inflammatory infiltrate is often present. Calcifications and metaplastic bone may also be seen. Some tumors have striking cytologic atypia (Figure 5.32C). In general, there is poor correlation between the histologic features and behavior; however, a recently described variant (termed

"epithelioid inflammatory myofibroblastic sarcoma") is highly aggressive and is characterized by epithelioid cells with prominent nucleoli, a unique nuclear membrane or perinuclear staining pattern of ALK, and a distinctive *RANBP2–ALK* gene fusion.

IMFTs are positive for SMA, and variably positive for desmin. Approximately 30% are immunopositive with keratin as well. Unlike GIST, they are negative for KIT and DOG1, as well as S100. Approximately half of tumors have an *ALK* gene rearrangement; the younger the patient, the more likely the tumor is to have this alteration. There is imperfect correlation between the gene rearrangement and ALK immunohistochemical positivity (Figure 5.32D), however. ALK staining is not specific to IMFT, and positivity has been reported in rhabdomyosarcomas and malignant peripheral nerve sheath tumors, although GISTs are ALK negative.

PEComa

PEComas, or perivascular epithelial cell tumors, are a family of related mesenchymal tumors that includes angiomyolipoma, lymphangiomyomatosis, and clear cell "sugar" tumor of lung. All share a distinctive perivascular epithelioid cell phenotype, with evidence of both smooth muscle and melanocytic differentiation. There is no known normal tissue counterpart. These tumors typically present in women of middle age, and can be found in the abdomen/pelvis, retroperitoneum, tubal gut, uterus, liver, and kidney. Rarely, they are associated with tuberous sclerosis. Histologically, tumors are spindled and/or epithelioid, with clear to granular eosinophilic "stringy" cytoplasm (Figure 5.33A–B). Admixed prominent blood vessels may be seen, as well as adipocytes. In some cases, alveolar nests of tumor cells are surrounded by delicate vasculature. Nuclear hyperchromasia and pleomorphism may be seen, and occasional cases have shown signet ring-like cells, strap-like cells, and multivacuolated cells resembling lipoblasts. Mitoses may be present but are typically not numerous, and necrosis may also be seen. Rare malignant PEComas have been reported.

PEComas, regardless of the site, are usually positive for SMA, and often for HMB-45 (Figure 5.33C), melan-A, and MiTF. Desmin immunoreactivity is variably present. Some tumors, especially epithelioid or clear cell variants, may lack SMA staining, however. There is focal S100 positivity in less than 10%. The presence of a spindle cell component, and the fact that the majority of PEComas mark with KIT, may lead to confusion with GIST.

Plexiform Fibromyxoma (Plexiform Angiomyxoid Myofibroblastic Tumor of Stomach)

These tumors are nearly exclusive to the gastric antrum, where they present as a mural mass in young to middle-aged adults that is often mistaken for GIST. These bland,

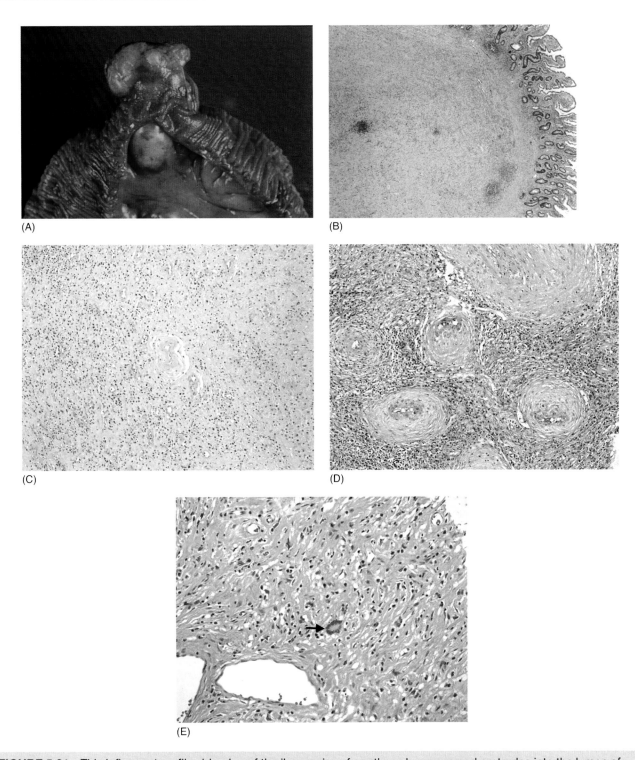

(A)

(B)

(C)

(D)

(E)

FIGURE 5.31 This inflammatory fibroid polyp of the ileum arises from the submucosa and protrudes into the lumen of the bowel (A). The interface between tumor and normal tissue is ill-defined, and may contain lymphoid aggregates. These lesions consist of a bland proliferation of spindle cells with prominent admixed inflammatory cells, especially eosinophils (B–C). Blood vessels are typically prominent, and may show surrounding "onion-skin" fibrosis (D). Occasionally, multinucleate giant cells are present (E, arrow).

multilobular spindle cell tumors are sharply circumscribed, have a plexiform growth pattern, and contain abundant myxoid stroma with prominent small blood vessels (Figure 5.34A–B). Vascular invasion is common. These tumors are positive for SMA and variably with desmin; they are negative for KIT, DOG1, and S100. Plexiform fibromyxomas are rare, and thus knowledge of natural history is limited, but they appear to behave in a benign fashion.

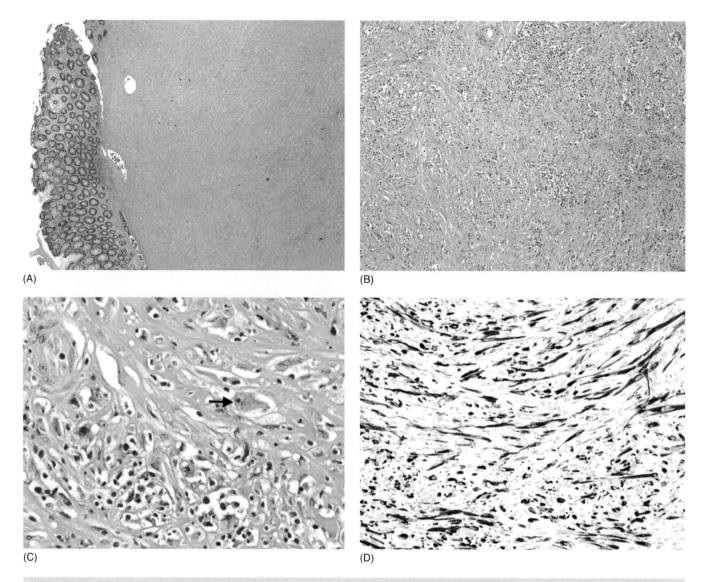

FIGURE 5.32 This solitary IMFT in the colon consists of interlacing bundles of spindled cells with an admixed prominent inflammatory infiltrate containing numerous plasma cells (A–B). The spindle cells typically have ovoid to tapering nuclei and pale eosinophilic cytoplasm. Approximately half contain ganglion-like cells, and there may be significant nuclear atypia (C). ALK positivity is often seen in IMFT, but is not specific for these tumors (D, courtesy of Dr. Andrew Folpe).

Gangliocytic Paraganglioma

Gangliocytic paragangliomas are triphasic tumors composed of a mixture of epithelioid and spindle cells along with ganglion cells (see also Chapters 3 and 9). They have a predilection for the second part of the duodenum. They typically present as polypoid submucosal masses, and they may be associated with NF1. Histologically, tumors consist of anastomosing cords and nests of spindled cells with admixed nests and clusters of epithelioid (neuroendocrine) cells, ganglion cells, and occasionally neuroendocrine cells (Figure 5.35A–B). Tumor cells stain with chromogranin A, and spindled cells will stain with S100. These tumors typically behave in a benign fashion.

Leiomyosarcoma

This is a rare smooth muscle tumor, accounting for only about 1% of GI mesenchymal tumors. This tumor can occur anywhere in the GI tract, and symptoms vary with location. They can present as polypoid lesions, or involve the entire thickness of the wall of the bowel. The overlying mucosa may be ulcerated, as mucosal invasion by tumor is typical. Tumors are grossly fleshy masses with necrosis and hemorrhage. They are histologically identical to leiomyosarcomas elsewhere, featuring highly cellular fascicles of spindle cells containing elongated nuclei and brightly eosinophilic cytoplasm (Figure 5.36). Nuclear pleomorphism is usually prominent, and

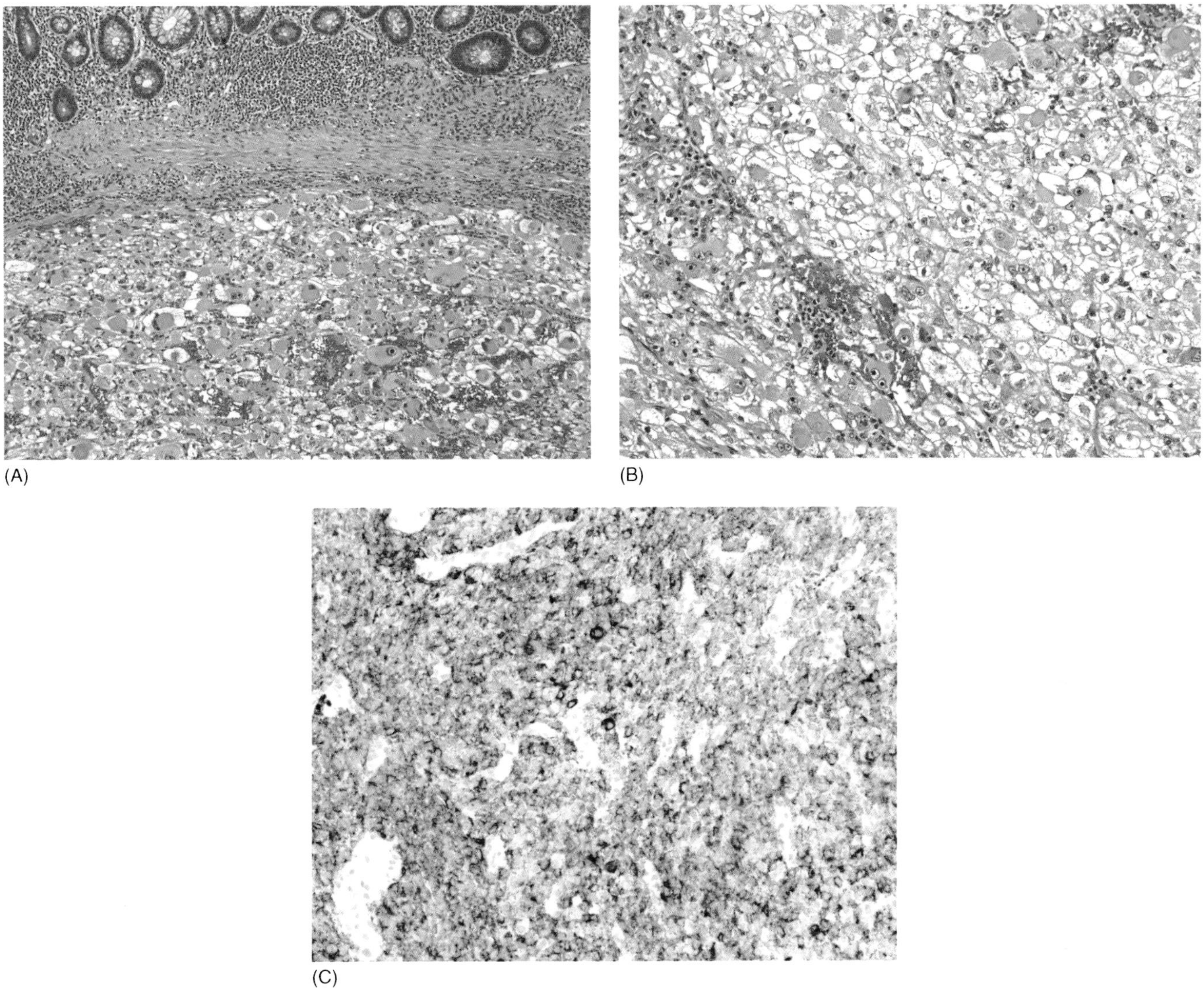

(A)

(B)

(C)

FIGURE 5.33 This colonic PEComa consists of a proliferation of epithelioid cells with clear to granular eosinophilic cytoplasm (A–B, courtesy of Dr. Andrew Folpe). Admixed prominent blood vessels may be seen, as well as adipocytes. Nuclear hyperchromasia and pleomorphism are present as well. HMB-45 is characteristically positive (C, courtesy of Dr. Andrew Folpe).

mitotic activity is brisk, typically around 50/50 HPF, with atypical mitoses. Unlike GISTs, leiomyosarcomas are negative for KIT and DOG1, and routinely show strong SMA expression. Desmin expression varies and may be lost in some higher grade tumors. Because these tumors are so rare, and many previous series mistakenly included high-grade GISTs, clinical behavior has not been well-defined.

True primary liposarcomas (LPSs) of the bowel are exceedingly rare, but dedifferentiated LPS, the most common sarcoma of the retroperitoneum, often involves the tubal gut by invading into the wall from an external location (Figure 5.37).

Other unusual mesenchymal tumors that rarely occur in the GI tract include solitary fibrous tumor, clear cell

sarcoma-like tumor of the GI tract (malignant GI neuroectodermal tumor), synovial sarcoma, alveolar soft parts sarcoma, rhabdomyosarcoma, and other small round blue cell tumors such as desmoplastic small round blue cell tumor.

SPECIFIC ILLUSTRATIVE EXAMPLES

Case 1

A 46-year-old woman presented with vague epigastric pain and nausea. Upper endoscopy was essentially normal, but CT scan revealed a 4 cm tumor in the body of the stomach. The patient underwent partial gastrectomy, and a firm, fleshy, white–tan tumor was resected

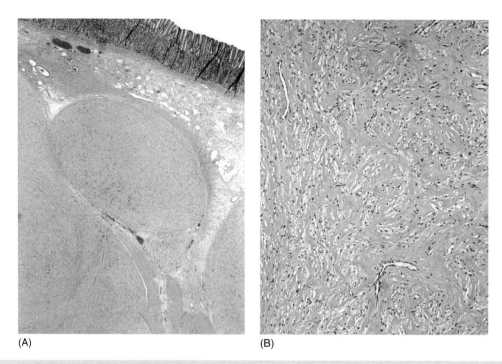

(A)   (B)

FIGURE 5.34   This gastric antral plexiform fibromyxoma is a bland, multilobular spindle cell lesion with a sharply circumscribed border and myxoid stroma (A). Small blood vessels are prominent (B).

that appeared to be arising from the muscularis propria. The tumor had epithelioid morphology (Figure 5.38A), with myxoid stroma and a very low mitotic count. Upon immunohistochemical staining, however, the tumor was essentially KIT negative (Figure 5.38B), but DOG1 was strongly and diffusely positive (Figure 5.38C).

This tumor emphasizes that the majority of KIT-negative GISTs mark with DOG1, including almost 80% of PDGFRA-positive GISTs. The fact that this tumor is an

epithelioid GIST from the stomach, with myxoid stroma, suggests that this tumor may well have a PDGFRA mutation, and thus mutational analysis would be useful as this subset of GISTs has a lower potential for malignant behavior.

Case 2

A 30-year-old woman underwent a CT scan as part of a workup for chronic pelvic pain. A 2 cm mass was found in

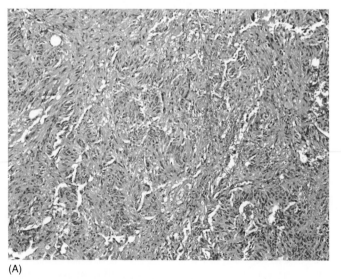

(A)

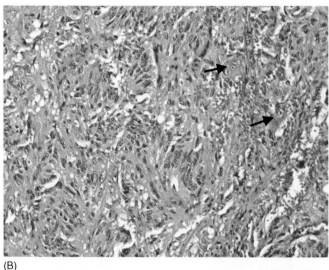

(B)

FIGURE 5.35   Gangliocytic paragangliomas consist of cords and nests of spindled and epithelioid cells (A) with admixed ganglion cells (B, arrows).

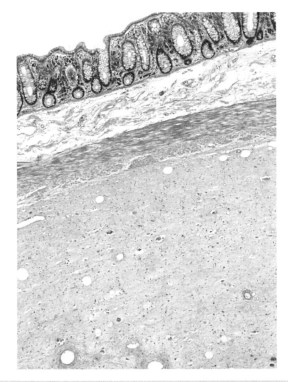

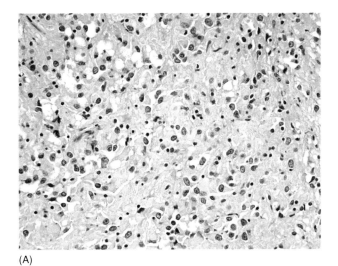

(A)

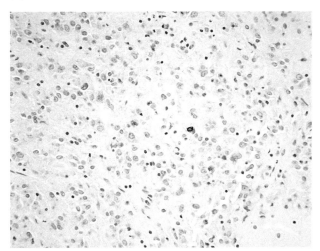

(B)

FIGURE 5.36 Gastrointestinal leiomyosarcomas are similar to their counterparts elsewhere, with highly cellular fascicles of spindle cells containing elongated nuclei with prominent pleomorphism, brightly eosinophilic cytoplasm, and brisk mitotic activity.

the colon, which was subsequently resected. The tumor was composed of plump eosinophilic cells with focal nuclear pleomorphism (Figure 5.39A–B), admixed with cells with clear cytoplasm. An initial panel of immunostains showed that the tumor was KIT positive, and thus it was initially thought to be a pleomorphic GIST. However, additional

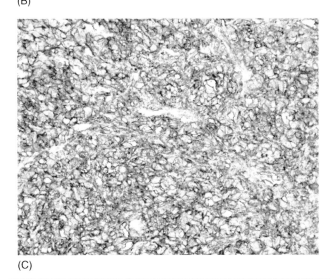

(C)

FIGURE 5.38 This gastric GIST has prominent epithelioid morphology with abundant myxoid stroma and a very low mitotic count (A, courtesy of Dr. Jason Hornick). It is also essentially KIT negative (B, courtesy of Dr. Jason Hornick) but strongly and diffusely DOG1 positive (C, courtesy of Dr. Jason Hornick). The epithelioid morphology, gastric location, and myxoid stroma suggest that this tumor may have a *PDGFRA* mutation.

FIGURE 5.37 This retroperitoneal liposarcoma extends into the wall of the colon. Note the overlying melanosis coli.

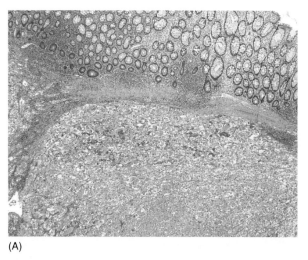

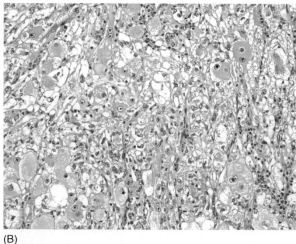

(A)   (B)

FIGURE 5.39   This colonic PEComa is composed of plump eosinophilic cells with nuclear pleomorphism and prominent nucleoli (A, courtesy of Dr. Andrew Folpe). Other cells have clear to granular cytoplasm (B, courtesy of Dr. Andrew Folpe). It would be unusual for a GIST to have this degree of nuclear pleomorphism,

stains revealed that the tumor was negative for DOG1, and positive for HMB-45 and SMA, characteristic of a PEComa.

This case illustrates the confusion that may arise between PEComa (especially those with a prominent spindle cell component) and GIST, due to the fact that both are KIT positive. As previously discussed in the section on PEComa, additional immunostains are helpful in resolving the differential diagnosis. In addition, it is unusual for a GIST to have this degree of nuclear pleomorphism and prominence of nucleoli.

SELECTED REFERENCES

Gastrointestinal Stromal Tumors

Abraham SC, Krasinskas AM, Hofstetter WL, et al. "Seedling" mesenchymal tumors (gastrointestinal stromal tumors and leiomyomas) are common incidental tumors of the esophagogastric junction. *Am J Surg Pathol.* 2007;31:1629–1635.

Antonescu CR, Romeo S, Zhang L, et al. Dedifferentiation in gastrointestinal stromal tumor to an anaplastaic KIT-negative phenotype: a diagnostic pitfall. *Am J Surg Pathol.* 2013;37:385–392.

Carvalho N, Albergaria D, Lebre R, et al. Anal canal gastrointestinal stromal tumors: case report and literature review. *World J Gastroenterol.* 2014;20:319–322.

Corless CL. Gastrointestinal stromal tumors: what do we know now? *Mod Pathol.* 2014;27:S1–S16.

Dematteo RP, Gold JS, Saran L, et al. Tumor mitotic rate, size, and location independently predict recurrence after resection of primary gastrointestinal stromal tumor (GIST). *Cancer.* 2008;112(3):608–615.

Doyle LA, Nelson D, Heinrich MC, et al. Loss of succinate dehydrogenase subunit B (SDHB) expression is limited to a distinctive subset of gastric wild-type gastrointestinal stromal tumors: a comprehensive genotype-phenotype correlation study. *Histopathol.* 2012;61:801–809.

Dwight T, Benn DE, Clarkson A, et al. Loss of SDHA expression identifies SDHA mutations in succinate dehydrogenase-deficient gastrointestinal stromal tumors. *Am J Surg Pathol.* 2013;37:226–233.

Gill AJ, Chou A, Vilain R, et al. Immunohistochemistry for SDHB divides gastrointestinal stromal tumors into 2 distinct types. *Am J Surg Pathol.* 2010;34:636–644.

Joensuu H, Roberts PJ, Sarlomo-Rikala M, et al. Effect of the tyrosine kinase inhibitor STI571 in a patient with a metastatic gastrointestinal stromal tumor. *N Engl J Med.* 2001;344:1052–1056.

Lasota J, Dansonka-Mieszkowska A, Sobin LH, Miettinen M. A great majority of GISTs with PDGFRA mutations represent gastric tumors of low or no malignant potential. *Lab Invest.* 2004;84:874–883.

Miettinen M, Killian JK, Wang ZF, et al. Immunohistochemical loss of succinate dehydrogenase subunit A (SDHA) in gastrointestinal stromal tumors (GISTs) signals SDHA germline mutation. *Am J Surg Pathol.* 2013;37:234–240.

Miettinen M, Lasota J. Histopathology of gastrointestinal stromal tumor. *J Surg Oncol.* 2011;104:865–873.

Miettinen M, Sarloma-Rikala M, Sobin LH, Lasota J. Esophageal stromal tumors: a clinicopathologic, immunohistochemical, and molecular genetic study of 17 cases and comparison with esophageal leiomyomas and leiomyosarcomas. *Am J Surg Pathol.* 2000;24:211–222.

Miettinen M, Sobin LH, Lasota J, Gastrointestinal stromal tumors of the stomach. A clinicopathologic, immunohistochemical, and molecular genetic study of 1765 cases with long term follow up. *Am J Surg Pathol.* 2005;29:52–68.

Miettinen M, Sobin LH, Lasota J. Gastrointestinal stromal tumors presenting as omental masses: a clinicopathologic analysis of 95 cases. *Am J Surg Pathol.* 2009;33:1267–1275.

Miettinen M, Wang ZF, Sarlomo-Rikala M, et al. Succinate dehydrogenase-deficient GISTs: a clinicopathologic, immunohistochemical, and molecular genetic study of 66 gastric GISTs with predilection to young age. *Am J Surg Pathol.* 2011;35(11):1712–1721.

Miettinien M, Sarlomo-Rikala M, Lasota J. Gastrointestinal stromal tumors: recent advances in understanding of their biology. *Hum Pathol.* 1999;30:1213–1220.

Patil DT, Rubin BP. Gastrointestinal stromal tumor: advances in diagnosis and management. *Arch Pathol Lab Med.* 2011;135:1298–1310.

Wagner AJ, Remillard SP, Zhang YX, et al. Loss of expression of SDHA predicts SDHA mutations in gastrointestinal stromal tumors. *Mod Pathol.* 2013;26:289–294.

Yantiss RK, Rosenberg AE, Sarran L, et al. Multiple gastrointestinal stromal tumors in type I neurofibromatosis: a pathologic and molecular study. *Mod Pathol.* 2005;18:475–484.

Immunohistochemistry

Espinosa I, Lee CH, Kim MK, et al. A novel monoclonal antibody against DOG1 is a sensitive and specific marker for gastrointestinal stromal tumors. *Am J Surg Pathol.* 2008;32:210–218.

Guler ML, Daniels JA, Abraham SC, Montgonery EA. Melanoma antigens in epithelioid gastrointestinal stromal tumors: a potential diagnostic pitfall. *Arch Pathol Lab Med.* 2008;132:1302–1306.

Hemminger J, Iwenofu OH. Discovered on gastrointestinal stromal tumours 1(DOG1) expression in non-gastrointestinal stromal tumour (GIST) neoplasms. *Histopathol.* 2012; 61:170–177.

Hornick JL. Novel uses of immunohistochemistry in the diagnosis and classification of soft tissue tumors. *Mod Pathol.* 2014;27:S47–S63.

Miettinen M, Lasota J. Gastrointestinal stromal tumors: pathology and prognosis at different sites. *Semin Diag Pathol.* 2006;23:70–83.

Miettinen M, Lasota J. KIT (CD117): a review on expression in normal and neoplastic tissues, and mutations and their clinicopathologic correlation. *Appl Immunohistochem Mol Morphol.* 2005;13(3):205–220.

Miettinen M, Want ZF, Lasota J. DOG1 antibody in the differential diagnosis of gastrointestinal stromal tumors: a study of 1840 cases. *Am J Surg Pathol.* 2009;33:1401–1408.

West RB, Corless CL, Chen X, et al. The novel marker, DOG1, is expressed ubiquitously in gastrointestinal stromal tumors irrespective of KIT or PDGFRA mutation status. *Am J Pathol.* 2004;165:107–113.

Molecular Evaluation

Corless CL, Barnett CM, Heinrich MC. Gastrointestinal stromal tumors: origin and molecular oncology. *Cancer.* 2011;11:865–878.

Corless CL, Schroeder A, Griffith D, et al. PDGFRA mutations in gastrointestinal stromal tumors: frequency, spectrum, and in vitro sensitivity to imatinib. *J Clin Oncol.* 2005;23:5357–5364.

Heinrich MC, Corless CL, Blanke CD, et al. Molecular correlates of imatinib resistance in gastrointestinal stromal tumors. *J Clin Oncol.* 2006;24:4764–4774.

Heinrich MC, Corless CL, Duensang A, et al. PDGFRA activating mutations in gastrointestinal stromal tumors. *Science.* 2003;299:708–710.

Heinrich MC, Owzar K, Corless CL, et al. Correlation of kinase genotype and clinical outcome in the North American Intergroup Phase II trial of imatinib mesylate for treatment of advanced gastrointestinal stromal tumor: CALGB 150105 study by Cancer and Leukemia Group B and Southwest Oncology Group. *J Clin Oncol.* 2008;26:5360–5367.

Hostein I, Faur N, Primois C, et al. BRAF mutation status in gastrointestinal stromal tumors. *Am J Clin Pathol.* 2010;133:141–148.

Lasota J, Dansonka-Mieszkowska A, Sobin LH, Miettinen M. A great majority of GISTs with PDGFRA mutations represent gastric tumors of low or no malignant potential. *Lab Invest.* 2004;84:874–883.

Lasota J, Stachura J, Miettinen M. GISTs with PDGFRA exon 14 mutations represent subset of clinically favorable gastric tumors with epithelioid morphology. *Lab Invest.* 2006;86:94–100.

Oudijk L, Gaal J, Korpershoek E, et al. SDHA mutations in adult and pediatric wild-type gastrointestinal stromal tumors. *Mod Pathol.* 2013;26:456–463.

Plesec TP. Gastrointestinal mesenchymal neoplasms other than gastrointestinal stromal tumors: focusing on their molecular aspects. *Pathol Res Intl.* 2011;2011:1–10.

Smooth Muscle Tumors

Bisceglia M, Galliani CA, Pizzolitto S, et al. Selected case from the Arkadi M. Rywlin International Pathology Slide Series: leiomyomatosis peritonealis disseminata: report of 3 cases with extensive review of the literature. *Adv Anat Pathol.* 2014;21:201–215.

Miettinen M, Furlong M, Sarloma-Rikala M, et al. Gastrointestinal stromal tumors, intramural leiomyomas, and leimyosarcomas in the rectum and anus. A clinicopathologic, immunohistochemical, and molecular genetic study of 144 cases. *Am J Surg Pathol.* 2001;25:1121–1133.

Miettinen M, Sarloma-Rikala M, Sobin LH. Mesenchymal tumors of muscularis mucosa of colon and rectum are benign leiomyomas that should be separated from gastrointestinal stromal tumors–a clinicopathological and immunohistochemical study of eighty-eight cases. *Mod Pathol.* 2001;14:950–956.

Mutrie CJ, Donahue DM, Wain JC, et al. Esophageal leiomyoma: a 40-year experience. *Ann Thorac Surg.* 2005;79:1122–1125.

Yamamoto H, Handa M, Tobo T, et al. Clinicopathologic features of primary leiomyosarcoma of the gastrointestinal tract following recognition of gastrointestinal stromal tumors. *Histopathol.* 2013;63:194–207.

Schwannoma

Hou YY, Tan YS, Xu JF, et al. Schwannoma of the gastrointestinal tract: a clinicopathological, immunohistochemical, and ultrastructural study of 33 cases. *Histopathol.* 2006;48:536–545.

Leigl B, Bennett MW, Fletcher CDM. Microcystic/reticular schwannoma: a distinct variant with predilection for visceral locations. *Am J Surg Pathol.* 2008;32:1080–1087.

Voltaggio L, Murray R, Lasota J, Miettinen M. Gastric schwannoma: a clinicopathologic study of 51 cases and critical review of the literature. *Hum Pathol.* 2012;43:650–659.

Benign Neural Polyps

Agaimy A, Vassos N, Croner RS. Gastrointestinal manifestations of neurofibromatosis type 1 (Recklinghausens's disease): clinicopathologic spectrum with pathogenetic considerations. *Int J Clin Exp Pathol.* 2012;5:852–862.

Eslami-Varzaneh F, Washington K, Robert ME, et al. Benign fibroblastic polyps of the colon: a histologic, immunohistochemical, and ultrastructural study. *Am J Surg Pathol.* 2004;28:374–378.

Fuller CE, Williams GT. Gastrointestinal manifestations of type 1 neurofibromatosis (von Recklinghausen's disease). *Histopathol.* 1991;19:1–11.

Gibson JA, Hornick JL. Mucosal Schwann cell "hamartoma:" clinicopathologic study of 26 neural colorectal polyps distinct from neurofibromas and mucosal neuromas. *Am J Surg Pathol.* 2009;33:781–787.

Groisman GM, Hershkovitz D, Vieth M, Sabo E. Colonic perineuriomas with and without crypt serrations: a comparative study. *Am J Surg Pathol.* 2013;37:745–751.

Groisman GM, Polak-Charcon S. Fibroblastic polyp of the colon and colonic perineurioma: 2 names for a single entity? *Am J Surg Pathol.* 2008;32, 1088–1094.

Hornick JL, Fletcher CDM. Intesitnal perineuriomas: clinicopathologic definition of a new anatomic subset in a series of 10 cases. *Am J Surg Pathol.* 2005;29:859–865.

Johnston J, Helwig EB. Granular cell tumors of the gastrointestinal tract and perianal region: a study of 74 cases. *Dig Dis Sci.* 1981;26:807–816.

Lee NC, Norton JA. Multiple endocrine neoplasia type 2B-genetic basis and clinical expression. *Surg Oncol.* 2000;9:111–118.

Pai RK, Mojtahed A, Rouse RV, et al. Histologic and molecular analyses of colonic perineurial-like proliferations in serrated polyps: perineurial-like stromal proliferations are seen in sessile serrated adenomas. *Am J Surg Pathol.* 2011 35(9):1373–1380.

Shekitka KM, Sobin LH. Ganglioneuromas of the gastrointestinal tract. Relation to von Recklinghausen's disease and other multiple tumor syndromes. *Am J Surg Pathol.* 1994;18:250–257.

Singhi AD, Montgomery EA. Colorectal granular cell tumor: a clinico-pathologic study of 26 cases. *Am J Surg Pathol.* 2010;34:1186–1192.

Desmoid Tumors

Montgomery E, Torbenson MS, Kaushal MK, et al. Beta catenin immu-nohistochemistry separates mesenteric fibromatosis from gastro-intestinal stromal tumor and sclerosing mesenteritis. *Am J Surg Pathol.* 2002;26;1296–1301.

Yantiss RK, Spiro IJ, Compton CC, Rosenberg AE. Gastrointestinal stromal tumor versus intra-abdominal fibromatosis of the bowel wall: a clinically important differential diagnosis. *Am J Surg Pathol.* 2000; 24:947–957.

Glomus Tumor

Kang G, Park HJ, Kim JY, et al. Glomus tumor of the stomach: a clini-copathologic analysis of 10 cases and review of the literature. *Gut Liver.* 2012;6:52–57.

Miettinen M, Paal E, Lasota J, Sobin LH. Gastrointestinal glomus tumors: a clinicopathologic, immunohistochemical, and molecular genetic study of 32 cases. *Am J Surg Pathol.* 2002;26:301–311.

Inflammatory Fibroid Polyp

Lasota J, Wang ZF, Sobin LH, Miettinen M. Gain-of-function PDGFRA mutations, earlier reported in gastrointestinal stromal tumors, are common in small intestinal inflammatory fibroid polyps. A study of 60 cases. *Mod Pathol.* 2009; 22(8):1049–1056.

Liu TC, Lin MT, Montgomery EA, Singhi AD. Inflammatory fibroid polyps of the gastrointestinal tract: spectrum of clinical, mor-phologic, and immunohistochemistry features. *Am J Surg Pathol.* 2013;37(4):586–592.

Ozolek JA, Sasatomi E, Swalsky PA, et al. Inflammatory fibroid pol-yps of the gastrointestinal tract: clinical, pathologic, and molec-ular characteristics. *Appl Immunohistochemist Mol Morph.* 2004;12:59–66.

Inflammatory Myofibroblastic Tumor

Coffin CM, Watterson J, Priest JR, et al. Extrapulmonary inflamma-tory myofibroblastic tumor (inflammatory pseudotumor). A clini-copathologic and immunohistochemical study of 84 cases. *Am J Surg Pathol.* 1995;19:859–872.

Cook JR, Dehner LP, Collins MH, et al. Anaplastic lymphoma kinase (ALK) expression in the inflammatory myofibroblastic tumor: a comparative immunohistochemical study. *Am J Surg Pathol.* 2001;25:1364–1371.

Makhlouf HR, Sobin LH. Inflammatory myofibroblastic tumors (inflammatory pseudotumors) of the gastrointestinal tract: how closely are they related to inflammatory fibroid polyps? *Hum Pathol.* 2002;33:307–315.

Marino-Enriquez A, Wang WL, Roy A, et al. An aggressive intra-abdominal variant of inflammatory myofibroblastic tumor with nuclear membrane or perinuclear ALK. *Am J Surg Pathol.* 2011;35:135–144.

Sanders BM, West KW, Gingalewski C, et al. Inflammatory pseudo-tumor of the alimentary tract: clinical and surgical experience. *J Pediatr Surg.* 2001;36:169–173.

PEComa

Bleeker JS, Quevedo JF, Folpe AL. "Malignant" perivascular epithe-lioid cell neoplasm: risk stratification and treatment strategies. *Sarcoma.* 2012; 2012:541626.

Doyle LA, Hornick JL, Fletcher CDM. PEComa of the gastrointestinal tract: clinicopathologic study of 35 cases with evaluation of prog-nostic parameters. *Am J Surg Pathol.* 2013;37:1769–1782.

Maluf H, Dieckgraefe B. Angiomyolipoma of the large intestine: report of a case. *Mod Pathol.* 1999;12:1132–1136.

Ryan P, Nguyen VH, Gholoum S, et al. Polypoid PEComa in the rectum of a 15-year-old girl. Case report and review of PEComa in the gastrointestinal tract. *Am J Surg Pathol.* 2009;33:475–482.

Yamamoto H, Oda Y, Tao T, et al. Malignant perivascular epithelioid cell tumor of the colon: report of a case with molecular analysis. *Path Intl.* 2006;56:46–50.

Plexiform Fibromyxoma

Miettinen M, Makhlouf HR, Sobin LH, Lasota J. Plexiform fibromyx-oma: a distinctive benign gastric antral neoplasm not to be con-fused with a myxoid GIST. *Am J Surg Pathol.* 2009;33:1624–1632.

Takahashi Y, Shimizu S, Ishida T, et al. Plexiform angiomyx-oid myofibroblastic tumor of the stomach. *Am J Surg Pathol.* 2007;31:724–728.

Gangliocytic Paraganglioma

Hamid QA, Bishop AE, Rode J, et al. Duodenal gangliocytic paragan-glioma: a study of 10 cases with immunocytochemical neuroendo-crine markers. *Hum Pathol.* 1986;17:1151–1157.

Okubo Y, Yokose T, tuchiya M, et al. Duodenal gangliocytic paragan-glioma showing lymph node metastasis: a rare case report. *Diagn Pathol.* 2012;5:27.

Scheithauer BW, Nora FE, Lechago J, et al. Duodenal gangliocytic para-ganglioma. Clinicopathologic and immunocytochemical study of 11 cases. *Am J Clin Pathol.* 1986;58:1720–1735.

Others

Akram S, Pardi DS, Schaffner JA, Smyrk TC. Sclerosing mesenteri-tis: clinical features, treatment, and outcome in 92 patients. *Clin Gastroenterol Hepatol.* 2007;5:589–596.

Company Campins MM, Morales R, Dolz C, et al. Primary monophasic synovial sarcoma of the duodenum confirmed by cytogenetic anal-ysis with demonstration of t(X;18); a case report. *J Gastrointestin Liver Dis.* 2009;18:89–93.

Emory TS, Monihan JM, Carr NJ, et al. Sclerosing mesenteritis, mes-enteric panniculitis, and mesenteric lipodystrophy: a single entity? *Am J Surg Pathol.* 1997;21:392–398.

Liu YQ, Yue JQ. Intramural solitary fibrous tumor of the ileum: a case report and review of the literature. *J Cancer Res Ther.* 2013;9:724–726.

Lyle PL, Amato CM, Fitzpatrick JE, Robinson WA. Gastrointestinal melanoma or clear cell sarcoma? Molecular evaluation of 7 cases previously diagnosed as malignant meloma. *Am J Surg Pathol.* 2008;32:858–866.

Stockman DL, Miettinen M, Suster S, et al. Malignant gastrointestinal neuroectodermal tumor: clinicopathologic, immunohistochemical, ultrastructural, and molecular analysis of 16 cases with a reap-praisal of clear cell sarcoma-like tumors of the gastrointestinal tract. *Am J Surg Pathol.* 2012;36:857–868.

6

Approach to Hereditary Cancer Syndromes

RHONDA K. YANTISS

INTRODUCTION

Several inherited disorders are associated with increased gastrointestinal cancer risk. Most of these cause epithelial gastrointestinal polyposis, although the severity of the polyposis is variable. Others, such as multiple endocrine neoplasia type 1 and type 1 neurofibromatosis, are associated with epithelial, endocrine, and mesenchymal tumors of the gastrointestinal tract. Polyposis disorders can be broadly classified into two groups: adenomatous and hamartomatous polyposes. The former includes entities such as familial adenomatous polyposis (FAP), *MUTYH*-associated polyposis, and Lynch syndrome, whereas Peutz–Jeghers syndrome, juvenile polyposis syndrome, and PTEN hamartoma tumor syndrome comprise the latter. Recent advances have provided important insight into the pathogenesis of all of these disorders and their relationships to cancer, although application of pathologic, clinical, and molecular criteria still fails to identify all patients with heritable cancer syndromes.

The purpose of this chapter is to discuss the clinicopathologic features and differential diagnoses of the most common heritable cancer syndromes, and provide pathologists with a framework for the evaluation of these entities. A comprehensive discussion of all tumor syndromes that may have gastrointestinal manifestations is beyond the scope of this chapter, which will focus on epithelial and hamartomatous polyposis disorders.

ADENOMATOUS POLYPOSES

Familial Adenomatous Polyposis

Overview of Molecular Alterations

FAP is an autosomal dominant condition characterized by the presence of hundreds to thousands of adenomatous polyps in the colorectum (Figure 6.1). The risk for colorectal cancer approaches 100% by 40 years of age among patients with this disorder, although less than 1% of colorectal carcinomas arise in patients with FAP. Patients with FAP have germline *APC* mutations, which develop at a rate of 1 per 10,000–15,000 live births and result in an overall disease prevalence of 2.3 to 3.2 per 100,000 individuals. Up to 50% of affected newborns have either de novo germline mutations or parents with germline *APC* mosaicism, in which case the mutant allele is limited to germ cells of the unaffected parent and manifests disease in the offspring. Patients carrying a germline *APC* mutation in one copy of the gene develop a "second hit" that inactivates the other allele and abolishes the tumor suppressor function of cytoplasmic APC. Inactivation of each allele does not occur as two random independent events. Rather, the nature of the somatic (second) mutation depends on the site of the germline alteration, such that one allele harbors a mutation near codon 1300. Selection for a mutation in this region ensures that the resultant APC protein retains some functionality such that it may

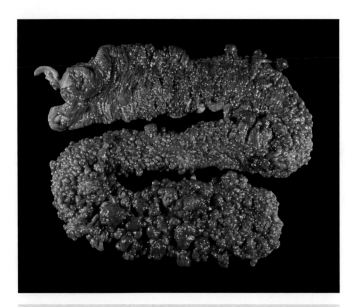

FIGURE 6.1 A resected colon from a patient with familial adenomatous polyposis contains innumerable adenomas that vary from only a few millimeters to several centimeters in diameter. Patients with extensive disease, such as this, are at high risk for cancer development.

bind β-catenin. Some patients with milder forms of disease (ie, attenuated FAP) inherit mutations at the extreme 3′ or 5′ prime ends of *APC* that lead to partially functional proteins, resulting in fewer polyps and a slightly lower lifetime cancer risk. The molecular features of FAP are further discussed in Chapter 14.

Clinical Features

The type of inherited *APC* mutation dictates the extent and severity of the gastrointestinal polyposis. Although most patients develop innumerable polyps and have a 100% risk of colorectal cancer if not treated by prophylactic proctocolectomy, those with attenuated FAP generally develop fewer than 100 colorectal polyps and have a slightly lower lifetime colorectal cancer risk of approximately 80%.

Extraintestinal manifestations are also related to the nature of the underlying germline mutations. Several named variants describe specific combinations of phenotypic characteristics. *Gardner syndrome* denotes the constellation of osteomas, mesenteric fibromatosis, cutaneous cysts, lipomas, and dental abnormalities that occur in addition to polyposis. This form of disease is commonly associated with germline *APC* mutations in codons 1395 to 1493. Patients with *Crail syndrome* have gastrointestinal polyposis in combination with medulloblastomas, ependymomas, or astrocytomas. Extracolonic manifestations of the disease are numerous and include increased

risk for gastric and small bowel adenocarcinoma (0.5% and 5%, respectively), hepatoblastoma (1.5%), adrenal cortical adenoma, nasopharyngeal angiofibroma, and papillary thyroid carcinoma (2%), particularly the cribriform morular variant. Congenital hyperpigmentation of the retinal pigmented epithelium is associated with mutations between codons 311 and 1444.

Pathologic Features and Diagnostic Considerations

Patients with FAP develop conventional tubular, villous, and tubulovillous adenomas of the colorectum that are indistinguishable from sporadic adenomas (Figure 6.2). Although untreated patients ultimately develop hundreds to thousands of colorectal adenomas, the increased use of genetic counseling and molecular testing has improved early detection and, as a result, most colectomy specimens now contain far fewer polyps than those removed in the past (Figure 6.3). These resection specimens should be carefully evaluated for the number of polyps present in order to facilitate classification of the disease and document the extent of polyposis, particularly when patients have not yet been evaluated with germline testing. In our practice, we entirely submit all polyps spanning at least 1 cm and obtain representative sections of smaller lesions at a rate of one section every 5 to 10 cm of the colon. Any lesions suspicious for invasive adenocarcinoma are sampled similar to sporadic colorectal carcinomas, and the regional lymph nodes are evaluated.

Patients with FAP also develop polyposis of the upper gastrointestinal tract. Gastric polyps include adenomas and fundic gland polyps, the latter of which frequently

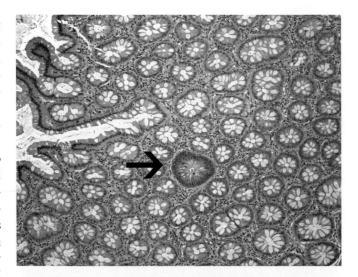

FIGURE 6.2 Cross sections through the colonic mucosa of patients with familial adenomatous polyposis can reveal single dysplastic crypts (arrow) that represent the earliest identifiable histologic stage of adenoma development.

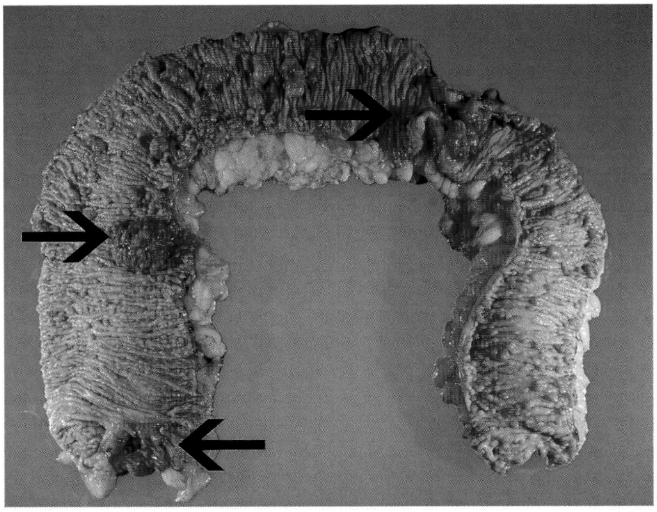

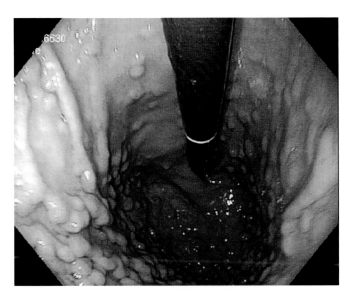

FIGURE 6.3 Patients with familial adenomatous polyposis may come to clinical attention before the entire colonic mucosa is carpeted by adenomas. This patient already has several tiny polyps that stud the mucosa, as well as three synchronous cancers (arrows).

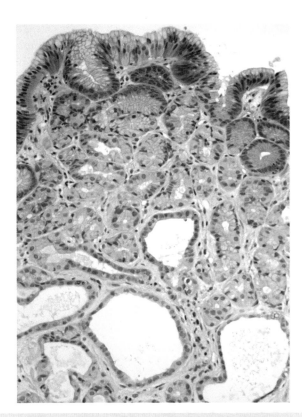

FIGURE 6.5 More than half of the patients with FAP and fundic gland polyps have dysplasia in some of the fundic gland polyps. The dysplasia is usually low-grade with enlarged, hyperchromatic nuclei and nuclear pseudostratification.

show dysplasia (Figure 6.4). Indeed, approximately 50% of patients with FAP have dysplasia in some of their fundic gland polyps. The dysplasia in these cases is typically low-grade and focal, although occasional polyps show more extensive abnormalities or high-grade dysplasia (Figure 6.5). The biologic risk of this finding is quite low and, thus, patients can be safely monitored with surveillance endoscopy and regular removal of large lesions without prophylactic gastrectomy. Nonsyndromic fundic

gland polyps show dysplasia much less frequently (less than 5%) than those associated with FAP. Thus, pathologists may suggest the possibility of a polyposis disorder when fundic gland polyps with dysplasia are encountered, particularly if the patient has multiple gastric polyps.

Adenomas of the small bowel are more common among patients with *APC* mutations between codons 976 and 1067. They show a predilection for the ampulla and nonampullary duodenum as well as the proximal jejunum. Development of nonampullary adenomas of the duodenum is extremely uncommon in the sporadic setting and, in fact, the pathologist should raise the possibility of FAP when these lesions are encountered, particularly if they are multiple.

Differential Diagnosis

The diagnosis of FAP is generally straightforward when patients have typical disease manifestations. Other disorders associated with gastrointestinal polyps can simulate the endoscopic appearance of FAP, however. These include lymphomatoid polyposis, inflammatory bowel disease with pseudopolyps, and hamartomatous polyposes,

FIGURE 6.4 Patients with familial adenomatous polyposis commonly develop multiple fundic gland polyps. This patient has numerous sessile nodules in the gastric body and fundus.

although all of these entities are readily distinguishable on biopsy analysis. The differential diagnosis of multiple gastrointestinal adenomas is more problematic. Attenuated FAP and *MUTYH*-associated polyposis manifest with similar numbers of colorectal adenomas that are histologically indistinguishable, and require germline analysis for diagnosis. However, patients with *MUTYH*-associated polyposis may present with nondysplastic and dysplastic serrated polyps, both of which are generally lacking in patients with FAP. Some patients with Lynch syndrome have multiple colorectal adenomas, as well as adenomas of the small bowel and periampullary region. One may suspect Lynch syndrome if adenomas contain increased intraepithelial lymphocytes or show high-grade features despite relatively small size. Immunohistochemical stains for DNA mismatch repair proteins may show loss of staining typical of Lynch syndrome when adenomas are large, located in the proximal colon, or show high-grade dysplasia. Carcinomas that develop in patients with Lynch syndrome show morphologic heterogeneity, tumor infiltrating lymphocytes, and a Crohn-like lymphoid response.

MUTYH-Associated Polyposis

Overview of Molecular Alterations

Some patients with gastrointestinal polyposis have an autosomal recessive disease that results from biallelic inactivating mutations in the base excision repair gene, *MUTYH*, on chromosome 1p32-34. Patients with these inactivating *MUTYH* mutations have a predilection for acquiring somatic *APC* mutations and, as a result, develop numerous colorectal polyps that simulate the phenotype of attenuated FAP. Patients can also develop transversion mutations or spontaneous promoter methylation affecting *MLH1*, so resultant tumors may have either chromosomal or microsatellite instability (MSI). Patients with polyposis due to *MUTYH* mutations have a lifetime colorectal cancer risk of approximately 80%. Recommended surveillance mirrors that of patients with attenuated FAP; patients should undergo complete biannual colonoscopy beginning at 18 to 20 years of age and upper endoscopic examination beginning at age 25 to 30 years.

Clinical Features

The incidence of *MUTYH*-associated polyposis is approximately 1 in 10,000 persons based on the 2% estimated prevalence of heterozygous mutations in Caucasian populations. This disorder accounts for less than 1% of colorectal carcinomas, but approximately one-third of patients with colorectal polyposis and wild-type *APC* have this syndrome. Nearly 20% of patients with *MUTYH*-associated polyposis develop duodenal adenomas. These patients have a 4% lifetime risk of duodenal carcinoma, and a substantial number have fundic gland polyps and/or

gastric adenomas. Other associated malignancies include carcinomas of skin, breast, ovary, and urinary bladder. Some patients develop sebaceous tumors in combination with the polyposis, thereby mimicking the features of the Muir–Torre variant of Lynch syndrome.

Pathologic Features and Diagnostic Considerations

MUTYH-associated polyposis was first described in 2002 and, thus, the full spectrum of phenotypic and molecular alterations has not been elucidated. Most patients have between 10 and 100 colorectal polyps, although rare individuals have several hundred polyps and some present with colorectal carcinoma in the absence of other lesions. Most adenomas are conventional intestinal-type adenomas with low-grade dysplasia that simulate FAP, but hyperplastic polyps and sessile serrated adenomas also occur. Furthermore, *MUTYH* mutations may underlie the development of serrated (hyperplastic) polyposis in some cases. Carcinomas associated with *MUTYH*-associated polyposis show a predilection for the proximal colon.

Differential Diagnosis

The differential diagnosis of *MUTYH*-associated polyposis includes attenuated FAP, Lynch syndrome, and serrated polyposis. Although germline mutational testing conclusively distinguishes between these entities, other clinicopathologic features can be helpful. Attenuated FAP is not associated with increased numbers of serrated polyps, whereas this finding is commonly present in *MUTYH*-associated polyposis. The latter has not been reported in combination with tumors of the central nervous system, mesenteric fibromatosis, or other extraintestinal manifestations of Gardner syndrome. Both *MUTYH*-associated polyposis and Lynch syndrome may be associated with the development of MSI-H colorectal carcinomas. Thus far, those associated with *MUTYH*-associated polyposis show *MLH1* deficiencies, either in the form of promoter methylation or mutations.

Lynch Syndrome (Hereditary Non-Polyposis Colon Cancer)

Overview of Molecular Alterations

Lynch syndrome is an autosomal dominant disorder characterized by early-onset colonic carcinoma due to inactivating germline mutations in mismatch repair genes. These genes (*MLH1, MSH2, MSH6,* and *PMS2*) encode proteins that form complexes and patrol the genome to correct DNA mismatches. Microsatellites are prone to mismatch repair errors owing to the tendency for DNA polymerase to slip over repetitive sequences in these areas. Failure of the mismatch repair system to correct errors results in their propagation, such that subsequent microsatellite sequences show expansion or contraction of length in tumor DNA compared to that of non-neoplastic tissues from the same patient.

Most laboratories now use quasimonomorphic mononucleotide markers (BAT25, BAT26, NR-1, NR-24, MONO-27) to assess for MSI. Tumors with instability at two or more markers are classified as showing MSI-H, whereas those without MSI at any marker are classified as microsatellite stable and those with MSI at one marker are considered to be indeterminate. Other rare causes of Lynch syndrome include heritable epigenetic inactivation of *MLH1* through *MLH1* germline promoter methylation, and a germline deletion affecting *TACSTD1 (EPCAM)* that eliminates the *TACSTD1* stop codon, leading to the formation of EPCAM–MSH2 fusion transcripts and *MSH2* inactivation. The molecular mechanisms underlying MSI are discussed more fully in Chapter 14. Immunohistochemical stains for mismatch repair proteins may be used as a surrogate marker of MSI, with the added benefit of identifying the deficient gene based on the pattern of staining (see Table 6.1), as discussed further in Chapter 13.

Clinical Features

Lynch syndrome accounts for 2% to 4% of all colorectal carcinomas, and affected patients have an 80% lifetime risk of colorectal carcinoma. Most tumors develop approximately 20 years earlier than they do in the general population (mean age at onset: 44 years), so affected patients undergo screening colonoscopy at age 20 to 25 years with surveillance examinations every 1 to 2 years thereafter. Lynch syndrome is also associated with an increased risk for extracolonic cancers of the endometrium, ovary, renal pelvis and ureter, small intestine, stomach, and hepatobiliary tract. Muir–Torre syndrome and Turcot syndrome represent named variants of Lynch syndrome. *Muir–Torre syndrome* features internal malignancies associated with sebaceous neoplasms, whereas patients with *Turcot syndrome* have glioblastoma multiforme in combination with intestinal neoplasms.

Rare patients have germline mutations affecting two mismatch repair genes, either in the form of homozygous biallelic loss or compound heterozygosity usually affecting

PMS2 or *MSH6*. These patients with constitutional mismatch repair deficiency develop Lynch-syndrome-related cancers in late adolescence or early adulthood and often have multiple colorectal polyps, thereby mimicking FAP. Extracolonic manifestations of constitutional mismatch repair deficiency include *cafè au lait* spots, leukemia or lymphoma, gliomas, and extracolonic gastrointestinal malignancies.

Pathologic Features and Diagnostic Considerations

Colorectal carcinomas with MSI-H characteristically occur in the proximal colon, where they form large, bulky masses (Figure 6.6). Tumors tend to have a circumscribed, rather than infiltrative, invasive front and show histologic heterogeneity, which may include combinations of conventional carcinoma admixed with areas of medullary growth, mucinous differentiation, or signet ring cells (Figure 6.7A–C). Approximately 50% of mucinous colorectal carcinomas are MSI-H, whereas nearly 90% of medullary carcinomas of the colon are MSI-H. These cancers are often associated with tumor infiltrating lymphocytes (Figure 6.7D) or the presence of lymphoid aggregates at the periphery of the tumor (Figure 6.7E). Both intraepithelial lymphocytes and the Crohn-like lymphoid response likely represent a host immune response to neoantigens elaborated as a result of MSI-H.

Patients with Lynch syndrome can sometimes initially present with extracolonic malignancies, in which case the diagnosis is rarely a clinical consideration. Gastric and

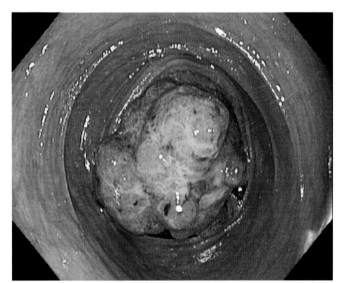

FIGURE 6.6 A 59-year-old male underwent colonoscopy after presenting with occult blood loss. He was found to have a nearly obstructing, fungating mass in the transverse colon. Biopsies revealed a mucinous carcinoma that proved to be *MLH1* deficient due to a germline mutation.

TABLE 6.1 Interpretation of Mismatch Repair Protein Immunohistochemistry

Immunostaining Profile	Defective Gene	Microsatellite Status
Loss of MLH1 and PMS2	*MLH1*	MSI-H
Loss of MSH2 and MSH6	*MSH2* or *TACSTD1 (EPCAM)*	MSI-H
Loss of PMS2	*PMS2*	MSI-H
Loss of MSH6	*MSH6*	MSI-H or MSS

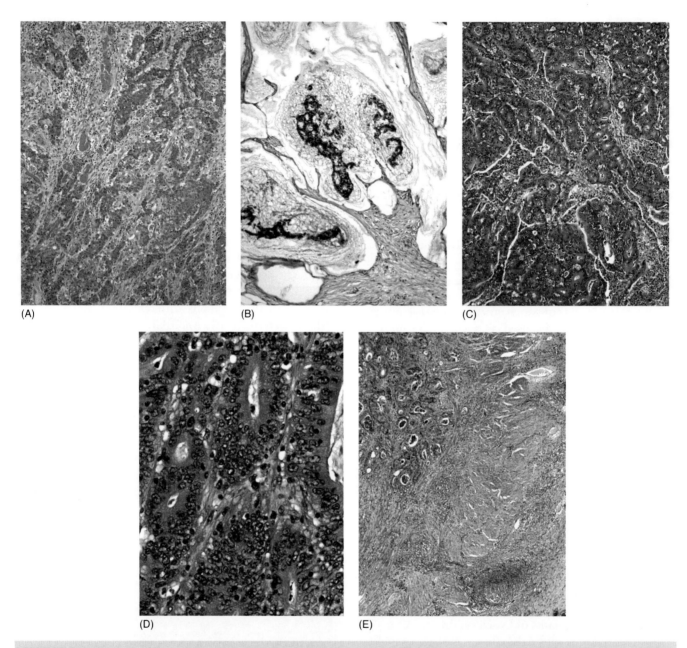

FIGURE 6.7 Microsatellite unstable carcinomas may display a variety of growth patterns, often in combination. Medullary carcinomas are composed of tumor cells arranged in trabeculae without overt gland formation (A). Mucinous carcinomas contain lace-like arrangements of neoplastic epithelial cells floating within pools of mucin (B). Some tumors have a conventional appearance with fused or cribriform glands (C). Intraepithelial lymphocytes are characteristic of tumors with MSI-H, regardless of the morphologic appearance of the lesion (D), and lymphoid aggregates at the periphery of the tumor may also be seen (E).

small intestinal adenocarcinomas associated with Lynch syndrome frequently show morphologic heterogeneity with high-grade areas or foci of mucinous differentiation. Tumor infiltrating lymphocytes are variably present, but when detected, should prompt pathologists to consider the possibility of MSI-H and Lynch syndrome.

The precursor lesion of Lynch-syndrome-associated carcinoma is a conventional adenoma, not a serrated neoplasm. Adenomas of affected patients show inactivation

of *APC* or *CTNNB1* mutations and develop MSI-H late in their evolution. These features have important clinical implications. Patients or clinicians may ask pathologists to evaluate adenomas for possible Lynch syndrome when multiple colorectal polyps are present, but this may not yield meaningful results. For example, Lynch syndrome is unlikely to be present in patients with multiple serrated polyps. Nondysplastic serrated polyps do not show MSI-H and dysplastic serrated polyps with MSI-H develop via

MLH1 promoter methylation, not germline mutations. Additionally, assessment of adenomas for Lynch syndrome often yields unreliable results, even among patients who carry a mutation. MSI develops late in adenoma progression and, thus, failure to detect mismatch deficiency in an adenoma does not necessarily exclude the possibility of Lynch syndrome in a given patient. Most data suggest that screening adenomas among unselected young patients (less than 40 years of age) has a very low yield for detecting Lynch patients owing to the relatively high prevalence of sporadic adenomas in this patient population. For these reasons, universal testing of adenomas for Lynch syndrome is not recommended. However, it is reasonable to assess large, or proximally located, adenomas for mismatch repair protein expression when there is a clinical suspicion for a heritable cancer syndrome.

Differential Diagnosis

The differential diagnosis of Lynch syndrome includes attenuated FAP and *MUTYH*-associated polyposis when patients have colorectal cancer in combination with colonic adenomas. The distinction is straightforward in most cases, as cancers associated with Lynch syndrome show typical morphologic features as well as immunohistochemical loss of one or more DNA mismatch repair proteins. The more problematic differential diagnosis lies with sporadic MSI-H colorectal cancers. Most sporadic MSI-H colorectal cancers develop as a result of *MLH1* promoter

hypermethylation and show loss of immunostaining for MLH1 and PMS2, similar to *MLH1* deficient carcinomas of Lynch syndrome. In fact, sporadic MSI-H carcinomas are indistinguishable from Lynch-related *MLH1* deficient tumors based on polymerase chain reaction (PCR) for MSI and immunohistochemistry alone. However, approximately 50% of sporadic MSI-H cancers also show *BRAF* V600E mutations, whereas this abnormality is not typical of *MLH1*-deficient tumors in Lynch syndrome. Mutations in *BRAF* may be detected in extracted tumoral DNA or with recently available immunohistochemical stains directed against the mutant protein. The molecular and immunohistochemical diagnosis of Lynch syndrome is further discussed in Chapters 11, 13, and 14.

HAMARTOMATOUS POLYPOSES

Peutz–Jeghers Syndrome

Overview of Molecular Features

Peutz–Jeghers syndrome is an autosomal dominant hereditary hamartomatous polyposis syndrome characterized by generalized gastrointestinal polyposis in combination with a variety of extraintestinal manifestations (see Table 6.2). Approximately 70% of patients have detectable mutations in *LKB1* (*STK11*), which is located on chromosome 19p13.3. This tumor suppressor gene encodes serine/threonine kinase 11, alternatively termed liver kinase

TABLE 6.2   Classic Features of Hamartomatous Polyposis Syndromes of the Gastrointestinal Tract

	Peutz–Jeghers Syndrome	Juvenile Polyposis Syndrome	PTEN Hamartoma Tumor Syndrome
Mutant gene	*LKB1* (*STK11*)	*SMAD4* *BMBR1A*	*PTEN* *SDHB* or *SDHD* *KLLN* *PIK3CA* *AKT1*
Gene function	Serine threonine kinase regulates adenine monophosphate activated protein kinase (AMPK)	TGF-β mediated signal transduction	Tumor suppressor gene
Mucocutaneous manifestations	Perioral, buccal, and conjunctival pigmentation; perioral pigment fades with age, but buccal and conjunctival lesions persist		Oral papillomas, tricholemmomas, acral keratoses
Other abnormalities	Ovarian tumors (sex cord–stromal tumor with annular tubules) Cervical cancer (adenoma malignum) Testicular tumors (large cell calcifying Sertoli cell tumor) Mammary carcinoma Pancreatic ductal adenocarcinoma	Cranial and cardiac abnormalities Cleft palate Polydactyly Intestinal malrotation Hereditary hemorrhagic telangiectasia Vascular malformations Hypertrophic osteoarthropathy	Thyroid disease: autoimmune thyroiditis and carcinoma Breast disease: fibrocystic breast disease and carcinoma Macrocephaly Mental impairment Glycogenic acanthosis of esophagus
Gastrointestinal polyp location	Small intestine most affected, followed by colon and stomach	Colon most affected, followed by stomach and small bowel	Colon most affected, followed by stomach and small bowel
Gastrointestinal carcinomas	Colorectum most affected, followed by stomach and small bowel	Colorectum most affected, followed by stomach and small bowel	Colorectum most affected, followed by stomach

B1, which normally maintains cell polarity and inhibits cell growth by activating other kinases and regulating the activity of adenine monophosphate activated protein kinase (AMPK). Phosphorylation of AMPK by STK11 leads to its activation, which is important to cell metabolism and homeostasis. Loss of *STK11* results in cellular disorganization and facilitates tumor growth. The disease phenotype tends to be more severe in patients with truncating mutations compared to those who have missense mutations.

Clinical Features

Peutz–Jeghers syndrome affects one in 200,000 persons in the United States and is characterized by gastrointestinal hamartomatous polyps, mucocutaneous pigmentation, and an increased risk of malignancy affecting multiple organ systems. Clinical criteria for the diagnosis include (a) at least three Peutz–Jeghers polyps; (b) any number of Peutz–Jeghers polyps in a patient with afflicted family members; (c) mucocutaneous pigmentation in a patient with afflicted family members; or (d) any number of Peutz–Jeghers polyps occurring in a patient with mucocutaneous pigmentation.

Peutz–Jeghers polyps are most numerous in the small intestine, where they are prone to cause intermittent intussusception. Virtually all patients with hamartomas of the colon, stomach, and appendix also have involvement of the small bowel. Polyps are round with smooth surfaces that may be eroded or, more commonly, resemble the background mucosa (Figure 6.8A–B). Pedunculated polyps tend to have thick stalks that may be much longer than

those of adenomas. Patients with Peutz–Jeghers syndrome are at markedly increased risk for gastrointestinal and extraintestinal cancers; more than 90% of the patients will develop some type of malignancy by 65 years of age. The lifetime risk of colorectal cancer is 35% to 40%, followed in decreasing frequency by pancreatic cancer (35%), gastric cancer (28%), and small bowel cancer (10%–15%). Children and young adults usually present with abdominal pain or bleeding, whereas malignant complications are more common among older adults.

Pathologic Features and Diagnostic Considerations

Solitary hamartomatous polyps that resemble Peutz–Jeghers polyps have been described as sporadic lesions in the older literature. However, increased use of molecular testing and improved clinical assessment have shown that virtually all solitary polyps with features of Peutz–Jeghers polyps occur in patients with germline *STK11* mutations or those with clinical features suggestive of Peutz–Jeghers syndrome. Thus, solitary Peutz–Jeghers polyps should be considered a forme fruste of the syndrome until proven otherwise, and prompt evaluation for a heritable syndrome.

Peutz–Jeghers polyps contain lobules of nondysplastic epithelium and associated lamina propria in the submucosa, and up to 10% of small bowel polyps are associated with aggregates of mucosa distributed in all layers of the wall (Figure 6.9A–E). These mucosal elements are surrounded by prominent bundles of smooth muscle cells that display a pronounced, arborizing pattern, particularly in polyps of the small intestine. Slightly more than 10% of

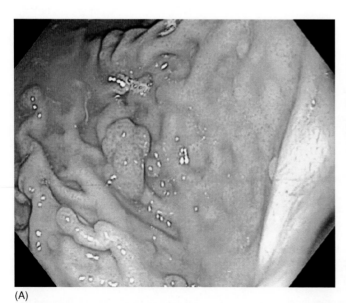

(A)

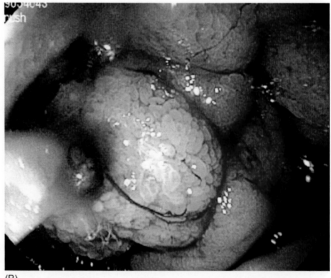

(B)

FIGURE 6.8 A gastric Peutz–Jeghers polyp forms an irregular, lobulated excrescence on a mucosal fold (A). The same patient had a multinodular, nearly obstructing hamartoma in the fourth part of the duodenum (B).

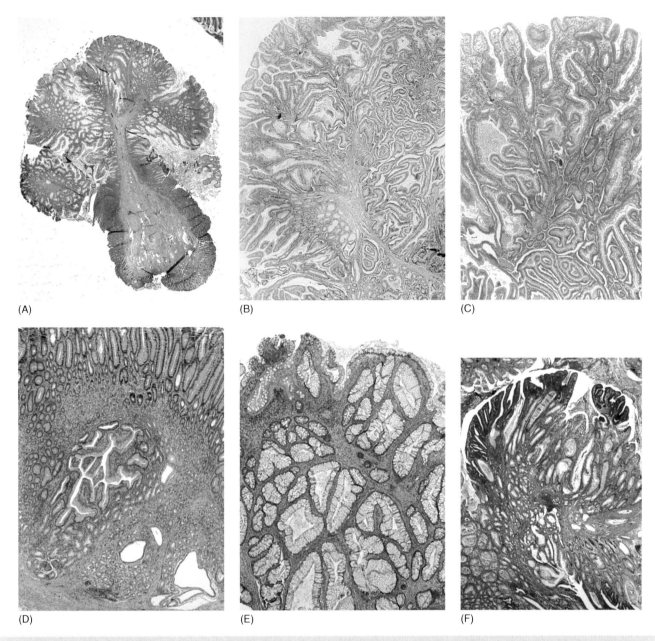

(A)   (B)   (C)

(D)   (E)   (F)

FIGURE 6.9 Peutz–Jeghers polyps develop throughout the gastrointestinal tract. Characteristic Peutz–Jeghers polyps, as seen here in the small bowel, contain lobules of mucosal elements surrounded by bundles of arborizing smooth muscle (A–C). However, these features are less well-developed in gastric polyps (D). This colonic Peutz–Jeghers polyp contains lobules of non-neoplastic mucosal elements surrounded by bundles of smooth muscle cells (E). Some lesions contain areas of dysplasia similar to that seen in tubular or villous adenomas (F).

Peutz–Jeghers polyps show dysplasia, which is usually low-grade and more commonly encountered in lesions of the colorectum (Figure 6.9F). Carcinomas may develop in either the polypoid or nonpolypoid mucosa and resemble sporadic colorectal carcinomas.

Differential Diagnosis

Peutz–Jeghers polyps most commonly simulate other types of hamartomatous polyps. The diagnosis of a Peutz–Jeghers polyp of the small intestine is straightforward, whereas gastric and colonic polyps are more problematic because they lack well-developed arborizing bundles of smooth muscle cells. Gastric Peutz–Jeghers polyps have a lobular architecture and usually lack the cystically dilated glands and pits typical of juvenile polyps and hyperplastic polyps. They also contain normal-appearing lamina propria, rather than the edematous, inflamed stroma of hyperplastic polyps and juvenile polyps. Colonic Peutz–Jeghers polyps contain rounded aggregates of epithelium and lamina propria without prominent crypt dilation, which is more typical of juvenile polyps, and there can be substantial morphologic overlap that causes diagnostic confusion. Stromal edema with inflammation and mucosal cysts are sometimes present in Peutz–Jeghers polyps of the colon to such an extent that they may not be discernible from juvenile polyps based on histologic evaluation alone.

Peutz–Jeghers polyps can also simulate the features of mucosal prolapse polyps, adenomas with misplaced epithelium, and invasive adenocarcinomas. Mucosal prolapse polyps contain prominent bundles of smooth muscle cells emanating from the muscularis mucosae, but also show other distinguishing features, such as erosions, crypt regeneration, and hyperplasia, ischemic injury, and inflammation. Lobules of mucosal elements in the bowel wall simulate epithelial misplacement in adenomas, although Peutz–Jeghers polyps contain non-neoplastic epithelium and lack hemosiderin deposits, extruded mucin, hemorrhage, fibrosis, and other features of trauma. Hamartomatous elements in the bowel wall may simulate invasive adenocarcinoma, particularly when they contain dysplastic epithelium. Helpful diagnostic features include the lobular arrangement of non-neoplastic, or low-grade dysplastic, and presence of epithelium invested with lamina propria, rather than the desmoplastic stroma of an invasive carcinoma.

Juvenile Polyposis Syndrome

Overview of Molecular Features

Juvenile polyposis syndrome is an autosomal dominant hereditary hamartomatous polyposis syndrome resulting from defects in the signal transduction pathway initiated by TGF-β. Approximately 20% of patients prove to have germline mutations in *SMAD4,* located on chromosome 18q21.1, and 20% to 25% of patients have mutations in *BMBR1A*, located on chromosome 10q22.3. As is the case in other hereditary polyposis disorders, specific mutations give rise to phenotypically different patterns of disease. Polyposis of the upper gastrointestinal tract is more common among patients with *SMAD4* mutations, whereas cardiac defects are more common among patients with germline *BMPR1A* mutations. Large deletions that encompass *BMBR1A* and *PTEN*, two contiguous tumor suppressor genes, have been described in infantile juvenile polyposis. Of note, less than 50% of patients with juvenile polyposis syndrome have a family history of the disease.

Clinical Features

Sporadic juvenile polyps are relatively common, affecting 1% to 2% of pediatric patients. They are smooth, somewhat friable mucosal-based polyps that may be pedunculated or sessile. Most sporadic juvenile polyps develop in the rectum, though they infrequently develop proximal

to the splenic flexure. Signs and symptoms usually reflect gastrointestinal bleeding, and include heme-positive stools, anemia, and passage of blood or tissue (autoamputated polyps) per rectum.

Juvenile polyposis syndrome affects one in 100,000 persons in the United States and shows variably severe disease depending on the type of mutation present. Infantile juvenile polyposis presents within the first two years of life in patients without a family history of juvenile polyposis syndrome. Manifestations include generalized gastrointestinal polyposis with bleeding, malabsorptive diarrhea, and protein-losing enteropathy, which can be life-threatening. Hamartomatous polyps are limited to the colons of patients with juvenile polyposis coli. Generalized juvenile polyposis manifests with numerous gastrointestinal polyps of the stomach, small intestine, and colon. Diagnostic criteria include (a) three or more colorectal juvenile polyps, (b) any number of extracolonic juvenile polyps, or (c) any number of juvenile polyps in patients with a family history of the syndrome.

Extraintestinal congenital abnormalities can be found in 10% to 20% of patients with juvenile polyposis syndrome. Some patients with *SMAD4* mutations develop hereditary hemorrhagic telangiectasia characterized by systemic vascular malformations, and pulmonary arteriovenous malformations as well as hypertrophic osteoarthropathy. Although patients with juvenile polyposis syndrome have gastrointestinal hamartomas, they are at increased risk for carcinomas of the colorectum (cumulative risk of nearly 70% by 60 years of age), stomach, pancreas, and proximal small intestine.

Patients with juvenile polyposis syndrome develop numerous colorectal polyps, ranging from a few to several hundred lesions (Figure 6.10A–C). Small intestinal and gastric polyps also occur in patients with generalized juvenile polyposis. Small lesions are sessile and erythematous polyps that resemble hyperplastic polyps, whereas larger polyps are usually pedunculated with erosions or ulcers (Figure 6.10D). Some juvenile polyps have a mulberry-like appearance and these have been termed "atypical juvenile polyps." Atypical juvenile polyps occur only in association with juvenile polyposis syndrome.

Pathologic Features and Diagnostic Considerations

Juvenile polyps are round, smooth lesions with surface erythema reflecting the presence of inflamed, eosinophil-rich stroma and frequent erosions (Figure 6.11A–B). Cross sections reveal numerous cysts that correspond to dilated crypts (colon) or glands (stomach) in the polyp head. Some polyps also contain clusters of ganglion cells in the mucosa. Sporadic and syndromic juvenile polyps can be indistinguishable, although many syndromic polyps display less crypt dilation and stromal edema. Atypical juvenile polyps occur exclusively in association with the syndrome

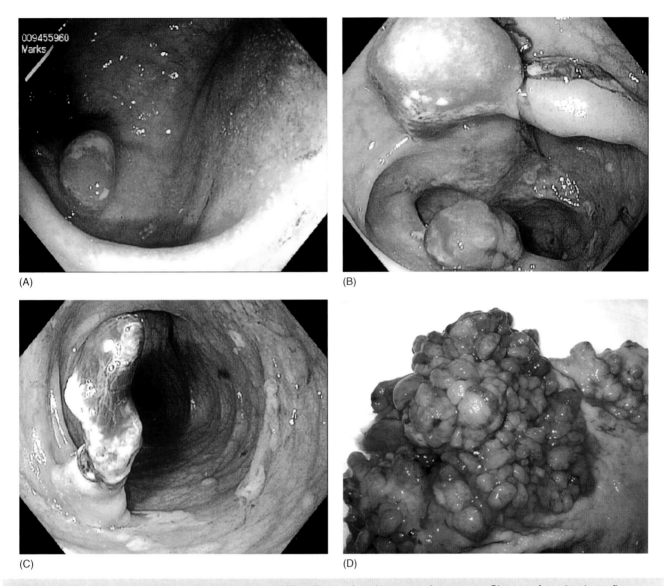

(A) (B) (C) (D)

FIGURE 6.10 A 3-year-old girl presented with anal bleeding and underwent colonoscopy. She was found to have five polyps, including three in the rectum and two in the abdominal colon, all of which proved to be juvenile polyps. All were smooth, sessile polyps with surface erythema and erosions (A). A 4-year-old girl was evaluated for hematochezia and proved to have juvenile polyposis coli. Multiple large polyps were present in the rectosigmoid colon, with stigmata of recent bleeding (B). The same patient had an irregular, pedunculated polyp in the sigmoid colon (C). Another patient with juvenile polyposis syndrome underwent a gastric resection. Juvenile polyps carpet the mucosa and simulate the appearance of Ménétrier disease (D).

and usually develop in the colon (Figure 6.11C). They contain crowded, irregularly shaped crypts with little intervening stroma. Some atypical juvenile polyps display areas of dysplasia, which is usually low-grade (Figure 6.11D). Carcinomas can develop in either polypoid or nonpolypoid mucosa.

Differential Diagnosis

Juvenile polyposis syndrome simulates other hamartomatous syndromes and inflammatory conditions. Fascicles of smooth muscle cells may be prominent and simulate

the appearance of Peutz–Jeghers polyps, although juvenile polyps with this finding also typically contain cystically dilated crypts and inflamed stroma, both of which are less frequent in Peutz–Jeghers polyps. Distinction between juvenile polyposis syndrome and inflammatory-type polyps due to other conditions is more problematic. Colonic juvenile polyps may be histologically indistinguishable from polyps seen in inflammatory bowel disease, inflammatory "cap" polyposis, and Cronkhite–Canada syndrome, whereas gastric involvement can mimic hyperplastic polyps or Ménétrier disease, particularly in biopsy samples. All of these disorders display inflammatory

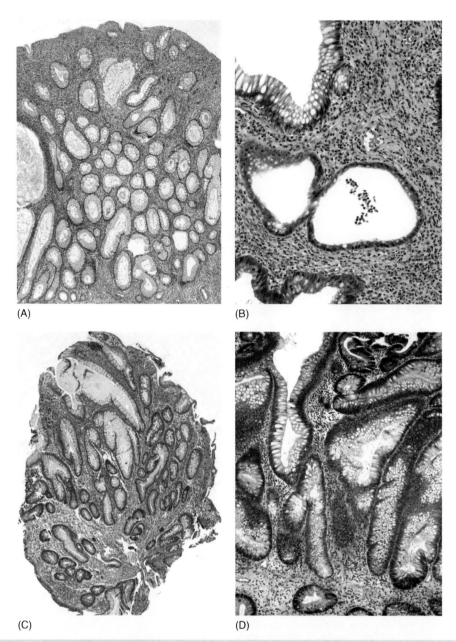

(A)   (B)

(C)   (D)

FIGURE 6.11   Juvenile polyps contain cystically dilated crypts that are irregularly dispersed in inflamed stroma (A), which contains a mixed inflammatory cell infiltrate rich in eosinophils (B). Atypical juvenile polyps display crowded crypts with less conspicuous cysts and stroma, thereby more closely resembling inflammatory polyps that develop in other conditions, such as inflammatory bowel disease (C). Atypical juvenile polyps may contain areas of dysplasia, which is often low-grade and similar to that seen in tubular or villous adenomas (D).

changes in the nonpolypoid mucosa, which is normal in patients with juvenile polyposis syndrome.

PTEN Hamartoma Tumor Syndrome

Overview of Molecular Features

PTEN hamartoma tumor syndrome is an autosomal dominant cancer syndrome that encompasses the previously named entities Cowden syndrome, Lhermitte–Duclos syndrome, and Bannayan–Ruvalcaba–Riley syndrome, as well as related disorders that develop as a result of germline *PTEN* mutations. This gene encodes phosphatase and tensin homolog, which is a 403 amino acid phosphatase with tumor suppressor activity. The PTEN protein plays key regulatory roles in cell cycling and migration, apoptosis, and genomic stability. Patients who have phenotypic manifestations of disease but lack *PTEN* mutations may harbor other germline alterations, including mutations in succinyl dehydrogenase complex subunits B (*SDHB*) on 1p35-36 or D (*SDHD*) on 11q23, hypermethylation of the *KLLN* promoter, and *PIK3CA* or *AKT1* mutations.

Clinical and Endoscopic Features

PTEN hamartoma tumor syndrome affects approximately one in 200,000 persons. Between 35% and 40% of patients develop numerous hamartomatous polyps throughout the gastrointestinal tract in combination with a variety of extraintestinal abnormalities. Gastrointestinal manifestations include glycogenic acanthosis, hyperplastic and inflammatory polyps, adenomas, and mesenchymal polyps (Figure 6.12). Breast and thyroid disease are the most common extraintestinal abnormalities. Female patients develop fibrocystic breast disease and breast cancer at a much higher rate and at an earlier age than women in the general population (estimated lifetime cancer risk of 25% to 50% compared to 10%). Hashimoto thyroiditis is relatively common and the lifetime risk for thyroid cancer is nearly 10%. Other extraintestinal manifestations include oral papillomas, cutaneous trichilemmomas, and acral keratoses, macrocephaly, and mental impairment.

The above-mentioned features are characteristic of Cowden syndrome, although several phenotypic variants exist. Patients with Lhermitte–Duclos disease have some of these findings in addition to dysplastic gangliocytomas of the cerebellum. Patients with Bannayan–Ruvalcaba–Riley syndrome develop hamartomas in combination with lipomatosis, hemagiomas, and mixed vascular and fatty tumors involving skin and viscera. Additional craniofacial features include downslanting palpebral fissures, ocular hypertelorism, pseudopapilledema and prominent corneal nerves, café au lait spots, acanthosis nigricans, and wart-like lesions. Most affected males have pigmented macules on the shaft and glans penis. Musculoskeletal abnormalities are present in more than 50% of patients and usually reflect hypotonia of proximal muscles due to abnormal lipid storage, although hyperextensible joints, scoliosis, and pectus excavatum are common. Autism spectrum disorder with macrocephaly, Proteus syndrome, and VATER with macrocephaly have also been reported in association with PTEN mutations.

Pathologic Features

Diffuse glycogenic acanthosis of the esophagus develops in 20% to 80% of affected patients (Figure 6.12A). The endoscopic features of gastrointestinal polyps are variable, depending on the relative amounts of epithelium, stroma, and inflammation present in the lesions. Adenomas may appear as sessile or pedunculated mucosa-based polyps similar to sporadic polyps, whereas mesenchymal lesions are dome-shaped, smooth polyps surfaced by normal mucosa and those with inflammatory changes display erythema or erosions. Gastric lesions mimic hyperplastic polyps and contain cystically dilated pits lined by mucin-depleted or hypermucinous epithelium. Intestinal lesions contain cystic crypts within an expanded and inflamed lamina propria similar to juvenile polyps (Figure 6.12B–C). Some PTEN hamartomatous polyps contain bundles of myofibroblastic spindle cells (Figure 6.12D), ganglion cells, or fat in the polyp head, all of which may be helpful diagnostic features. Lipomas, ganglioneuromas, and lymphoid nodules are often detected as small, incidental lesions upon colonoscopic examination. Indeed, one should consider the possibility of PTEN hamartoma tumor syndrome in any patient with multiple mesenchymal lesions or "hyperplastic" polyps that contain fat or spindle cells in the lamina propria.

Differential Diagnosis

Diffuse esophageal glycogenic acanthosis is virtually pathognomonic of PTEN hamartoma tumor syndrome, and essentially has no histologic differential diagnosis, although the endoscopic appearance may simulate either eosinophilic esophagitis or Candida infection. Syndromic hamartomatous polyps with prominent spindle cells can be indistinguishable from sporadic leiomyomas, benign stromal/epithelial polyps (ie, perineurioma), and ganglioneuromas, but the presence of multiple lesions is strongly suggestive of PTEN hamartoma tumor syndrome. Other gastrointestinal hamartomas that develop in association with PTEN hamartoma tumor syndrome bear a resemblance to inflammatory-type polyps and display variably dilated crypts or pits enmeshed in inflamed lamina propria, thereby simulating juvenile polyposis and Cronkhite–Canada syndrome, as well as inflammatory-type polyps unassociated with polyposis syndromes. Isolated gastric hyperplastic polyps and mucosal abnormalities of Ménétrier disease simulate the features of gastric hamartomas, whereas the differential diagnosis of colorectal lesions includes inflammatory-type polyps associated with mucosal prolapse, inflammatory cap polyposis, or inflammatory bowel disease.

The distribution of disease in the gastrointestinal tract aids distinction of PTEN hamartoma tumor syndrome from inflammatory conditions that may be considered in the differential diagnosis. The intervening nonpolypoid mucosa of patients with PTEN hamartoma tumor syndrome is essentially normal, whereas many of the entities in the differential diagnosis (inflammatory bowel disease or Cronkhite–Canada syndrome, for example) have inflamed intervening nonpolypoid mucosa. The PTEN hamartoma tumor syndrome should be considered in any patient with multiple inflammatory-type polyps, especially if they occur in combination with adenomas and mesenchymal polyps, or contain a myofibroblastic spindle cell proliferation in the lamina propria. However, many PTEN hamartomas lack distinctive features, so evaluation of patients with multiple juvenile or inflammatory-type polyps should include molecular testing for this possibility.

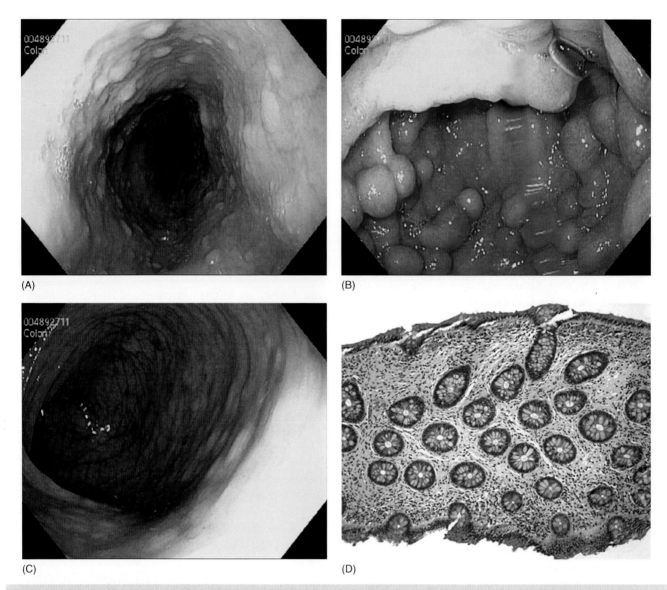

FIGURE 6.12 A 25-year-old woman underwent surveillance endoscopy for Cowden syndrome. Glycogenic acanthosis appears as numerous white plaques throughout the esophagus (A). Numerous hamartomas form smooth, round nodules in the duodenum (B). Colonic hamartomas appear as subtle excrescences surfaced by normal mucosa (C). This hamartomatous colon polyp consists of normal-appearing epithelium and a spindle-cell-rich cellular proliferation in the lamina propria (D).

SUMMARY AND CONCLUSIONS

Pathologists play a major role in guiding patient management and endoscopic surveillance of patients with suspected heritable cancer syndromes. Many affected patients do not have known genetic alterations at the time of initial evaluation, and disease manifestations are often variable. Careful pathologic assessment of morphologic features and distribution of disease is vital to the evaluation of patients with multiple gastrointestinal polyps. The distinction between subtypes of adenomatous polyposis coli is best made through germline mutational testing, although some histologic clues are typical of lesions associated with Lynch syndrome, such as tumor heterogeneity

and intraepithelial lymphocytes. However, the onset of MSI-H is a relatively late event in Lynch-related neoplasia, so its absence from an adenoma (or preservation of mismatch repair protein staining) does not necessarily exclude the possibility of Lynch syndrome.

Histologically similar hamartomatous polyps can occur in patients with different types of syndromic polyposis (see also Table 6.2). Key features in the past medical history should alert pathologists to the possibility of a hamartomatous disorder. These include the presence of hyperplastic and inflammatory-type polyps, particularly if they are multiple, affect the upper and lower gastrointestinal tract, or develop in the proximal small bowel where such lesions are uncommon. Multiple diagnoses of ganglioneuroma, perineurioma, and lipoma in biopsies from a single patient should also arouse suspicion, particularly if they occur in combination with hyperplastic polyps or adenomas.

SPECIFIC ILLUSTRATIVE EXAMPLES

Case 1

A 45-year-old man with no significant past medical history presented to his primary care physician with rectal bleeding and abdominal pain. Colonoscopy demonstrated an extensive polyposis, with lesions ranging from a few millimeters to 3 cm. Snare polypectomy of one of the larger lesions located in the distal transverse colon revealed a tubulovillous adenoma (Figure 6.13A), while biopsy of

a flat lesion in the right colon revealed a sessile serrated polyp (Figure 6.13B). There was no known cancer history in the patient's parents or grandparents. An upper endoscopy was negative. The patient underwent a total proctocolectomy for what was deemed to be a polyposis not amenable to endoscopic management.

Gross examination of the colectomy specimen revealed 85 to 95 polyps, ranging in size from 0.1 to 3 cm (Figure 6.13C), which were right-side predominant (Figure 6.13D). All of the polyps greater than 1 cm in size were entirely submitted; 15 additional polyps from throughout the colon were sampled in five cassettes. The larger polyps represented adenomas, while several sessile serrated polyps and hyperplastic polyps were also noted.

The patient was referred to a genetic counselor and *APC* mutation testing was pursued, which failed to

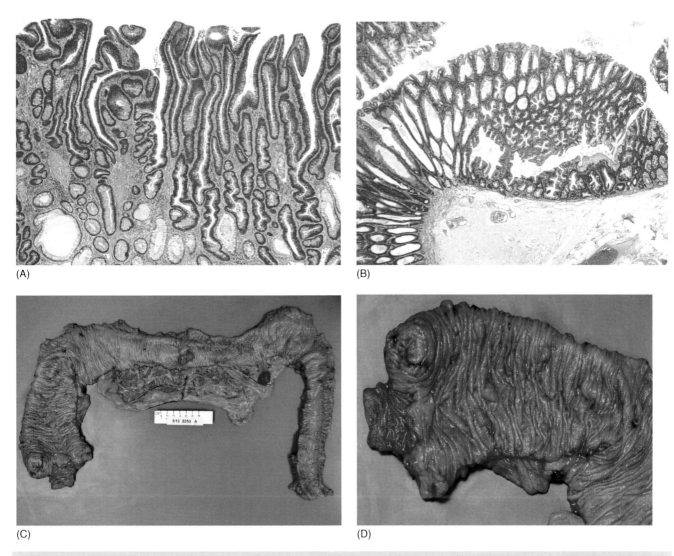

(A)

(B)

(C)

(D)

FIGURE 6.13 A 45-year-old man with *MUTYH*-associated polyposis had an attenuated polyposis characterized by a combination of adenomas (A) and serrated polyps (B). The colectomy specimen contained fewer than 100 polyps, ranging in size from 0.1 to 3 cm (C). The polyps were right-side predominant (D).

demonstrate a germline mutation. This was followed by *MUTYH* mutation testing, and the patient was found to be a Y179C/G396D compound heterozygote. Genetic testing was offered to the patient's four siblings, each of whom was found to have a 25% risk of being affected.

Because *MUTYH*-associated polyposis was fairly recently described, the full spectrum of phenotypic and molecular alterations has not been elucidated, and this disease is often overlooked or mistaken for other polyposis syndromes. This case highlights the phenotypic overlap of *MUTYH*-associated polyposis with other hereditary cancer syndromes, particularly attenuated FAP, which complicates its recognition. In both conditions, patients typically present with 10 to 100 adenomas (ie, attenuated polyposis), and some patients with *MUTYH*-associated polyposis have serrated polyps as well. A significant minority of patients with *MUTYH*-associated polyposis also have, congenital hypertrophy of retinal pigment epithelium, osteomas, and especially duodenal adenomas, the latter of which are found in up to 25%. Approximately 15% to 20% of affected patients with *MUTYH*-associated polyposis have multiple serrated polyps and, in fact, meet diagnostic criteria for serrated polyposis. In addition, some patients present with colon cancer, typically at a relatively young age, in the absence of overt polyposis; this presentation can mimic Lynch syndrome. *MUTYH*-associated polyposis should be considered in patients with attenuated polyposis and a family history suggestive of autosomal recessive inheritance. In cases with apparent autosomal dominant inheritance, FAP should be considered first, though *MUTYH* testing may be helpful in patients in whom an *APC* mutation is not detected.

Case 2

A 40-year-old man presented to the emergency department in a rural hospital with upper gastrointestinal bleeding. He had no significant past medical history and no previous episodes of bleeding or gastrointestinal symptoms. Upon upper and lower endoscopy, the patient was found to have multiple polyps of the stomach, small bowel, and colon. The endoscopist noted that the polyps did not look like "regular" adenomatous polyps. Several were resected from the stomach and small and large bowel. The gastric polyps were ulcerated and contained dilated glands within inflamed stroma (Figure 6.14A–B). Some intestinal polyps were similar to the gastric polyps, containing enlarged, dilated glands with inspissated mucus and inflammation within prominent, markedly inflamed stroma (Figure 6.14C–D). Other intestinal polyps contained irregular, crowded crypts with much less inflammation and intervening stroma (Figure 6.14E–F). Several of the gastric and the intestinal polyps contained foci of dysplasia (Figure 6.14G–J). Upon questioning, the patient did not have a history of polyposis or cancer in his family, but he was not a good historian. Genetic testing revealed a mutation in *SMAD4*, confirming juvenile polyposis syndrome.

As previously discussed in the section on juvenile polyposis, the hamartomatous polyps of juvenile polyposis have an extensive differential diagnosis (particularly the gastric polyps), including Peutz–Jeghers polyps, inflammatory polyps, Cronkhite–Canada syndrome, and even Ménétrier disease. Genetic testing is important not only for diagnostic purposes but also in determining future surveillance and risk assessment for both

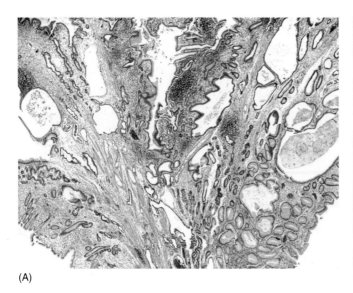

(A)

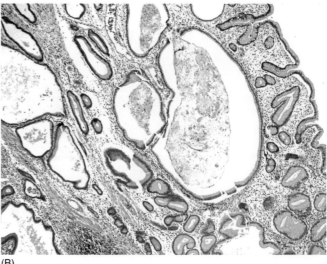

(B)

FIGURE 6.14 This gastric polyp from a patient with juvenile polyposis syndrome shows dilated, focally cystic glands containing inspissated mucus and inflammation, within inflamed stroma (A–B). (*continued*)

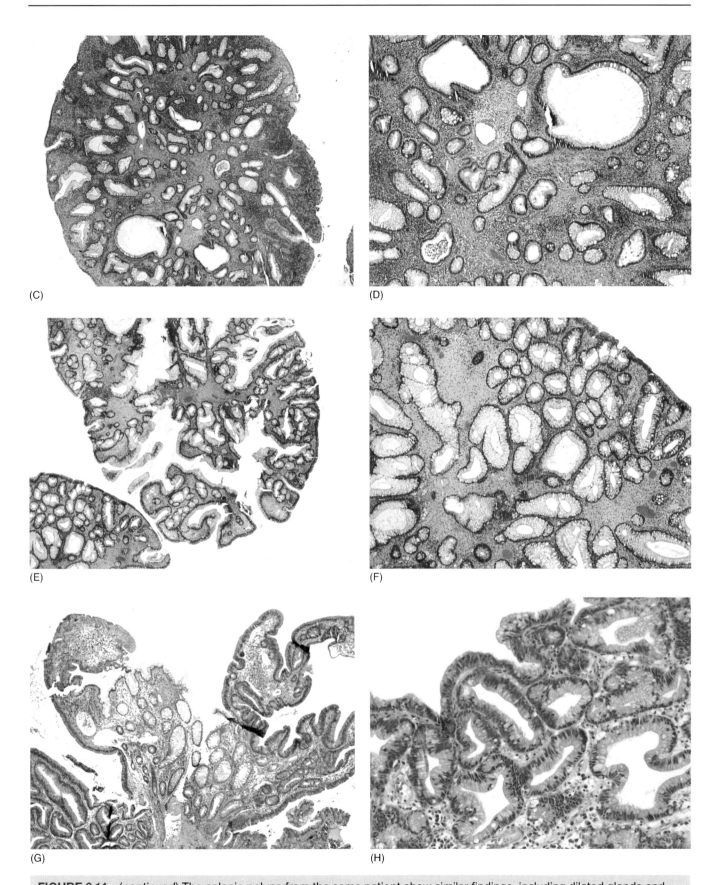

FIGURE 6.14 (*continued*) The colonic polyps from the same patient show similar findings, including dilated glands and a prominent, markedly inflamed stroma (C–D). Other intestinal polyps contained irregular, crowded crypts with much less inflammation and intervening stroma (E–F). (*continued*)

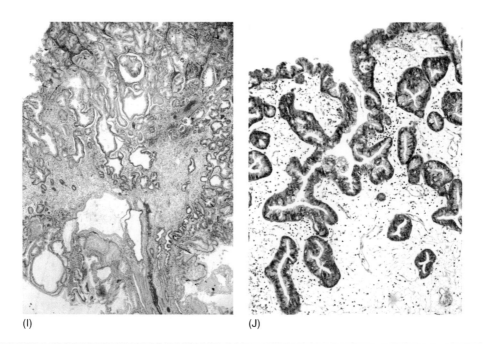

(I)   (J)

FIGURE 6.14 *(continued)* Several of the intestinal (G–H) and gastric (I–J) polyps contained foci of dysplasia.

gastrointestinal and nongastrointestinal cancers in both the patient and their family members. It is also important to note that only 20% to 50% of juvenile polyposis syndrome patients will have a family history of polyps; so lack of a history of polyposis does not exclude this diagnosis.

Case 3

A 35-year-old woman presented to her primary care physician complaining of abdominal pain and nausea. She was initially treated with proton pump inhibitor therapy, but her symptoms did not improve, and in fact worsened. She was eventually referred to a gastroenterologist. Upon endoscopy, the gastroenterologist did not see any definite lesions but took random biopsies to rule out *Helicobacter pylori*. Biopsies showed small, subtle foci of in situ signet ring cell adenocarcinoma (Figure 6.15A–C). The patient's maternal grandfather had a history of gastric cancer, and she thought that one other maternal family member had a history of breast cancer. Mutational analysis revealed a germline mutation in the *E-cadherin/CDH1* gene, and the patient was counseled regarding prophylactic gastrectomy.

Familial diffuse gastric carcinoma will be further discussed in Chapter 8, but this case illustrates several important issues that are pertinent to the discussion of hereditary cancer syndromes. This is a relatively rare condition, that poses diagnostic and therapeutic

challenges for pathologists, gastroenterologists, and surgeons. Indeed, our clinical colleagues are often surprised at the poor correlation between histologic findings and their endoscopic impressions and may have reservations regarding the value of prophylactic gastrectomy in affected patients. However, the lifetime risk for developing gastric adenocarcinoma is extremely high (greater than 80% by age 80), and women with *CDH1* germline mutations also have an increased risk of developing lobular breast cancer. Because of this increased risk, as well as the difficulty in detecting early lesions in these patients (as illustrated by this case), prophylactic gastrectomy is usually advised after age 20. Indications for genetic testing are somewhat controversial, but recent criteria suggest that the following scenarios should prompt genetic testing for this disease:

- Families with two or more cases of gastric cancer in first- or second-degree relatives, with one diffuse cancer diagnosed in a patient younger than 50 years
- Personal or family history of diffuse gastric cancer and lobular breast cancer, with one patient under the age of 50
- Three cases of diffuse gastric cancer in first- or second-degree relatives, regardless of age
- Patients diagnosed with diffuse gastric cancer before age 40, especially in a low incidence population (such as those in the United States and Canada)

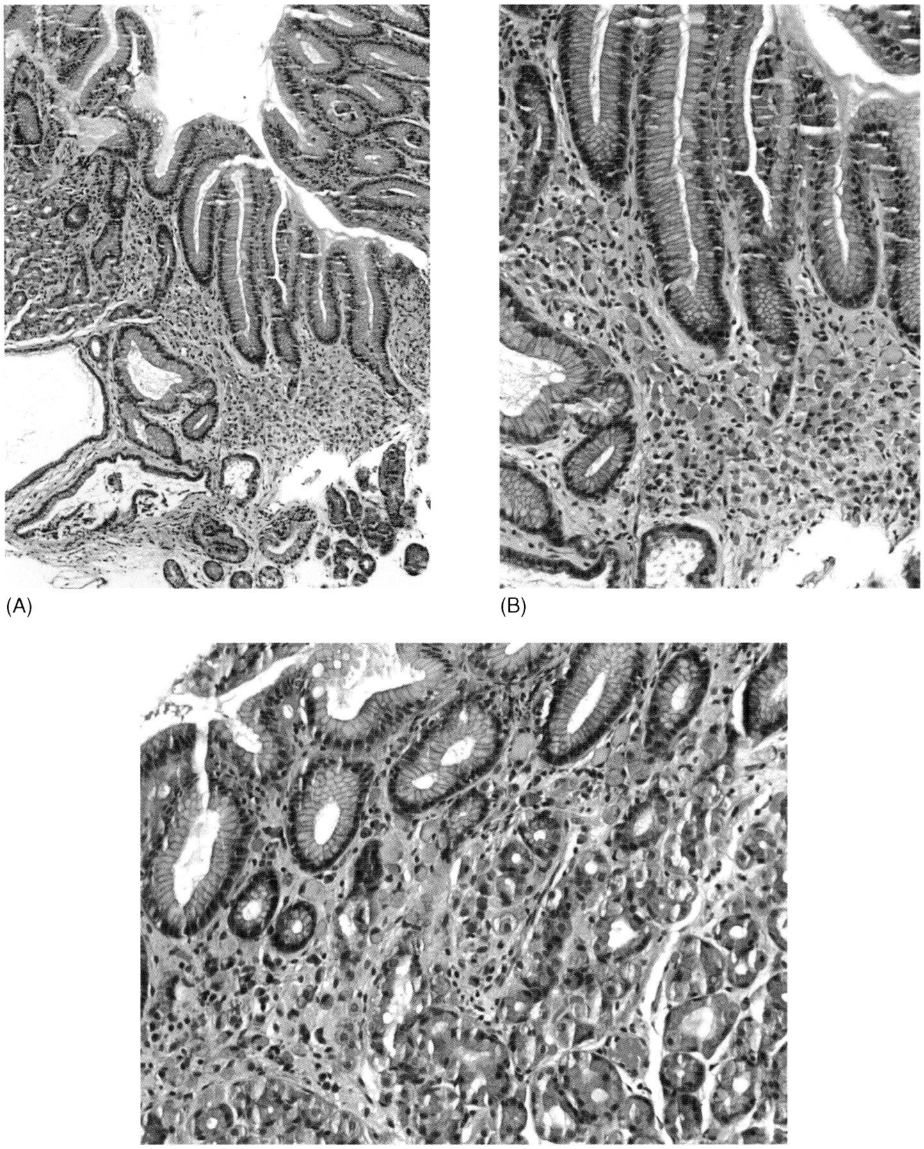

FIGURE 6.15 Gastric biopsies in patients with *CDH1* mutations often show multiple foci of in situ signet ring cell carcinoma, without corresponding macroscopically visible lesions (A–C).

SELECTED REFERENCES

General

Baron TH, Smyrk TC, Rex DK. Recommended intervals between screening and surveillance colonoscopies. *Mayo Clin Proc.* 2013;88(8):854–858.

Burn J, Mathers J, Bishop DT. Genetics, inheritance and strategies for prevention in populations at high risk of colorectal cancer (CRC). *Recent Results Cancer Res.* 2013;191:157–183.

Hegde M, Ferber M, Mao R, Samowitz W, Ganguly A. ACMG technical standards and guidelines for genetic testing for inherited colorectal cancer (Lynch syndrome, familial adenomatous polyposis, and MYH-associated polyposis). *Genet Med.* 2014;16(1):101–116.

Jasperson KW. Genetic testing by cancer site: colon (polyposis syndromes). *Cancer J.* 2012;18(4):328–333.

Lucci-Cordisco E, Risio M, Venesio T, Genuardi M. The growing complexity of the intestinal polyposis syndromes. *Am J Med Genet A.* 2013;161A(11):2777–2787.

Patel SG, Ahnen DJ. Familial colon cancer syndromes: an update of a rapidly evolving field. *Curr Gastroenterol Rep.* 2012;14(5):428–438.

Shia J, Yantiss RK. Molecular mechanisms of colorectal carcinogenesis. In: Yantiss RK, ed. *Colorectal carcinoma and tumors of the vermiform appendix.* Philadelphia, PA: Wolters Kluwer Lippincott Williams & Wilkins; 2014:191–203.

Familial Adenomatous Polyposis and Related Syndromes

Kerr SE, Thomas CB, Thibodeau SN, Ferber MJ, Halling KC. APC germline mutations in individuals being evaluated for familial adenomatous polyposis: a review of the Mayo Clinic experience with 1591 consecutive tests. *J Mol Diagn.* 2013;15(1):31–43.

Liang J, Lin C, Hu F, et al. APC polymorphisms and the risk of colorectal neoplasia: a HuGE review and meta-analysis. *Am J Epidemiol.* 2013;177(11):1169–1179.

Pavicic W, Nieminen TT, Gylling A, et al. Promoter-specific alterations of APC are a rare cause for mutation-negative familial adenomatous polyposis. *Genes, Chromosomes Cancer*. 2014;53(10):857–864.

MUTYH-Associated Polyposis

Aretz S, Uhlhaas S, Goergens H, et al. MUTYH-associated polyposis: 70 of 71 patients with biallelic mutations present with an attenuated or atypical phenotype. *Intl J Cancer*. 2006;119(4):807–814.

Nielsen M, Franken PF, Reinards TH, et al. Multiplicity in polyp count and extracolonic manifestations in 40 Dutch patients with MYH associated polyposis coli (MAP). *J Med Genet*. 2005;42(9):e54.

Nielsen M, Joerink-van de Beld MC, Jones N, et al. Analysis of MUTYH genotypes and colorectal phenotypes in patients With MUTYH-associated polyposis. *Gastroenterol*. 2009;136(2):471–476.

Vogt S, Jones N, Christian D, et al. Expanded extracolonic tumor spectrum in MUTYH-associated polyposis. *Gastroenterol*. 2009;137(6):1976–1985 e1–e10.

Lynch Syndrome

Campbell PT, Curtin K, Ulrich CM, et al. Mismatch repair polymorphisms and risk of colon cancer, tumour microsatellite instability and interactions with lifestyle factors. *Gut*. 2009;58(5):661–667.

Geiersbach KB, Samowitz WS. Microsatellite instability and colorectal cancer. *Arch Pathol Lab Med*. 2011;135(10):1269–1277.

Gudgeon JM, Williams JL, Burt RW, et al. Lynch syndrome screening implementation: business analysis by a healthcare system. *Am J Managed Care*. 2011;17(8):e288–e300.

Jasperson KW, Samowitz WS, Burt RW. Constitutional mismatch repair-deficiency syndrome presenting as colonic adenomatous polyposis: clues from the skin. *Clin Genet*. 2011;80(4):394–397.

Kerber RA, Neklason DW, Samowitz WS, Burt RW. Frequency of familial colon cancer and hereditary nonpolyposis colorectal cancer (Lynch syndrome) in a large population database. *Fam Cancer*. 2005;4(3):239–244.

Rasmussen LJ, Heinen CD, Royer-Pokora B, et al. Pathological assessment of mismatch repair gene variants in Lynch syndrome: past, present, and future. *Hum Mutat*. 2012;33(12):1617–1625.

Samowitz WS, Curtin K, Wolff RK, et al. Microsatellite instability and survival in rectal cancer. *Cancer Causes Control*. 2009;20(9):1763–1768.

Shia J, Holck S, Depetris G, et al. Lynch syndrome-associated neoplasms: a discussion on histopathology and immunohistochemistry. *Fam Cancer*. 2013;12(2):241–260.

Shia J, Stadler Z, Weiser MR, et al. Immunohistochemical staining for DNA mismatch repair proteins in intestinal tract carcinoma: how reliable are biopsy samples? *Am J Surg Pathol*. 2011;35(3):447–454.

Steinhagen E, Shia J, Markowitz AJ, et al. Systematic immunohistochemistry screening for Lynch syndrome in early age-of-onset colorectal cancer patients undergoing surgical resection. *J Am Coll Surg*. 2012;214(1):61–67.

Steinke V, Holzapfel S, Loeffler M, et al. Evaluating the performance of clinical criteria for predicting mismatch repair gene mutations in Lynch syndrome: a comprehensive analysis of 3,671 families. *Int J Cancer*. 2014;135(1):69–77.

Vaughn CP, Baker CL, Samowitz WS, Swensen JJ. The frequency of previously undetectable deletions involving 3′ exons of the PMS2 gene. *Genes, Chromosomes Cancer*. 2013;52(1):107–112.

Hamartomatous Polyposes

Bennett KL, Mester J, Eng C. Germline epigenetic regulation of KILLIN in Cowden and Cowden-like syndrome. *JAMA*. 2010;304(24):2724–2731.

Canzonieri C, Centenara L, Ornati F, et al. Endoscopic evaluation of gastrointestinal tract in patients with hereditary hemorrhagic telangiectasia and correlation with their genotypes. *Genet Med*. 2014;16(1):3–10.

Heald B, Mester J, Rybicki L, Orloff MS, Burke CA, Eng C. Frequent gastrointestinal polyps and colorectal adenocarcinomas in a prospective series of PTEN mutation carriers. *Gastroenterol*. 2010;139(6):1927–1933.

Hiljadnikova Bajro M, Sukarova-Angelovska E, Adelaide J, et al. A new case with 10q23 interstitial deletion encompassing both PTEN and BMPR1A narrows the genetic region deleted in juvenile polyposis syndrome. *J Appl Genet*. 2013;54(1):43–47.

Jee MJ, Yoon SM, Kim EJ, et al. A novel germline mutation in exon 10 of the SMAD4 gene in a familial juvenile polyposis. *Gut Liver*. 2013;7(6):747–751.

Lachlan KL. Cowden syndrome and the PTEN hamartoma tumor syndrome: how to define rare genetic syndromes. *J Natl Cancer Inst*. 2013;105(21):1595–1597.

Latchford AR, Neale K, Phillips RK, Clark SK. Juvenile polyposis syndrome: a study of genotype, phenotype, and long-term outcome. *Dis Col Rect*. 2012;55(10):1038–1043.

Marsh Durban V, Jansen M, Davies EJ, et al. Epithelial-specific loss of PTEN results in colorectal juvenile polyp formation and invasive cancer. *Am J Pathol*. 2014;184(1):86–91.

Mester JL, Moore RA, Eng C. PTEN germline mutations in patients initially tested for other hereditary cancer syndromes: would use of risk assessment tools reduce genetic testing? *The Oncologist*. 2013;18(10):1083–1090.

Ni Y, Zbuk KM, Sadler T, et al. Germline mutations and variants in the succinate dehydrogenase genes in Cowden and Cowden-like syndromes. *Am J Hum Genet*. 2008;83(2):261–268.

Orloff MS, He X, Peterson C, et al. Germline PIK3CA and AKT1 mutations in Cowden and Cowden-like syndromes. *Am J Hum Genet*. 2013;92(1):76–80.

Pilarski R, Burt R, Kohlman W, Pho L, Shannon KM, Swisher E. Cowden syndrome and the PTEN hamartoma tumor syndrome: systematic review and revised diagnostic criteria. *J Natl Cancer Inst*. 2013;105(21):1607–1616.

Septer S, Zhang L, Lawson CE, et al. Aggressive juvenile polyposis in children with chromosome 10q23 deletion. *World J Gastroenterol*. 2013;19(14):2286–2292.

Tse JY, Wu S, Shinagare SA, et al. Peutz-Jeghers syndrome: a critical look at colonic Peutz-Jeghers polyps. *Mod Pathol*. 2013;26(9):1235–1240.

Wain KE, Ellingson MS, McDonald J, et al. Appreciating the broad clinical features of SMAD4 mutation carriers: a multicenter chart review. *Genet Med*. 2014;16(8):588–593.

White BD, Chien AJ, Dawson DW. Dysregulation of Wnt/beta-catenin signaling in gastrointestinal cancers. *Gastroenterol*. 2012;142(2):219–232.

Yantiss RK. Hamartomatous polyps and polyposis syndromes. In: Yantiss RK, ed. *Colorectal carcinoma and tumors of the vermiform appendix*. Philadelphia, PA: Wolters Kluwer Lippincott Williams & Wilkins; 2014:33–56.

7

Neoplasms of the Esophagus

RHONDA K. YANTISS

INTRODUCTION

A variety of benign and malignant neoplasms occur in the esophagus; these can be broadly classified as epithelial, mesenchymal, and lymphoid proliferations (Table 7.1). In the esophagus, epithelial tumors (both benign and malignant) are far more common than those of mesenchymal or lymphoid origin. Indeed, benign lymphoid proliferations and lymphomas are exceedingly rare primary esophageal lesions; most cases represent secondary esophageal involvement in the setting of systemic disease. The purpose of this chapter is to discuss the most common tumors and tumor-like lesions of the esophagus. Diseases that can affect any part of the gastrointestinal tract, but infrequently affect the esophagus, are discussed elsewhere.

INFLAMMATORY AND NON-NEOPLASTIC LESIONS

Gastroenterologists frequently identify and sample endoscopically apparent polyps and excrescences in the esophagus, most of which are clinically inconsequential. Polyps, plaques, and nodules of the proximal esophagus generally reflect small islands of heterotopic tissue, whereas those of the distal esophagus tend to be reactive lesions related to gastroesophageal reflux disease or other forms of esophagitis. The latter may contain squamous epithelium, glandular mucosa, or both, thereby mimicking either squamous or glandular neoplasms. For this reason, a brief discussion of these entities is warranted.

Glycogenic Acanthosis

Glycogenic acanthosis appears as one or more white mucosal plaques spanning only a few millimeters. Solitary or scattered lesions are common and of no clinical importance, whereas diffuse esophageal glycogenic acanthosis resembling candidiasis is a relatively specific manifestation of PTEN hamartoma tumor (Cowden) syndrome. Lesions reflect nodular expansion of the epithelium by increased numbers of keratinocytes that contain abundant cytoplasmic glycogen, which can be highlighted with a periodic acid–Schiff (PAS) stain (Figure 7.1A–B). Glycogenic acanthosis is best appreciated when both lesional and nonlesional tissues are included in the biopsy. Occasionally, gastroenterologists may also mistake glycogenic acanthosis for the white plaques seen in eosinophilic esophagitis.

Squamous Papilloma

Squamous papillomas are very common and have a reported prevalence of 1% in the general population, although it is likely that many reported cases are best considered to be inflammatory-type polyps. Squamous papillomas are classified as endophytic, exophytic, and spiked. Endophytic papillomas are almost exclusively located in the distal esophagus. They are most common among patients with gastroesophageal reflux disease or other types of esophagitis, but are not consistently associated with human papillomavirus (HPV) infection. For this reason, some pathologists classify these lesions as inflammatory-type polyps, rather than papillomas, in order to

TABLE 7.1　Classification of Esophageal Neoplasms According to the World Health Organization

Epithelial Tumors	Mesenchymal Tumors
Premalignant lesions	Granular cell tumor
Squamous dysplasia (intraepithelial neoplasia)	Hemangioma
Low-grade	Leiomyoma
High-grade	Lipoma
Glandular dysplasia (intraepithelial neoplasia)	Gastrointestinal stromal tumor
Low-grade	Kaposi sarcoma
High-grade	Leiomyosarcoma
Carcinoma	Melanoma
Squamous cell carcinoma	Rhabdomyosarcoma
Basaloid squamous cell carcinoma	Synovial sarcoma
Spindle cell (sarcomatoid) carcinoma	
Verrucous squamous cell carcinoma	**Lymphoma**
Adenocarcinoma	
Adenosquamous carcinoma	**Secondary malignancies**
Mucoepidermoid carcinoma	
Adenoid cystic carcinoma	
Undifferentiated carcinoma	
(Neuro)Endocrine neoplasms	
Well-differentiated (neuro)endocrine tumor	
G1	
G2	
Poorly differentiated (neuro)endocrine carcinoma	
Large cell variant	
Small cell variant	
Mixed adeno(neuro)endocrine carcinoma	

avoid unnecessary concern on the part of the clinician and/or patient. Endophytic squamous papillomas have smooth, rounded contours and are surfaced by variably thick squamous epithelium that is usually inflamed or even ulcerated (Figure 7.2A). The papillae are elongated with expansion of the basal zone, intercellular edema, and inflamed granulation tissue in the lamina propria (Figure 7.2B).

Exophytic papillomas contain broad, finger-like projections of lamina propria lined by hyperplastic squamous epithelium. The cells display minimal, if any, cytologic atypia and convincing viral cytopathic changes are typically lacking (Figure 7.2C). Historical studies demonstrated HPV DNA in nearly 80% of cases, although these older experiments may have been compromised by contaminant DNA in study samples. More recent reports have failed to identify a clear association between squamous papillomas and HPV. Similar to endophytic lesions, exophytic papillomas show a predilection for the distal esophagus and are more commonly observed in patients with esophagitis. They may be multiple, but do not have an established association with squamous dysplasia or squamous cell carcinoma of the esophagus.

Spiked papillomas are morphologically distinct and comprise the least common subtype of squamous papilloma. They may display hyperkeratosis with a verrucous appearance and occur anywhere in the esophagus (Figure 7.2D). Squamous hyperplasia with hyperkeratosis is typical and some cases do show a prominent granular cell layer with koilocytic features, similar to cutaneous verrucae. Unlike other subtypes, spiked papillomas frequently harbor HPV DNA. They have not been associated with increased risk of squamous dysplasia or squamous cell carcinoma.

Inflammatory-Type Polyp

Most esophageal inflammatory-type polyps occur in close proximity to the gastroesophageal junction. They are frequently encountered in patients with esophagitis, including erosive gastroesophageal reflux disease, pill esophagitis, prior surgery, and infection. Those that develop in the squamous-lined esophagus have been

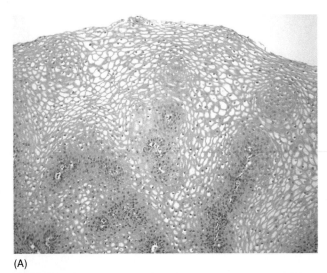
(A)

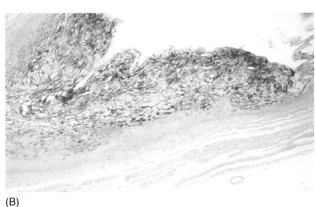
(B)

FIGURE 7.1　Glycogenic acanthosis produces pale white mucosal plaques that reflect accumulation of glycogen within squamous epithelial cells. Enlarged cells have abundant colorless cytoplasm and expand the full thickness of the epithelium (A). PAS stain highlights the cytoplasmic glycogen (B).

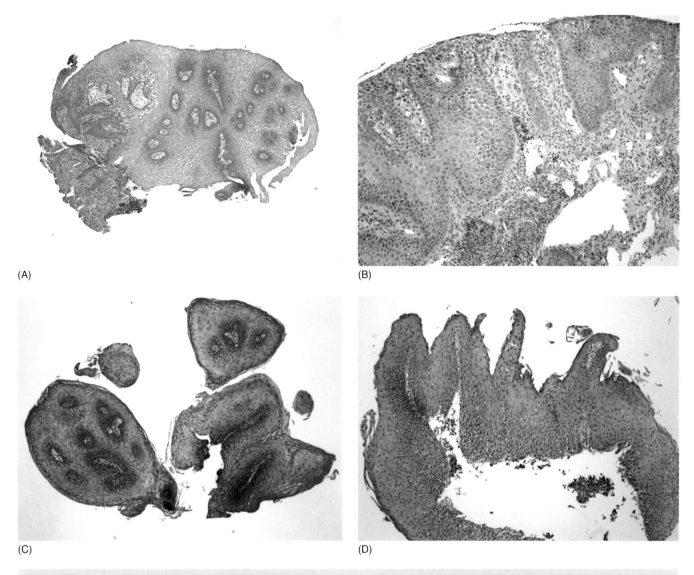

(A)

(B)

(C)

(D)

FIGURE 7.2 Endophytic squamous papillomas have a nodular appearance and are composed of hyperplastic squamous mucosa with inflamed, edematous lamina propria (A). This endophytic papilloma shows mild reactive cytologic atypia and intraepithelial neutrophils (B). Exophytic squamous papillomas consist of frond-like projections of hyperplastic squamous epithelium and edematous lamina propria (C). Spiked squamous papillomas contain proliferating squamous cells with a verrucous appearance (D).

termed "endophytic squamous papillomas," as described in the preceding paragraphs. Inflammatory-type polyps of the gastroesophageal junction and gastric cardia contain glandular mucosa at the surface. These hyperplastic, or regenerative, polyps contain an edematous lamina propria covered by either hypermucinous or mucin-depleted foveolar epithelium (Figure 7.3A–C). They may display a villous or serrated appearance at low magnification, similar to hyperplastic/regenerative polyps of the gastric mucosa.

Esophageal Heterotopias

At least 10% of patients undergoing upper endoscopic evaluation have islands of ectopic mucosa in the proximal to mid esophagus. Most of these lesions consist of gastric mucosa. Clinicians refer to them as "inlet patches" because they appear as pink plaques at the inlet of the esophagus. Gastric heterotopias may contain antral-type mucosa, oxyntic glands, or a combination of both. They are generally asymptomatic, although large lesions may secrete enough acid to produce heartburn, dysphagia, or bleeding, and some become colonized by *Helicobacter pylori*. Transformation to adenocarcinoma is extremely rare. Heterotopias may also consist of sebaceous glands (Figure 7.4); these lesions are known as Fordyce spots. They appear as solitary yellow plaques or nodules owing to the presence of parakeratotic debris overlying sebaceous glands, as well as abundant lipid within glands.

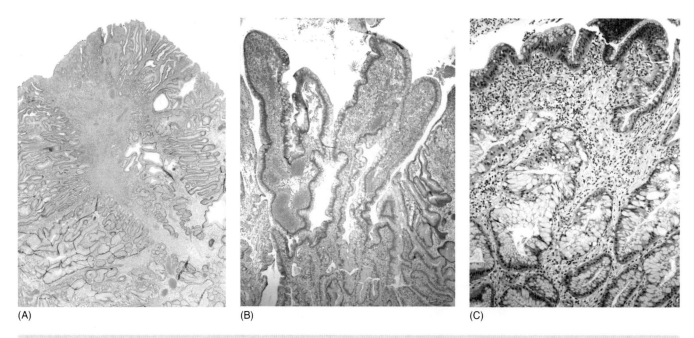

(A)   (B)   (C)

FIGURE 7.3 Inflammatory polyps at the gastroesophageal junction resemble gastric hyperplastic polyps. Finger-like projections of inflamed lamina propria support hypermucinous epithelial cells (A–B). Slightly convoluted pits are enmeshed in inflamed lamina propria and lined by distended mucinous cells (C), and mucin-depleted foveolar epithelium may also be present on the polyp surface.

Heterotopic pancreatic tissue is a common finding in biopsy samples of the gastroesophageal junction, reportedly present in up to 25% of normal patients. Pancreatic heterotopias consist of tightly packed lobules of acini lined by polarized cells with basally located nuclei and granular, luminally oriented cytoplasm (Figure 7.5A–B). Although this finding has historically been considered a metaplastic response to gastroesophageal reflux disease,

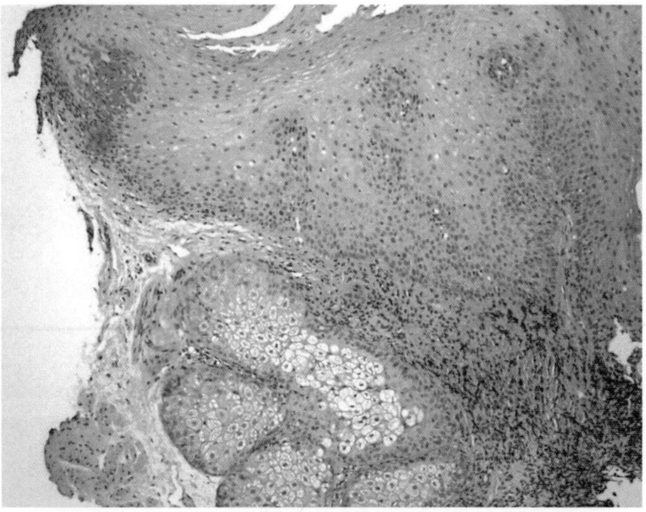

FIGURE 7.4 This sebaceous heterotopia produced an endoscopically evident yellow plaque in the midesophagus. Lobules of mature sebaceous glands are present beneath the squamous mucosa.

its frequent occurrence among both pediatric patients and healthy individuals with normal pH probe studies argues against this viewpoint.

EPITHELIAL NEOPLASMS

Squamous Dysplasia and Squamous Cell Carcinoma

Epidemiology and Pathogenesis

Squamous cell carcinoma is the most common malignant tumor of the esophagus worldwide, yet its incidence varies depending on several factors. Most patients are older adults, and men are affected more frequently than women. Areas of highest incidence include China, Iran, South America, and South Africa, where risk is associated with lower socioeconomic status, dietary nitrates, and vitamin deficiencies. Risk factors for squamous cell carcinoma in Europe and the United States include alcohol use, smoking, and radiation, although the incidence of disease has been decreasing in these regions over the past several decades. Patients with squamous dysplasia, underlying achalasia, Plummer–Vinson syndrome, chronic esophagitis, or strictures are at particularly increased risk, as are those with tylosis palmaris et plantaris, a hereditary disorder resulting from a defect in *RHBDF2*, which encodes a serine protease important to epithelial integrity. Epidemiologic features of squamous dysplasia are similar to those of squamous cell carcinoma.

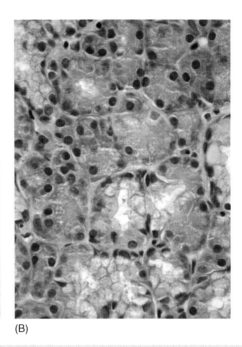

(A)   (B)

FIGURE 7.5 Pancreatic heterotopias are commonly encountered in biopsy samples of the gastroesophageal junction, but do not produce an endoscopically apparent lesion in most cases. Lobules of exocrine glands are associated with neutral mucin-containing glands (A). The cuboidal cells contain finely granular eosinophilic cytoplasm and, unlike parietal cells, are polarized with basally located nuclei (B).

Early data suggested a causal role of HPV in the development of squamous cell carcinoma, although this hypothesis has been largely disproven. More than 70 studies have evaluated the role of HPV in human esophageal carcinoma and many with positive results describe the presence of cutaneous viral types that are not oncogenic. None have demonstrated any relationship between esophageal squamous cell carcinoma and other factors that may implicate HPV, such as sexual behavior, immunosuppression, and other HPV-related malignancies. Furthermore, recent studies performed under stringent conditions have failed to demonstrate a relationship between HPV infection and either squamous cell carcinoma or dysplasia, even in extremely high-risk areas of China. Thus, HPV likely plays a limited, if any, role in the development of esophageal squamous cell carcinoma.

Clinical and Endoscopic Features

Squamous dysplasia is asymptomatic; most cases are identified in patients who undergo endoscopic examination for other reasons or undergo surveillance due to presumed cancer risk. Endoscopic manifestations of dysplasia are often subtle and many cases are not visible by white light examination. Some lesions appear as an erosion or area of erythema, whereas others cause slight mucosal irregularity. Abnormal keratin or parakeratosis on the surface of dysplasia can produce a white plaque or patch (Figure 7.6). Enhancing techniques, such as iodine

application, chromoendoscopy, narrow band imaging, and confocal laser endomicroscopy exploit properties unique to dysplasia and improve its endoscopic detection.

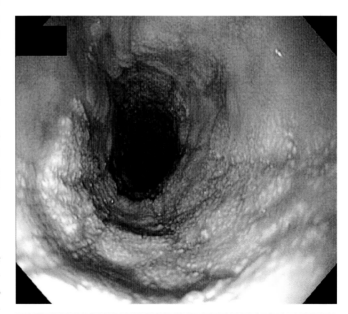

FIGURE 7.6 A 69-year-old male underwent surveillance endoscopy for high-grade squamous dysplasia. Diffuse mucosal abnormalities, including circumferential yellow–white plaques, extensively involve the midesophagus. Biopsy sampling revealed low- and high-grade squamous dysplasia.

Invasive squamous cell carcinomas usually cause obstructive-type symptoms, such as progressive dysphagia from solids to liquids, although occult bleeding and weight loss are not uncommon. Slightly more than half (60%) of cases occur in the midesophagus; those remaining are evenly distributed in the upper and lower esophagus. Squamous carcinomas typically develop on a background of multifocal, or extensive, squamous dysplasia and produce clinically evident mass lesions. Early cancers appear as nodules or plaques, whereas locally advanced tumors circumferentially involve the esophageal wall and produce luminal narrowing (Figure 7.7A–B). Some specific subtypes of squamous cell carcinoma characteristically produce polypoid luminal masses, as discussed in the section on macroscopic and microscopic features of squamous cell carcinoma.

Management and Prognostic Factors

Squamous dysplasia, especially high-grade dysplasia, is a major risk factor for the development of invasive squamous cell carcinoma. Patients with low-grade dysplasia have a cancer risk 3- to 8-fold higher than that of the general population, and the risk increases to 28- to 34-fold among patients with high-grade dysplasia. Thus, foci of dysplasia are removed or ablated and followed by endoscopic surveillance. Improved endoscopic techniques, such as endoscopic mucosal resection, are increasingly used to remove relatively large lesions and, as a result, esophagectomy is generally reserved for patients who are not candidates for endoscopic management. Ablative

therapies are utilized in debilitated patients, as discussed in subsequent sections.

Tumor stage, as determined by the tumor, node, metastasis (TNM) staging system, is the most important prognostic factor among patients with esophageal squamous cell carcinoma. Tumors confined to the mucosa have a low (less than 5%) risk of regional lymph node metastasis, but metastatic risk increases with progressive depth of invasion. Current data suggest that slightly more than 50% of tumors confined to the deep submucosa do not have associated regional lymph node metastases and, thus, may be treated with endoscopic resection in selected patients. These early lesions are usually detected in regions of high-disease prevalence where screening and surveillance programs are widely utilized. Unfortunately, such programs in the United States are limited to select patient groups due to the low prevalence of the disease. As a result, most patients in this country have locally advanced disease at the time of diagnosis and may not be surgical candidates. Overall 5-year survival rates for esophageal squamous cell carcinoma range from 5% to 10% in the United States and improve to only 35% among patients treated with curative surgical resection. In a subset of patients, resectability and overall survival may be improved through the use of neoadjuvant therapy.

Macroscopic and Microscopic Features

Squamous dysplasia is generally treated by endoscopic techniques, rather than surgery, so most resection specimens consist of small pieces of mucosa and a variable

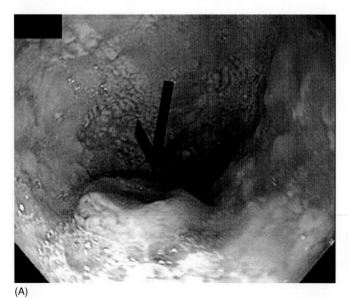

(A)

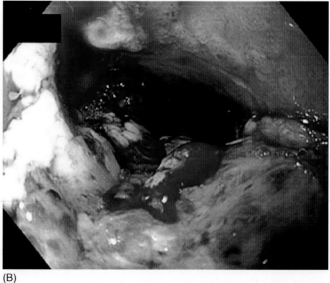

(B)

FIGURE 7.7 An early squamous cell carcinoma appears as an umbilicated nodule (A, arrow). The background mucosa shows multifocal dysplasia characterized by numerous white plaques. A more advanced lesion is nearly circumferential and narrows the esophageal lumen. The tumor is surfaced by gray–white plaques and displays stigmata of recent hemorrhage (B).

amount of submucosa. These specimens are often oriented by gastroenterologists to ensure optimal tissue processing and histologic evaluation. The deep and lateral aspects of endoscopic excisional specimens represent resection margins that should be inked prior to perpendicular sectioning of the tissue. Dysplastic foci are also frequently present in esophagectomy specimens that contain invasive squamous cell carcinoma. Similar to their endoscopic appearances, dysplastic areas may be erythematous, ulcerated, or white, reflecting abnormal accumulation of keratin (Figure 7.8). Some cases have a diffuse corrugated appearance that reflects abnormal keratinization and expansion of the mucosal thickness.

At low power, there is an abrupt transition between foci of dysplasia and adjacent non-neoplastic mucosa in histologic sections (Figure 7.9A). Features of dysplasia include crowded, immature cells with nuclear enlargement, nuclear membrane irregularities, hyperchromasia, and increased mitotic activity. Most cases do not show striking keratinization, but some have overlying ortho- or parakeratosis and show intense cytoplasmic eosinophilia. Squamous dysplasia is graded based on a two-tiered

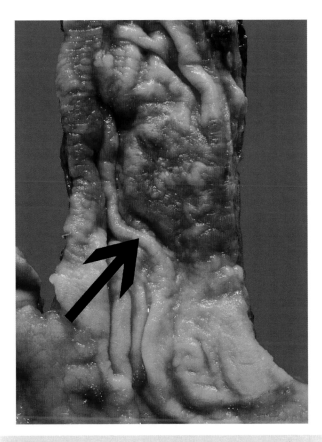

FIGURE 7.8 This archival resection specimen contains extensive low- and high-grade squamous dysplasia. The area of high-grade dysplasia is erythematous (arrow). The background mucosa is slightly thick, reflecting squamous hyperplasia.

system. Low-grade dysplasia is defined by the presence of neoplastic cells limited to the lower half of the epithelial thickness, whereas the presence of neoplastic cells occupying more than 50% of the epithelial thickness is classified as high-grade dysplasia (Figure 7.9B–C). The latter category encompasses squamous cell carcinoma in situ, which is no longer a preferred term in gastrointestinal neoplasia.

Epidermoid metaplasia has been recently described as a harbinger of squamous cell carcinoma in the esophagus, and likened to leukoplakia of the oral mucosa. Lesions typically develop in patients with risk factors for esophageal squamous cell carcinoma, namely exposure to tobacco smoke and alcohol, and nearly 20% of patients have concomitant squamous dysplasia or carcinoma at endoscopy. Epidermoid metaplasia may also be observed in resected esophagi containing invasive squamous cell carcinoma. Lesions are sharply demarcated from adjacent normal mucosa and characterized by squamous hyperplasia, expansion of the basal zone, acanthosis, prominence of the granular cell layer, and hyperorthokeratosis (Figure 7.9D). Although its prognostic significance is not clear at this point, epidermoid metaplasia may represent a mature-appearing variant of dysplasia, similar to that occurring in the oropharynx.

The gross appearance of squamous cell carcinoma varies depending on the stage of the disease. Early tumors appear as small, pearly white nodules or ulcers (Figure 7.10A–B). Superficial cancers may be removed by endoscopic mucosal resection or endoscopic submucosal dissection. Similar to endoscopically removed foci of squamous dysplasia, the deep and lateral aspects of excision specimens should be denoted as resection margins at the time of gross examination, and serially sectioned perpendicularly to the deep margin. Endoscopically removed carcinomas are submitted entirely for histologic evaluation and the depth of invasion into the submucosa and proximity of the tumor to the margin reported. Multifocal and advanced tumors may be treated with esophagectomy (Figure 7.10C), provided the disease is limited to the esophagus and regional lymph nodes. Resected cancers are characteristically fungating, nearly circumferential masses with surface ulceration and nodularity, although those treated with neoadjuvant therapy may show some regression in the form of mural fibrosis or a residual ulcer (Figure 7.10D). Tumors should be sampled to assess the depth of invasion as well as the extent of therapeutic response in cases treated with neoadjuvant therapy.

The microscopic features of esophageal squamous cell carcinoma are similar to those of squamous carcinomas at other sites. Irregular sheets and nests of overtly malignant cells are associated with keratin pearls and desmoplastic stroma (Figure 7.11A). Tumor cells are typically large and contain abundant, densely eosinophilic cytoplasm. Nuclei are centrally located and display irregular contours, coarse chromatin, and prominent nucleoli. Mitotic figures, including abnormal ones, are readily

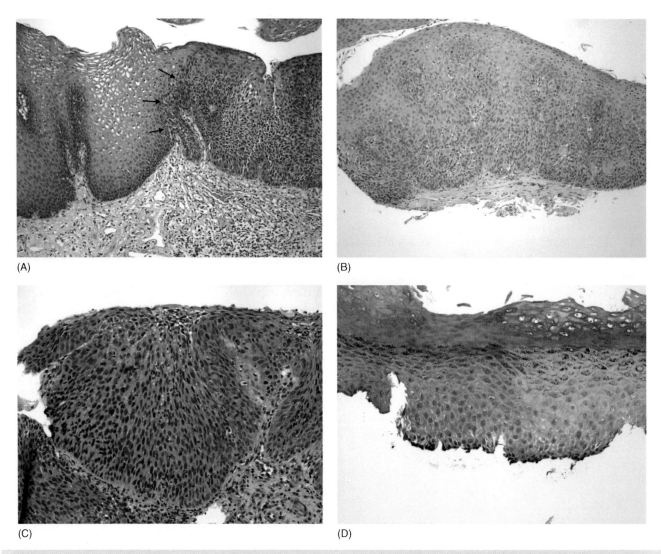

FIGURE 7.9 Squamous dysplasia (right) is sharply demarcated from the adjacent nondysplastic squamous epithelium (A, arrows). Lesional cells contain enlarged, hyperchromatic nuclei. In low-grade dysplasia, the dysplastic cells are limited to the lower half of the squamous mucosa. The basal layer is disorganized, and increased mitotic activity is present up to the midlevel of the epithelium (B). High-grade dysplasia displays full-thickness cytologic atypia with numerous mitotic figures (C). Epidermoid metaplasia consists of mature-appearing epithelium with an abnormal granular cell layer and parakeratosis (D).

apparent and cellular necrosis is frequently present. Not uncommonly, basaloid cells with hyperchromatic nuclei and scant cytoplasm occupy the peripheries of tumor cell nests and seem to mature toward their centers. High-grade features include the presence of single infiltrating cells, delicate trabeculae of neoplastic cells, and sheet-like growth of nonkeratinizing, basaloid cells (Figure 7.11B). Striking pleomorphism and multinucleated cells may be encountered. Of note, tumors treated with neoadjuvant therapy should be assessed for therapeutic response, as greater tumor regression is associated with better survival. However, nonviable tumor (ie, keratin debris and fibrosis) in the esophagus or regional lymph nodes should not be counted toward tumor extent when assigning TNM stage, as discussed subsequently.

There are several morphologic variants of esophageal squamous cell carcinoma, but all have similar clinical features, treatment, and stage-dependent outcomes. Extremely well-differentiated verrucous carcinomas feature minimal nuclear atypia and well-developed acanthosis with hyperkeratosis (Figure 7.12A–C). These tumors can be difficult to recognize because invasion occurs across a broad smooth front, rather than overtly infiltrating single cells and clusters, and thus may not be apparent in superficial biopsy samples. High-grade variants include basaloid squamous cell carcinoma and spindle cell (sarcomatoid) carcinoma. The former show a predilection for the mid- and distal esophagus and contain tumor cells with large nuclei, finely granular chromatin, small nucleoli, and scant cytoplasm arranged in lobules,

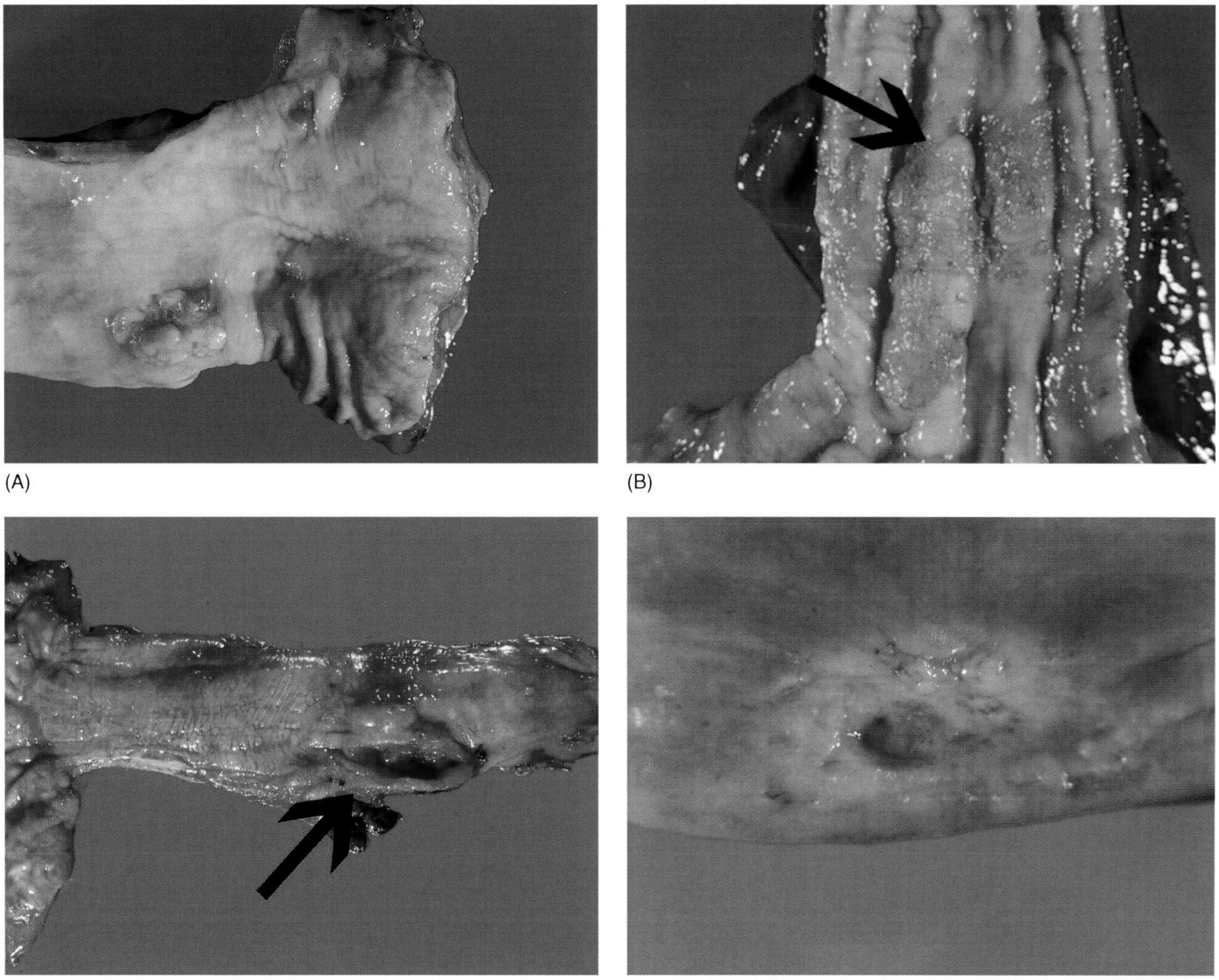

FIGURE 7.10 An early invasive squamous cell carcinoma forms an irregular, pearly-white nodule in the squamous mucosa above the level of the gastroesophageal junction (A). Another example of squamous cell carcinoma forms an irregular plaque (arrow) on a background of squamous dysplasia (B). An advanced cancer forms an ulcerated mass (arrow) in the upper esophagus (C). Neoadjuvant treatment may cause tumor regression, leaving behind an ulcer on a background of atrophic mucosa (D).

nests, and cords (Figure 7.12D–E). Lobules frequently display peripheral nuclear palisading and central necrosis that simulate the appearance of high-grade neuroendocrine carcinoma. They may also show a cribriform growth pattern and contain faintly eosinophilic, hyalinized, basement membrane-like material reminiscent of adenoid cystic carcinoma (Figure 7.12E). In fact, most reported cases of esophageal adenoid cystic carcinoma likely represent basaloid squamous cell carcinomas. Spindle cell carcinoma (Figure 7.12F–I) is an unusual variant of squamous cell carcinoma that typically grows as a polypoid, intraluminal mass, rather than an infiltrative lesion. Variable numbers of epithelioid and spindle cells comprise the tumors, although epithelioid cells may be scarce or limited to the in situ component. Spindle cells display a spectrum of cytologic abnormalities and may

closely resemble fibroblasts in some cases. They contain ovoid, or elongated, nuclei and bipolar cytoplasmic tails. Nucleoli and nuclear hyperchromasia are variable, and pleomorphic tumor giant cells are seen in some cases. Spindle cell carcinomas may also contain bone, cartilage, or other heterologous elements that raise the possibility of a sarcoma. However, primary osteosarcoma, chondrosarcoma, and rhabdomyosarcoma are exceedingly rare in the esophagus, so consideration for spindle cell carcinoma must be given prior to rendering a diagnosis of sarcoma.

Ancillary Studies

Squamous dysplasia and squamous cell carcinoma show similar molecular abnormalities, consistent with the theory that squamous carcinogenesis is a progressive, multistep

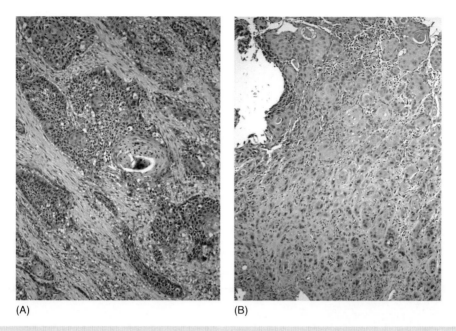

FIGURE 7.11 A well-differentiated squamous cell carcinoma displays keratin pearls in the invasive component (A). Note the associated desmoplastic stroma. A higher grade squamous cell carcinoma infiltrates as single cells, cords, and small nests (B).

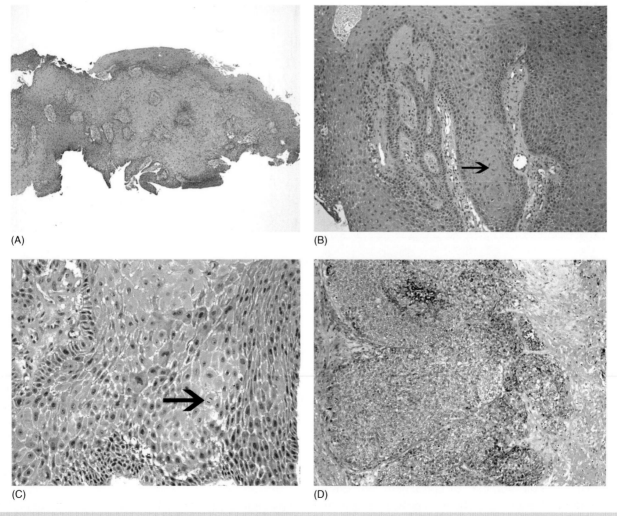

(A) (B) (C) (D)

FIGURE 7.12 (*continued*)

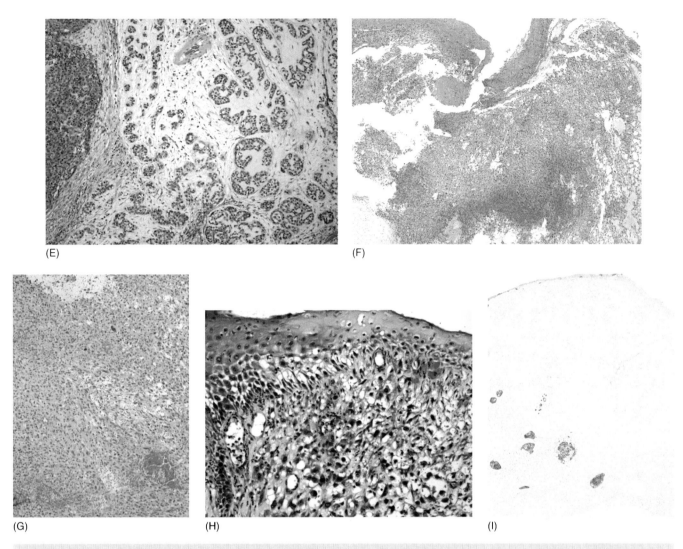

FIGURE 7.12 (*continued*) Extremely well-differentiated verrucous carcinomas pose diagnostic challenges in biopsy samples. This patient had a nearly circumferential, fungating mass, but biopsy samples showed only an extremely well-differentiated proliferation of squamous cells with overlying thick parakeratosis (A). Thick, irregular projections of squamous cells extend from the deep aspect of the epithelium and scattered dyskeratotic cells are present (arrow) in an abnormal location (B). Enlarged, but mature, squamous cells are also present in this region, some of which show mitotic activity (arrow) and nuclear enlargement (C). Basaloid squamous cell carcinomas are high-grade malignancies that often show sheet-like growth (D). However, some cases contain round aggregates of tumor cells associated with basement membrane-like material that simulates adenoid cystic carcinoma (E). Esophageal spindle cell carcinomas are composed of a diffuse proliferation of malignant spindle cells that may resemble a sarcoma (F–G). Plump, stellate tumor cells with enlarged, hyperchromatic nuclei undermine the mucosa (H). Similar to spindle cell carcinomas at other sites, these tumors may show an absence, or near lack, of keratin staining (I).

process. Early changes present in dysplasia include alterations in telomerase activity, loss of heterozygosity (LOH), increased cyclin D1 expression, and hypermethylation of *INK4/CDKNA* (p16), whereas *TP53* mutations accompany onset of high-grade cytologic abnormalities. Increased expression of epidermal growth factor receptor (EGFR) has been described in at least 50% of carcinomas and abnormal expression of cell cycle regulatory proteins is common. Studies have implicated other biomarkers as important players in the evolution of esophageal squamous

cell carcinoma, but none have proven to be clinically useful for diagnostic or therapeutic purposes.

Diagnostic Challenges

Biopsy samples from patients with inflammatory conditions of the esophagus may contain epithelial regenerative changes that mimic dysplasia, particularly when ulcers are present. Squamous cell hyperplasia, nuclear enlargement and hyperchromasia, nucleolar prominence, and increased

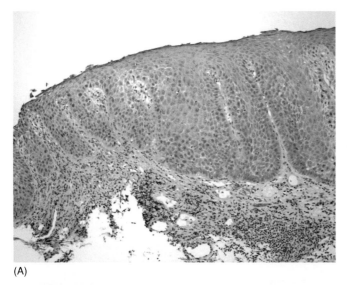

(A)

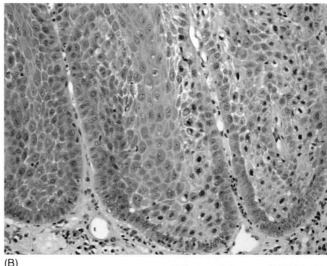

(B)

FIGURE 7.13 Reactive squamous epithelial changes may mimic low-grade dysplasia. Cytologic atypia tends to be more pronounced near the base of the epithelium in reactive mucosa (A). Mitotic figures are increased, but basal keratinocytes maintain their polarity and show maturation (B).

mitotic activity are all features of reparative atypia that mimic dysplasia. These inflammatory changes tend to be uniform and show a gradual transition to more normal-appearing areas, whereas dysplasia is sharply demarcated from adjacent non-neoplastic mucosa. Benign epithelial hyperplasia shows regular papillary elongation and protrusions of basal keratinocytes into the lamina propria, and reactive atypia is largely confined to the basal epithelium (Figure 7.13A–B). Most reparative changes that are severe enough to mimic dysplasia are also associated with intraepithelial neutrophilic inflammation. In contrast, the interface between dysplastic squamous epithelium and the lamina propria tends to be irregular with broad, or fused, projections from the base of the epithelium. Cytologic atypia is heterogeneous, varying from one cell to the next, and intraepithelial inflammation is less common than in reactive atypia. Chemotherapeutic agents and radiation can produce severe abnormalities that simulate neoplasia, including nuclear enlargement and hyperchromasia with membrane irregularities. However, the epithelium usually appears attenuated, rather than proliferative, and affected cells contain vacuolated cytoplasm while maintaining their nuclear-to-cytoplasmic ratios (Figure 7.14).

The diagnosis of invasive squamous cell carcinoma is generally straightforward, although challenges occur in some situations. "Pseudoepitheliomatous" hyperplasia adjacent to erosions or overlying a granular cell tumor is a well-recognized mimic of squamous cell carcinoma, especially in superficial biopsies (Figure 7.15A–B). Features favoring a diagnosis of benign hyperplasia include the presence of only mild cytologic atypia and confinement of squamous cell nests to the superficial mucosa.

A more problematic issue is the failure to recognize invasive squamous cell carcinoma in superficial biopsy samples. Well-differentiated carcinomas may show a papillary growth pattern with apparent surface maturation that simulates the appearance of a squamous papilloma. Such tumors often have a broad, pushing type of invasion that does not elicit a striking desmoplastic stromal response. They also lack substantial mitotic activity beyond the basal regions of the epithelium, and show minimal cytologic atypia (Figure 7.16A–B). Fortunately,

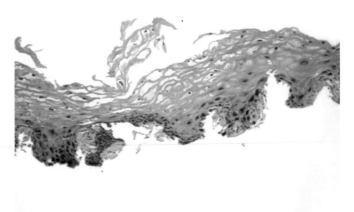

FIGURE 7.14 Chemotherapy induces cytologic atypia that may simulate neoplasia. However, the epithelium is attenuated, rather than proliferative, and atypical epithelial cells contain abundant cytoplasm.

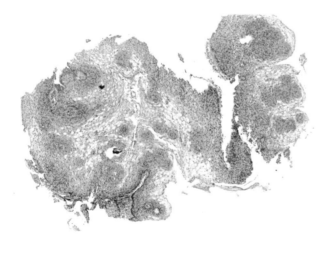

(A)

(B)

FIGURE 7.15 Granular cell tumors of the esophagus, as in other sites, are associated with pseudoepitheliomatous hyperplasia. Irregular nests of keratinizing squamous epithelium are present in the lamina propria (A). The subjacent granular cell tumor contains cells with abundant, faintly eosinophilic granular cytoplasm and pyknotic nuclei. Tumor cells are intimately associated with dense collagen bands (B).

the clinical appearance of such lesions is not at all that of a squamous papilloma, at least in most cases. Well-differentiated carcinomas tend to be quite large, destructive plaque-like lesions that may be circumferential, whereas papillomas appear as small verrucous plaques that rarely exceed 1.0 cm in diameter. Carcinomas also display an irregular interface with the subjacent stroma and show abnormal keratinization in the deep epithelium.

Finally, biopsy samples from an ulcer may contain unusually large endothelial cells and fibroblasts with an epithelioid or stellate appearance. These activated stromal cells contain abundant cytoplasm, as well as large nuclei and prominent nucleoli, and lack the clustered appearance of carcinoma cells (Figure 7.17A). Biopsy samples of ulcers may also contain sheets of activated lymphocytes, macrophages, and necrotic granulocytes in adherent exudates

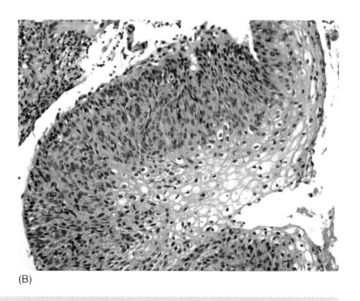

(A)

(B)

FIGURE 7.16 This biopsy from a patient with dysphagia was initially interpreted as an atypical squamous papilloma before the macroscopic description of a large, destructive mass lesion was obtained. At low power, the tumor cells show surface maturation, and lack an infiltrating growth pattern (A). At higher power, there is focal loss of nuclear polarity, but the surface maturation is maintained and the broad, pushing invasive front is deceptively bland (B).

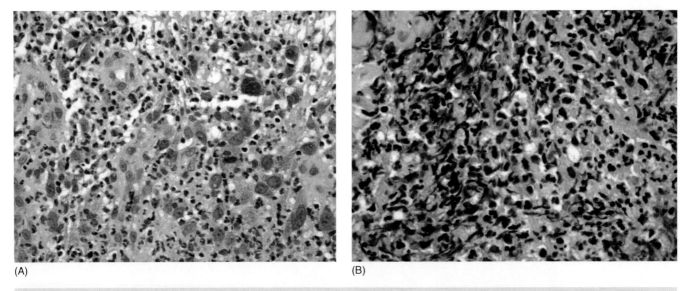

(A)   (B)

FIGURE 7.17   Biopsy samples of an esophageal ulcer contain activated fibroblasts and endothelial cells with enlarged, slightly hyperchromatic nuclei with smooth contours dispersed in granulation tissue (A). Ulcer debris contains necrotic inflammatory cells that may simulate the appearance of lymphoma. This case also contains embedded crystalline iron reflecting a drug-related injury (B).

that can be misinterpreted as lymphoma. However, the atypical cells do not infiltrate the tissue and often contain small, convoluted nuclei, even in degenerated material (Figure 7.17B).

Adenocarcinoma, Dysplasia, and Barrett Esophagus

Barrett Esophagus

Barrett esophagus is relatively common, affecting nearly 6% in the general population and 11% of patients with a history of heartburn. Males are affected more than females and prevalence increases with age. Risk factors include gastroesophageal reflux disease, hiatal hernia, central obesity, delayed esophageal clearance, and decreased resting tone of the lower esophageal sphincter. Barrett esophagus is a premalignant condition characterized by replacement of the normal squamous epithelium by non-neoplastic, but genetically unstable, glandular mucosa in the distal esophagus. Persistent gastroesophageal reflux disease leads to inflammation-related injury and cumulative molecular events in the metaplastic epithelium, placing the patient at risk for progressive dysplasia and adenocarcinoma. The American Gastroenterology Association defines Barrett esophagus as (a) the presence of endoscopically apparent metaplasia of the distal esophagus (columnar-lined esophagus) that (b) shows intestinal metaplasia (goblet cells) on histology. However, this definition is not accepted in some countries, including the United Kingdom and Japan, where a diagnosis of Barrett esophagus can be based on the presence of *any* glandular epithelium in the distal esophagus, even if intestinal metaplasia is lacking (ie, columnar-lined esophagus). The overall cancer risk of patients with intestinal metaplasia in the esophagus is less than 2% and increases with the extent of the disease. However, evidence substantiating the biologic risk of nongoblet glandular metaplasia is not yet available. For this reason, most practitioners in the United States still require goblet cells to establish a diagnosis of Barrett esophagus. Patients with Barrett esophagus are usually treated with aggressive antireflux medications followed by regular surveillance endoscopy with four-quadrant sampling every 1 to 2 cm of the length of affected mucosa.

Barrett esophagus is classified as long (greater than 3 cm), short (1–3 cm), and ultrashort (less than 1 cm) segments, depending upon its extent. Small areas of metaplasia near the gastroesophageal junction may appear as a mucosal irregularity or produce no abnormalities, making it difficult to establish a diagnosis of ultrashort segment Barrett esophagus. Extensive metaplasia produces salmon-pink, velvety mucosal tongues that emanate from the gastroesophageal junction into the distal esophagus (Figure 7.18A). Corresponding biopsy samples contain goblet cells interspersed on a background of nongoblet columnar (ie, foveolar) epithelial cells filled with faintly eosinophilic neutral mucin (Figure 7.18B). Occasional oxyntic glands, absorptive cells, Paneth cells, and endocrine cells may be present, and the mucosa is often inflamed. Importantly, many patients with Barrett esophagus develop duplication of the muscularis mucosae, in which case the most superficial layer consists of haphazardly arranged discontinuous bundles of smooth muscle

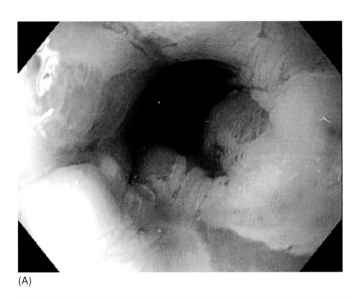
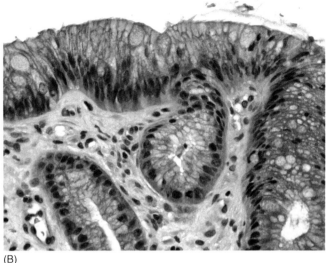

(A)

(B)

FIGURE 7.18 Barrett esophagus appears as erythematous tongues of glandular mucosa that emanate into the distal esophagus (A). Gray–blue, barrel-shaped goblet cells are interspersed in a background of foveolar-type epithelium (B).

cells and lies within lamina propria. The deeper, second layer is better organized with compact bundles of smooth muscle cells (Figure 7.19A–B). This layer represents the true muscularis mucosae and delineates the deepest aspect of the mucosa. Failure to recognize duplication of the muscularis mucosae may pose a problem to pathologists when assessing for depth of invasion in biopsies of early adenocarcinomas, as the thickened muscularis mucosae may be mistaken for muscularis propria.

Epidemiology and Pathogenesis of Barrett-Esophagus-Related Neoplasia

There has been a six-fold increase in the incidence of esophageal adenocarcinoma over the past three decades, as well as a seven-fold increase in disease-related mortality during the same time period. Virtually all cases of glandular dysplasia and invasive adenocarcinoma develop in patients with Barrett esophagus, and thus the epidemiology of

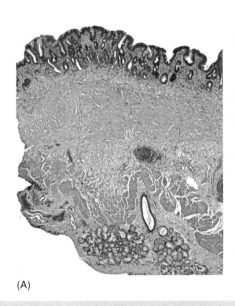
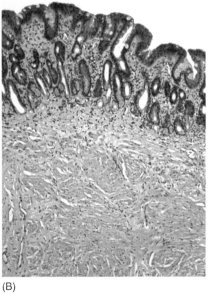

(A)

(B)

FIGURE 7.19 Barrett esophagus often displays duplication of the muscularis mucosae. In this example, submucosal glands are present deep to an organized layer of smooth muscle cells, which represents the true muscularis mucosae. A thick band of smooth muscle cells is also present directly subjacent to the mucosa (A). Higher magnification of the same area demonstrates the haphazard arrangement of smooth muscle cells in the duplicated muscularis mucosae. This layer is present in the lamina propria (B).

these disorders is the same as that of Barrett esophagus. Rare tumors derived from gastric heterotopias and submucosal glands do occur, but these lesions are so rare that their representation in the literature consists of case reports and extremely small series. Carcinomas associated with Barrett esophagus typically occur in older adults, and males are affected more than females. The presence of glandular dysplasia is the most important risk factor for cancer development in patients with Barrett esophagus.

Clinical and Endoscopic Features of Barrett Esophagus and Glandular Neoplasia

Although patients with Barrett esophagus may have symptoms related to chronic gastroesophageal reflux disease, metaplasia and dysplasia of the esophageal mucosa are asymptomatic. As a result, many patients with Barrett esophagus or dysplasia in the United States never participate in surveillance programs. Such individuals only come to clinical attention when they develop symptoms related to advanced adenocarcinoma, such as progressive dysphagia to solids and liquids, pain, and weight loss. Indeed, approximately 80% of patients in this country have locally advanced cancers and 50% have metastases at the time of diagnosis.

Glandular dysplasia occurs in a multifocal fashion, reflecting a field effect in Barrett mucosa. Most foci of dysplasia are endoscopically inapparent by white light examination, and because of this surveillance protocols have historically called for random four-quadrant mucosal biopsies every 2 cm from the gastroesophageal junction to the neo-squamocolumnar junction (Figure 7.20). Recent advances in endoscopic imaging techniques, such

as chromoendoscopy with indigo carmine, high-resolution magnification with narrow band imaging, and confocal laser endomicroscopy, enhance detection of dysplasia with improved sensitivity and specificity. Some cases of glandular dysplasia produce subtle areas of erythema or raised plaques that can also be better visualized with enhancing techniques. Early cancers usually produce an endoscopically evident abnormality, such as a polypoid or plaque-like configuration, ulcer, or a subtle mucosal irregularity (Figure 7.21A–B). The presence of an ulcer, polyp, or plaque in the context of Barrett esophagus is much more likely to represent a cancer than dysplasia. Advanced tumors form bulky, friable masses that show ulceration or obstruct the lumen (Figure 7.21B).

Management and Prognostic Features

Cancer risk increases with progressive dysplasia among patients with Barrett esophagus: approximately 5% to 10% of patients with low-grade dysplasia develop carcinoma, compared to 15% to 30% of patients with high-grade dysplasia. Treatment of dysplasia generally consists of endoscopic mucosal resection, although a variety of ablative techniques may be considered in debilitated or elderly patients. These include photodynamic therapy, radiofrequency ablation, laser ablation, and argon plasma coagulation. Esophagectomy is limited to specific situations as determined by patient circumstances.

Slightly more than 20% of submucosally invasive tumors metastasize to regional lymph nodes, compared to only 1.3% of tumors confined to the mucosa. For this reason, early lesions limited to the superficial submucosa can be managed with endoscopic mucosal resection, whereas cancers that infiltrate the deeper submucosa may be amenable to endoscopic submucosal dissection. Survival of patients with invasive adenocarcinoma is determined by tumor stage. Five-year survival rates exceed 80% among tumors limited to the mucosa or submucosa without regional lymph node metastases, but patients with unresectable disease have a poor prognosis with 5-year survival rates of less than 5%. Treatment of esophageal adenocarcinoma is stage-dependent. Virtually all patients with locally advanced disease receive preoperative neoadjuvant therapy to improve resectability and survival.

Macroscopic and Microscopic Features of Barrett-Esophagus-Related Neoplasia

Glandular Dysplasia

Dysplasia is defined as a neoplastic proliferation of epithelial cells confined to the basement membrane of the epithelium in which it developed. Biopsy samples from patients with Barrett esophagus are designated as negative for dysplasia, positive for dysplasia, or indefinite for dysplasia. Cases classified as positive for dysplasia are graded using

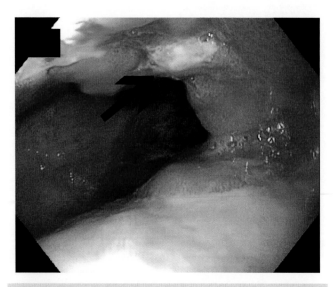

FIGURE 7.20 This patient with long segment Barrett esophagus underwent thermal ablation of the metaplastic mucosa. At the time of the procedure, he was noted to have a small ulcer (arrow), which was sampled and proved to be high-grade dysplasia.

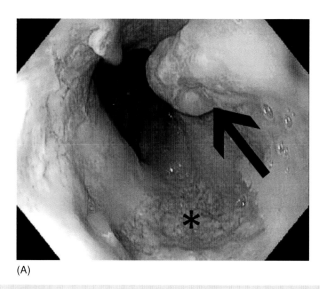
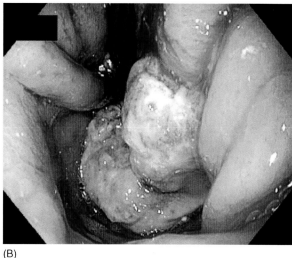

(A)

(B)

FIGURE 7.21 This elderly patient was found to have an irregular nodule (arrow) on a background of Barrett esophagus (asterisk). Biopsy and subsequent endoscopic submucosal dissection revealed a superficially invasive cancer (A). Another patient with dysphagia was found to have a nearly obstructing friable mass in the distal esophagus that proved to be a high-grade invasive adenocarcinoma (B).

a two-tiered system (low- and high-grade dysplasia). Cases with cytologic atypia that do not reach the threshold of dysplasia, or for which limited sampling or a background of inflammation are confounding factors, may be considered indefinite for dysplasia. Most problematic cases labeled as indefinite for dysplasia show cytologic atypia limited to the crypts, or atypical features in mucosa that is also inflamed.

There is often a sharp demarcation between foci of dysplasia and adjacent nondysplastic epithelium. Foci of dysplasia are characterized by the presence of the same population of atypical cells in both deep glands and surface epithelium, and a concomitant lack of surface maturation. Most cases of dysplasia display an overall increase in gland density at low magnification that reflects their proliferative nature, although the crowding is generally mild in cases of low-grade dysplasia. Most cases of low-grade dysplasia have an intestinal phenotype with cytologic abnormalities similar to those seen in intestinal

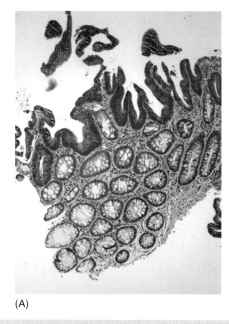
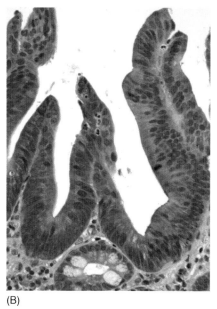

(A)

(B)

FIGURE 7.22 Foci of low-grade dysplasia are typically sharply demarcated from the background glands of Barrett esophagus (A). Crowded, mucin-depleted cells are present at the surface and show mild cytologic atypia that is morphologically similar to intestinal adenomas. Enlarged, hyperchromatic nuclei maintain their polarity with respect to the basement membrane (B). A small amount of active inflammation is present, but is not enough to account for the cytologic abnormalities.

adenomas (Figure 7.22A). Dysplastic cells contain ovoid or elongated hyperchromatic nuclei with membrane irregularities, but maintain their polarity in low-grade dysplasia (Figure 7.22B).

High-grade dysplasia shows severe cytologic atypia often in combination with architectural abnormalities of the dysplastic glands. Most cases have an intestinal phenotype and consist of crowded, irregularly shaped glands, cribriform glands, and/or villous or papillary projections on the surface (Figure 7.23A–B). Cytologically, the cells of high-grade dysplasia have a complete loss of cell polarity, pronounced nuclear membrane irregularities,

open or dispersed chromatin, and conspicuous nucleoli (Figure 7.23C–D). Mitotic figures, including atypical ones, and necrotic cellular debris are common and may be seen at all levels within the mucosa (Figure 7.23E). The distinction between high-grade dysplasia and intramucosal carcinoma in the setting of Barrett esophagus can be very challenging, and is discussed in the subsequent Diagnostic Challenges section.

The term "foveolar dysplasia" refers to cases with a papillary or "tufted" growth pattern at the surface and/or dilated glands, or microglands, in the deep mucosa (Figure 7.24). The dysplastic cells in these cases are

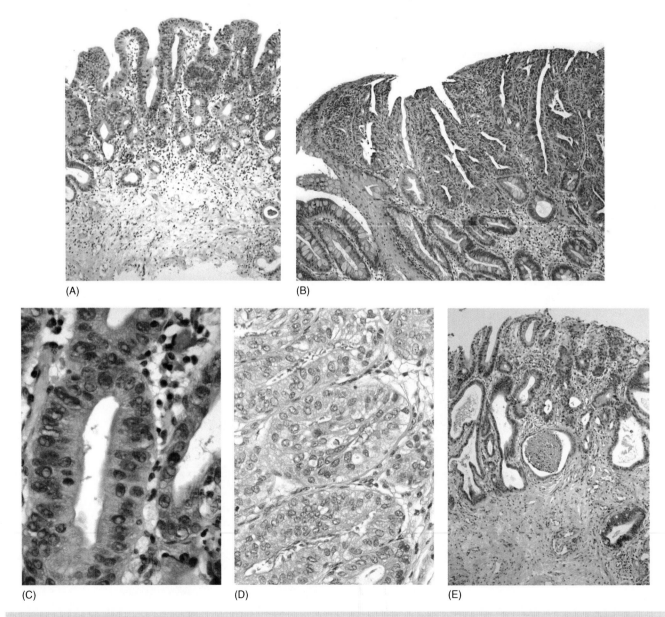

(A)   (B)

(C)   (D)   (E)

FIGURE 7.23 High-grade dysplasia typically features both architecturally abnormal glands and high-grade cytologic atypia (A). Architectural abnormalities include irregularly branched, fused, and dilated glands, as well as microlumina or cribriform glands (B). Closer examination of this area demonstrates high-grade nuclear abnormalities, including round nuclei with dispersed chromatin, irregular membranes, and prominent nucleoli. Many cells have lost their polarity to the basement membrane (C–D). Some glands may contain necrotic luminal debris (E).

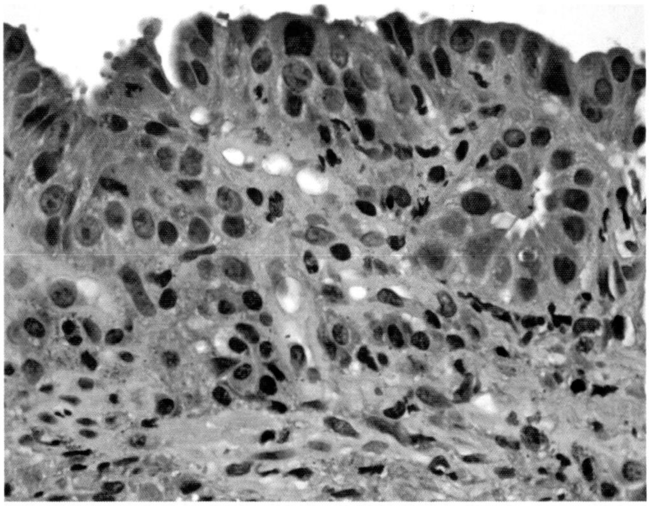

FIGURE 7.24 Cases of foveolar dysplasia feature a highly atypical proliferation of cells at the mucosal surface. The nuclei are large and ovoid with irregular contours, open chromatin, and macronucleoli, and the cytoplasm is often eosinophilic. Mitotic figures are readily identified.

polygonal, with eosinophilic or clear cytoplasm. They typically contain large round nuclei with irregular contours, vesicular chromatin, and macronucleoli, and are often designated as high-grade dysplasia.

"Crypt dysplasia" is a term used to define cytologic atypia (often high-grade) confined to the deep glands, in association with apparent surface maturation (Figure 7.25A–D). This finding has been postulated to represent a precursor to invasive adenocarcinoma, similar to other types of dysplasia. However, most available data regarding the biologic importance of this finding are based on small retrospective studies that include a disproportionate number of high-risk patients with concomitant overt dysplasia or carcinoma. To date, there are no controlled prospective studies assessing the significance of crypt dysplasia in patients with Barrett esophagus. From a practical standpoint, problematic cases with marked cytologic atypia limited to the glands may be designated as indefinite for dysplasia. However, most pathologists consider low-grade atypia confined to the crypts to be negative for dysplasia. It is important to remember that true high-grade dysplasia may occasionally be confined to the deep glands, and lack overlying surface maturation.

Barrett adenoma is a historical term used to denote the presence of polypoid dysplasia in the setting of Barrett esophagus. Such lesions often have an intestinal phenotype similar to tubular or villous adenomas of the colorectum, and may contain areas of low- or high-grade dysplasia. This terminology has fallen out of favor in the modern era because such lesions arise from a background of "at-risk" Barrett mucosa or even multifocal dysplasia, which is more analogous to dysplasia in the

setting of inflammatory bowel disease than a sporadic adenoma. Neoplastic polyps that develop in Barrett esophagus are better classified as polypoid dysplasias. The term "adenoma" should be reserved for the (very rare) benign neoplasm derived from submucosal glands in the esophagus or lesions that develop near the gastro-esophageal junction in the setting of familial adenomatous polyposis.

Glandular dysplasia is increasingly treated by endoscopic techniques, and thus resection specimens generally consist of excisional specimens rather than esophagectomy specimens. The deep and lateral aspects of these specimens comprise the resection margins, and they should be inked prior to processing, similar to excisional specimens for squamous dysplasia, as previously described in that section. Specimens should be submitted entirely for histologic evaluation. Esophagectomy is rarely performed for high-grade dysplasia alone in the current era.

Esophageal Adenocarcinoma

Currently, the majority of superficially invasive adenocarcinomas are managed endoscopically, so esophagectomies are usually performed for advanced tumors (Figure 7.26A). Locally advanced adenocarcinomas may be treated with neoadjuvant chemoradiotherapy in an effort to improve tumor resectability and overall survival. Similar to rectal carcinomas, neoadjuvant treatment can cause substantial tumor regression that may produce an apparent ulcer surrounded by dense fibrosis (Figure 7.26B). We recommend submitting the entire ulcerated area with perpendicular sections to the radial (adventitial) margin to evaluate for residual tumor. However, cases that show an essentially unaltered tumor mass or an obvious carcinoma are evaluated with representative sections of the tumor and margin.

Most invasive esophageal adenocarcinomas have an intestinal phenotype, or at least demonstrate prominent glandular differentiation (Figure 7.27A–D). Variants including signet ring cell carcinoma, mucinous carcinoma, and lymphoepithelioma-like carcinoma (see the section on uncommon types of esophageal adenocarcinoma) can also develop at this site, although they are much less common. Most of these less common variants display at least some degree of sheet-like growth, and are usually considered high-grade neoplasms.

Treated tumor cells often show striking degenerative cytologic atypia that should not be taken into account when assigning tumor grade. Regressed tumors may also contain acellular mucin pools in the esophageal wall or regional lymph nodes (Figure 7.28), although only viable tumor cells should be considered when assigning pathologic tumor stage. Documentation of tumor regression is important in these cases because it is predictive of survival; extensive regression is associated with improved survival, whereas a limited tumor response predicts a poorer outcome.

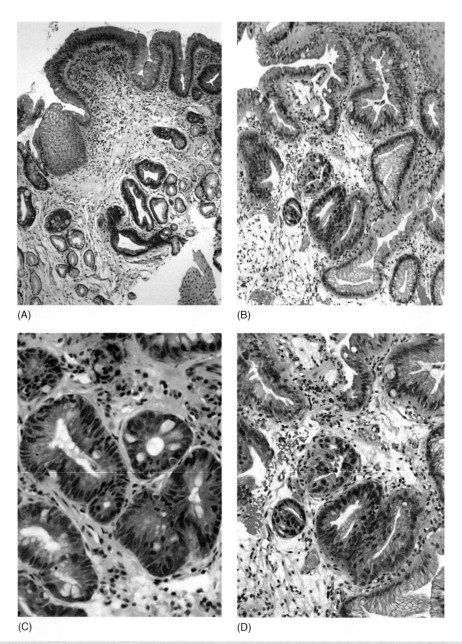

(A)   (B)

(C)   (D)

FIGURE 7.25 These biopsies of Barrett esophagus contain atypical glands in the deep mucosa that are associated with mature epithelium at the luminal surface (A–B). High magnification demonstrates marked cytologic atypia in the deep glands. The nuclei are large and hyperchromatic, but maintain their polarity to the basement membrane (C–D). Many pathologists would designate findings such as these as indefinite for dysplasia, although these changes have also been termed "crypt dysplasia."

Ancillary Studies

As previously mentioned, Barrett esophagus contains genetically unstable epithelial cells. Lesional epithelium harbors a variety of molecular abnormalities despite its morphologic similarities to gastric and intestinal epithelium. The majority (90%) of cases show *INK4/CDKNA* (p16) alterations. Aneuploid cell populations, cytogenetic abnormalities, LOH, DNA methylation, and *TP53* mutations may also be detected, even in cases that lack dysplasia. Aneuploidy, LOH at 17p and 9p, and inactivation of

p16 through *INK4/CDKNA* methylation are associated with progression to high-grade dysplasia and/or esophageal adenocarcinoma, but none of these biomarkers are superior to histologic evaluation in predicting progression of Barrett esophagus. Some investigators have shown that immunohistochemical stains for AMACR and p53 may identify cases of low-grade dysplasia that are more likely to progress to high-grade dysplasia or cancer, but these markers are of limited value in distinguishing nondysplastic glandular epithelium from dysplasia.

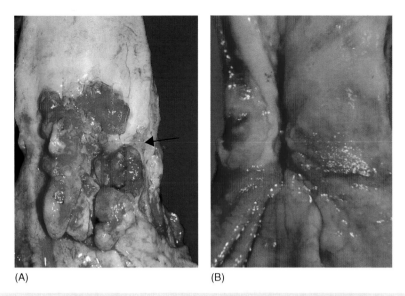

(A)   (B)

FIGURE 7.26   This esophagectomy specimen contains a large, friable mass located above the gastroesophageal junction. A small amount of residual Barrett mucosa is present at the right (A, arrow). Neoadjuvant therapy induces tumor regression. Resection specimens usually lack a luminal mass, but show ulcers in association with mural fibrosis (B).

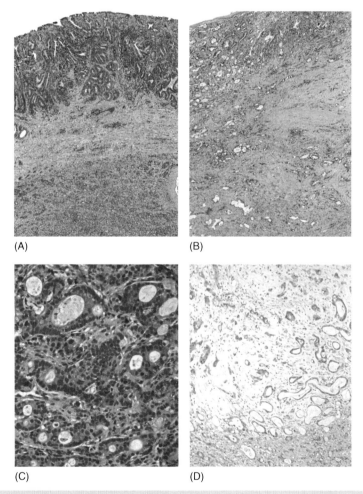

(A)   (B)

(C)   (D)

FIGURE 7.27   Invasive adenocarcinomas of the esophagus usually show glandular differentiation. This resection specimen shows a poorly differentiated adenocarcinoma, in which some degree of gland formation is still visible, beneath an area of extensive high-grade dysplasia (A). Note the thickened muscularis mucosae. A second example features irregular, infiltrating glands extending from the mucosa into the muscularis propria (B). At high power, this example contains both glands and single infiltrating tumor cells (C). This high-grade carcinoma contains numerous infiltrating signet ring cells, in addition to glands (D).

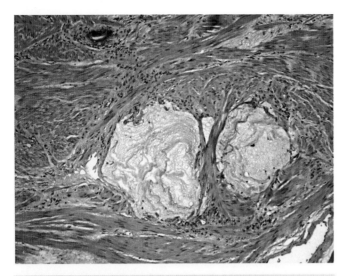

FIGURE 7.28 Neoadjuvant therapy causes a variable degree of tumor regression. Residual pools of acellular mucin are present in the esophageal wall of this case.

Many esophageal adenocarcinomas harbor molecular alterations that represent potential targets of directed medical therapies that have a synergistic effect when used in combination with conventional adjuvant therapy. These tumors frequently overexpress transmembrane tyrosine kinase growth factor receptors, including those of the EGFR family, such as HER2. Approximately 25% to 30% of esophageal and gastroesophageal junctional adenocarcinomas, especially intestinal-type tumors,

overexpress HER2. This receptor is targeted by trastuzumab, a humanized monoclonal antibody that binds its extracellular domain. Treatment with this agent in combination with conventional chemotherapy results in a 26% reduced risk of cancer-related death compared to conventional therapy alone. Other emerging targeted therapies include the EGFR inhibitor cetuximab and lapatinib, an orally administered small molecule tyrosine kinase inhibitor with activity against HER2 and EGFR. Bevacizumab, sunitinib, and sorafenib are new agents with anti-VEGF activity that may have applications in the future.

Diagnostic Challenges

Biopsy samples from Barrett esophagus often display reparative cytologic changes due to persistent gastroesophageal reflux disease which, in some cases, may mimic dysplasia. Features of regenerative atypia include variable mucin depletion, slight nuclear enlargement with dense chromatin, prominent nucleoli, and increased mitotic activity. In contrast to dysplasia, however, regenerative changes are usually more pronounced in the deep glands compared to the surface epithelium, and show a gradual (rather than sharply demarcated) transition to regions that are clearly non-neoplastic. In general, one may consider a diagnosis of "indefinite for dysplasia" when cytologic atypia is limited to the gland region (see also preceding section on crypt dysplasia), or when abundant neutrophilic inflammation is present in immature-appearing surface epithelium (Figure 7.29A–B). However, complex architectural

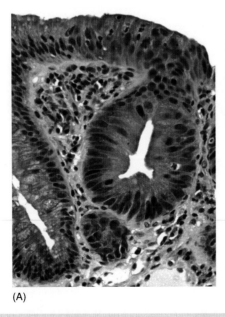
(A)

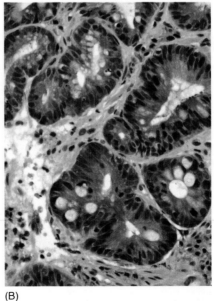
(B)

FIGURE 7.29 This case of Barrett esophagus shows a mildly atypical proliferation of glandular epithelium at the luminal surface with associated neutrophilic inflammation (A). Another case displays cytologically atypical cells in the deep glands that meet criteria of low-grade dysplasia, but are associated with mature epithelium on the surface (B). Both cases may be considered to be indefinite for dysplasia.

abnormalities cannot be adequately explained by either a location within the deep gland region or the presence of neutrophils. Thus, fused or cribriform glands, papillary or micropapillary projections, and microglands are evidence of high-grade dysplasia, regardless of inflammation or confinement of atypical epithelium to the deep mucosa.

Recognition of invasive carcinoma within the mucosa is important because these tumors have a small but definite risk of spread through lymphatic vessels to regional lymph nodes. For this reason, intramucosal carcinoma of the esophagus is assigned a pathologic stage of pT1a, whereas similar lesions in the colon are regarded as essentially equivalent to carcinoma in situ.

The distinction between high-grade glandular dysplasia and invasive adenocarcinoma can be challenging, especially in biopsy samples. Superficial biopsies of invasive adenocarcinoma generally do not show desmoplasia, because tumors rarely elicit a stromal reaction when they invade the mucosa. However, there are several features of intramucosal carcinoma in the esophagus that serve as helpful diagnostic clues (Figure 7.30A–F). Architecturally complex anastomosing or cribriform glands that expand the lamina propria are highly suggestive of carcinoma, as are single infiltrating tumor cells in the lamina propria and angulated glands that lack a connection to clearly noninvasive glands. Pagetoid spread of tumor cells in the adjacent, non-neoplastic squamous mucosa can be a very helpful distinguishing feature as well when the differential diagnosis includes high-grade dysplasia and adenocarcinoma, as this finding is not seen in high-grade dysplasia.

Recently, two groups have published criteria advocating for a category intermediate between high-grade dysplasia and intramucosal carcinoma, referred to as "high-grade dysplasia with marked glandular architectural distortion, cannot exclude intramucosal carcinoma" or "high-grade dysplasia with features 'suspicious' for invasive carcinoma." These authors suggest that cases with three or more glands with luminal debris or single cell infiltration of the lamina propria are more likely to have invasive adenocarcinoma on resection. However, this designation has not been widely accepted in general practice.

The differential diagnosis of invasive carcinoma in the submucosa is more straightforward. Dysplasia may colonize deep mucosal and submucosal esophageal glands and simulate the appearance of invasive adenocarcinoma in rare cases. Unlike invasive adenocarcinoma in the submucosa, colonization of glands by dysplasia does not show a destructive growth pattern or a desmoplastic tissue reaction, and the benign submucosal glands are tightly clustered in lobules.

The increased use of advanced endoscopic techniques has led to greater expectations of pathologists with respect to tumor reporting in small specimens. Excisional specimens often show artifactual erosion of the surface epithelium that results from suction of the sample into a plastic cap during the procedure. Cautery on the deep and lateral margins may cause challenges when evaluating for adequacy of excision as well. Assessing the depth of tumor invasion in these limited specimens can also be particularly problematic when the muscularis mucosae is duplicated. Penetration through the deeper layer is required in order to render a diagnosis of submucosal invasion, whereas tumors that transgress the duplicated superficial layer are classified as intramucosal cancers.

Less Common Types of Esophageal Carcinoma

Some esophageal carcinomas resemble those of salivary gland origin, particularly adenoid cystic or mucoepidermoid carcinomas, and have been labeled as such in the older literature. Although it is possible that salivary-type tumors could arise from submucosal glands, most cancers with these features develop in association with Barrett esophagus or squamous neoplasia and contain elements of adenocarcinoma or squamous cell carcinoma. The vast majority of esophageal tumors classified as adenoid cystic carcinoma are more appropriately considered to be high-grade, basaloid squamous carcinomas and pursue a clinical course comparable to that of squamous cell carcinoma; biologically indolent adenoid cystic carcinomas are exceedingly rare in the esophagus. Similarly, cancers that display divergent differentiation with glandular and squamous elements do not behave in an indolent fashion typical of mucoepidermoid carcinoma. Most of these lesions are probably best considered as adenosquamous carcinomas because they pursue a clinical course comparable to that of esophageal adenocarcinoma and squamous cell carcinoma (Figure 7.31). Lymphoepithelioma-like carcinomas of the esophagus contain syncytial sheets of malignant cells intimately admixed with mononuclear cell-rich infiltrates and tumor infiltrating lymphocytes. The neoplastic cells harbor large nuclei with thick, irregular membranes and one or more prominent nucleoli, as well as faintly eosinophilic cytoplasm. Some lymphoepithelioma-like carcinomas contain areas of either squamous cell carcinoma or adenocarcinoma and may show microsatellite instability. Pagetoid spread of tumor cells in non-neoplastic squamous epithelium of the esophagus can occur in patients with invasive squamous cell carcinoma, adenocarcinoma, or Paget disease derived from submucosal gland ducts.

Neuroendocrine Tumors of the Esophagus

Early investigators postulated that the diffuse endocrine system of the gastrointestinal tract was derived from the neural crest and, thus, classified tumors composed of similar cells as neuroendocrine neoplasms. Others later noted that these cells, and tumors that simulated their appearance, contained ultrastructural dense core granules, which they interpreted to reflect a "neurosecretory" nature, and

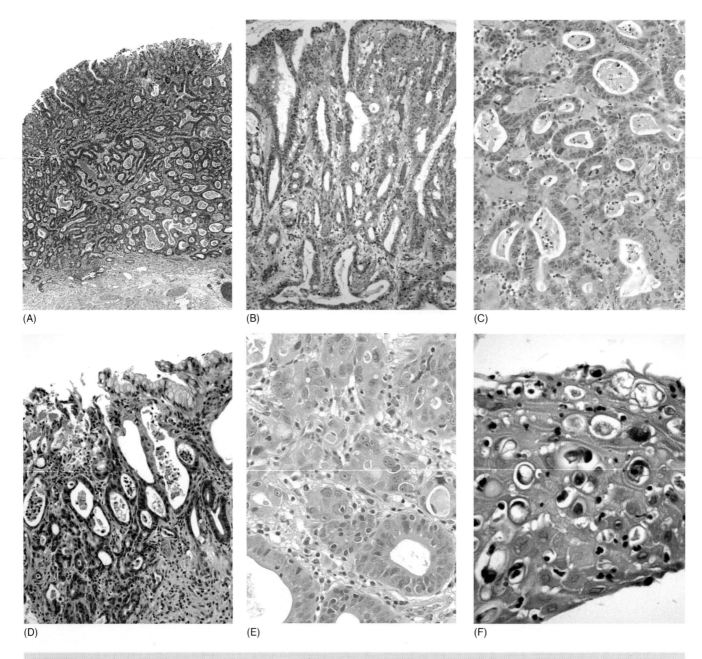

FIGURE 7.30 Features that suggest the presence of intramucosal carcinoma include complex, fused, and irregularly shaped glands, sometimes referred to as the "never-ending gland pattern," (A–C), detached, proliferating glands with dilation and luminal necrotic debris (D), single infiltrating tumor cells (E), and pagetoid spread of cells in squamous epithelium (F).

showed a "neuroendocrine" phenotype with immunopositivity for chromogranin A, neuron specific enolase, CD56, and synaptophysin. We now know that endocrine cells of the gastrointestinal tract have no relationship to the neural crest. They are derived from epithelial stem cells with potential for divergent differentiation into endocrine cells, Paneth cells, goblet cells, and absorptive cells, and neoplasms with similar features are also derived from multipotent stem cells. Endocrine cells of the gastrointestinal tract contain dense core secretory granules that reflect the

normal secretory function of these hormone-producing cells. Importantly, chromogranin A is a prohormone that is cleaved to produce functionally active peptides, so it is better considered a marker of endocrine, rather than neural, differentiation. It is interesting that, while many authors accept that endocrine cells comprise the diffuse endocrine system of the gastrointestinal tract, they advocate "neuroendocrine" to denote neoplasms that are phenotypically similar. At this point, "endocrine" and "neuroendocrine" are used synonymously to describe gastrointestinal tumors

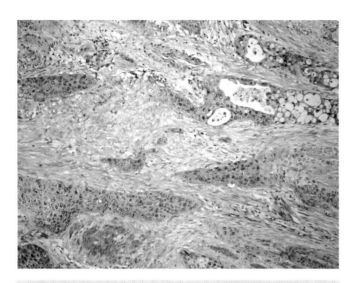

FIGURE 7.31   Adenosquamous carcinomas contain nests of squamoid tumor cells admixed with areas of glandular differentiation.

that elaborate hormones and express endocrine markers and synaptophysin.

Primary neuroendocrine tumors of the esophagus are uncommon, and account for less than 1% of epithelial tumors at this site. Similar to other organs of the gastrointestinal tract, they are classified as well-differentiated and poorly differentiated based upon the extent to which the tumor cells resemble endocrine cells normally present in the gastrointestinal tract (see also Chapter 3). By convention, well-differentiated tumors are subclassified as low (G1) or intermediate (G2) grade based on a combination of mitotic activity (less than 2 versus 2–10 mitotic figures/10 high-power fields) and Ki-67 immunolabeling (less than 3% versus 3%–20% immunopositivity). However, well-differentiated neuroendocrine tumors of the esophagus are so uncommon that their clinicopathologic features have not been well described. Like similar tumors of the stomach and intestines, they display an organoid, or nested, growth pattern of tumor cells within collagenous stroma. Tumor cells contain pale, or faintly eosinophilic, cytoplasm and round nuclei with stippled chromatin and small nucleoli.

Poorly differentiated neuroendocrine tumors are more common than well-differentiated tumors in the esophagus. These bulky, exophytic malignancies are high-grade (G3) carcinomas that typically present at an advanced stage in older adults (particularly males) and pursue an aggressive course with a mean survival of less than 1 year. Most of these tumors have a small cell phenotype similar to their counterparts in the lung, and contain nests and sheets of overtly malignant cells with scant cytoplasm and angulated, irregular nuclei, although large cell variants also occur (Figure 7.32A–C). Mitotic activity is generally brisk (greater than 20 mitotic figures/10 high-power fields) and

cellular necrosis is readily identified. Immunostains for Ki-67 demonstrate a large proportion of positive tumor cells, often approaching 80%. Some cases are associated with a variable component of invasive squamous cell carcinoma or high-grade squamous dysplasia in the surface epithelium. The major differential diagnosis in these types of tumors is extension into the esophagus from a small cell carcinoma of the lung, although occasionally the dyscohesive nature of these tumors raises the possibility of lymphoma.

GRADING AND STAGING OF ESOPHAGEAL CARCINOMA

The World Health Organization and TNM staging system do not provide useful guidance to pathologists regarding grade assignment to esophageal carcinomas. Some subtypes, including lymphoepithelioma-like, basaloid squamous, spindle cell (sarcomatoid), signet ring cell, mucinous, and neuroendocrine carcinomas, are generally regarded as high-grade malignancies, but criteria for grading of conventional squamous cell carcinoma and adenocarcinoma are lacking. This issue is particularly problematic with respect to pathologic stage classification since tumor grade is incorporated into the overall stage assignment for both tumor subtypes. In our practice, we generally limit the definition of well-differentiated squamous cell carcinoma to examples of verrucous carcinoma and those that are mostly keratinizing with few basaloid cells. With respect to adenocarcinomas, we endorse a two-tiered system that combines well-to-moderately differentiated (G1–G2) tumors in the low-grade category and groups those with less than 25% glandular differentiation as high-grade (G3–G4), similar to grading systems applied to other gastrointestinal malignancies.

Pathologic tumor staging of esophageal carcinoma is performed in accordance with the TNM staging manual of the American Joint Committee on Cancer (Table 7.2). Similar to the rest of the gastrointestinal tract, the local extent of the disease is assessed in the T category, whereas regional lymph node and distant metastases are classified in the N and M categories, respectively. Although this staging system assigns a tumor stage to dysplasia (pTis), many pathologists do not include this information in pathology reports of endoscopic mucosal resections, as the biologic risk of this finding is essentially nil provided that the lesional area is completely removed.

Although the same criteria are used for pathologic stage assessment of squamous cell carcinoma and adenocarcinoma, the overall stage groupings of these entities are separate. Stage groupings for invasive squamous cell carcinoma incorporate information regarding the primary tumor stage, regional lymph nodes, and distant

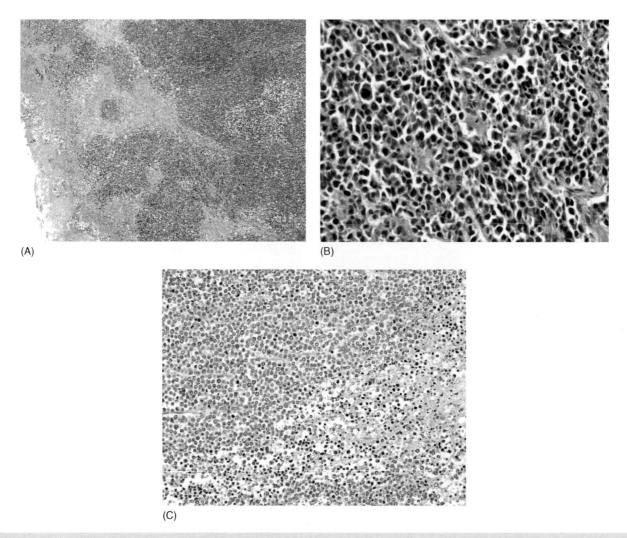

(A)

(B)

(C)

FIGURE 7.32   This high-grade neuroendocrine carcinoma of the esophagus has a sheet-like growth pattern and extensive necrosis. The overlying surface is completely ulcerated (A). At higher power, the tumor contains sheets of dyscohesive tumor cells with large round nuclei, stippled chromatin, and numerous mitotic figures, and a rim of amphophilic cytoplasm (B). Necrosis and karyorrhectic nuclear debris are common, and numerous mitoses are easily seen (C).

TABLE 7.2   Pathologic Staging Criteria of Esophageal and Gastroesophageal Junctional Carcinomas

Primary tumor (pT)	
TX	Primary tumor cannot be assessed
T0	No evidence of primary tumor
Tis	High-grade dysplasia
T1a	Tumor invades lamina propria or muscularis mucosae
T1b	Tumor invades submucosa
T2	Tumor invades muscularis propria
T3	Tumor invades adventitia
T4	Tumor invades adjacent structures
T4a	Resectable tumor invading pleura, pericardium, or diaphragm
T4b	Unresectable tumor invading other adjacent structures
Regional lymph nodes (pN)	
NX	Regional lymph nodes cannot be assessed
N0	No regional lymph node metastases
N1	Metastasis in 1–2 regional lymph nodes
N2	Metastasis in 3–6 regional lymph nodes
N3	Metastasis in 7 or more regional lymph nodes
Distant metastases (pM)	
M0	No distant metastases
M1	Distant metastases

TABLE 7.3   Anatomic Stage Groupings of Esophageal Squamous Cell Carcinoma

Stage	T	N	M	Grade	Location
0	Tis	N0	M0	1, X	Any
IA	T1	N0	M0	1, X	Any
IB	T1	N0	M0	2, 3	Any
	T2, T3	N0	M0	1, X	Lower, X
IIA	T2, T3	N0	M0	1, X	Upper, Middle
	T2, T3	N0	M0	2, 3	Lower, X
IIB	T2, T3	N0	M0	2, 3	Upper, Middle
	T1, T2	N1	M0	Any	Any
IIIA	T1, T2	N2	M0	Any	Any
	T3	N1	M0	Any	Any
	T4a	N0	M0	Any	Any
IIIB	T3	N2	M0	Any	Any
IIIC	T4a	N1, N2	M0	Any	Any
	T4b	Any	M0	Any	Any
	Any	N3	M0	Any	Any
IV	Any	Any	M1	Any	Any

metastases as well as anatomic tumor location and tumor grade (Table 7.3). Well-differentiated squamous cell carcinoma is generally assigned a lower overall stage compared to moderate-to-poorly differentiated tumors in cases without metastatic disease. Similarly, overall stage groupings of esophageal adenocarcinoma also incorporate tumor grade (Table 7.4). The distinction between low-grade (G1–G2) and high-grade (G3–G4) is considered most relevant, so the use of either a two- or four-tiered system is appropriate.

The increased use of endoscopic techniques for the management of dysplasia and early invasive carcinoma has resulted in a shift among pathologists with respect to pathologic reporting of endoscopically removed lesions. As it turns out, the depth of tumor invasion in the mucosa and submucosa predicts the likelihood of regional lymph node metastasis of both squamous cell carcinoma and adenocarcinoma. Thus, pathologists should report the depth of tumor invasion in endoscopic excision specimens.

Tumor invasion of the mucosa (pT1a) can be subclassified based on tumor extent: m1 denotes neoplasia confined to the basement membrane (ie, high-grade dysplasia), m2 is defined as tumor limited to the lamina propria, and m3 describes tumor that invades, but is limited to, the muscularis mucosae. Although it lacks anatomic landmarks, invasion of the submucosa (pT1b) can be similarly divided into inner (sm1), middle (sm2), and outer (sm3) thirds.

MESENCHYMAL TUMORS OF THE ESOPHAGUS

Granular Cell Tumor

Granular cell tumors may occur anywhere in the gastrointestinal tract, but are most common in the esophagus (see also Chapter 5). Benign tumors are often multifocal, and

TABLE 7.4   Anatomic Stage Groupings of Esophageal Adenocarcinoma

Stage	T	N	M	Grade
0	Tis	N0	M0	1, X
IA	T1	N0	M0	1, 2, X
IB	T1	N0	M0	3
	T2	N0	M0	1, 2, X
IIA	T2	N0	M0	3
IIB	T3	N0	M0	Any
	T1, T2	N1	M0	Any
IIIA	T1, T2	N2	M0	Any
	T3	N1	M0	Any
	T4a	N0	M0	Any
IIIB	T3	N2	M0	Any
IIIC	T4a	N1, N2	M0	Any
	T4b	Any	M0	Any
	Any	N3	M0	Any
IV	Any	Any	M1	Any

can be deeply infiltrative, but these features do not imply malignancy. Granular cell tumors usually occur in older adults, are slightly more common in women, and affect African Americans more frequently than Caucasians. Most tumors are incidentally discovered at the time of endoscopy and appear as firm, pale yellow polyps or plaques limited to the mucosa and submucosa of the distal esophagus. However, large lesions that extensively involve the muscularis propria may cause dysphagia.

Granular cell tumors consist of sheets and nests of cells with infiltrative borders that are intimately associated with thick bands of collagen (Figure 7.15B). Tumor cells are closely related to Schwann cells and show strong, diffuse S100 immunopositivity. They contain abundant faintly eosinophilic, granular cytoplasm that reflects the presence of myelin-filled lysosomes. Occasional PASD-positive eosinophilic globules are present in most cases. Granular cell tumors display minimal cytologic atypia; nuclei may appear to be pyknotic and mitotic figures are sparse. Some granular cell tumors elicit a peculiar pattern of pseudo-epitheliomatous squamous hyperplasia in the overlying epithelium, which may simulate the appearance of invasive squamous cell carcinoma. For this reason, one should carefully examine the lamina propria and submucosa before rendering a diagnosis of squamous cell carcinoma, especially in cases without a clinical suspicion for malignancy. Malignant granular cell tumors are extremely rare and show atypical cytologic features, nuclear enlargement, increased mitotic activity, and cellular necrosis, similar to malignant mesenchymal neoplasms elsewhere.

Gastrointestinal Stromal Tumor

Less than 1% of all gastrointestinal stromal tumors arise from the esophagus. These tumors usually occur in older adults and cause symptoms of obstruction, dysphagia, or occult blood loss. Most esophageal stromal tumors are biologically aggressive with high-risk features including large size and relatively brisk mitotic activity (greater than 5 mitoses/50 high-power fields). They have a fleshy appearance with hemorrhage, necrosis, and cystic degeneration, rather than the firm, whorled appearance of a leiomyoma. Gastrointestinal stromal tumors are highly cellular with long, sweeping fascicles of spindle cells that intersect at oblique angles. Lesional cells contain abundant eosinophilic cytoplasm and tapered nuclei with coarse chromatin and show strong immunopositivity for KIT and DOG1. The topic of gastrointestinal stromal tumors is discussed further in Chapter 5.

Leiomyoma and Leiomyomatosis

Leiomyomas are the most common mesenchymal tumors of the esophagus. They occur equally among men and women and are multifocal in nearly 25% of patients.

Historic data suggested that nearly 80% occurred in the distal esophagus and arose from the inner circular layer of the muscularis propria, whereas only 20% developed from the muscularis mucosae. However, more recent experience in the endoscopic era suggests that tumors of the muscularis mucosae are more common than previously believed. Tiny multifocal tumors have been termed *seedling leiomyomata,* and multiple large tumors are considered to represent *leiomyomatosis.* Tumors derived from the muscularis propria produce irregular thickening and may attain a large size that causes symptoms of obstruction. Leiomyomas have smooth, rounded contours and homogeneous echogenicity by endoscopic ultrasound. Small tumors of the muscularis mucosae can be endoscopically excised, whereas larger lesions are treated with surgical enucleation. Esophagectomy is reserved for patients with extremely large, or multiple, tumors.

Leiomyomas are firm, unencapsulated nodules with a pale, whorled cut surface. Paucicellular fascicles of bland smooth muscle cells intersect at right angles. The tumor cells contain densely eosinophilic cytoplasm and ovoid, blunt-ended nuclei (Figure 7.33A–B). A small amount of coagulative necrosis may be present in large tumors, but any substantial necrosis or mitotic activity should raise concern for a leiomyosarcoma. Tumor cells show strong diffuse immunohistochemical staining for actins, desmin, and caldesmon, but are uniformly negative for KIT. Some tumors do contain KIT-positive mast cells that should not be misinterpreted as evidence of a gastrointestinal stromal tumor (Figure 7.33B).

Leiomyosarcoma

Many reports of esophageal leiomyosarcoma predate the recognition of gastrointestinal stromal tumor, which is now believed to account for most malignant mesenchymal tumors of this site. Leiomyosarcoma is a tumor that develops almost exclusively in older adults. Most cases are high-grade spindle cell neoplasms with overt features of malignancy, including brisk mitotic activity, cellular necrosis, and severe cytologic atypia. Esophageal tumors share a similar immunophenotype with leiomyomas and are negative for KIT.

Giant Fibrovascular Polyp

Fibrovascular polyps are intriguing, but rare, lesions of the proximal esophagus. Virtually all cases occur in adults and originate near the cricopharyngeus muscle. Presumably, polyp formation is the result of prolapsing redundant mucosal folds that become increasingly distorted due to elevated intraluminal pressures in the upper esophageal sphincter region. Most patients complain of progressive dysphagia that reflects gradual enlargement of the polyp. However, some polyps are clinically silent

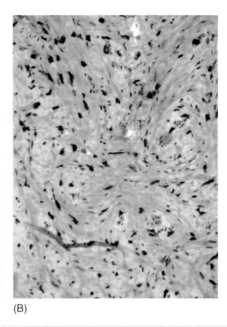

(A)   (B)

FIGURE 7.33 Leiomyomas contain sweeping fascicles of bland smooth muscle cells and display negligible mitotic activity (A). They do contain mast cells that show immunopositivity for KIT (B), which should not be mistaken as evidence of a GIST.

until they obstruct the larynx, or are regurgitated into the posterior hypopharynx. Such cases produce symptoms of acute respiratory distress, vomiting, belching, coughing, or even sudden death by asphyxiation.

Fibrovascular polyps have a sausage-like, multilobulated appearance. They tend to be large and protrude into the lumen on a broad stalk. The squamous mucosal surface is often inflamed or eroded, owing to local trauma, and the lamina propria and submucosa contain variable amounts of loose, edematous myxoid tissue, extracellular collagen, and mature adipose tissue (Figure 7.34A–D). Most polyps are inflamed and harbor proliferating fibroblasts, some of which may contain bizarre nuclei with prominent nucleoli, especially in areas of ulceration. Vessels are prominent, and often have thick walls and surrounding fibrosis. Fibrovascular polyps are benign and cured by simple excision. Of note, some atypical lipomas may develop in the esophagus and closely simulate the appearance of a giant fibrovascular polyp.

OTHER ESOPHAGEAL NEOPLASMS

Pyloric Gland Adenoma

Pyloric gland adenomas rarely develop at the gastroesophageal junction where they can form esophageal polyps, but they are more commonly encountered in the stomach. Most are incidentally discovered in patients undergoing endoscopic evaluation for symptoms related to the upper gastrointestinal tract. Pyloric gland adenomas contain tightly packed lobules of small round glands with little intervening stroma. Cuboidal epithelial cells harbor neutral mucin and basally oriented nuclei with minimal cytologic atypia. Unlike hyperplastic polyps, pyloric gland adenomas show strong immunohistochemical staining for MUC6 and contain foveolar epithelial cells that are largely limited to the polyp surface. Preliminary data suggest that at least 50% of pyloric gland adenomas near the gastroesophageal junction develop in association with intestinal metaplasia, many of which can show dysplasia.

Metastases to the Esophagus

Secondary malignancies involve the esophagus by direct extension from adjacent organs or hematogenous metastasis. Most commonly, carcinomas of the respiratory tract invade the thoracic esophagus, causing symptoms of dysphagia, hematemesis, or pneumonitis due to fistulizing disease. These tumors typically display squamous or glandular differentiation. Invasive squamous cell carcinomas of pulmonary origin are morphologically and immunohistochemically indistinguishable from those of the esophagus, although the differential diagnosis between pulmonary and esophageal adenocarcinoma can usually be resolved. Tumor location above the level of the gastroesophageal junction and an absence of Barrett esophagus are useful pathologic features that should suggest secondary involvement of the esophagus by adenocarcinoma. Immunostains for pulmonary markers, such as TTF-1, are typically negative in esophageal adenocarcinomas. Napsin does not reliably distinguish between tumors of pulmonary and esophageal origin.

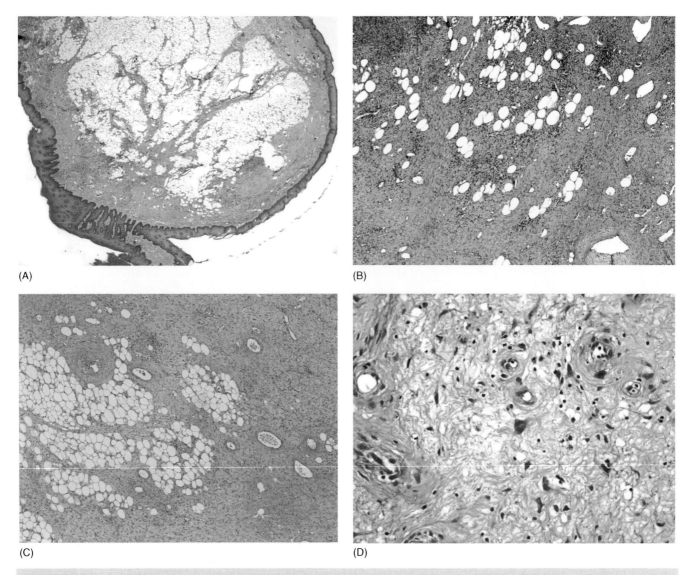

FIGURE 7.34 Giant fibrovascular polyps contain both mesenchymal and epithelial elements. This polyp contains abundant fat and fibrous tissue with chronic inflammation, lymphoid aggregates, and normal squamous epithelium (A–B; A, courtesy of Dr. Elizabeth Montgomery). Vessels are prominent, and may be thick-walled with surrounding fibrosis (C). Occasional atypical stromal stellate cells are seen, enmeshed in collagen (D, courtesy of Dr. Elizabeth Montgomery).

Any advanced malignancy may metastasize to the esophagus, although esophageal metastases are much less common than those to other organs of the tubular gut. Patients with metastatic disease typically present with symptoms similar to those of individuals with primary malignancies, namely dysphagia, coughing, vomiting, and occult blood loss or hematemesis. Tumors that show a predilection for the gastrointestinal tract include carcinomas of the lung, breast, and kidney, as well as malignant melanoma. Features suggesting the possibility of a metastasis include tumor multifocality, location of adenocarcinoma in the upper or midesophagus, and the presence of extensive lymphovascular invasion in biopsy samples.

Malignant Melanoma

Primary malignant melanoma of the esophagus is extremely rare and accounts for less than 0.1% of all esophageal neoplasms. Patients are older adults who present with progressive dysphagia, obstruction, hemorrhage, cough, or pain due to locally advanced tumors. The prognosis is dismal with a mean survival of less than 1 year. Esophageal melanoma is unassociated with any identifiable risk factors and has no apparent relationship with cutaneous melanoma. The background mucosa may show melanosis, although a causal role for this finding has not been established. Tumors typically appear

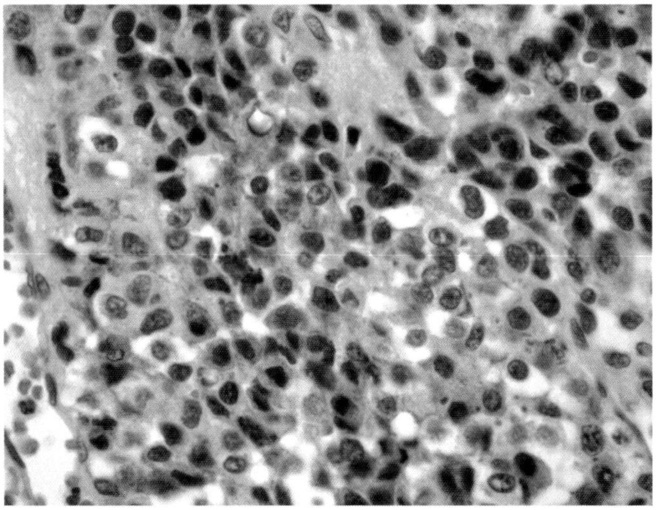

FIGURE 7.35 This primary malignant melanoma of the esophagus contains sheets of neoplastic cells, some of which are pigmented. Lesional cells contain abundant cytoplasm and have a vaguely plasmacytoid appearance, although they show nuclear variability.

as a polypoid intraluminal mass. Similar to malignant melanoma of other organs, esophageal tumors may be pigmented or amelanotic, and display either spindle or epithelioid cells with an organoid arrangement. Tumor cells contain eosinophilic or amphophilic cytoplasm and large, often eccentric nuclei that impart a plasma-cytoid appearance. Intranuclear inclusions and nucleoli may be prominent (Figure 7.35). Esophageal melanomas express melanocytic markers, including S100, A103, and HMB-45, although high-grade and spindle cell lesions may show loss of immunostaining for one, or more, antibodies.

SELECTED REFERENCES

General

Barker N, Clevers H. Lineage tracing in the intestinal epithelium. *Curr Protoc Stem Cell Biol.* 2010;Chapter 5:Unit5A 4.

Jemal A, Bray F, Center MM, et al. Global cancer statistics. *CA Cancer J Clin.* 2011;61(2):69–90.

Rice TW, Blackstone EH, Rusch VW. Esophagus and esophagogastric junction. In: Edge SB, Byrd DR, Compton CC, Fritz AG, Greene FL, Trotti A, eds. *AJCC Cancer Staging Manual.* 7th ed. New York, NY: Springer;2010:103–115.

Wang KK, Prasad G, Tian J. Endoscopic mucosal resection and endoscopic submucosal dissection in esophageal and gastric cancers. *Curr Opin Gastroenterol.* 2010;26(5):453–458.

Inflammatory and Non-Neoplastic Lesions

Abe T, Hosokawa M, Kusumi T, et al. Adenocarcinoma arising from ectopic gastric mucosa in the cervical esophagus. *Am J Clin Oncol.* 2004;27(6):644–645.

Abraham SC, Singh VK, Yardley JH, Wu TT. Hyperplastic polyps of the esophagus and esophagogastric junction: histologic and clinicopathologic findings. *Am J Surg Pathol.* 2001;25(9):1180–1187.

Akiyama J, Bertele A, Brock C, et al. Benign and precursor lesions in the esophagus. *Ann NY Acad Sci.* 2014;1325(1):226–241.

Squamous Dysplasia and Squamous Cell Carcinoma

Cao W, Chen X, Dai H, et al. Mutational spectra of p53 in geographically localized esophageal squamous cell carcinoma groups in China. *Cancer.* 2004 15;101(4):834–844.

Denlinger CE, Thompson RK. Molecular basis of esophageal cancer development and progression. *Surg Clin North Am.* 2012;92(5):1089–1103.

Devlin S, Falck V, Urbanski SJ, et al. Verrucous carcinoma of the esophagus eluding multiple sets of endoscopic biopsies and endoscopic ultrasound: a case report and review of the literature. *Can J Gastroenterol.* 2004;18(7):459–462.

Kwatra KS, Prabhakar BR, Jain S, Grewal JS. Sarcomatoid carcinoma (carcinosarcoma) of the esophagus with extensive areas of osseous differentiation: a case report. *Indian J Pathol Microbiol.* 2003;46(1):49–51.

Lauwers GY, Grant LD, Scott GV, et al. Spindle cell squamous carcinoma of the esophagus: analysis of ploidy and tumor proliferative activity in a series of 13 cases. *Hum Pathol.* 1998;29(8):863–868.

Liu H, Li YQ, Yu T, et al. Confocal endomicroscopy for in vivo detection of microvascular architecture in normal and malignant lesions of upper gastrointestinal tract. *J Gastroenterol and Hepatol.* 2008;23(1):56–61.

Metzger R, Schneider PM, Warnecke-Eberz U, et al. Molecular biology of esophageal cancer. *Onkologie.* 2004;27(2):200–206.

Singhi AD, Arnold CA, Crowder CD, et al. Esophageal leukoplakia or epidermoid metaplasia: a clinicopathological study of 18 patients. *Mod Pathol.* 2014;27(1):38–43.

Teng H, Li X, Liu X, et al. The absence of human papillomavirus in esophageal squamous cell carcinoma in East China. *Int J Clin Exp Pathol.* 2014;7(7):4184–4193.

Uedo N, Fujishiro M, Goda K, et al. Role of narrow band imaging for diagnosis of early-stage esophagogastric cancer: current consensus of experienced endoscopists in Asia-Pacific region. *Dig Endosc.* 2011;23 Suppl 1:58–71.

Wang GQ, Abnet CC, Shen Q, et al. Histological precursors of oesophageal squamous cell carcinoma: results from a 13 year prospective follow up study in a high risk population. *Gut.* 2005;54(2):187–192.

Zhang XH, Sun GQ, Zhou XJ, et al. Basaloid squamous carcinoma of esophagus:a clinicopathological, immunohistochemical and electron microscopic study of sixteen cases. *World J Gastroenterol.* 1998;4(5):397–403.

Adenocarcinoma, Glandular Dysplasia, and Barrett Esophagus

Abraham SC, Krasinskas AM, Correa AM, et al. Duplication of the muscularis mucosae in Barrett esophagus: an underrecognized feature and its implication for staging of adenocarcinoma. *Am J Surg Pathol.* 2007;31(11):1719–1725.

Anaparthy R, Sharma P. Progression of Barrett oesophagus: role of endoscopic and histological predictors. *Nat Rev Gastroenterol Hepatol.* 2014;11(9):525–534.

Angulo-Pernett F, Smythe WR. Primary lymphoepithelioma of the esophagus. *Ann Thorac Surg.* 2003;76(2):603–605.

Appelman HD, Matejcic M, Parker MI, et al. Progression of esophageal dysplasia to cancer. *Ann NY Acad Sci.* 2014;1325(1):96–107.

Bang YJ, Van Cutsem E, Feyereislova A, et al. Trastuzumab in combination with chemotherapy versus chemotherapy alone for treatment of HER2-positive advanced gastric or gastro-oesophageal junction cancer (ToGA): a phase 3, open-label, randomised controlled trial. *Lancet*. 2010;376(9742):687–697.

Chen S, Chen Y, Yang J, et al. Primary mucoepidermoid carcinoma of the esophagus. *J Thorac Oncol*. 2011;6(8):1426–1431.

Davies AR, Gossage JA, Zylstra J, et al. Tumor stage after neoadjuvant chemotherapy determines survival after surgery for adenocarcinoma of the esophagus and esophagogastric junction. *J Clin Oncol*. 2014;32(27):2983–2990.

Davydov CE, Delektorskaya VV, Kuvshinov YP, et al. Superficial and early cancers of the esophagus. *Ann NY Acad Sci*. 2014;1325(1):159–169.

Downs-Kelly E, Mendelin JE, Bennett AE, et al. Poor interobserver agreement in the distinction of high grade dysplasia and adenocarcinoma in pretreatment Barrett's esophagus biopsies. *Am J Gastroenterol*. 2008;103:2333–2340.

Estrella JS, Hofstetter WL, Correa AM, et al. Duplicated muscularis mucosae invasion has similar risk of lymph node metastasis and recurrence-free survival as intramucosal esophageal adenocarcinoma. *Am J Surg Pathol*. 2011;35(7):1045–1053.

Flejou JF, Odze RD, Montgomery E, et al. Adenocarcinoma of the oesophagus. In: Bosman FT, Carneiro F, Hruban RH, Theise ND, eds. *WHO Classification of Tumours of the Digestive System*. 4th ed. Lyon: International Agency for Research on Cancer; 2010:25–31.

Hagen CE, Lauwers GY, Mino-Kenudson M. Barrett esophagus: diagnostic challenges. *Semin Diagn Pathol*. 2014;31(2):100–113.

Hermann RM, Horstmann O, Haller F, et al. Histomorphological tumor regression grading of esophageal carcinoma after neoadjuvant radiochemotherapy: which score to use? *Dis Esophagus*. 2006;19(5):329–334.

Hobel S, Dautel P, Baumbach R, et al. Single center experience of endoscopic submucosal dissection (ESD) in early Barrett s adenocarcinoma. *Surg Endosc*. 2014. [Epub ahead of print]

Leers JM, DeMeester SR, Oezcelik A, et al. The prevalence of lymph node metastases in patients with T1 esophageal adenocarcinoma a retrospective review of esophagectomy specimens. *Ann Surg*. 2011;253(2):271–278.

Lomo LC, Blount PL, Sanchez CA, et al. Crypt dysplasia with surface maturation: a clinical, pathologic, and molecular study of a Barrett's esophagus cohort. *Am J Surg Pathol*. 2006;30(4):423–435.

Menezes A, Tierney A, Yang YX, et al. Adherence to the 2011 American Gastroenterological Association medical position statement for the diagnosis and management of Barrett's esophagus. *Dis Esophagus*. 2014. [Epub ahead of print]

Merlo LM, Shah NA, Li X, et al. A comprehensive survey of clonal diversity measures in Barrett's esophagus as biomarkers of progression to esophageal adenocarcinoma. *Cancer Prev Res*. 2010;3(11):1388–1397.

Noble F, Nolan L, Bateman AC, et al. Refining pathological evaluation of neoadjuvant therapy for adenocarcinoma of the esophagus. *World J Gastroenterol*. 2013;19(48):9282–9293.

Okines A, Cunningham D, Chau I. Targeting the human EGFR family in esophagogastric cancer. *Nat Rev Clin Oncol*. 2011;8(8):492–503.

Patil DT, Golblum JR, Rybicki L, et al. Prediction of adenocarcinoma in esophagectomy specimens based upon analysis of preresection biopsies of Barrett esophagus with at least high trade dysplasia: a comparison of two systems. *Am J Surg Pathol*. 2012;36:134–141.

Sami SS, Subramanian V, Butt WM, et al. High definition versus standard definition white light endoscopy for detecting dysplasia in patients with Barrett's esophagus. *Dis Esophagus*. 2014. [Epub ahead of print]

Sampliner RE. Updated guidelines for the diagnosis, surveillance, and therapy of Barrett's esophagus. *Am J Gastroenterol*. 2002;97(8):1888–1895.

Schnell TG, Sontag SJ, Chejfec G, et al. Long-term nonsurgical management of Barrett's esophagus with high-grade dysplasia. *Gastroenterol*. 2001;120(7):1607–1619.

Skacel M, Petras RE, Gramlich TL, Sigel JE, Richter JE, Goldblum JR. The diagnosis of low-grade dysplasia in Barrett's esophagus and its implications for disease progression. *Am J Gastroenterol*. 2000;95(12):3383–3387.

Spechler SJ, Souza RF. Barrett's esophagus. *N Engl J Med*. 2014;371(9):836–845.

Verbeek RE, Leenders M, Ten Kate FJ, et al. Surveillance of Barrett's esophagus and mortality from esophageal adenocarcinoma: a population-based cohort study. *Am J Gastroenterol*. 2014;109(8):1215–1222.

Wainberg ZA, Anghel A, Desai AJ, et al. Lapatinib, a dual EGFR and HER2 kinase inhibitor, selectively inhibits HER2-amplified human gastric cancer cells and is synergistic with trastuzumab in vitro and in vivo. *Clin Cancer Res*. 2010;16(5):1509–1519.

Weston AP, Sharma P, Mathur S, et al. Risk stratification of Barrett's esophagus: updated prospective multivariate analysis. *Am J Gastroenterol*. 2004;99(9):1657–1666.

Yantiss RK. Diagnostic challenges in the pathologic evaluation of Barrett esophagus. *Arch Pathol Lab Med*. 2010;134(11):1589–1600.

Zhu W, Appelman HD, Greenson JK, et al. A histologically defined subset of high-grade dysplasia in Barrett mucosa is predictive of associated carcinoma. *Am J Clin Pathol*. 2009;132(1):94–100.

Neuroendocrine Tumors

Helle KB. Chromogranins A and B and secretogranin II as prohormones for regulatory peptides from the diffuse neuroendocrine system. *Results Probl Cell Differ*. 2010;50:21–44.

Hoang MP, Hobbs CM, Sobin LH, Albores-Saavedra J. Carcinoid tumor of the esophagus: a clinicopathologic study of four cases. *Am J Surg Pathol*. 2002;26(4):517–522.

Pearse AG, Polak JM. Neural crest origin of the endocrine polypeptide (APUD) cells of the gastrointestinal tract and pancreas. *Gut*. 1971;12(10):783–788.

Mesenchymal Tumors

Fei BY, Yang JM, Zhao ZS. Differential clinical and pathological characteristics of esophageal stromal tumors and leiomyomata. *Dis Esophagus*. 2014;27(1):30–35.

Goldblum JR, Rice TW, Zuccaro G, Richter JE. Granular cell tumors of the esophagus: a clinical and pathologic study of 13 cases. *Ann Thorac Surg*. 1996;62(3):860–865.

Miettinen M, Sarlomo-Rikala M, Sobin LH, Lasota J. Esophageal stromal tumors: a clinicopathologic, immunohistochemical, and molecular genetic study of 17 cases and comparison with esophageal leiomyomas and leiomyosarcomas. *Am J Surg Pathol*. 2000;24(2):211–222.

Miscellaneous Other Tumors

Bisceglia M, Perri F, Tucci A, et al. Primary malignant melanoma of the esophagus: a clinicopathologic study of a case with comprehensive literature review. *Adv Anat Pathol*. 2011;18(3):235–252.

Chen ZM, Scudiere JR, Abraham SC, Montgomery E. Pyloric gland adenoma: an entity distinct from gastric foveolar type adenoma. *Am J Surg Pathol*. 2009;33(2):186–193.

8

Neoplasms of the Stomach

LAURA W. LAMPS AND SCOTT R. OWENS

INTRODUCTION

A wide variety of benign and malignant neoplasms arise in the stomach; they can be broadly classified as epithelial, neuroendocrine, mesenchymal, and hematolymphoid (Table 8.1). Gastric adenocarcinoma remains the second most common malignancy worldwide, although there has been a decline in its incidence over the past five decades. Well differentiated neuroendocrine tumors (NETs) have comprised less than 1% of gastric neoplasms in the past; this number is likely a significant underestimate, and has increased in recent years due to awareness of these types of tumors and improved imaging and endoscopic techniques. Although mesenchymal tumors reportedly account for less than 1.0% of gastrointestinal (GI) malignancies overall, most of these are gastrointestinal stromal tumors (GISTs), many of which (60%–70%) arise in the stomach. Gastric lymphoma accounts for approximately 5% to 10% of gastric malignancies. This chapter will address the most commonly encountered tumors of the stomach; neoplasms that can affect any part of the GI tract, but infrequently affect the stomach, are discussed elsewhere.

INFLAMMATORY AND NON-NEOPLASTIC LESIONS

Gastroenterologists commonly biopsy inflammatory or non-neoplastic gastric lesions and polyps that are found incidentally at endoscopy. Some of these mimic or enter into the differential diagnosis of other gastric neoplasms, or have an associated risk of developing dysplasia, and thus will be discussed here briefly.

Inflammatory Polyps

There are no well-defined criteria for inflammatory polyps in the stomach. Some pathologists use this term to refer to polypoid granulation tissue, or synonymously with "polypoid gastritis," to reflect marked chronic gastritis that produces nodular or polypoid inflammatory lesions. This most often happens in the context of *Helicobacter pylori* infection, although it has also been described in association with chronic atrophic gastritis.

Hyperplastic Polyps

Hyperplastic polyps are reportedly the second most common gastric polyp after fundic gland polyps (FGPs), although diagnostic criteria have not been clearly defined in the past (see discussion in subsequent paragraphs). Most are discovered incidentally during upper endoscopy for another reason. They have been associated with autoimmune gastritis and with longstanding *H. pylori*-associated gastritis, as well as other inflammatory conditions. Historically, entities termed hyperplastic polyp have represented a very heterogeneous group of polyps that also include inflammatory polyps, foveolar hyperplasia, and gastric mucosal prolapse polyps. Numerous hyperplastic polyps may raise the possibility of gastric hyperplastic polyposis, although neither the clinical nor the pathologic criteria for this rare disorder have been well elucidated.

More recent criteria suggest classifying lesions consisting of a sharply localized focus of elongated foveolar glands without cystic changes, significant inflammation, or architectural derangement as "polypoid foveolar hyperplasia" (Figure 8.1A–B). Hyperplastic polyps, in contrast,

173

TABLE 8.1   Classification of Gastric Neoplasms According to the 2010 World Health Organization

Epithelial Tumors
Premalignant Lesions
Adenoma
Intraepithelial neoplasia, low grade
Intraepithelial neoplasia, high grade
Carcinoma
Adenocarcinoma
  Papillary
  Tubular
  Mucinous
  Poorly cohesive (including signet ring cell carcinoma)
  Mixed
Adenosquamous carcinoma
Medullary carcinoma
Hepatoid adenocarcinoma
Squamous cell carcinoma
Undifferentiated carcinoma
Neuroendocrine Neoplasms
Neuroendocrine tumor (NET)
  G1 (carcinoid)
  G2
Neuroendocrine carcinoma (NEC)
  Large cell NEC
  Small cell NEC
Mixed adenoneuroendocrine tumor (MANEC)
Enterochromaffin (EC) cell, serotonin producing NET
Gastrinoma (gastrin-producing NET)
Mesenchymal Tumors
Glomus tumor
Granular cell tumor
Leiomyoma
Plexiform fibromyxoma
Inflammatory myofibroblastic tumor
Gastrointestinal stromal tumors (GIST)
Kaposi sarcoma
Leiomyosarcoma
Synovial sarcoma
Lymphoma
Secondary Tumors

Source: Data adapted from *WHO Classification of Tumors of the Digestive System*, 4th Edition, 2010.

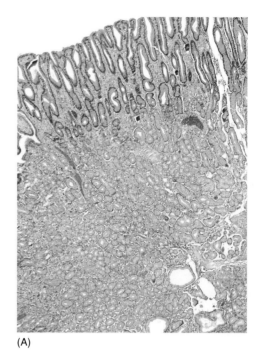

(A)

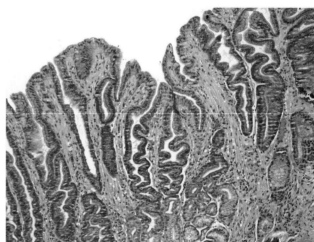

(B)

FIGURE 8.1   Polypoid foveolar hyperplasia features elongated, tortuous foveolar glands without cystic changes or significant inflammation (A–B). Mucin depletion is common in the epithelium.

feature elongation of the pit region imparting a corkscrew appearance, branching and cystic dilatation of glands, lamina propria edema and inflammation, and variably present surface erosions (Figure 8.2A–C). Pseudogoblet cells, or distended mucinous cells, are frequently seen as well (Figure 8.2D). Although there may be thin strands of smooth muscle, the thick bundles of muscle typically seen in hamartomatous polyps are not a feature of hyperplastic polyps. Hyperplastic polyps can be pedunculated or sessile, and range in size from a few millimeters to 3 cm or more. They are most common in the antrum, but can be found anywhere in the stomach, and are often multiple. Hyperplastic polyps and polypoid foveolar hyperplasia may well represent related lesions along a spectrum of regenerative/reactive polyps, and both lesions can be seen in the context of reactive gastropathy, *H. pylori* infection,

or nonspecific chronic inactive gastritis. Because the majority of hyperplastic polyps are associated with some form of gastritis, biopsy of intervening nonpolypoid mucosa is strongly recommended. Many hyperplastic polyps regress with treatment of the background gastritis, but recurrence is common.

Hyperplastic polyps often contain foci of intestinal metaplasia, but intestinal metaplasia is even more likely to be found in the mucosa adjacent to hyperplastic polyps. There is an associated very low (approximately 4%) but well-recognized risk of dysplasia, especially when hyperplastic polyps are large (over 2 cm) (Figure 8.2E–F).

Gastric Mucosal Prolapse Polyps

Gastric mucosal prolapse polyps are a more recently described inflammatory lesion typically seen in the antrum and pylorus of middle-aged patients. They may be sessile, papular, or pedunculated, and range in size from a few millimeters to over 3 cm. Similar to hyperplastic polyps, mucosal prolapse polyps show elongation and cystic dilatation of the gastric pits, but also feature bundles of arborizing smooth muscle and thick-walled, prominent vessels

(Figure 8.3A–B). A prominent basal glandular component consisting of tightly packed, back-to-back glands is another distinguishing feature.

Heterotopic Pancreas/Adenomyoma

Pancreatic rests or pancreatic heterotopias are congenital lesions that represent separation of portions of pancreatic tissue during rotation of the foregut. They present in a variety of ways, ranging from asymptomatic incidental findings

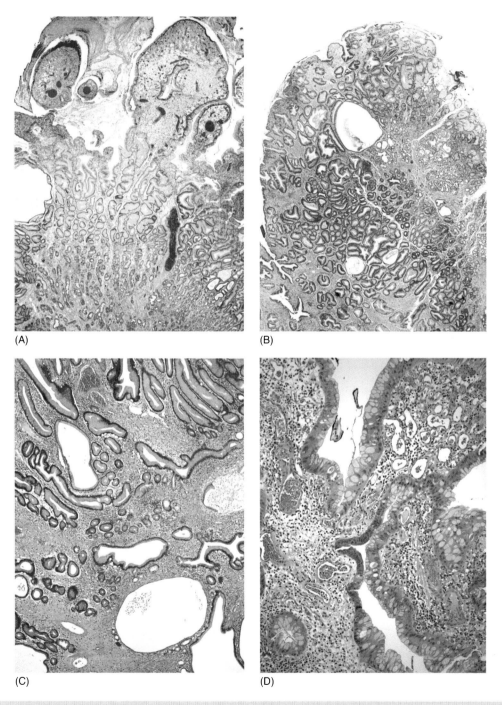

(A)

(B)

(C)

(D)

FIGURE 8.2 Hyperplastic polyps feature elongation of the pit region (A [courtesy Dr. Rhonda Yantiss] and B), imparting a corkscrew appearance, along with branching and cystic dilatation of glands and lamina propria edema and inflammation (C). Pseudogoblet cells are frequently seen as well (D, courtesy Dr. Rhonda Yantiss). (*continued*)

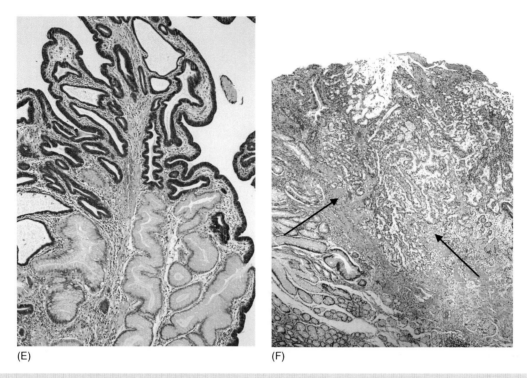

(E)   (F)

FIGURE 8.2 (*continued*) There is a low but well-recognized risk of dysplasia in hyperplastic polyps, especially in those greater than 2 cm (E, low-grade dysplasia [courtesy Dr. Rhonda Yantiss]; F [arrow], high grade dysplasia/carcinoma in situ).

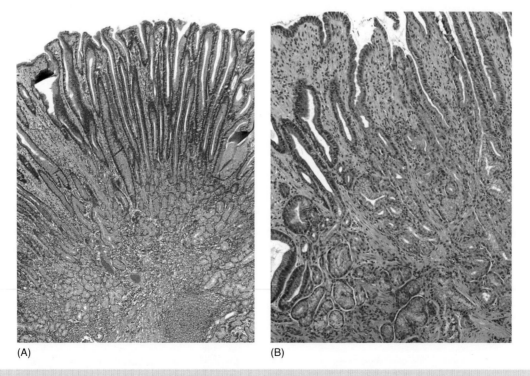

(A)   (B)

FIGURE 8.3 Mucosal prolapse polyps show elongation and variable dilatation of the gastric pits, as well as prominent bundles of arborizing smooth muscle and prominent vessels (A–B). A prominent basal glandular component consisting of tightly packed, back-to-back glands is another distinguishing feature.

to ulceration with associated GI bleeding. The classic endoscopic appearance is that of a bulging dome-shaped mass with a broad base, smooth surface, and central umbilication (Figure 8.4A). In the stomach, pancreatic heterotopias are most often located in the antrum.

Although usually asymptomatic, pancreatic heterotopias have several clinically important sequelae. They may present with localized inflammation and ulceration that leads to bleeding, and more rarely, they cause pyloric obstruction or intussusception due to mass effect. Rare cases of malignant transformation (both adenocarcinoma and well-differentiated NETs) have been reported.

Histologically, pancreatic heterotopia consists of irregularly dilated cystic glands lined by cuboidal epithelium, resembling biliary epithelium. These ductal structures are arranged in a lobular pattern, with surrounding dense fibromuscular stroma and (usually) pancreatic exocrine and endocrine cells, including islets of Langerhans (Figure 8.4B–C). Occasionally, however, only ductal epithelium is present (sometimes called an "adenomyoma"), which may mimic invasive adenocarcinoma, particularly on frozen section. In addition, lesions with prominent islet cells can occasionally mimic NET in a biopsy specimen.

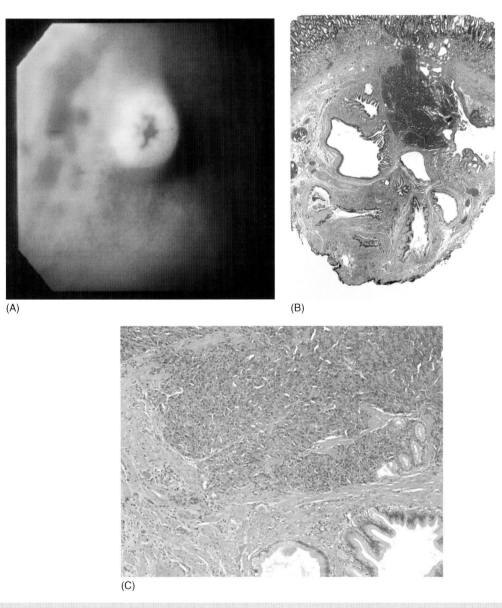

(A)

(B)

(C)

FIGURE 8.4 Macroscopically, pancreatic heterotopia often appears as an umbilicated nodule (A). The lesion is composed of ducts arranged in a lobular pattern (B), with surrounding dense fibromuscular stroma and pancreatic exocrine and endocrine cells, including islets of Langerhans (C).

Diagnostic Challenges

Hyperplastic polyps and inflammatory-type polyps present two distinct diagnostic challenges in terms of differential diagnosis. The first is differentiating between a hyperplastic or inflammatory lesion with marked regenerative/reparative changes, and dysplasia. Nuclear enlargement and hyperchromasia, prominent nucleoli, and increased mitotic activity are all features of reparative atypia that can mimic dysplasia. Most reparative changes that are severe enough to mimic dysplasia are also associated with marked acute inflammation and/or mucosal ulceration, and therefore cytologic atypia in association with marked inflammation and/or ulceration should be interpreted with caution. It is also important to remember that immunostains such as p53 may be positive in areas of marked regeneration as well. Inflammatory changes tend to be uniform and show a gradual transition to more normal-appearing mucosa, whereas dysplasia is sharply demarcated from the adjacent non-neoplastic mucosa.

The second challenge is distinguishing between hyperplastic polyps and other entities in the differential diagnosis, including hamartomatous polyps and Ménétrier disease. Gastric Peutz–Jeghers polyps (PJPs) typically have well-developed lobular architecture, and lack the cystically dilated, tortuous glands and pits as well as the edematous, inflamed stroma typical of hyperplastic polyps. Hyperplastic polyps also typically lack the well-developed smooth muscle component often seen in Peutz–Jeghers polyps. Gastric hyperplastic polyps and gastric juvenile polyps can have substantial histologic overlap, and thus clinical and family history as well as endoscopic information may be necessary to distinguish these lesions. Gastric hyperplastic polyps can also mimic Ménétrier disease and Cronkhite–Canada syndrome, particularly if only a small biopsy of a larger endoscopic lesion is available for evaluation. Knowledge of the clinical history and endoscopic findings is essential in this circumstance as well. Gastritis cystica profunda/polyposis may also mimic hyperplastic polyps. This condition typically develops in patients who are status-post surgery, particularly if bile reflux is present. If the lesion is polypoid and intraluminal, then the *polyposa* moniker is used; if the lesions are intramural, then *profunda* is used. Patients develop polypoid lesions that are similar to hyperplastic polyps or prolapse polyps; in addition, as in colitis cystica profunda, entrapped benign gastric epithelium is often present beneath the mucosal surface.

EPITHELIAL NEOPLASMS

Hamartomatous Polyps

Several types of hamartomatous polyps occur in the stomach, including polyps associated with Peutz–Jeghers

syndrome (PJS), juvenile polyposis syndromes (JPS), and Cowden disease; these are discussed in more detail in Chapter 6.

Fundic Gland Polyps

Fundic gland polyps (FGPs) are the most common hamartomatous gastric polyp, and one of the most common types of gastric polyp overall. These polyps may be syndromic (most commonly associated with familial adenomatous polyposis [FAP]) or sporadic. FGPs are also associated with Zollinger–Ellison syndrome and with the rare entity known as sporadic fundic gland polyposis, defined as multiple fundic gland polyps in patients without FAP or related syndromes. FGPs in sporadic fundic gland polyposis are histologically identical to solitary sporadic FGP, but demonstrate frequent somatic activating mutations in exon 3 of *CTNNB1*, which encodes β-catenin.

FGPs are smooth, sessile lesions that by definition occur in a background of gastric oxyntic mucosa. They may be single or multiple, and are often multiple in the context of FAP. Typically these are small lesions (less than 1.0 cm), but may grow to 2 cm to 3 cm. Histologically, FGPs are composed of oxyntic as well as foveolar epithelium (Figure 8.5A–B). There is frequently cystic dilatation of glands, as well as prominent epithelial budding. Inflammation is not prominent. The overlying surface foveolae are shortened. Patients on protein pump inhibitor (PPI) therapy may show parietal cell hypertrophy and hyperplasia, with tufting of cells into the lumen as well as vacuolization of the cytoplasm (Figure 8.5C).

Sporadic FGPs are increasing in incidence, which is most likely a reflection of increasing PPI use as these drugs have been implicated in the pathogenesis of sporadic FGPs. Women are more likely to develop sporadic FGPs, whereas syndromic FGPs show no gender predilection. Sporadic FGPs have essentially no malignant potential, and dysplasia occurs in less than 1.0% of sporadic lesions.

Approximately 90% of patients with FAP have FGPs, which frequently show dysplasia (Figure 8.6A–B). In this context, dysplasia is associated with larger polyp size, antral gastritis, and increased severity of duodenal polyposis; PPI therapy appears to be protective against the development of dysplasia. The dysplasia is typically low-grade and focal, although occasional polyps show more extensive abnormalities or high-grade dysplasia. The biologic risk of developing gastric adenocarcinoma from these lesions is quite low, and thus patients are usually monitored with surveillance endoscopy and regular removal of large lesions without prophylactic gastrectomy. Pathologists may suggest the possibility of a polyposis disorder when FGPs with dysplasia are encountered, particularly when multiple, or if FGPs are detected in children who have not been exposed to PPIs.

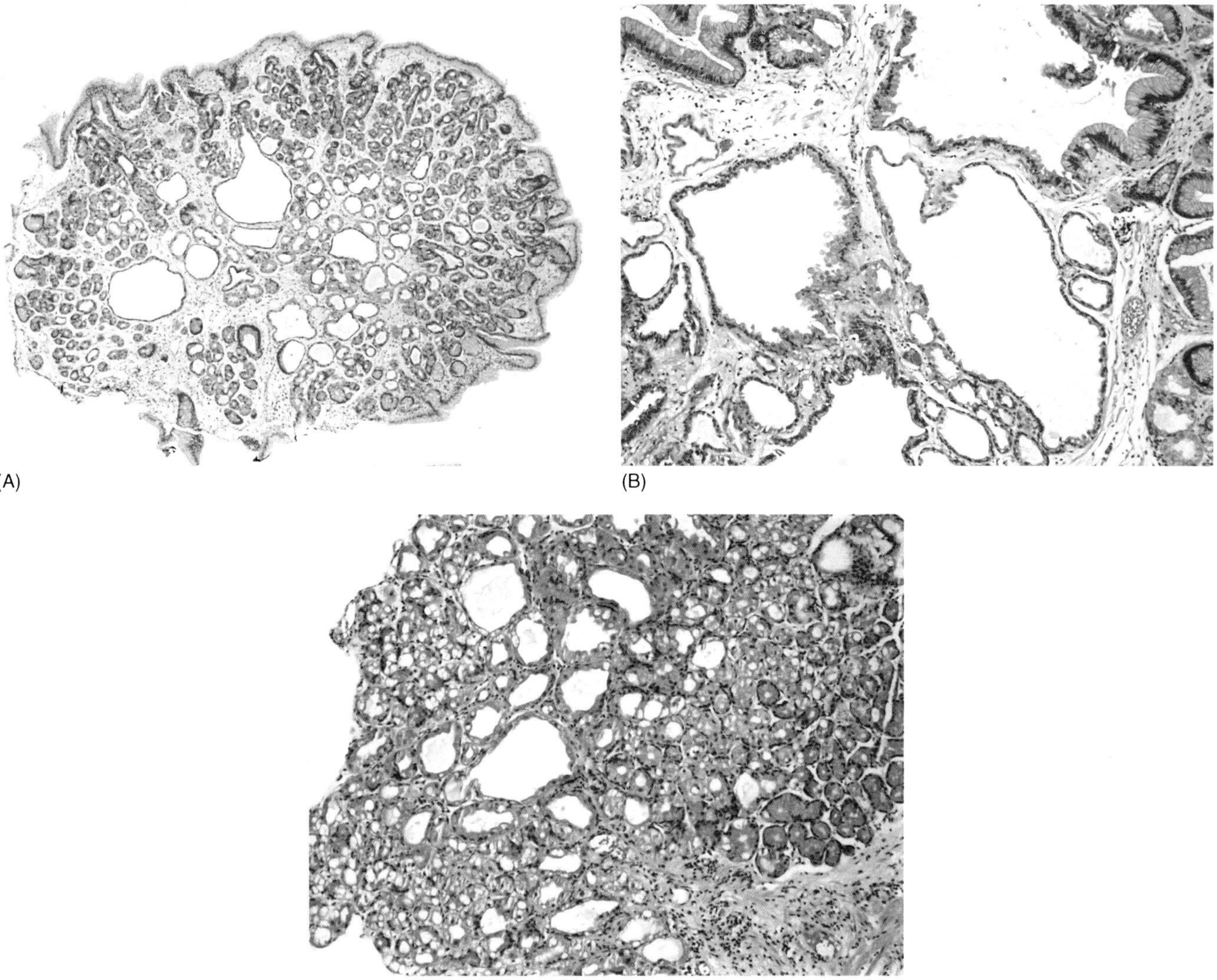

(A)

(B)

(C)

FIGURE 8.5 Fundic gland polyps are composed of a mixture of oxyntic as well as foveolar epithelium (A–B). There is frequently cystic dilatation of glands, and inflammation is not prominent. Fundic gland polyps from patients on PPIs may show parietal cell hypertrophy and hyperplasia, with tufting of cells into the lumen and vacuolization of the cytoplasm (C).

Peutz–Jeghers Syndrome

Peutz-Jeghers syndrome (PJS) is an inherited syndrome characterized by a germline mutation of the tumor suppressor gene *STK11/LKB1*. Patients typically have polyps throughout the GI tract, as well as mucocutaneous melanocytic pigmentation. The polyps preferentially affect the small intestine, but are seen in the stomach in 25% to 50% of patients. Gastric PJPs are typically small and asymptomatic, and macroscopically similar to PJ polyps elsewhere in the GI tract with a villiform or papillary surface. Histologically, PJ polyps show irregular arborizing bundles of smooth muscle that extend upward from the muscularis mucosae to separate the epithelial components into lobules (Figure 8.7A–B). Surface and foveolar hyperplasia is common, along with cystic dilatation of glands.

As noted in the preceding paragraphs, gastric PJPs are very similar histologically to hyperplastic polyps, and the only distinguishing features may be a more prominent smooth muscle component and less prominent cystically dilated glands. Gastric PJPs also contain normal-appearing lamina propria, rather than the edematous, inflamed stroma typical of hyperplastic polyps and juvenile polyps. In many cases, however, histologic distinction from hyperplastic polyps is impossible, and the diagnosis rests on the knowledge that the patient has PJS. Patients with McCune–Albright syndrome may also have polyps that are identical to PJPs.

Although some literature cites the development of gastric dysplasia and adenocarcinoma in PJS as rare, more recent studies indicate a 29% lifetime risk of developing gastric cancer. It is recommended that patients with PJS

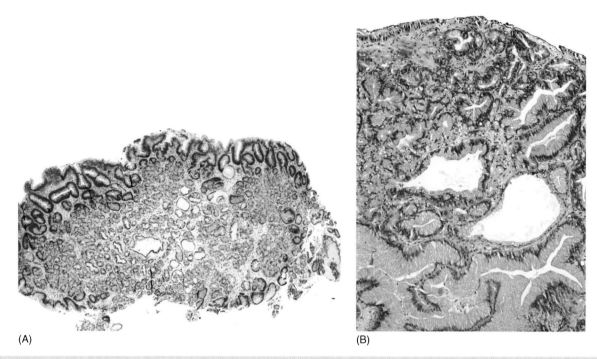

FIGURE 8.6   These fundic gland polyps from patients with familial adenomatous polyposis show low-grade dysplasia at the surface of the polyp (A [courtesy Dr. Rhonda Yantiss]–B).

begin surveillance of the upper and lower GI tracts at age 8; if no polyps are seen, then re-evaluation is recommended at age 18 and every 3 years thereafter. If polyps are seen, evaluation every 3 years is recommended.

Juvenile Polyps

Juvenile polyps may be either sporadic or syndromic, but sporadic polyps are very rare in the stomach. Gastric

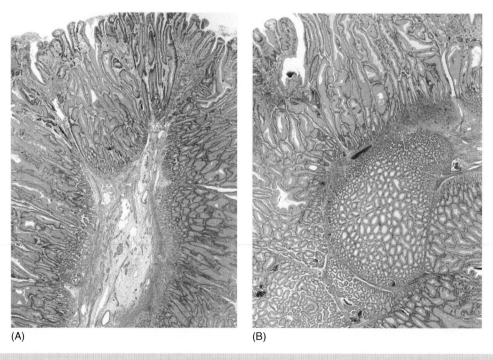

FIGURE 8.7   Peutz–Jeghers polyps are composed of irregular arborizing bundles of smooth muscle that extend upward from the muscularis mucosae to separate the epithelial components into lobules (A). Surface and foveolar hyperplasia is common, along with cystic dilatation of glands (B).

juvenile polyps typically occur as part of generalized JPS or the rare subtype that is limited to the stomach. JPS is characterized by a germline mutation in the *SMAD4* or *BMPR1A* gene, and 20% to 50% of patients with JPS have gastric polyps. In addition to the increased risk of developing colorectal cancer, JPS patients are also at risk for small intestinal, gastric, and possibly pancreatic cancer. Surveillance recommendations for JPS include beginning upper endoscopy and colonoscopy at ages 12 to 15, and repeating every 1 to 3 years depending on symptoms and findings.

Gastric JP range from a few millimeters to several centimeters in size, and histologically feature cystic dilatation of glands within an edematous, inflamed stroma. Foveolar hyperplasia and smooth muscle hyperplasia may also be present (Figure 8.8A). Gastric JP can mimic hyperplastic polyps or Ménétrier disease, particularly in biopsy samples. Because of the histologic overlap with hyperplastic polyps and other hamartomatous polyps, knowledge of the clinical history is essential. Syndromic gastric juvenile polyps may also develop dysplasia (Figure 8.8B), and thus patients are at increased risk for the development of gastric adenocarcinoma as well.

Cronkhite–Canada Syndrome

Cronkhite–Canada Syndrome (CCS) is a very rare, nonhereditary generalized polyposis disorder that involves the stomach, small bowel, and colorectum. The pathogenesis remains unclear, although an autoimmune etiology has been proposed. Unlike most polyposis syndromes, which present in childhood or young adulthood, CCS typically presents in middle-aged adults. Patients with CCS have numerous GI polyps, as well as diarrhea, weight loss, anorexia, abdominal pain, and GI bleeding. Extraintestinal manifestations include skin hyperpigmentation, vitiligo, alopecia, and nail atrophy. The mortality rate is quite high (approximately 50%), most often due to anemia and chronic malnutrition. In addition, patients have an increased risk of adenocarcinoma in the stomach as well as other parts of the GI tract. The increased risk of malignancy is not directly related to the presence of the polyps, apparently, as cancers may develop in the polyps or in nonpolypoid mucosa.

In the stomach, CCS features diffuse but irregular hypertrophy of the gastric rugae. Polyps typically measure between 5 and 15 mm, and are superimposed on the hypertrophic rugae. A very helpful feature of CCS is that the histologic changes involve both the polypoid and nonpolypoid mucosa, and include marked surface and foveolar hyperplasia with cystic dilatation as well as atrophy of glands (Figure 8.9A–B). The lamina propria is edematous and inflamed, often with prominent eosinophils, but intestinal metaplasia is not a typical feature. The nonpolypoid mucosa shows similar alternating areas of hyperplasia and atrophy with cystic changes, which can help differentiate CCS from histologically similar lesions such as juvenile polyps, in which the nonpolypoid mucosa is typically normal. The microscopic differential diagnosis also includes Ménétrier disease, hyperplastic polyps, and other hamartomatous polyps, and thus knowledge of the clinical history is essential. In contrast to Ménétrier disease, CCS involves the entire stomach and is not limited to the body and fundus.

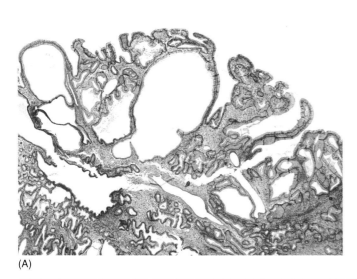

(A)

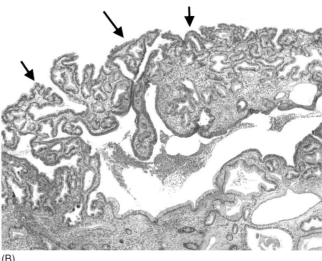

(B)

FIGURE 8.8 Gastric juvenile polyps feature cystic dilatation of glands within edematous, inflamed stroma (A). Syndromic gastric juvenile polyps may also develop dysplasia, as seen here at the surface of a large juvenile polyp (B, arrows); note the adjacent cystically dilated glands and inflamed, edematous stroma.

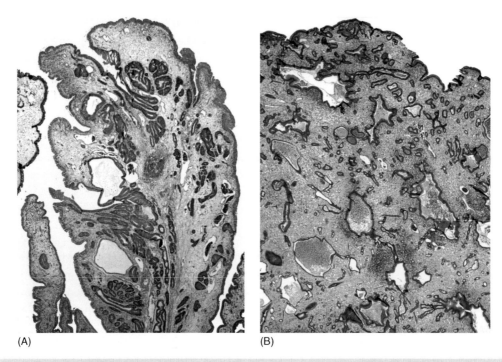

(A)   (B)

FIGURE 8.9   The polyps in gastric Cronkhite–Canada syndrome show marked surface and foveolar hyperplasia with cystic dilatation as well as atrophy of glands, similar to hyperplastic polyps (A). The lamina propria is edematous and mildly inflamed. The nonpolypoid mucosa shows similar alternating areas of hyperplasia and atrophy with cystic changes (B). Courtesy Dr. Rhonda Yantiss.

GASTRIC DYSPLASIA

Gastric epithelial dysplasia is widely accepted as an important precursor lesion to gastric adenocarcinoma, as well as a marker of increased risk of synchronous adenocarcinoma elsewhere in the stomach. The prevalence varies widely depending on population, with rates ranging between 0.5 and 3.75% in Western countries, but much higher (ranging from 9%–20%) in high-risk geographic areas such as Korea, China, Japan, and Colombia. Historically, polypoid dysplasias are referred to as adenomas in the United States and Europe, whereas flat, sessile, or depressed lesions are more often referred to as flat or nonpolypoid dysplasia, or simply dysplasia. In Japan, however, the term "adenoma" includes all gross types of dysplasia including polypoid, flat, or depressed lesions. Regardless of configuration, the histologic features are essentially identical, and therefore some authors recommend grouping all of these dysplastic lesions into the term "gastric intra-epithelial neoplasia/dysplasia."

Risk factors for the development of gastric epithelial dysplasia include, most prominently, *H. pylori* infection (particularly if intestinal metaplasia/atrophy is present), and atrophic gastritis. Cigarette smoking, low serum vitamin C levels, high salt consumption, and malnutrition have been implicated as risk factors as well. Gastric adenomas are also found in up to 15% of patients with FAP.

Gastric dysplasia is morphologically classified as either adenomatous/intestinal or foveolar/gastric, based on histologic characteristics. The adenomatous/intestinal type resembles intestinal-type colonic adenomas, with columnar cells containing hyperchromatic, pencillate, pseudostratified nuclei (Figure 8.10A–D). In contrast, the foveolar type consists of cuboidal to columnar cells with clear to eosinophilic cytoplasm and hyperchromatic round to ovoid nuclei (Figure 8.11A–B). Some gastric dysplasias consist of a mixture of both types. Either type can be associated with intestinal metaplasia, as well as the development of high-grade dysplasia and adenocarcinoma; the rates of development of high-grade dysplasia and/or carcinoma vary widely in the literature, most likely based on the patient population studied, the presence of *H. pylori* infection, and genetic predisposition. Adenomas themselves (and flat dysplasia) are almost always asymptomatic and found incidentally on endoscopy. However, as they often occur in a background of chronic gastritis, patients may present with melena, abdominal pain, nausea and vomiting, or anemia.

Macroscopically, adenomas and flat dysplasia can be located anywhere in the stomach. Polypoid adenomas are most commonly found in the antrum, and the vast majority are solitary. Most measure less than 2.0 cm, and grossly they may have either a pedunculated, nodular, or sessile configuration. Flat or depressed dysplastic foci may be

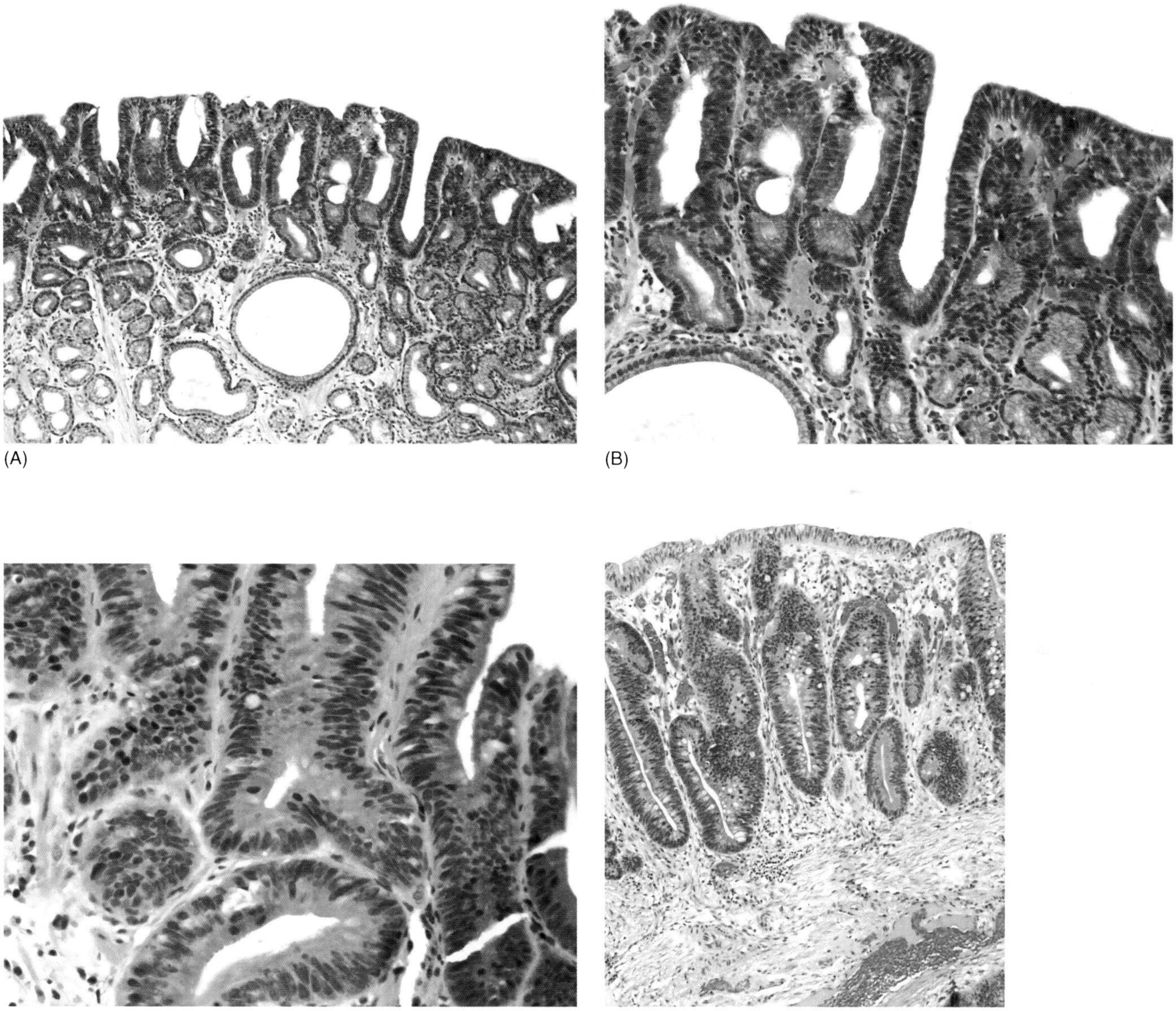

FIGURE 8.10 The adenomatous or intestinal type of gastric dysplasia resembles colonic adenomas, and is composed of columnar cells containing hyperchromatic, pencillate, pseudostratified nuclei (A–B). Neuroendocrine cells are common (C), as are goblet cells (D).

very difficult to detect with conventional endoscopy, but may have an irregular appearance on chromoendoscopy.

As discussed in the previous paragraphs, gastric intestinal type dysplasia resembles a colonic adenoma, and this type of dysplasia comprises the majority of dysplastic lesions in the stomach. Goblet cells, Paneth cells, and neuroendocrine cells are often seen (Figure 8.10C–D). Foveolar dysplasia (Figure 8.11A–B), in contrast, lacks goblet and Paneth cells, and is composed of round or cuboidal to columnar cells with clear to eosinophilic cytoplasm and hyperchromatic round to oval nuclei.

Similar to colonic adenomas, gastric dysplasia (both intestinal and foveolar types) is classified as either low or high grade in Western countries. High-grade dysplasia

features more complex architecture (such as cribriforming or budding of glands) and high-grade nuclear features with prominent nucleoli and loss of nuclear polarity (Figure 8.12A–C). However, classification of dysplasia differs in other parts of the world, particularly Japan. The most significant difference between Western and Japanese classifications is that Western pathologists require lamina propria invasion to establish a diagnosis of intramucosal adenocarcinoma, whereas Japanese pathologists place greater emphasis on cytologic features of malignancy. For these reasons, cases diagnosed as high-grade dysplasia in Western countries may well be classified as adenocarcinoma by Japanese pathologists. There are also multiple international grading schemes for the classification of

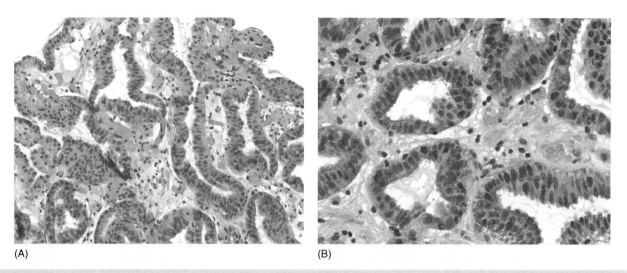

(A)   (B)

FIGURE 8.11   Foveolar-type gastric dysplasia consists of cuboidal to columnar cells with clear to eosinophilic cytoplasm and hyperchromatic, round to oval nuclei (A–B). Neuroendocrine cells and goblet cells are typically absent.

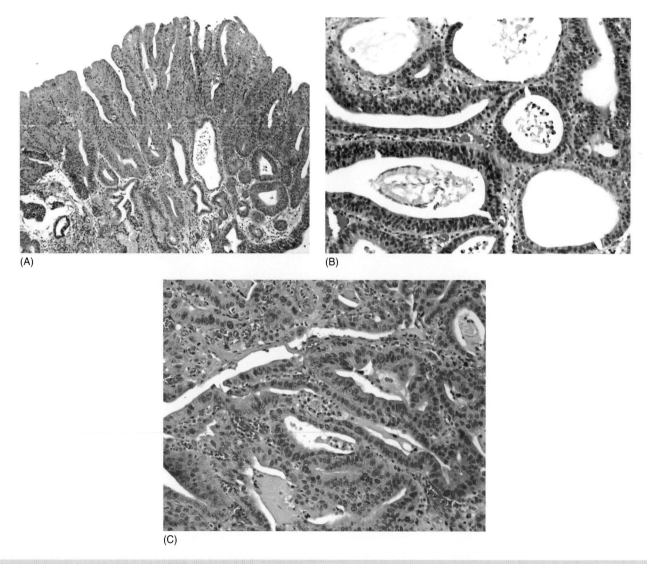

(A)   (B)

(C)

FIGURE 8.12   High-grade dysplasia features more complex architecture (A) and high-grade nuclear features with prominent nucleoli, loss of nuclear polarity, and nuclear stratification extending to the luminal surface (B–C).

gastric dysplasia; the Vienna classification is the most widely used in the United States.

The progression from dysplasia to carcinoma is variable, but reportedly over 20% of low-grade lesions progress to carcinoma within 10 to 48 months, and up to 85% of high-grade lesions progress over a similar period. The risk of neoplastic transformation of adenomas increases with size, particularly once the lesion exceeds 2.0 cm.

Because of the high risk of development of adenocarcinoma, all dysplastic lesions should be completely removed and submitted for pathologic evaluation. In addition, the remainder of the stomach should be carefully evaluated and biopsied for additional lesions, particularly flat dysplasia. First-line treatment options include endoscopic polypectomy for pedunculated polyps, and endoscopic mucosal resection (EMR) or endoscopic submucosal dissection (ESD) for large and/or sessile polyps. Lesions that are not amenable to polypectomy or local excision

(due to size, location, etc.) should be managed surgically. Eradication of *H. pylori* in patients with gastric dysplasia as well as careful clinical follow-up with regular endoscopy and biopsy is recommended due to the risk of developing subsequent lesions.

Differential Diagnosis and Diagnostic Challenges

The most problematic issue in the differential diagnosis of gastric dysplasia is differentiation from marked regenerative/reparative atypia. Reactive changes may be particularly worrisome in the context of chronic bile reflux in a postoperative stomach, as these patients are at risk for gastric dysplasia/carcinoma. Caution should be exercised in this situation, as the reactive changes induced by bile reflux can be very striking (Figure 8.13A–C). True dysplasia should extend to the surface of the gastric mucosa in

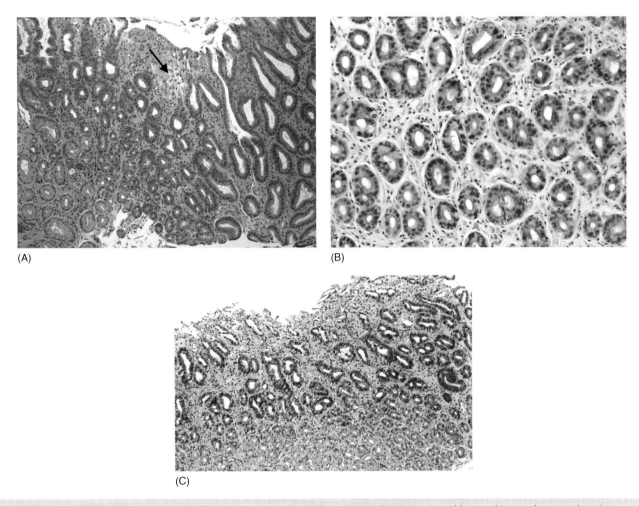

(A)

(B)

(C)

FIGURE 8.13 Reactive gastric epithelium may show marked nuclear enlargement and hyperchromasia, prominent nucleoli, and increased mitotic activity that may mimic dysplasia, as shown here in a case of erosive gastritis (A, arrow denotes focus of muciphages; courtesy Dr. Rhonda Yantiss). Similar nuclear changes are seen in this case of bile reflux (B). The changes are associated with mucosal erosion, however, and do not extend to the surface (C). In addition, dysplasia is sharply demarcated from the adjacent non-neoplastic mucosa, whereas reactive changes show a more gradual transition to normal mucosa.

both intestinal- and foveolar-type dysplasia. Furthermore, most reparative changes that are severe enough to mimic dysplasia are also associated with marked acute inflammation and/or mucosal ulceration. Reactive changes tend to be uniform and show a gradual transition to more normal-appearing mucosa, whereas dysplasia is sharply demarcated from the adjacent non-neoplastic mucosa. It is important to remember, as in other parts of the GI tract, that immunostains such as p53 may be positive in areas of marked regeneration as well as foci of dysplasia. Epithelial lesions worrisome for dysplasia, but for which the diagnosis cannot be made with certainty, may be interpreted as "indefinite for dysplasia." Similar issues may arise in biopsies of gastric ulcer beds when marked inflammatory and regenerative changes, including exuberant granulation tissue, mimic dysplasia and neoplasia.

Chemotherapeutic agents and radiation, including gastric injury secondary to microsphere radioembolization, can also produce severe epithelial abnormalities that mimic dysplasia (Figure 8.14A–C). Although these changes include nuclear enlargement and hyperchromasia with membrane irregularities, affected cells often contain vacuolated cytoplasm, and although there is nuclear enlargement the nuclear-to-cytoplasmic ratio is maintained.

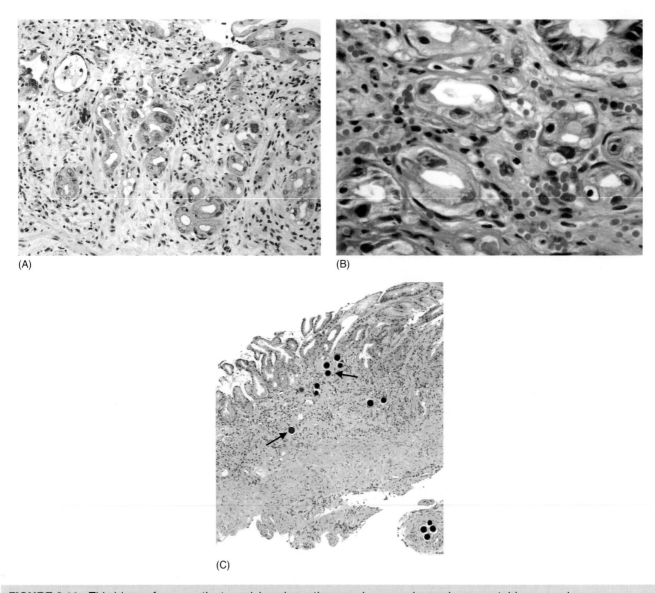

(A)

(B)

(C)

FIGURE 8.14 This biopsy from a patient receiving chemotherapy shows nuclear enlargement, bizarre nuclear pleomorphism, and loss of nuclear polarity. However, the affected cells have vacuolated cytoplasm, and the nuclear-to-cytoplasmic ratio is maintained (A). Similar changes are seen in this biopsy from a patient who had undergone radiation therapy (B, courtesy Dr. Rhonda Yantiss). Gastric injury secondary to microsphere radioembolization can also produce severe reactive abnormalities that mimic dysplasia (C, courtesy Dr. Shawn Kinsey).

Other entities in the differential diagnosis of gastric adenomas include FGPs, hyperplastic polyps, or other types of hamartomatous polyps with dysplasia. The background changes in these lesions typically help distinguish them from true gastric adenomas. In addition, the dysplasia in these other types of polyps is typically focal. Finally, dysplasia is unusual in FGPs and other types of hamartomatous polyps that are not associated with a polyposis syndrome.

OTHER EPITHELIAL POLYPS

Pyloric Gland Adenomas

Pyloric gland adenoma (PGA) is a rare type of adenoma that most often involves the stomach; they account for less than 3% of all gastric polyps, reportedly, but are likely underrecognized. Gastric PGAs tend to arise in elderly patients and are more common in women. Most arise in the body, but they may occur anywhere in the stomach. The surrounding gastric mucosa usually shows evidence of autoimmune gastritis or *H. pylori* gastritis.

PGAs are often relatively large at the time of diagnosis, with a mean diameter of 1.6 cm. They are composed of closely packed pyloric-type tubules or glands lined by a single layer of columnar or cuboidal epithelium (Figure 8.15A–B). The cytoplasm is eosinophilic or amphophilic, and often has a "ground-glass" appearance. Apical mucin caps are absent. Nuclei are characteristically round, and may or may not contain easily identifiable nucleoli. By immunohistochemistry, PGAs characteristically express MUC6 (a marker of pyloric gland mucin)

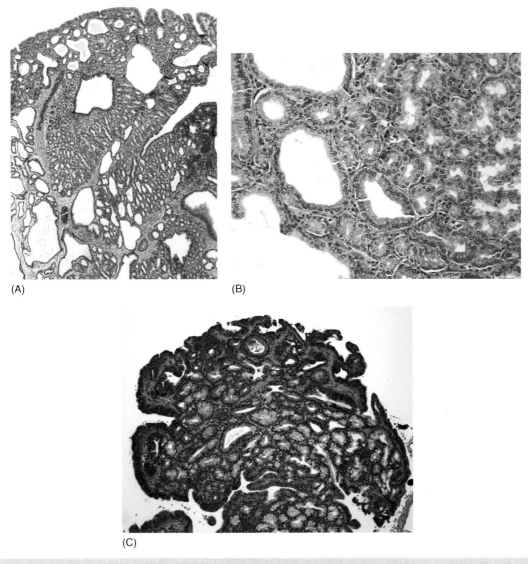

(A)   (B)

(C)

FIGURE 8.15 Pyloric gland adenomas are composed of closely packed pyloric-type tubules or glands (A) lined by a single layer of columnar or cuboidal epithelium. The cytoplasm is eosinophilic or amphophilic, and often has a "ground-glass" appearance. Apical mucin caps are absent. Nuclei are characteristically round, and may or may not contain easily identifiable nucleoli (B). Dysplasia is a common finding in these lesions (C, courtesy Dr. Rhonda Yantiss).

and MUC5AC (a foveolar mucin marker). The intestinal mucin MUC2 and the intestinal marker CDX2 are generally not expressed in PGAs.

The term "pyloric gland adenoma" has been criticized, because the name "adenoma" is used to describe a lesion that does not a priori have conventional-type dysplasia. However, dysplasia is quite common in these lesions (Figure 8.15C). Dysplasia (both low and high grades) has been reported in up to 40% of PGAs, and there has also been a reported frequency of adenocarcinoma in up to 30%. Little is known regarding prognosis, due to limited clinical and follow-up data. However, complete removal with subsequent close clinical follow-up and endoscopic surveillance is recommended.

Differential Diagnosis

PGAs are likely underrecognized as they are often confused with other types of polyps, particularly hyperplastic polyps. PGAs lack the marked elongation, branching, and tortuosity of the glands seen in hyperplastic polyps, and also typically lack the inflammatory stroma. In addition, PGAs are composed of pyloric-type glands rather than foveolar-type cells, and lack the apical mucin droplet characteristic of foveolar epithelium. MUC6 should be absent in foveolar epithelium, as well. Occasionally, foveolar-type gastric adenomas may be confused with PGAs. As discussed in the preceding section on foveolar-type dysplasia, these also are composed of cells resembling foveolar epithelium, with different cytologic features and by definition at least low-grade cytologic dysplasia.

Oxyntic Gland Polyp/Adenoma

Nodular mucosa-based lesions composed of oxyntic mucosa have had several names, including chief cell hyperplasia, oxyntic mucosa pseudopolyp, and oxyntic gland polyp/adenoma, reflecting the confusion as to whether or not these represent mucosal hyperplasia or true neoplasia. Some cases have also been termed adenocarcinoma with chief cell differentiation, although this term should probably be avoided given the apparent lack of recurrence of metastasis of these lesions, as well as the lack of associated desmoplasia, perineural invasion, and lymphovascular invasion.

These lesions are composed of a mixture of parietal and chief cells (Figure 8.16A–C), although some are almost exclusively composed of chief cells; they are most often solitary and found in the body and fundus of the stomach. Admixed mucus neck cells may also be present, and may be quite prominent. They are centered in the mucosa, and do not extend into the submucosa. The cells are arranged in tightly packed clusters, tubules, and cords

of cells, which can have notable nuclear hyperchromasia, pleomorphism, anisocytosis, and enlargement. MUC6 is characteristically positive, whereas MUC5AC and MUC2 are negative. Oxyntic gland polyps lack the cystic dilatation and admixed foveolar cells typically seen in FGPs, and FGPs lack the nuclear atypia seen in oxyntic gland polyps.

ADENOCARCINOMA

Epidemiology

Gastric adenocarcinoma accounts for approximately 7% to 10% of cancers and is the second most common type of cancer worldwide; however, there is a striking geographical heterogeneity due to a variety of genetic and environmental factors. This heterogeneity is further underscored by the wide spectrum of macroscopic and histologic findings in these tumors. High-incidence areas include eastern Asia, central and eastern Europe, Latin America, and South America, and antral and pyloric tumors are more common in these regions. Low-incidence areas include North America, northern Europe, most of Africa, and southeast Asia, and proximal stomach/gastroesophageal (GE) junction tumors are more common in these areas. The diffuse type of gastric carcinoma does not vary with region, and is more common in younger patients.

Of note, there has been a declining overall incidence of gastric carcinoma over the past five decades, although there has been an increase in proximal and GE junction carcinomas since the 1980s that parallels the increase in esophageal adenocarcinoma. This increase appears restricted to low-incidence areas, and has not been observed in areas that are at high risk for the development of gastric carcinoma, such as Japan. The reason for the increase is controversial, in part because of the lack of consensus as to the definition of the gastric cardia, and in part because widespread use of endoscopy for surveillance has most likely resulted in increased detection of these tumors. Regardless, there are clear differences between gastric cardia carcinomas and those in the more distal stomach, including a greater incidence in men and Caucasians. Whether or not the risk factors associated with esophageal carcinoma (obesity, reflux, smoking, alcohol use) are also implicated in the pathogenesis of gastric cardiac cancers remains controversial, as does the significance of gastric cardiac intestinal metaplasia, and thus patients with intestinal metaplasia in the gastric cardia do not undergo rigorous surveillance as do patients with Barrett's esophagus.

More than 80% of cases of gastric carcinoma are sporadic, and appear to develop via a progression from chronic gastritis to atrophic gastritis to intestinal metaplasia, dysplasia, and carcinoma (the Correa cascade). A number of

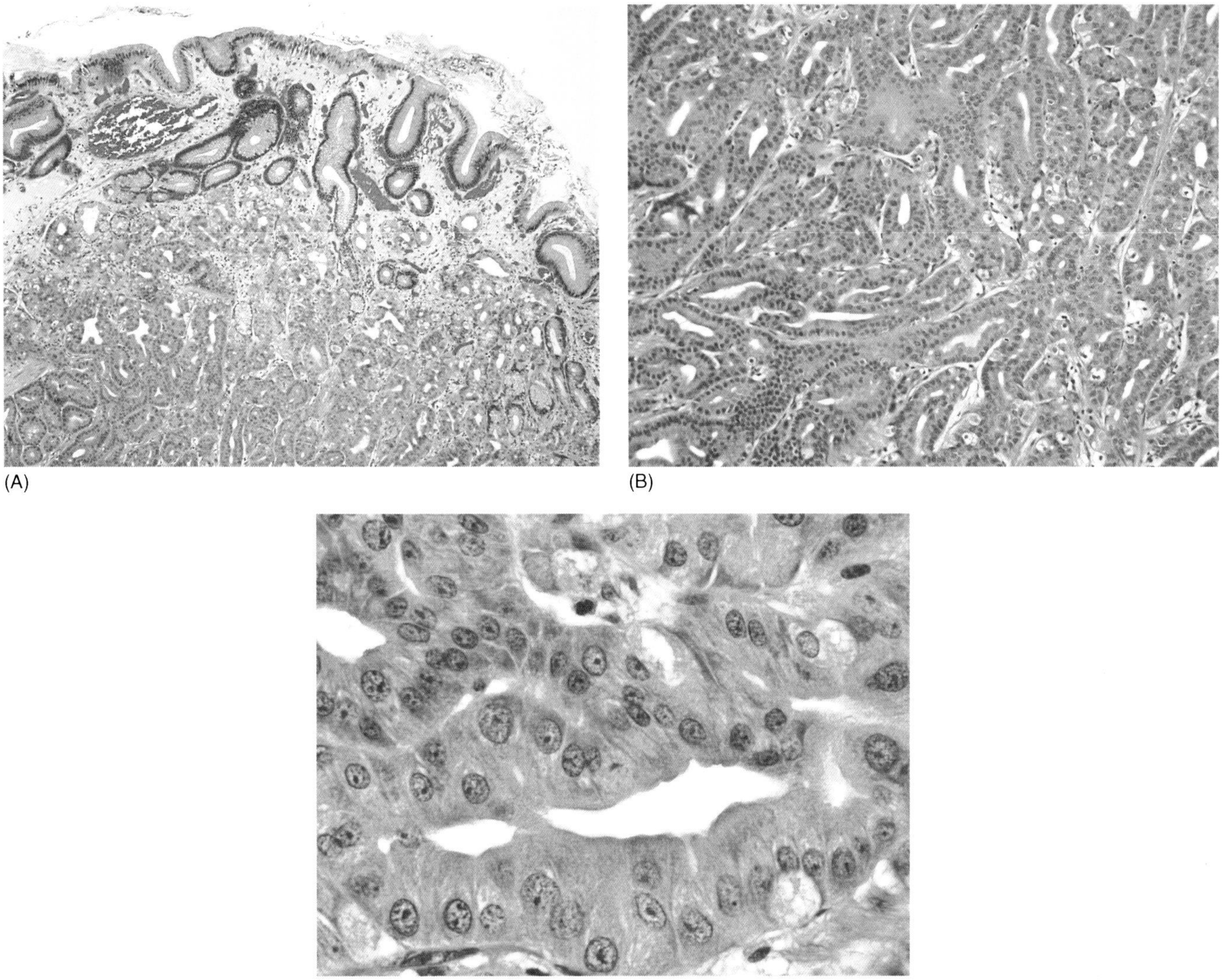

FIGURE 8.16   This oxyntic gland adenoma is composed of a mixture of parietal and chief cells (A). The cells are arranged in tightly packed tubules (B), and have notable nuclear hyperchromasia, pleomorphism, anisocytosis, and enlargement (C). Courtesy Dr. Elizabeth Montgomery.

risk factors, associated diseases, and precancerous conditions are associated with gastric cancer (particularly the intestinal type), including chronic *H. pylori* infection, autoimmune gastritis, Ménétrier disease, and long-standing chemical gastropathy/bile reflux, especially in patients who have undergone distal gastrectomy and a Billroth II procedure. High salt diets and nutrient-poor diets have been implicated, as they are believed to lead to the formation of intraluminal carcinogens such as N-nitroso compounds. The diffuse type of gastric cancer is associated more strongly with genetic abnormalities than environmental factors, however (see subsequent paragraphs). A minority of gastric cancers have a well-defined genetic abnormality; these are also discussed subsequently.

Clinical Features

Gastric carcinomas are typically divided into two general categories: early gastric cancer (EGC) and advanced gastric cancer (AGC). EGC is defined as carcinoma limited to the mucosa or submucosa, regardless of lymph node status, whereas AGC is defined as a lesion that invades beyond the submucosa. EGC accounts for 15% to 20% of gastric carcinomas in Western countries, but more than half of cases in Japan, in large part due to the use of aggressive surveillance and different diagnostic definitions of carcinoma in high-risk areas (see preceding section on gastric dysplasia). EGCs are most often seen in male patients over the age of 50, the majority of whom are asymptomatic. When symptomatic, patients typically present with

TABLE 8.2 Endoscopic Classification of Early Gastric Cancers

	Appearance	Significance	Additional Macroscopic Features
Type I	Protruding	Low rate of lymph node metastases	
Type II	Superficial	Most common, especially IIa	
Type IIa	Elevated	Low rate of lymph node metastases	Twice as thick as adjacent normal mucosa; hard to detect endoscopically
Type IIb	Flat	Majority of tumors that are smaller than 0.5 cm	
Type IIc	Depressed	More likely to be poorly differentiated	Mimics benign gastric ulcer
Type III	Excavating	More likely to be poorly differentiated	

dyspepsia, epigastric pain, anemia, or melena. AGCs are also more common in men over the age of 50. Symptoms include epigastric pain, weight loss, dyspepsia, GI bleeding, anemia, and evidence of gastric outlet obstruction.

Pathologic Features

EGCs are usually relatively small (2–5 cm) and present on the lesser curvature near the angularis. They are most often solitary. A macroscopic classification of early gastric neoplasia was developed in Japan in the 1960s (see Table 8.2); however, this classification scheme is not widely used in Western countries.

Histologically, ECGs are usually well-differentiated, and have glandular or papillary morphology that may be difficult to distinguish from adjacent high-grade dysplasia (Figure 8.17). Poorly differentiated and/or signet ring cell morphology is unusual in this context.

AGCs are typically solitary, and are located in the antrum or antropylorus. Half measure 2 to 6 cm in greatest dimension, and approximately 30% measure up to 10 cm. Only a minority of gastric carcinomas measure over

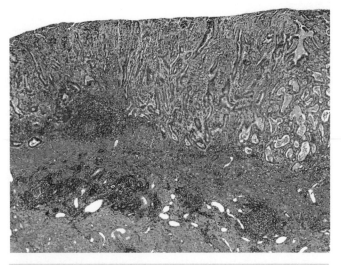

FIGURE 8.17 This early gastric carcinoma has a tubular pattern, and is confined to the mucosa.

10 cm at presentation. There are a variety of macroscopic appearances, including a polypoid or exophytic mass; an ulcerating lesion; an infiltrating lesion (including diffusely infiltrating or linitis plastica); and combined. (Figure 8.18A–D).

The architectural and cytologic morphologic heterogeneity in gastric cancer has resulted in many different histologic classifications and grading schemes, none of which is universally accepted. The Lauren classification is most widely used by pathologists, and it classifies tumors histologically as intestinal, diffuse, or indeterminate/unclassified. The World Health Organization (WHO) classification recognizes several other types and variants (see Table 8.1), in addition to those delineated in the Lauren classification. Other classification schemes have also been proposed, including the Goseki system, which is based on gland formation and mucin production, and a relatively new phenotypic classification scheme based on mucin immunohistochemistry.

Intestinal-type adenocarcinomas (Figure 8.19A–B), as the name implies, are composed of neoplastic tubules and/or papillary structures with varying degrees of differentiation. Nuclear atypia is common, and mucin and necroinflammatory luminal debris are variably present. The tubular or glandular type is associated with older patient age, the formation of a mass lesion in the antrum, chronic H. pylori infection, gastric atrophy, and hematogenous spread. Papillary carcinomas (Figure 8.19C–D) are also more common in older patients and are associated with hematogenous spread, especially to the liver, as well as with a high rate of lymph node metastases.

Poorly cohesive carcinomas (including signet ring cell carcinoma, which should have at least 50% signet ring cells) are composed of infiltrating small nests or single cells (Figure 8.19E–F). This type is more often found in the gastric body and in younger patients; there is also an association with H. pylori infection, although the relationship between H. pylori and poorly cohesive carcinomas is not well understood. As in other sites in the GI tract, the cells have pale cytoplasm and an eccentrically placed nucleus.

Mucinous gastric adenocarcinomas should be at least 50% mucinous. Similar to the colon, these carcinomas

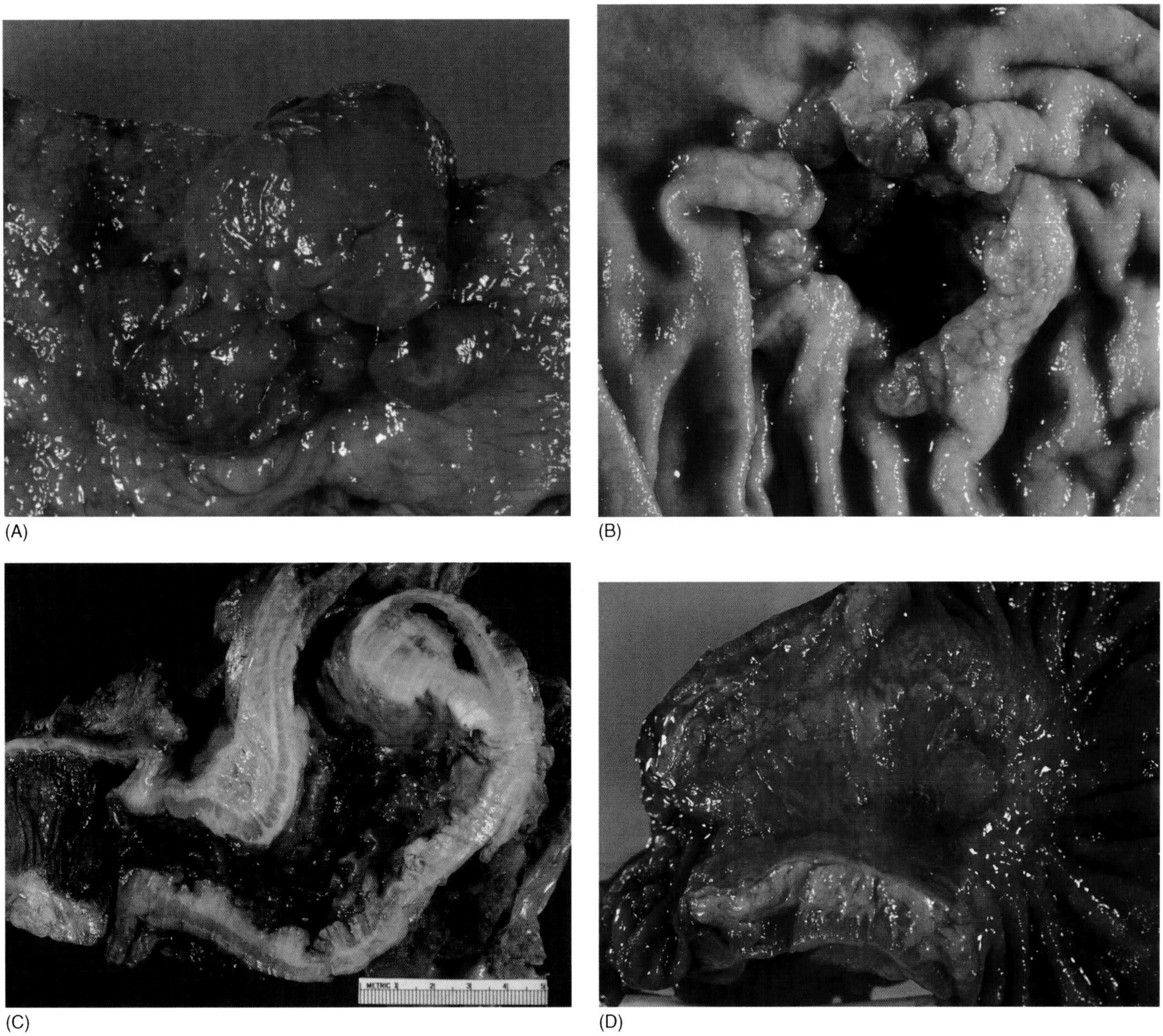

FIGURE 8.18 Advanced gastric adenocarcinomas have a wide variety of macroscopic appearances, including a polypoid or exophytic mass (A), an ulcerating lesion (B), an infiltrating lesion, including linitis plastica or diffuse infiltration of the gastric wall by tumor cells (C), or combined forms, such as this combined ulcerative and infiltrative tumor (D).

consist of pools of mucin that contain floating strips or clusters of neoplastic epithelium, or single cells.

Undifferentiated carcinomas lack morphologic and cytologic differentiation entirely. This type most often enters into the differential diagnosis with lymphoma, melanoma, or another type of tumor.

There are several rare morphologic subtypes of gastric adenocarcinoma that comprise a small minority of cases. Adenosquamous carcinoma of the stomach must have a neoplastic squamous component that comprises at least 25% in addition to the glandular component. Pure squamous carcinomas of the stomach have been reported as well, but metastases must be rigorously excluded in this circumstance. Both the adenosquamous and squamous subtypes have a very poor prognosis.

Gastric choriocarcinomas often feature a mixture of trophoblastic elements with other morphologic types of gastric carcinoma. Tumors are typically very necrotic and hemorrhagic (Figure 8.20A–B), and both immunohistochemical expression of β-HCG and elevated serum levels are characteristic. These very rare tumors have an extremely poor prognosis.

Hepatoid and alpha feto-protein (AFP)-producing carcinomas are characterized by AFP production in the context of either morphologic features that resemble hepatocellular carcinoma (hepatoid), or a well-differentiated

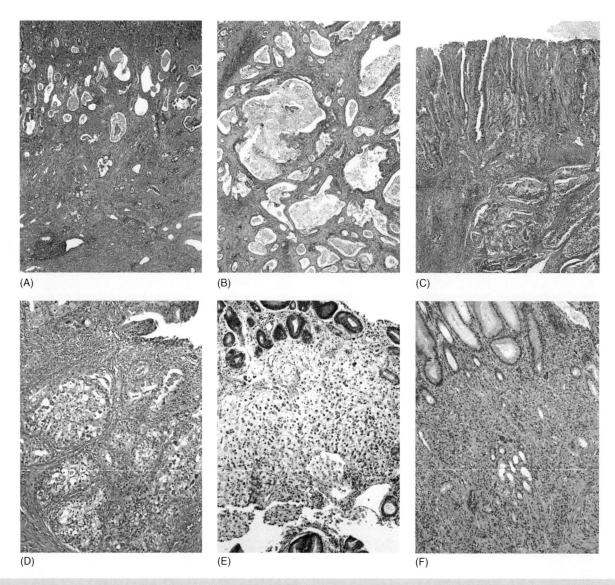

FIGURE 8.19 This intestinal (tubular) type adenocarcinoma features well-differentiated tubules extending through the gastric wall (A). Another example shows greater nuclear atypia and luminal necroinflammatory debris (B). This papillary gastric adenocarcinoma forms papillary structures with prominent clear cell change, which is frequently seen in this type (C–D). Signet ring cell carcinomas should have at least 50% signet ring cells; the neoplastic cells have clear cytoplasm and an eccentrically placed nucleus (E). This poorly cohesive adenocarcinoma is composed of infiltrating cords of single cells that fill the lamina propria (F).

tubulopapillary carcinoma with clear cell features and AFP production. The former closely resembles neoplastic liver (Figure 8.20C–D), and variably expresses hepatocyte antigen, AFP, and glypican-3. The morphology and immunophenotype can lead to diagnostic confusion, particularly when evaluating liver metastases or the possibility of a primary liver tumor that has invaded the stomach. Both morphologic types may be associated with high serum levels of AFP, and both have an extremely poor prognosis.

Medullary carcinoma (also known as lymphoepithelioma-like carcinoma or gastric carcinoma with lymphoid stroma) is strongly associated with Epstein–Barr virus

(EBV) infection, although the actual role of EBV in carcinogenesis is controversial. Morphologically, these somewhat nodular tumors have a pushing border, and are composed of sheets of cells with eosinophilic cytoplasm and numerous tumor infiltrating lymphocytes (Figure 8.20E–F). These tumors are more common in the proximal stomach of Hispanic males, and although controversial, are believed to have a better prognosis. This subtype is also associated with previous subtotal gastrectomy.

Other unusual subtypes include carcinosarcoma, parietal cell carcinoma, Paneth cell carcinoma, and malignant rhabdoid tumor.

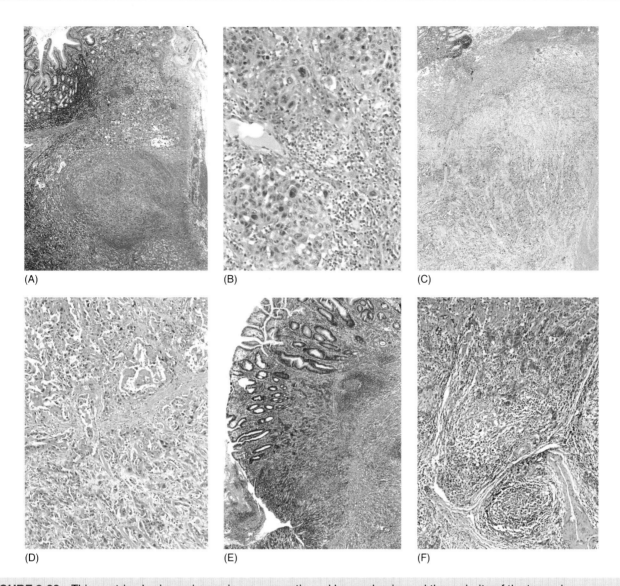

FIGURE 8.20 This gastric choriocarcinoma is very necrotic and hemorrhagic, and the majority of the tumor is composed of choriocarcinoma (A–B). The patient had markedly elevated serum β-HCG, and the tumor stained with β-HCG as well. This hepatoid subtype of gastric adenocarcinoma closely resembles neoplastic liver (C–D). Medullary carcinomas feature nodules or clusters of tumor cells with numerous intratumoral lymphocytes (E–F). Peripheral lymphoid aggregates are commonly seen at the edges of the tumor.

HEREDITARY DIFFUSE GASTRIC CANCER AND OTHER GENETIC ASSOCIATIONS

Hereditary diffuse gastric cancer is an autosomal dominant cancer syndrome characterized by signet ring cell carcinoma of the stomach, often in combination with lobular breast carcinoma in women (see also Chapters 6 and 14). Families with the syndrome are defined by the presence of two or more documented cases of diffuse gastric cancer in first- or second-degree relatives, at least one of whom is diagnosed before age 50 years; or three or more cases of diffuse gastric cancer in first- or second-degree relatives,

regardless of age. The presence of either of these features, in addition to a diagnosis of diffuse gastric cancer at a young age (less than 40 years), or a family history of both lobular breast cancer and diffuse gastric cancer, should prompt evaluation for germline CDH1 mutations, as they underlie a substantial proportion (30%–40%) of cases. Patients with suspected hereditary diffuse gastric cancer require evaluation of peripheral blood DNA, usually in the form of direct sequencing.

Patients with hereditary diffuse gastric cancer usually have normal or near-normal upper endoscopic evaluations, and often the microscopic lesions do not correlate with a more visible or impressive lesion endoscopically. Furthermore, gastroenterologists must biopsy widely, as microscopic foci of malignancy are typically present within a macroscopically normal stomach. Lesions typically consist of in situ foci of signet ring cell carcinoma, as well as surface signet ring cell change in some cases (Figure 8.21A–B). Of note, both familial and sporadic diffuse gastric cancers may show decreased, or absent, E-cadherin expression on immunohistochemistry, so this technique cannot be reliably used to identify patients with germline mutations. The fact that there are no impressive gross lesions may cause some clinicians to be cautious about recommending prophylactic gastrectomy. However, the lifetime risk for developing gastric adenocarcinoma is extremely high (greater than 80% by age 80), and women with *CDH1* germline mutations also have an increased risk of developing lobular breast cancer. Because of this increased risk, as well as the difficulty in detecting early lesions in these patients, prophylactic gastrectomy is usually advised after age 20.

Gastric adenocarcinoma is also associated with hereditary nonpolyposis cancer syndrome (more commonly in Asian patients); FAP (also more common in Asian patients); Peutz–Jeghers syndrome; Li–Fraumeni syndrome, and gastric hyperplastic polyposis.

Ancillary Studies

The molecular features of gastric carcinoma and targeted molecular therapies are discussed in detail in Chapters 13 and 14. In brief, the molecular features of gastric adenocarcinoma are variable and related to tumor morphology. Intestinal-type carcinomas generally have molecular alterations similar to those of colorectal carcinomas, including loss of heterozygosity or mutations affecting *APC* (30%–40%), *DCC* (60%), *KRAS* (up to 30%), and *TP53* (25%–40%). In contrast, abnormalities affecting these genes are detected in less than 2% of diffuse-type carcinomas. Up to 20% of cases of gastric cancer show increased *EGFR* copy number by in situ hybridization, reflecting gene amplification or polysomy of chromosome 7. In addition, approximately 25% of intestinal-type tumors overexpress HER2, compared to only 5% of diffuse-type carcinomas and 10% of tumors containing mixed intestinal and diffuse areas.

Epigenetic alterations and promoter methylation are also more common among intestinal-type gastric adenocarcinomas, and high-frequency microsatellite instability (MSI-H) is more frequently encountered in intestinal-type carcinomas. Virtually all sporadic carcinomas with MSI-H develop via hypermethylation of the *MLH1* promoter, similar to MSI-H colon cancers. However, gastric adenocarcinoma may also be a manifestation of Lynch syndrome, and similar to their counterparts in the colon, morphologic features associated with gastric MSI-H tumors include tumor heterogeneity, abundant lymphoid stroma with intraepithelial lymphocytes (ie, medullary carcinoma), and mucinous differentiation.

Although diffuse-type gastric adenocarcinomas have not been as extensively studied, more than 50% of diffuse-type gastric adenocarcinomas show diminished

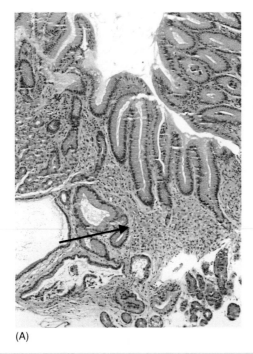 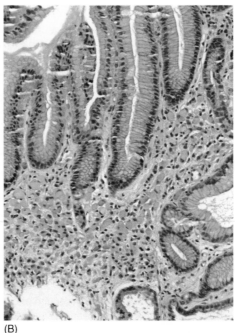

(A)   (B)

FIGURE 8.21 Patients with hereditary diffuse gastric cancer typically have in situ foci of signet ring cell carcinoma, as seen here in the lamina propria (A, arrow; B).

E-cadherin expression, reflecting abnormalities of *CDH1* located on chromosome 16q22.

HER2

Similar to adenocarcinomas of the esophagus and GE junction, trastuzumab improves survival of patients with AGCs that overexpress HER2 when used in combination with conventional chemotherapy. Although data from the ToGA trial suggested that immunohistochemical overexpression of HER2 correlates with response to trastuzumab better than in situ hybridization, several studies since have shown comparable predictive values of these assays and many laboratories now use either immunohistochemistry, in situ hybridization, or both to determine whether patients with AGC should receive trastuzumab.

There are two key differences between HER2 immunohistochemical testing in GE cancer and breast cancer. The first is that there is more frequent HER2 staining heterogeneity in GE tumors. The second is that GE cases may demonstrate basolateral (U-shaped) or lateral membrane staining rather than complete membrane staining, yet some of these cases are HER2-amplified by FISH. Because of the heterogeneity, there are different scoring criteria for GE biopsies and resections, and any amount of 2+ or 3+ staining in a biopsy is considered equivocal or positive, respectively, in esophagogastric cancers. Because cases with basolateral and lateral membrane staining may be HER2-amplified, the strict requirement for "complete membrane staining" that applies in breast cancer is relaxed.

Management and Prognosis

The two most important prognostic characteristics for EGCs are overall size of tumor, and depth of invasion. Although larger tumors have an increased risk of submucosal invasion, even very small tumors (less than 0.5 cm) have invasive potential. Lymph node metastases occur in 0% to 7% of intramucosal adenocarcinomas, but still have an excellent (approximately 100%) 5-year survival rate. EGCs with submucosal invasion have an 8% to 25% rate of lymph node metastasis, and the 5-year survival rate is slightly lower but still quite high (80%–90%).

EMR (or ESD) is the treatment of choice for EGCs, typically in concert with endoscopic ultrasound for optimal staging. Criteria for EGCs that are candidates for local excision include elevated lesions less than 2.0 cm; depressed lesions less than 1.0 cm that are not ulcerated; and documented absence of lymph node metastases. These specimens, similar to those from other sites in the GI tract, should be carefully evaluated grossly and entirely submitted with attention to margin status. When followed by surveillance alone, over half of EGCs progress to advanced carcinomas within 6 months to 7 years.

The most important independent prognostic indicator for AGCs remains the anatomic stage (see the following section on grading and staging), as depth of invasion and lymph node status are critical predictors of prognosis. Some workers have argued that distally located carcinomas have a better prognosis than proximal tumors, but this remains controversial.

Gastric adenocarcinomas spread by three primary mechanisms: metastasis, direct extension, and peritoneal spread. Diffuse-type carcinomas are more likely to spread throughout the peritoneum, whereas intestinal type tumors are more likely to spread hematogenously. The prognosis for gastric adenocarcinoma in the West is poor, with a 1-year overall survival rate of 63%, and a 10-year survival rate of only 10%. The survival rates are somewhat better in Japan, although earlier detection of lower-stage cancers may help to explain this difference. Female patients and younger patients also have a better prognosis overall.

AGCs are treated with complete surgical resection and lymph node dissection; partial versus complete gastrectomy depends on the size and location of the tumor. A controversial subject in the surgical management of gastric cancer is the recommended extent of lymph node dissection. Although more extended lymph node dissections result in more accurate staging and possibly survival due to removal of diseased nodes, there may be significantly increased morbidity and mortality with extended dissections. Many patients also undergo adjuvant chemotherapy and radiation.

Grading and Staging

There are many classification schemes for gastric carcinoma, none of which is universally used or accepted. From a practical perspective, many pathologists grade intestinal-type gastric adenocarcinomas similarly to colorectal adenocarcinomas, where well-differentiated tumors are composed of well-formed glands or papillae composed of more mature-appearing cells; moderately differentiated tumors are composed of more complex architecture; and poorly differentiated tumors have solid growth patterns, very poorly formed glands, or single cells. By definition, signet ring cell carcinomas and diffuse-type gastric carcinomas are considered poorly differentiated.

Pathologic tumor staging of gastric carcinoma is performed in accordance with the TNM staging manual of the American Joint Committee on Cancer (Table 8.3). The proximal 5 cm of stomach are included with and staged similarly to the esophagus (see Chapter 7). The proximal stomach is staged as detailed in Table 8.3, but well-differentiated NETs, lymphomas, and sarcomas are not included in this staging scheme.

Similar to the rest of the gastrointestinal tract, local extent of disease is assessed in the T category, whereas regional lymph node and distant metastases are classified in the N and M categories, respectively.

TABLE 8.3　Pathologic Staging Criteria of Gastric Carcinomas

Primary Tumor (pT)

TX	Primary tumor cannot be assessed
T0	No evidence of primary tumor
Tis	Carcinoma in situ: intraepithelial tumor without lamina propria invasion
T1a	Tumor invades lamina propria or muscularis mucosae
T1b	Tumor invades submucosa
T2	Tumor invades muscularis propria
T3	Tumor invades subserosal connective tissues, without involvement of visceral peritoneum or adjacent structures
T4	Tumor invades visceral peritoneum or adjacent structures
T4a	Tumor invades visceral peritoneum
T4b	Tumor invades adjacent structures

Regional Lymph Nodes (pN)

NX	Regional lymph nodes cannot be assessed
N0	No regional lymph node metastases
N1	Metastasis in 1–2 regional lymph nodes
N2	Metastasis in 3–6 regional lymph nodes
N3	Metastasis in 7 or more regional lymph nodes
N3a	Metastasis in 7–15 regional lymph nodes
N3b	Metastasis in 16 or more regional lymph nodes

Distant Metastases (pM)

M0	No distant metastases
M1	Distant metastases

Source: Adapted from *AJCC Cancer Staging Manual*, 7th Edition, 2010.

Because the depth of tumor invasion in early gastric carcinomas predicts the likelihood of regional lymph node metastasis, it is helpful to report the depth of tumor invasion (as well as the T level) in EMR and ESD specimens.

Differential Diagnosis and Diagnostic Challenges

The diagnosis of most cases of gastric adenocarcinoma is relatively straightforward, particularly those with intestinal morphology. Adenocarcinomas of other organs can occasionally metastasize to the stomach (see subsequent section on metastases), and correlation with imaging studies, patient history, and immunohistochemical studies is often helpful. Poorly differentiated gastric adenocarcinomas may be much more problematic, and entities such as melanoma, lymphoma, and epithelioid mesenchymal tumors may enter into the differential diagnosis. Most of these cases can also be resolved by a carefully selected panel of immunostains.

A number of reactive conditions can also mimic gastric adenocarcinoma. One of the most challenging is signet ring cell change a benign condition that morphologically mimics signet ring cell carcinoma, particularly in biopsy specimens. These cells have also been referred to as "pseudo-signet ring cells." They are believed to be degenerative/reactive in nature, and have been described in association with various types of gastritis and gastric ulcers. Distinguishing these entities is obviously critical, because misdiagnosis of signet ring cell carcinoma may lead to significant and irreversible therapeutic interventions such as surgery and/or chemoradiation.

Typically, signet ring cell change lacks nuclear atypia and mitotic activity, although this is not always the case, particularly in the context of highly reactive background mucosa (Figure 8.22A–B). Immunostains and special histochemical stains are somewhat helpful in the differential diagnosis, but there are numerous pitfalls. Neoplastic signet ring cells are mucin positive, but the cells of signet ring cell change may be either positive or negative for mucin. Cytokeratins (CK)

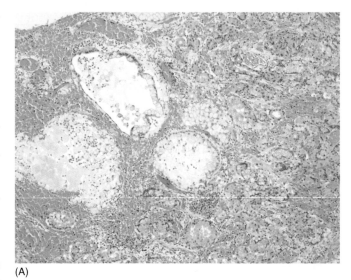

(A)

(B)

FIGURE 8.22　Signet ring cell change, or pseudo-signet ring cells, are seen in a biopsy of a hyperplastic gastric polyp with marked degenerative and inflammatory changes (A, B). Note that the dyscohesive atypical cells are all sloughing from glands, and none are present in areas of intact lamina propria.

will mark both neoplastic signet ring cells and signet ring cell change, as both are epithelial. In contrast to signet ring cell carcinoma, the cells of signet ring cell change are often strongly positive for E-cadherin and negative for p53. However, reactive epithelia may be strongly positive for proliferation markers, and E-cadherin stains may be difficult to interpret due to high background staining. If the atypical cells are confined to glands on reticulin stains this may also be helpful, as pseudo-signet ring cells typically are confined within glands and lack an infiltrating growth pattern into the lamina propria; however, reticulin may not be helpful if all the worrisome cells are detached, or if the worrisome cells are in the context of an ulcer where normal glandular architecture is severely disrupted. Occasionally, muciphages in the lamina propria may also mimic signet ring cell carcinoma, but the nuclei are typically small and uniform, and macrophage immunohistochemical markers make this a much easier distinction.

Several reactive conditions may also enter into the differential diagnosis with gastric adenocarcinoma. Ulcers often contain epithelial regenerative changes that mimic dysplasia, including nuclear enlargement and hyperchromasia, prominent nucleoli, and increased mitoses, particularly when there is marked acute inflammation. These inflammatory changes tend to be uniform and show a gradual transition to more normal-appearing areas, whereas dysplasia is sharply demarcated from adjacent non-neoplastic mucosa. In addition, exuberant granulation tissue with prominent endothelial cells can mimic a proliferation of malignant glands. For these reasons, caution should be used when entertaining a diagnosis of

malignancy in the context of a gastric ulcer with marked inflammation and granulation tissue. Gastritis cystica profunda can occasionally mimic well-differentiated adenocarcinoma as well. Similar to colitis cystica profunda, the benign appearance of the epithelium, surrounding lamina propria, and noninfiltrative rounded contours of the misplaced epithelium help to confirm a diagnosis of gastritis cystica profunda/polyposa (Figure 8.23A–B).

Metastases to the Stomach

Gastric metastases are relatively rare. However, when present, they tend to be solitary and produce either a large mural mass or ulcer, and thus may mimic a primary gastric malignancy. The most common tumors metastasizing to the stomach include melanoma (Figure 8.24A–B), breast carcinoma, and lung carcinoma, but metastases from virtually every site in the body have been reported in the literature. Metastatic breast carcinoma can be particularly problematic, as it can present with a diffuse growth pattern with signet ring cells that closely mimics gastric adenocarcinoma (Figure 8.25A–B). As breast carcinoma is positive for GATA3, GCDFP-15, ER, and PR, and negative for CDX2 and CK20, these markers can be helpful in making a diagnosis; however, it is important to remember that some gastric cancers are CK7+, and some do not mark with CK20 either. The presence of an adjacent dysplastic lesion favors a primary gastric cancer, but these may not be sampled or may be overgrown by the invasive component, so the absence of an adjacent dysplasia does not exclude a primary gastric tumor.

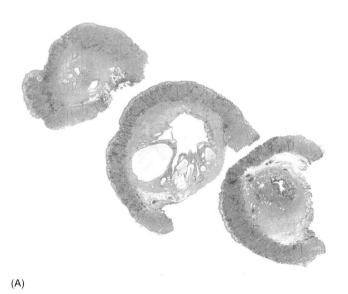

(A)

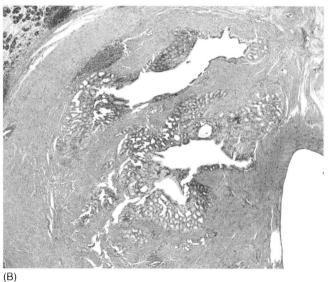

(B)

FIGURE 8.23 The entrapped submucosal epithelium seen in gastritis cystica profunda can occasionally mimic well-differentiated adenocarcinoma as well. Similar to colitis cystica profunda, the benign appearance of the epithelium, surrounding lamina propria, and noninfiltrative, rounded contours of the misplaced epithelium argue against a diagnosis of malignancy (A–B). Courtesy Dr. Andrew Bellizzi.

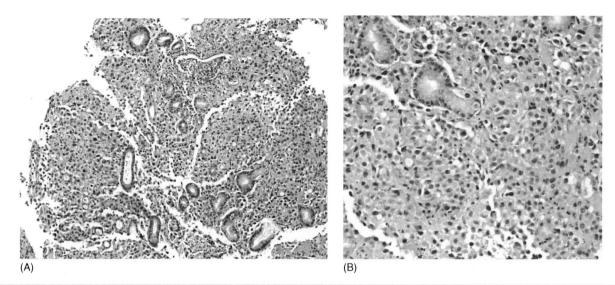

FIGURE 8.24   Metastatic malignant melanoma can closely mimic a poorly differentiated gastric adenocarcinoma (A–B).

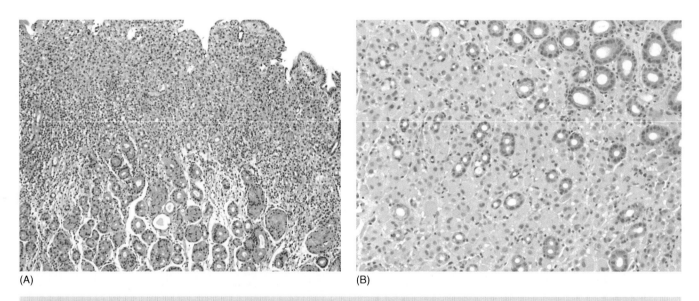

FIGURE 8.25   Metastatic breast carcinoma can closely mimic gastric adenocarcinoma. Tumor cells diffusely permeate the mucosa (A–B). The two can be indistinguishable histologically, thus ER and/or GATA3 immunostains may be very helpful.

NEUROENDOCRINE NEOPLASMS

Neuroendocrine neoplasms are discussed in detail in Chapter 3. This section will focus on aspects particular to gastric neuroendocrine neoplasia.

Terminology

Well-differentiated NENs (formerly known as carcinoid tumors in the tubular gut) are referred to as neuroendocrine tumors (NETs) in the 2010 World Health Organization Classification, and poorly differentiated NENs are referred to as neuroendocrine carcinomas (NECs). The term NEC encompasses small cell and large cell neuroendocrine carcinoma, as well as mixed small and large cell carcinomas. This classification scheme also contains the category "mixed adenoneuroendocrine carcinoma" (MANEC), defined as a mixed tumor with at least 30% of each component (malignant epithelial and neuroendocrine).

Epidemiology and Demographics

Approximately 6% of GI NETs arise in the stomach; the stomach is the second most common location within the GI tract, following jejunum/ileum and rectum. The incidence of NETs appears to be rising, as well, due at least in part to increased recognition and reporting. The male to female ratio is essentially equal for gastric NETs (0.9:1), and the median age at presentation is 63 for both men and women. Up to a quarter of extrapulmonary visceral NECs arise in the GI tract, and NECs reportedly account for 6% to 16% of gastric neuroendocrine neoplasms. NECs are more common in men, but the age of presentation is similar to that seen in gastric NET.

Clinical Features

Gastric NETs arise in three distinctive clinical settings, with implications for prognosis and management. Type I tumors, representing 70% to 80%, arise in the setting of autoimmune atrophic gastritis (Figure 8.26). Type II tumors (5%–10%) arise in association with MEN1–Zollinger–Ellison syndrome. Type III tumors (20%–25%) arise sporadically. Overall, the majority of gastric NET (76%) have localized disease at the time of presentation.

Type I and II tumors are found in the gastric body, typically confined to the mucosa or submucosa, and have a tendency to be multifocal. They are composed of ECL-cells (ie, histamine-producing) and are driven by hypergastrinemia. Hypergastrinemia-driven tumors, especially type I, are typically indolent (100% and 60%–90% five-year survival, respectively, for types I and II). Patients with small type I and II tumors may be managed with endoscopic removal and surveillance, while patients with type II tumors additionally benefit from removal of the gastrinoma, in which case their NET may spontaneously regress.

Type III tumors are nearly always solitary and may arise anywhere in the stomach. They, too, are generally

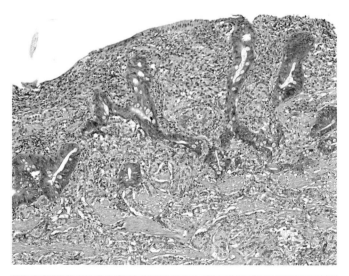

FIGURE 8.26 The majority of gastric NETs arise in the context of autoimmune atrophic gastritis; note the adjacent intestinal metaplasia and inflammation.

composed of ECL-cells, although approximately 25% are composed of alternative cell types (eg, gastrin, somatostatin, or serotonin-producing). Type III tumors are inherently aggressive (less than 50% five-year survival), and tend to invade the gastric wall and demonstrate frequent lymphovascular invasion. They are managed with resection, usually gastrectomy, and regional lymph node dissection. Occasionally, very small polypoid type III tumors can be followed with polypectomy and extremely rigorous clinical surveillance.

Pathologic Features

In the stomach, intramucosal tumors greater than 500 µm and submucosally invasive tumors are designated as NETs, while lesions measuring 150 to 500 µm are termed neuroendocrine dysplasias, and those less than 150 µm are classified as hyperplasias. The distinction of these seems arbitrary, as lesions as small as 200 µm have been shown to have neoplastic potential based on molecular studies.

Grossly, NETs are usually well-circumscribed, with a fleshy and homogeneous cut surface. The majority of the tumor is often in the submucosa and muscular wall, although polypoid lesions may be covered by mucosa and protrude into the lumen. Mucosal ulceration and necrosis may be macroscopic signs of aggressive behavior.

Histologically, NETs are characterized by a variety of organoid growth patterns (discussed and illustrated in detail in Chapter 3), including nested, trabecular, gyriform, glandular, tubuloacinar, pseudorosette-forming, solid, and mixed. The nuclear chromatin is typically granular and/or speckled, often referred to as "salt and pepper." Nucleoli are generally inconspicuous. Cells are typically monomorphic with moderate to abundant cytoplasm. The neuroendocrine nature of these neoplasms is usually evident on hematoxylin and eosin (H&E) staining, but can be confirmed with immunohistochemical staining for neuroendocrine markers.

NECs have morphologic features similar to those seen in other sites (see Chapter 3). Mitotic activity and necrosis are usually conspicuous, as is Azzopardi effect. Many gastric NECs have an admixed component of adenocarcinoma along with the neuroendocrine component, and adjacent epithelial dysplasia and/or intramucosal carcinoma is often present as well. As with NETs, the diagnosis can be supported with general neuroendocrine markers.

Most MANECs consist of NEC with a coexistent component of adenocarcinoma (Figure 8.27A–E). The WHO specifically states that adenocarcinomas in which scattered neuroendocrine cells are identified immunohistochemically are *not* considered to be MANECs. In addition, the non-neuroendocrine component must be overtly cytologically malignant, and care must be taken not to confuse entrapped glands with a glandular component.

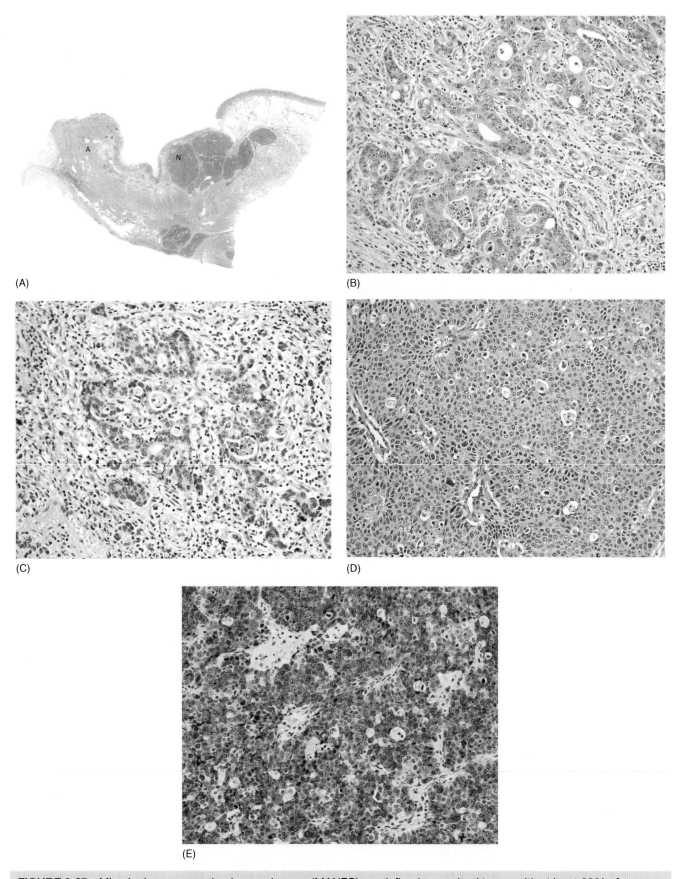

FIGURE 8.27   Mixed adenoneuroendocrine carcinomas (MANEC) are defined as a mixed tumor with at least 30% of adenocarcinoma and NEC (A). The adenocarcinoma component (B) is negative for chromogranin (C). Morphologically distinct areas of neuroendocrine differentiation (D) show strong, diffuse chromogranin positivity (E). Courtesy Dr. Andrew Bellizzi.

Grading and Staging

Grading of neuroendocrine neoplasms is discussed in detail in Chapter 3. Staging of gastric NET is summarized in Table 8.4. Staging of gastric NEC and MANEC is performed similarly to gastric adenocarcinomas (see previous section grading and staging on page 195).

Differential Diagnosis

The primary entities in the differential diagnosis of NET include non-NECs and (rarely) lymphoma; fortunately, the distinction can be made easily by immunohistochemistry in most cases. NETs with glandular, acinar, or pseudorosette patterns are most likely to mimic adenocarcinoma, whereas tumors with nested growth may be mistaken for squamous cell carcinoma or solid-pattern adenocarcinoma. It is also important to note that NETs may produce luminal or stromal mucin (Figure 8.28), a further mimic of adenocarcinoma. NETs are characterized by relative monomorphism and the characteristic nuclear chromatin pattern, while non-NECs tend to exhibit greater pleomorphism. When the diagnosis is in question, pathologists should consider NET and have a low threshold for ordering IHC for general neuroendocrine markers.

Gastric glomus tumors (see Chapter 5) may also be mistaken for neuroendocrine tumors, especially since they often express synaptophysin (albeit weakly). Glomus tumors are often multinodular and/or plexiform, and tend to grow within blood vessel walls (subendothelially).

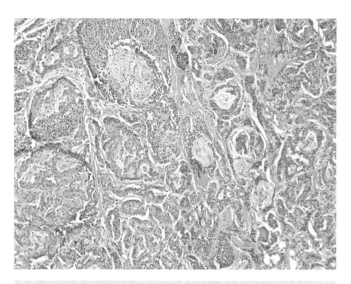

FIGURE 8.28 NETs can produce both stromal and luminal mucin, which can lead to confusion with gastric adenocarcinoma.

Tumor cells lack the classic "speckled" pattern of neuroendocrine chromatin as well. Demonstration of strong smooth muscle actin (SMA) expression is useful in securing the diagnosis of glomus tumor.

The primary entities in the differential diagnosis of NEC also include non-NECs, as well as other high-grade round blue cell tumors (including lymphoma, melanoma, and some sarcomas), and occasionally chronic inflammation in crushed specimens. NECs should feature characteristic cellular morphology and demonstrate diffuse expression of at least one general neuroendocrine marker in addition to broad-spectrum keratins, which may appear perinuclear or dot-like. Significant pleomorphism is more suggestive of non-NEC. CD45 is helpful in excluding lymphoma, and S100 for excluding melanoma. In crushed small biopsies, IHC for broad-spectrum keratins (and/or general neuroendocrine markers) and CD45 may be used to distinguish NEC from chronic inflammation.

MESENCHYMAL NEOPLASMS

Mesenchymal neoplasms, including the differential diagnoses and immunohistochemical and molecular features, are discussed in detail in Chapter 5. This section will focus on those mesenchymal tumors that are most common to the stomach.

Gastrointestinal Stromal Tumors

Gastrointestinal stromal tumors (GISTs) are the most common mesenchymal tumor of the GI tract, and the majority of them are located in the stomach (60%–70% of

TABLE 8.4 Staging of Well-Differentiated Gastric Neuroendocrine Tumors (NETs)

Primary Tumor (T)

TX	Primary tumor cannot be assessed
T0	No evidence of primary tumor
Tis	Tumor less than 0.5 cm, confined to mucosa
T1	Tumor invades lamina propria or submucosa and 1.0 cm or less in size
T2	Tumor invades muscularis propria or more than 1.0 cm in size
T3	Tumor penetrates subserosa
T4	Tumor invades visceral peritoneum (serosa) or other organs or adjacent structures

Regional Lymph Nodes (N)

NX	Nodes cannot be assessed
N0	No regional lymph node metastases
N1	Regional lymph node metastases

Distant Metastases (M)

M0	No distant metastases
M1	Distant metastases

Source: Adapted from *AJCC Cancer Staging Manual*, 7th Edition, 2010.

tumors). GISTs are believed to arise from the KIT-positive interstitial cells of Cajal, which are an innervated network of cells associated with Auerbach's plexus that coordinate peristalsis. Although symptoms may include nonspecific upper abdominal pain, GI bleeding, bloating, early satiety, and signs/symptoms of a mass, a significant proportion are incidental findings on imaging studies or procedures for unrelated conditions. In the stomach, GISTs are more likely to occur in older patients (median age 63).

A number of important genetic syndromes involve gastric GISTs. Carney triad includes epithelioid gastric GIST, pulmonary chondroma, and paragangliomas; GISTs in this context are wild-type, and believed to be part of the spectrum of succinate dehydrogenase (SDH) deficient GISTs. Patients with Carney–Stratakis syndrome have epithelioid gastric GISTs and paragangliomas; these patients also have germline *SDH* subunit gene mutations and thus are part of the spectrum of SDH-deficient GISTs as well.

Pathologic Features

Grossly, GISTs arise in the muscularis propria, and are usually somewhat centered in the wall of the stomach. They vary widely in size, ranging from 1.0 mm to more than 40 cm, with a median size of 6 cm in the stomach. Tumors may protrude into the lumen in a polypoid fashion, with overlying mucosal ulceration. The cut surface may show hemorrhage, calcification, or, less commonly, necrosis. GISTs are typically circumscribed, and although the overlying mucosa is often ulcerated, true invasion of the mucosa is uncommon, and is associated

with a worse prognosis. Gastric GISTs located in the fundus and cardia have a worse prognosis than those located in the antrum.

Morphologically, gastric GISTs have a spindle cell pattern approximately 50% of the time, an epithelioid phenotype approximately 40% of the time, and are mixed pattern 10% of the time. Nuclear palisading and cytoplasmic vacuolization are also more commonly seen in gastric GISTs (Figure 8.29A–B).

SDH-deficient GISTs (also known as pediatric GIST or type 2 GIST) typically occur in female children and adolescents with a peak age of onset in the second decade. Most tumors develop in the stomach or omentum. This subtype accounts for approximately 5% to 7% of gastric GISTs. The distinctive histology features a multinodular or plexiform growth pattern (Figure 8.30A), often with epithelioid morphology. These tumors are positive for KIT, but virtually all demonstrate a loss of SDHB staining by immunohistochemistry, and thus this stain is a good screening tool for this tumor. Only a minority of these tumors have an identifiable *SDH* mutation, however. Typical grading criteria are not applicable to this subtype (see the following section on grading and risk stratification), and they are often imatinib resistant. Additionally, this subtype is more likely to metastasize to lymph nodes, although this finding does not appear to affect prognosis.

There is also a subset of gastric GISTs with *PDGFRA* mutations (particularly exon 18) that have an extremely indolent course, even when large. These tumors typically are purely epithelioid or have an epithelioid component, and have low or no mitotic activity.

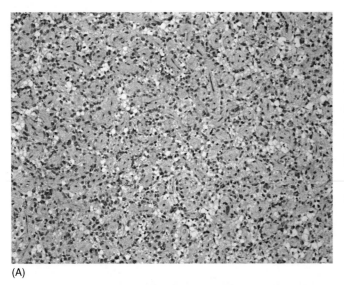

(A)

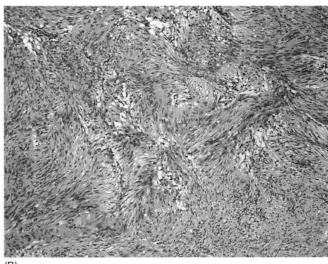

(B)

FIGURE 8.29 Gastric GISTs are more likely to be epithelioid, and perinuclear vacuoles are frequent (A). Nuclear palisading can be striking in gastric GISTs (B).

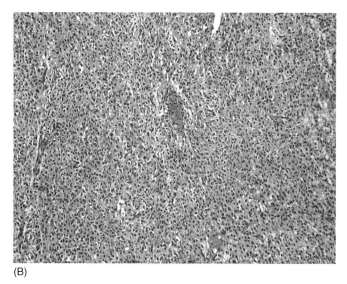

(A)

(B)

FIGURE 8.30 SDH-deficient GISTs have a distinctive multinodular or plexiform growth pattern (A), typically with epithelioid morphology (B).

Ancillary Studies

A detailed discussion of the immunohistochemical features of GISTs is presented elsewhere (Chapters 5, 13, and 14). In brief, 95% of GISTs are KIT-positive. Approximately 5% of GISTs are KIT-negative; the majority of these are epithelioid GISTs that have *PDGFRA* mutations, and these typically arise in the stomach (as noted in the preceding section on pathologic features) or are extraintestinal. Most GISTs (~99%) also mark with DOG1 (also known as ANO-1). The majority of KIT-negative GISTs stain with DOG1 as well, including 79% of those with *PDGFRA* mutations (as opposed to KIT which only stains 9% of GISTs that have a *PDGFRA* mutation). Caveats regarding the use of KIT and DOG1 are discussed in detail in Chapter 5.

Approximately 80% of GISTs have *KIT* mutations, and up to 20% contain wild-type *KIT*. Nearly 10% of the latter harbor mutations in *PDGFRA* (platelet-derived growth factor A). This subset of GISTs is more likely to occur in the stomach (as noted in the preceding section on pathologic features) or proximal small bowel, or to be extraintestinal. They are typically epithelioid and have an indolent clinical course. Immunohistochemistry for KIT in these tumors shows faint positive or negative staining. Because certain mutations (both *KIT* and *PDGFRA*) may affect prognosis, molecular analysis of GISTs is increasingly regarded as the standard of care.

Some wild-type GISTs lack both *KIT* and *PDGFRA* mutations; these include the SDH-deficient GIST described in the preceding section on pathologic features, as well as those occurring in the setting of NF1, Carney triad, and Carney–Stratakis syndrome. Some of these

harbor *BRAF V600E* mutations; these are KIT positive by immunohistochemistry.

Grading, Risk Stratification, and Prognosis

Grading, risk stratification, and prognosis are discussed in detail in Chapter 5. Of note, the risk of aggressive behavior in gastric GISTs is relatively low until tumors reach more than 10 cm in size. As mentioned previously, SDH-deficient GISTs have a tendency to metastasize to lymph nodes (approximately half of cases), yet overall their behavior is indolent even when lymph node metastases occur. Because of this unusual behavior, standard criteria for grading and risk stratification are probably not applicable to this subgroup of tumors, and it has been recommended that conventional criteria not be used in this specific context. Detailed discussions of therapy for GISTs are presented in Chapters 5, 13, and 14.

Differential Diagnosis

A detailed discussion of the differential diagnosis of GIST is presented in Chapter 5. In the stomach, the most common entity in the differential diagnosis is gastric schwannoma. Less common mesenchymal tumors that may enter into the differential diagnosis at this site include inflammatory fibroid polyp (IFP), glomus tumor, and plexiform angiomyxoid tumor. Leiomyomas, granular cell tumors, and benign neural polyps are rarely seen in the stomach, as are neurofibromas; the latter are typically seen in association with NF1. Desmoid tumors, PEComas, and inflammatory myofibroblastic tumors, which are also rare in the stomach, are discussed in detail in Chapter 5.

Schwannoma

The stomach is the most common site for GI schwannomas, and these lesions are more common in women. Grossly, schwannomas are circumscribed but unencapsulated tumors with a firm, rubbery, yellow–gray to tan cut surface. Cystic change and hemorrhage are not usually seen. Schwannomas are moderately cellular tumors; focal nuclear atypia is common, but mitotic figures should be rare to absent, and atypical mitoses should not be seen. Unlike soft tissue schwannomas, palisading is rare in the GI tract, as are foamy histiocytes. A notable feature in GI tract schwannomas (as opposed to those that occur in the soft tissues) is a dense lymphoplasmacytic cuff, often with germinal centers, present at the periphery of the tumor (Figure 8.31A–B). Numerous lymphocytes may also be seen admixed with tumor cells. Epithelioid foci are very rare in GI tract schwannomas. GI tract schwannomas express S100 and generally lack immunoreactivity for KIT, DOG1, SMA, desmin, and other smooth muscle markers; however, rare tumors can show focal expression of keratin, SMA, or desmin. In addition, unlike their soft tissue counterparts, GI tract schwannomas do not express calretinin.

Glomus Tumor

On the rare occasion when glomus tumors arise in the GI tract, they are most commonly seen in the antrum of the stomach. They typically arise in the muscularis propria, and feature cellular nodules or nests separated by bands of smooth muscle extending from the muscularis propria (see Chapter 5). Prominent slit-like and dilated vessels are common, and the tumor cells show a subendothelial growth pattern within walls of blood vessels. The cells are uniform and rounded, with clear to eosinophilic cytoplasm and sharply defined cell borders. The nucleus appears "punched out" and round, and is well demarcated from the surrounding cytoplasm. There is typically diffuse reactivity for SMA, but KIT and DOG1 are negative, in contrast to GIST. Calponin and caldesmon are typically positive as well, but desmin is often negative. Some tumors are focally positive with CD34 and synaptophysin, but chromogranin and keratin should be negative.

Inflammatory Fibroid Polyp

Inflammatory fibroid polyps (IFPs) are benign mesenchymal tumors that are commonly found in the antrum of the stomach or the ileum, and often present as a polyp. The neoplastic nature of these lesions has been debated, but some IFPs have been found to have activating mutations in *PDGFRA*, so they in fact may be neoplastic. They present in a wide age range but are typically seen in adults from 60 to 80 years old. These lesions arise from the submucosa, and the overlying mucosa is often ulcerated (Figure 8.32A–B). Tumors range in size from less than 0.5 cm to over 4.0 cm, with an average size of 1 to 2 cm. Histologically, they have ill-defined margins, and consist of a bland proliferation of spindle cells and stellate cells with prominent admixed inflammatory cells, particularly eosinophils. Blood vessels are usually prominent, and may show surrounding concentric "onion-skin" fibrosis. IFPs are positive for CD34 and variably positive for SMA; they are negative for KIT, desmin, and S100.

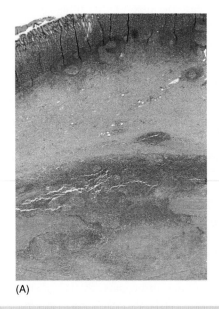
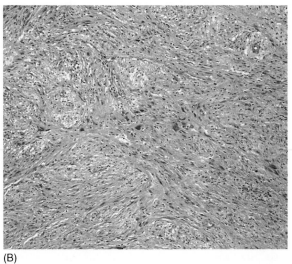

(A)   (B)

FIGURE 8.31 Gastric schwannomas feature a dense lymphoplasmacytic cuff present at the periphery of the tumor (A). Focal nuclear atypia is common, and numerous lymphocytes may also be seen admixed with tumor cells (B).

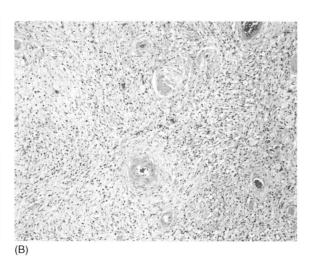

FIGURE 8.32 Inflammatory fibroid polyps arise from the submucosa (A), and typically have ill-defined margins. They consist of a bland proliferation of spindle cells with admixed inflammatory cells, particularly eosinophils, as well as prominent blood vessels that may show a surrounding cuff of plump lesional cells (B).

Plexiform Fibromyxoma (Plexiform Angiomyxoid Myofibroblastic Tumor of Stomach)

These tumors present as a mural mass in young to middle aged adults, are nearly exclusive to the gastric antrum, and are often mistaken for GISTs. They are bland, multilobular spindle cell tumors that are sharply circumscribed, have a plexiform growth pattern, and contain abundant myxoid stroma with prominent small blood vessels (Figure 8.33A–B). Vascular invasion is common. These tumors are positive for SMA and stain variably with desmin; they

are negative for KIT, DOG1, and S100. Plexiform fibromyxomas are rare, and thus knowledge of natural history is limited, but they appear to behave in a benign fashion.

HEMATOLYMPHOID NEOPLASMS

The stomach is the most common primary site for GI lymphomas to develop, and it may be involved by many of the lymphomas discussed throughout this text. In the stomach, as in the remainder of the GI tract, B cell

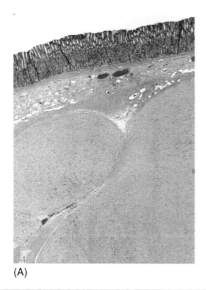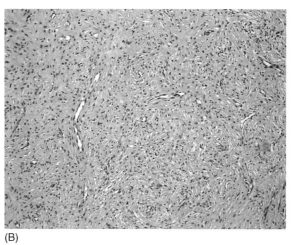

FIGURE 8.33 Plexiform fibromyxoid tumors are bland, multiolobular spindle cell tumors (A) that are sharply circumscribed, have a plexiform growth pattern, and contain abundant myxoid stroma with prominent small blood vessels (B).

lymphomas far outnumber their T cell counterparts. The two most important gastric hematolymphoid neoplasms are mucosa-associated lymphoid tissue (MALT) lymphoma and diffuse large B cell lymphoma (DLBCL); these will be discussed here in addition to important (if relatively rare) variants of these lymphomas.

MALT Lymphoma

This low-grade B cell lymphoma is more properly referred to as "extranodal marginal zone lymphoma of mucosa-associated lymphoid tissue" and was described by Isaacson and Wright in 1983. While MALT lymphoma can occur throughout the GI tract, the stomach is, by far, the most common site of involvement, with around 85% of all GI MALT lymphomas occurring here. In the stomach, most MALT lymphomas are intimately related to underlying infection with *H. pylori*, and arise from so-called "acquired" mucosa-associated lymphoid tissue, as discussed in Chapter 4. As such, the majority of cases can actually be treated by eradication of the underlying infection.

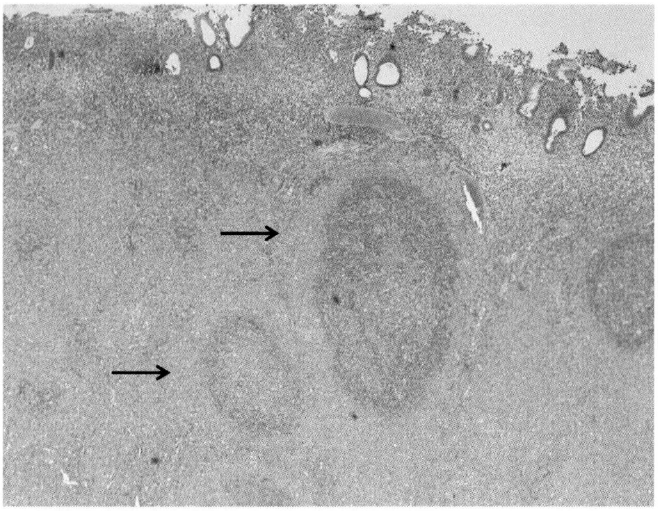

FIGURE 8.35 Arising most often in a background of *H. pylori* gastritis, MALT lymphoma frequently has admixed germinal centers, which can have a "moth-eaten" appearance when colonized by lymphoma cells. Note the prominent, expanded marginal zone composed of pale-staining cells around the germinal centers (arrows).

Pathologic Findings

The cells comprising MALT lymphomas are small, and may resemble either centrocytes of the follicle center, or have more abundant, pale cytoplasm and indented nuclei, giving them a "monocytoid" appearance (Figure 8.34). Most MALT lymphomas also contain some large cells resembling centroblasts, although these are in the minority

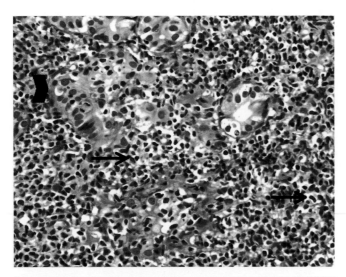

FIGURE 8.34 MALT lymphoma is usually composed of predominantly small lymphocytes, many of which have ample cytoplasm and indented nuclei (arrows), an appearance that has been termed "monocytoid." A number of gastric glands (arrowhead) are destroyed by infiltrating lymphoma cells.

and individually scattered. One may also see reactive germinal centers (similar to those seen in *H. pylori* gastritis), which are infiltrated or colonized by the lymphoma cells, sometimes creating a "moth-eaten" or "naked" appearance (Figure 8.35). In addition, the lymphoma cells commonly infiltrate and disrupt normal mucosal structures (glands and pits), creating lymphoepithelial lesions (Figure 8.36A–B). These are a characteristic feature of MALT lymphomas, although they are nonspecific, and similar destructive infiltration may be seen in other types of lymphoma. In addition, infiltration of the epithelium by benign lymphocytes can be seen in a variety of reactive conditions. While scattered large, centroblast-like cells are common in MALT lymphoma, large collections (greater than 20 or so together) or sheets of such cells should raise the diagnosis of DLBCL, which will be discussed in a subsequent section. Some cases of MALT lymphoma have plasmacytic differentiation, in which clonal plasma cells comprise a component of the infiltrate. Occasionally, there may be essentially complete plasmacytic differentiation, an appearance that can lead to diagnostic difficulty (Figure 8.37).

Ancillary Studies

Immunohistochemically, MALT lymphoma expresses pan-B cell markers such as CD20 and CD79a (Figure 8.38). Between 30% and 50% of MALT lymphomas are purported to aberrantly coexpress CD43 on the malignant B cells, though this is not specific, as it may be seen in other types of lymphoma including mantle cell lymphoma

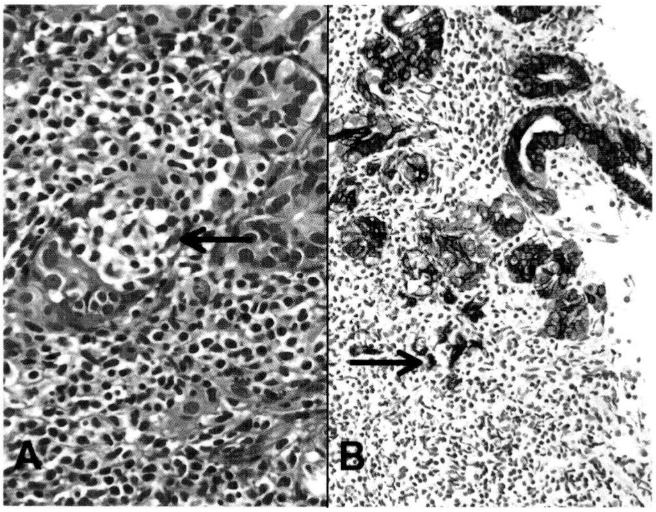

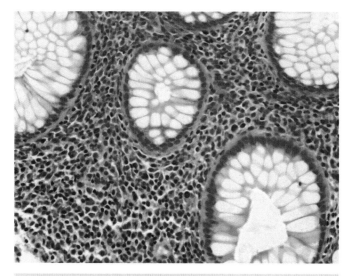

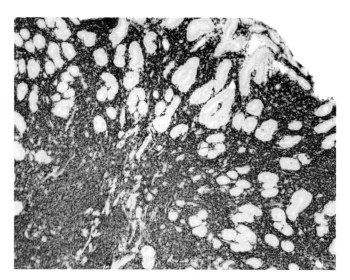

FIGURE 8.36   Though not specific to MALT lymphoma, lymphoepithelial lesions (LELs) are a hallmark, created when lymphoma cells invade and destroy the epithelial structures of mucosa, in this case, gastric glands (A, arrow). The use of a cytokeratin immunostain (B) highlights the destruction, revealing scattered remnant epithelial cells among the infiltrate (arrow). Courtesy Dr. Henry Appelman.

FIGURE 8.38   This CD20 immunostain highlights the diffuse infiltrate of neoplastic B cells in a gastric MALT lymphoma.

(MCL) and chronic lymphocytic leukemia/small lymphocytic lymphoma (CLL/SLL). In fact, there is no specific immunohistochemical marker for MALT lymphoma, meaning that the diagnosis relies fairly heavily on the morphologic impression. If there is a plasmacytic component

to the process, it will likely express either monotypic kappa or lambda light chain, which can be a helpful indicator of clonality when it is present (Figure 8.39).

While there is no specific immunohistochemical phenotype that points to MALT lymphoma, there are a number of associated molecular abnormalities that can be seen. The t(11;18)(q21;q21) translocation is the most common translocation found in GI MALT lymphomas, bringing together the *API2* gene on chromosome 11 and the *MALT1* gene on chromosome 18. This translocation may

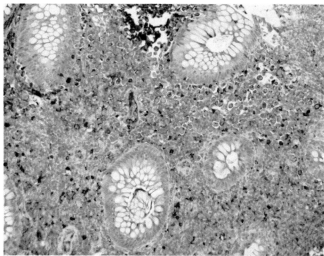

FIGURE 8.37   Some MALT lymphomas, in this case an example in the colon, have extensive or even complete plasmacytic differentiation. When the cells have the appearance of mature plasma cells like this, it can lead to diagnostic difficulty, being easily confused with a chronic inflammatory condition or a plasma cell neoplasm such as plasma cell myeloma.

FIGURE 8.39   This colonic MALT lymphoma had extensive plasmacytic differentiation, including many cells with crystallized immunoglobulin in their cytoplasm ("Mott cells"). This kappa light chain immunostain confirms their monotypic/clonal nature.

be seen in cases arising in the setting of *H. pylori* infection or in cases that are *H. pylori* negative, but in either case, its presence is associated with resistance of the lymphoma to conservative therapy aimed at eradication of the infection. Other molecular abnormalities reported in MALT lymphoma include t(14;18)(q32;q21) [*IgH/MALT1*], t(1;14)(p22;q32) [*BCL10/IgH*], and trisomy 3q27. There is debate about whether to test for the t(11;18) a priori when making a diagnosis of MALT lymphoma in order to predict the small subset of patients unlikely to respond to conservative therapy. There is currently no clear recommendation for or against this practice.

Differential Diagnosis and Diagnostic Challenges

The differential diagnosis for MALT lymphoma includes a number of small B cell neoplasms such as MCL (discussed in detail in Chapter 11) and follicular lymphoma (discussed in Chapter 9). Both can have a nodular pattern that can overlap with the appearance of the reactive germinal centers that can be seen in MALT lymphomas, though immunohistochemical stains are usually sufficient to make the distinction, with the cyclin-D1 expression of MCL and the BCL2 positivity of the neoplastic follicles in follicular lymphoma being most helpful. Plasmacytic differentiation in MALT lymphoma can lead to confusion with true plasma cell neoplasms, and this can be difficult to sort out when there is complete plasma cell differentiation. Correlation with other systemic manifestations of disease, such as a search for a monoclonal serum protein, may help to identify a plasma cell neoplasm like myeloma, but it may be necessary simply to provide a differential diagnosis in such situations.

Perhaps the most challenging situation is discerning when an intense *H. pylori* gastritis has "crossed the line" and become a lymphoma. Aberrant coexpression of CD43 by the B lymphocytes is useful but, unfortunately, there is no specific immunohistochemical marker for lymphoma; it thus is often a matter of morphologic evaluation and judgment. Molecular studies for B cell gene rearrangements may also be helpful, but the presence of clonality does not unequivocally imply a diagnosis of malignancy. In addition to the histologic evidence provided by a monotonous and destructive infiltrate of CD20-positive B cells, it is important to take into account the clinical impression. For example, a malignant-appearing ulcer or macroscopic evidence of an infiltrative process such as thickened mucosal folds may prove helpful in making the diagnosis. In addition, such findings give the endoscopist a "target" to assess on follow-up examinations after therapy.

The association with *H. pylori* infection makes MALT lymphoma amenable to conservative therapy aimed at eradication of the inciting infection. The vast majority of gastric MALT lymphomas will respond to this therapy, though those harboring the t(11;18) have a high prevalence of resistance, as described in the preceding section on MALT

lymphoma. Interestingly, there are reports of MALT lymphomas outside the stomach, including in the small intestine and even in the colon, responding to similar therapy. Importantly, while standard follow-up biopsies to assess eradication of *H. pylori* typically occur in the 4 to 6 week timeframe, the lymphoid infiltrate is likely to be unchanged at this point in time, even in patients who successfully undergo treatment and achieve remission. In fact, there are reports of complete resolution of the atypical lymphoid population taking many months, even more than a year. Thus, it is important to be sure that treating physicians are aware of this fact to avoid chemoradiation or other aggressive therapies for a lymphoma that would likely respond to conservative therapy if given enough time. Comparison of follow-up biopsies to the pretreatment tissue and/or to earlier follow-up samples can be very helpful, with a diagnosis such as "residual MALT lymphoma, improved from [DATE]" providing useful information to the clinician.

While it does not affect the stomach, there is a variant of MALT lymphoma affecting the small intestine that merits mention. Immunoproliferative small intestinal disease (IPSID) is a lymphoma with complete or nearly complete plasmacytic differentiation that preferentially involves the small intestine and causes malabsorption and weight loss (Figure 8.40). The plasma cells are CD138 positive, and are

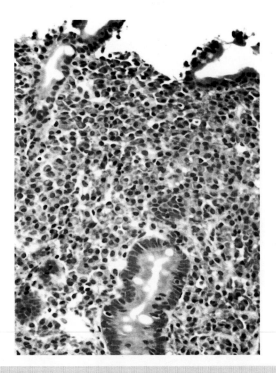

FIGURE 8.40 Immunoproliferative small intestinal disease (IPSID) is considered a variant of MALT lymphoma that may be associated with underlying *Campylobacter* infection. IPSID is composed almost entirely of plasma cells, at least in early stages of the process. Patients may also have a monoclonal serum protein, composed of a truncated IgA heavy chain and leading to the alternate name for the process, "IgA heavy chain disease."

often immunohistochemically positive for immunoglobulin A (IgA) heavy chain. In about half of the cases, there is an associated production of an abnormal, truncated IgA heavy chain that can be found in the serum, leading to the alternative name "IgA heavy chain disease." IPSID is most common in young men and has a strong geographic association, occurring in the Middle East, the Mediterranean region, and the Cape region of South Africa. It tends to be associated with low socioeconomic status and may result from a chronic infection, perhaps with a *Campylobacter* species; early cases have been shown to respond to broad-spectrum antibiotics. Many cases, however, present at advanced stage and IPSID may progress to a high-grade lymphoma indistinguishable from DLBCL.

Diffuse Large B Cell Lymphoma

DLBCL is the most common lymphoma affecting the GI tract, and the stomach is a common site of involvement. It may arise de novo, or evolve from a precursor low-grade lymphoma, such as follicular lymphoma or MALT lymphoma.

Pathologic Features

DLBCL is characterized morphologically by diffuse clusters (usually defined as more than 20 cells together) and/or sheets of large, dyscohesive cells with vesicular nuclei and one or more inconspicuous nucleoli (Figure 8.41). Occasionally, the cells of DLBCL will be more "intermediate" in size, which can cause some diagnostic confusion, though the other features such as a rapid proliferative

rate and immunohistochemical staining pattern should still be present. When judging cell size, endothelial cells in the vessels in and around a DLBCL are a convenient metric, as their nuclei are a good measure of "large" size (Figure 8.42). By definition, the cells of DLBCL should be at least the size of a macrophage nucleus and at least twice the size of a normal lymphocyte nucleus. DLBCL is a destructive neoplasm, in which the malignant cells infiltrate widely through the tissue, obliterating normal structures and, in the GI tract, often leading to a mucosal ulcer (Figure 8.43A–B). A large number of cases present at high stage, reflecting the aggressiveness of the process. In addition to the most common morphology described earlier in this paragraph (technically, the "centroblastic variant" due to the resemblance of the cells to normal centroblasts of the germinal center), there are two other fairly common morphologic variants. The first is the immunoblastic variant, in which the cells have a more uniform appearance with one large, centrally located nucleolus (Figure 8.44). DLBCL may also have an "anaplastic" appearance, with cells that are much more pleomorphic (Figure 8.45), though it is important to understand that this variant is unrelated to anaplastic large cell lymphoma, which is a T cell process. In elderly patients, a subtype of DLBCL can be associated with EBV in a manner analogous to EBV-driven lymphoproliferative disorders in immunosuppressed patients who have undergone organ transplants (so-called monomorphic post-transplant lymphoproliferative disorders). In both of these cases, the lymphoma is essentially indistinguishable from conventional DLBCL, though there can be relatively more immunoblast-like cells and even large atypical cells resembling Reed–Sternberg

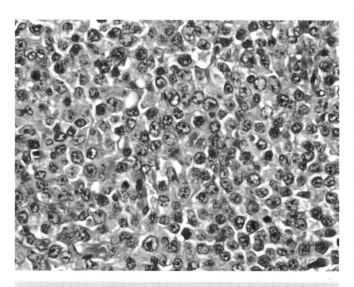

FIGURE 8.41 Diffuse large B cell lymphoma (DLBCL) is most frequently composed of large cells resembling the centroblasts of the normal germinal center, with vesicular nuclei and fairly inconspicuous nucleoli.

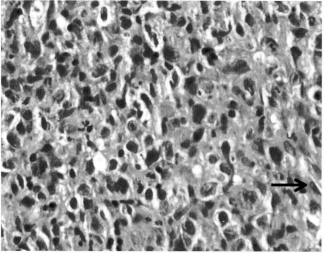

FIGURE 8.42 As an internal gauge of "large" cell size, endothelial cells from vessels admixed with a lymphoma provide a convenient comparison. Note the similarity of this endothelial nucleus (arrow) to the nuclei of the surrounding lymphoma cells.

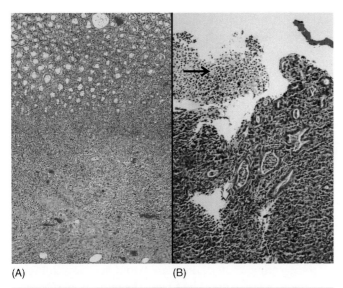

(A)   (B)

FIGURE 8.43   DLBCL is a destructive process,
obliterating normal structures of the wall of a viscus (A)
and often leading to mucosal ulcer (B) as evidenced by
overlying ulcer exudate (arrow).

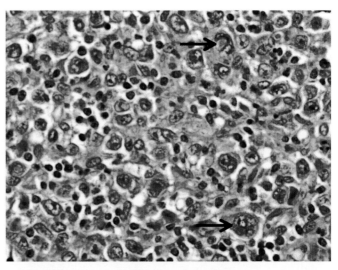

FIGURE 8.45   The anaplastic variant of DLBCL has very
pleomorphic cells, many of which show nuclear lobes
and/or indentation (arrows). While the morphology can
be similar, the anaplastic variant of DLBCL is completely
unrelated to anaplastic large cell lymphoma, which is a T
cell process.

cells in Hodgkin lymphoma (Figure 8.46). Evidence of
EBV involvement such as a positive EBV-encoded ribonucleic acid (EBER; in situ hybridization) probe is useful in
the diagnosis (Figure 8.46, inset).

Ancillary Studies

Immunohistochemically, most DLBCLs express pan-B
cell markers including CD20, PAX-5, and CD79a
(Figure 8.47). BLC-2 is commonly expressed as well, and

DLBCL may have a germinal center cell phenotype, with
expression of CD10 and/or BCL6, or a so-called "activated B cell" phenotype, with expression of MUM-1 and
other markers. Perhaps 10% of cases aberrantly coexpress
CD5, a T cell marker, which can lead to confusion with
the blastoid or pleomorphic variants of MCL, discussed in
detail in Chapter 11. Unlike MCL, DLBCL is negative for
cyclin-D1 expression.

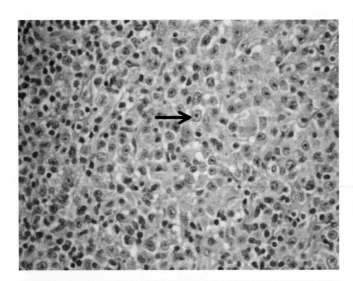

FIGURE 8.44   The immunoblastic variant of DLBCL
consists of somewhat uniform cells that have prominent,
central nucleoli (arrow), reminiscent of normal
immunoblasts.

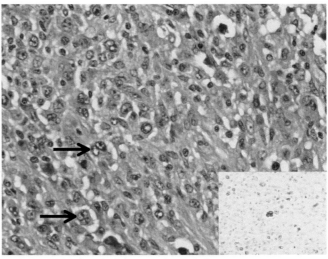

FIGURE 8.46   Scattered Reed–Sternberg-like cells
(arrows) are present in an EBV-driven lymphoma in an
elderly patient. A positive EBER probe (in situ hybridization
for EBV) confirms the diagnosis (inset).

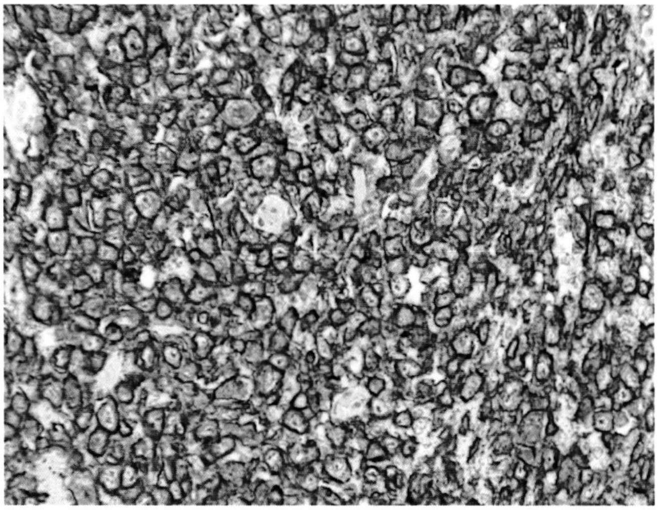

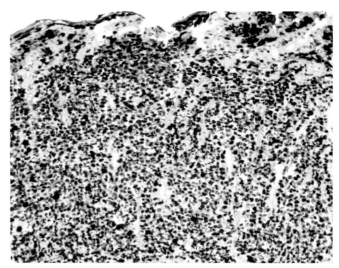

FIGURE 8.47 Immunostains for CD20 are diffusely positive in a DLBCL.

FIGURE 8.48 Strong nuclear staining for Ki-67 reveals a very high proliferative rate in this "double-hit" lymphoma.

From a molecular standpoint, DLBCL may harbor a number of abnormalities, often reflecting the presence of an underlying low-grade process. As such, the t(14;18) translocation characteristic of follicular lymphoma is present in up to one-third of cases. Other abnormalities include *BCL6* gene alterations (chromosome 3q27) and, for those with an activated B cell phenotype, molecular aberrancies along the NF-κB pathway, leading to constitutive activation and inhibition of apoptosis. As discussed in Chapters 4 and 9, a group of neoplasms with features intermediate between DLBCL and Burkitt lymphoma, the so-called "double-hit" lymphomas, have a germinal center immunophenotype with CD10 expression. They harbor abnormalities in *MYC*, along with *BCL2* and/or *BCL6*. Such cases usually have a high proliferative rate (Figure 8.48) and their distinction seems to be important from a prognostic, and possibly therapeutic, standpoint in younger patients, as there is a subset of cases with *MYC* and *BCL2* abnormalities that are treatment-refractory.

Differential Diagnosis and Diagnostic Challenges

The differential diagnosis of DLBCL includes a number of other B cell lymphoproliferative disorders. Perhaps most important is the differentiation from (or recognition of superimposition upon) an underlying low-grade lymphoma. This is crucial because de novo DLBCL, as an aggressive lymphoma, is potentially curable by appropriate therapy, while cases that evolve from a low-grade process may respond to therapy only to leave behind an incurable disease like follicular lymphoma. In addition, a common scenario in the stomach is the finding of DLBCL with an associated MALT lymphoma. Morphologically, MALT lymphomas may consist of cells that are large and have ample cytoplasm (Figure 8.49). Furthermore, scattered large cells are common in

MALT lymphoma, and distinction of early DLBCL can be diagnostically difficult. While a large collection or sheet(s) of large cells in the setting of something recognizable as MALT lymphoma was termed "high-grade MALT lymphoma" in the past, this designation is now out of date, and such an appearance should currently be diagnosed as DLBCL. Other entities in the differential diagnosis include blastoid or pleomorphic MCL as described in the preceding section on ancillary studies, Burkitt lymphoma (usually BCL2 negative and harboring *MYC* abnormalities), and B lymphoblastic leukemia/lymphoma, which expresses markers of immaturity such as CD34 and terminal deoxynucleotidyl

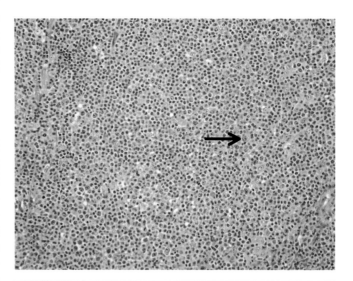

FIGURE 8.49 This MALT lymphoma has an abundance of somewhat larger cells and could be mistaken for a DLBCL at a cursory glance. Truly large, centroblast-like cells, however, are still individually scattered (arrow).

transferase (TdT). T cell lymphomas such as enteropathy-associated T cell lymphoma (see Chapter 9) and anaplastic large cell lymphoma may also resemble DLBCL, but their lack of B cell marker expression by immunohistochemistry is helpful in most cases.

The prognosis of DLBCL depends on the stage at presentation, including the involvement of regional lymph nodes. Like other aggressive lymphomas, it is potentially curable, though an underlying low-grade component should be recognized and mentioned in the diagnosis since it may persist even after the DLBCL is treated. Standard therapy for DLBCL has long been the "CHOP" regimen, consisting of cyclophosphamide, vincristine, doxorubicin, and dexamethasone. More recently, anti-CD20 immunotherapy with rituximab has been added successfully (R-CHOP) and is now the standard of care. Interestingly, some targeted therapies aimed at BCL2 inhibitors (in the case of germinal center B cell phenotype) and the NF-κB pathway (in the case of activated B cell phenotype) are under investigation. Additionally, there are some reports of DLBCLs of limited stage in the stomach that are associated with underlying *H. pylori* infection being amenable to very conservative therapy aimed at *H. pylori* eradication. In aggressive cases with large ulcers or intractable bleeding, surgical therapy may be required, though surgery is not generally considered front-line therapy for lymphoma.

SELECTED REFERENCES

General

Carneiro F, Lauwers GY. Epithelial tumors of the stomach. In: Shepherd NA, Warren BF, et al, eds. *Morson and Dawson's Gastrointestinal Pathology.* 5th ed. West Sussex: Wiley-Blackwell; 2013.

Chun N, Ford JM. Genetic testing by cancer site: stomach. *Cancer J.* 2012;18:355–363.

Correa P. Human gastric carcinogenesis: a multistep and multifactorial process. *Cancer Res.* 1992;52:6735–6740.

Lauwers GY. Epithelial Neoplasms of the stomach. In: Odze RD, Goldblum JR, eds. *Surgical Pathology of the GI Tract, Liver, Biliary Tract, and Pancreas.* 3rd ed. Philadelphia, PA: Elsevier; 2015.

Naymagon S, Warner RR, Patel K, et al. Gastroduodenal ulceration associated with radioembolization for the treatment of hepatic tumors: an institutional experience and review of the literature. *Dig Dis Sci.* 2010;55:2450–2458.

Park DY, Lauwers GY. Gastric polyps: classification and management. *Arch Pathol Lab Med.* 2008;132:633–640.

Syngal S, Brand RE, Church JM, et al. ACG clinical guideline: genetic testing and management of hereditary gastrointestinal cancer syndromes. *Am J Gastroenterol.* 2015;110:223–262.

Turner JR, Odze RD. Polyps of the stomach. In: Odze RD, Goldblum JR, eds. *Surgical Pathology of the GI Tract, Liver, Biliary Tract, and Pancreas.* 3rd ed. Philadelphia, PA: Elsevier, 2015.

Inflammatory Polyps, Hyperplastic Polyps, and Non-neoplastic Lesions

Abraham SC, Singh VK, Yardley JH, Wu TT. Hyperplastic polyps of the stomach: associations with histologic patterns of gastritis and gastric atrophy. *Am J Surg Pathol.* 2001;25:500–507.

Carmack SW, Genta RM, Schuler CM, Saboorian MH. The current spectrum of gastric polyps: a 1-year national study of over 120,000 patients. *Am J Gastroenterol.* 2009;104:1524–1532.

Carneiro F, David L, Seruca R, et al. Hyperplastic polyposis and diffuse carcinoma of the stomach. A study of a family. *Cancer.* 1993;72:323–329.

Gonzalez-Obeso E, Fujita H, Deshpande V, et al. Gastric hyperplastic polyps: a heterogeneous clinicopathologic group including a distinct subset best categorized as mucosal prolapse polyp. *Am J Surg Pathol.* 2011;35:670–677.

Hattori T. Morphological range of hyperplastic polyps and carcinomas arising in hyperplastic polyps of the stomach. *J Clin Pathol.* 1985;38:622–630.

Niv Y, Delpre G, Sperber AD, et al. Hyperplastic gastric polyposis, hypergastrinaemia, and colorectal neoplasia: a description of four cases. *Eur J Gastroenterol Hepatol.* 2003;15:1361–1366.

Ogata H, Oshio T, Ishibashi H, et al. Heterotopic pancreas in children: review of the literature and report of 12 cases. *Pediatr Surg Int.* 2008;24:271–275.

Rich A, Toro TZ, Tanksley J, et al. Distinguishing Menetrier's disease from its mimics. *Gut.* 2010;59:1617–1624.

Triffin A, Tarcoveanu E, Danciu M, et al. Gastric heterotopic pancreas: an unusual case and review of the literature. *J Gastrointest Liver Dis.* 2012;21:209–212.

Wei R, Want QB, Chen QH, et al. Upper gastrointestinal tract heterotopic pancreas: findings from CT and endoscopic imaging with histopathologic correlation. *Clin Imaging.* 2011;35:353–359.

Zea-Iriarte WL, Sekine I, Itsuno M, et al. Carcinoma in gastric hyperplastic polyps. A phenotypic study. *Dig Dis Sci.* 1996;41:377–386.

Hamartomatous Polyps

Amason T, Liang WY, Alfaro E, et al. Morphology and natural history of familial adenomatous polyposis-associated dysplastic fundic gland polyps. *Histopathology.* 2014;65:353–362.

Bettington M, Brown IS, Kumarasinghe MP, et al. The challenging diagnosis of Cronkhite-Canada syndrome in the upper gastrointestinal tract: a series of 7 cases with clinical follow-up. *Am J Surg Pathol.* 2014;38:215–233.

Bianchi LK, Burke CA, Bennett AE, et al. Fundic gland polyp dysplasia is common in familial adenomatous polyposis. *Clin Gastroenterol Hepatol.* 2008;6:180–185.

Burke AP, Sobin LH. The pathology of Cronkhite-Canada polyps. A comparison to juvenile polyps. *Am J Surg Pathol.* 1989;13:940–946.

Burt RW. Gastric fundic gland polyps. *Gastroenterology.* 2003;125:1462–1469.

Choudhry U, Boyce HW Jr., Coppola D. Proton pump inhibitor-associated gastric polyps: a retrospective analysis of their frequency, and endoscopic, histologic, and ultrastructural characteristics. *Am J Clin Pathol.* 1998;110:615–621.

Chow E, Macrae F. A review of juvenile polyposis syndrome. *J Gastroenterol Hepatol.* 2005;20:1634–1640.

Giardiello FM, Brensinger JD, Tersmette AC, et al. Very high risk of cancer in familial Peutz-Jeghers syndrome. *Gastroenterology.* 2000;119;1447–1453.

Hizawa K, Iida M, Yao T, et al. Juvenile polyposis of the stomach: clinicopathologic features and its malignant potential. *J Clin Pathol.* 1997;50:771–774.

Lam-Himlin D, Park JY, Cornish TC, et al. Morphologic characterization of syndromic gastric polyps. *Am J Surg Pathol.* 2010;34:1656–1662.

Latchford AR, Neale K, Phillips RK, Clark SK. Juvenile polyposis syndrome: a study of genotype, phenotype, and long-term outcome. *Dis Colon Rectum.* 2012;55(10):1038–1043.

Ma C, Giardiello FM, Montgomery EA. Upper tract juvenile polyps in juvenile polyposis patients: dysplasia and malignancy are associated with foveolar, intestinal, and pyloric differentiation. *Am J Surg Pathol.* 2014;38(12):1618–1626.

McAllister AJ, Richards KF. Peutz-Jeghers syndrome: experience with twenty patients in five generations. *Am J Surg*. 1977;134:717–720.

Odze RD, Marcial MA, Antonioli D. Gastric fundic gland polyps: a morphological study including mucin histochemistry, stereometry, and MIB-1 immunohistochemistry. *Hum Pathol*. 1996;27:896–903.

Pintiliciuc OG, Heresbach D, de-Lajarte-Thirouard AS, et al. Gastric involvement in juvenile polyposis associated with germline SMAD4 mutations: an entity characterized by a mixed hypertrophic and polypoid gastropathy. *Gastroenterol Clin Biol*. 2008;32 (5 Pt 1): 445–450.

Swwetser S, Ahlquist DA, Osborn NK, et al. Clinicopathologic features and treatment outcomes in Crokhite-Canada syndrome: support for autoimmunity. *Dig Dis Sci*. 2012;57:496–502.

Torbenson M, Lee HH, Cruz-Correa M, et al. Sporadic fundic gland polyposis: a clinical, histological, and molecular analysis. *Mod Pathol*. 2002;15:718–723.

Van Lier MG, Wagner A, Mathus-Vliegen EM, et al. High cancer risk in Peutz-Jeghers syndrome: a systematic review and surveillance recommendations. *Am J Gastroenterol*. 2010;105:1258–1264.

Zacharin M, Bajpai A, Chow CW, et al. Gastrointestinal polyps in McCune Albright syndrome. *J Med Genet*. 2011;48:458–461.

Zelter A, Fernandez JL, Bilder C, et al. Fundic gland polyps and association with proton pump inhibitor intake: a prospective study in 1780 endoscopies. *Dig Dis Sci*. 2011;56:1743–1748.

Gastric Adenomas and Flat Dysplasia

Abraham Sc, Montgomery EA, Singh VK, et al. Gastric adenomas: intestinal-type and gastric-type adenomas differ in the risk of adenocarcinoma and presence of background mucosal pathology. *Am J Surg Pathol*. 2002;26:1276–1285.

Baek DH, Kim GH, park do Y, et al. Gastric epithelial dysplasia: characteristics and long-term follow-up results after endoscopic resection according to morphological categorization. *BMC Gastroenterol*. 2015;15:249.

Bearzi I, Brancorsini D, Santinelli A, et al. Gastric dysplasia: a ten-year follow up study. *Pathol Res Pract*. 1994;190:61–68.

Everett SM, Axon AT. Early gastric cancer in Europe. *Gut*. 1997;41:142–150.

Farinati F, Rugge M, Di Mario F, et al. Early and advanced gastric cancer in the follow up of moderate and severe gastric dysplasia patients. A prospective study. I.G.G.E.D. Interdisciplinary Group on Gastric Epithelial Dysplasia. *Endoscopy*. 1993;25:261–264.

Jang JS, Choi SR, Qureshi W, et al. Long-term outcomes of endoscopic submucosal dissection in gastric neoplastic lesions at a single institution in South Korea. *Scand J Gastroenterol*. 2009;44:1315–1322.

Lauwers GY. Defining the pathology diagnosis of metaplasia, atrophy, dysplasia, and gastric adenocarcinoma. *J Clin Gastroenterol*. 2003;36:S37–S43.

Park DY, Srivastava A, Kim GH, et al. Adenomatous and foveolar gastric dysplasia: distinct patterns of mucin expression and background intestinal metaplasia. *Am J Surg Pathol*. 2008;32:524–533.

Rugge M, Capelle LG, Cappellesso R, et al. Precancerous lesions in the stomach: from biology to clinical patient management. *Best Practice Res Clin Gastroenterol*. 2013;27:205–223.

Salirao U, Lauwers GY, Vieth M, et al. Gastric high grade dysplasia can be associated with submucosal invasion: evaluation of its prevalence in a series of 121 endoscopically resected specimens. *Am J Surg Pathol*. 2014;38:1545–1550.

Schlemper RJ, Hirata I, Dixon MF. The macroscopic classification of early neoplasia of the digestive tract. *Endoscopy*. 2002;34:163–168.

Schlemper RJ, Riddell RH, Kato Y, et al. The Vienna classification of gastrointestinal epithelial neoplasia. *Gut*. 2000;47:251–255.

Yamada H, Ikegami M, Shimoda T, et al. Long term follow-up study of gastric adenoma/dysplasia. *Endoscopy*. 2004;36:390–396.

You WC, Zhang L, Chang YS, et al. Gastric dysplasia and gastric cancer: Helicobacter pylori, serum vitamin C, and other risk factors. *J Natl Cancer Inst*. 2000;92:1607–1612.

Pyloric Gland Adenoma

Chen ZM, Scudiere JR, Abraham SC, Montgomery E. Pyloric gland adenoma. An entity distinct from gastric foveolar type adenoma. *Am J Surg Pathol*. 2009;33:186–193.

Kushima R, Ruthlein HJ, Stolte M, et al. Pyloric gland-type adenoma arising in heterotopic gastric mucosa of the duodenum with dysplastic progression of the gastric type. *Virchows Arch*. 1999;435:452–457.

Vieth M, Kushima R, Borchard F, Stolte M. Pyloric gland adenoma: a clinicopathological analysis of 90 cases. *Virchows Arch*. 2003;442:317–321.

Vieth M, Montgomery EA. Some observations on pyloric gland adenoma: an uncommon and long ignored entity! *J Clin Pathol*. 2014;67:883–890.

Oxyntic Gland Polyp/Adenoma

Singhi AD, Lazenby AJ, Montgomery EA. Gastric adenocarcinoma with chief cell differentiation: a proposal for reclassification as oxyntic gland polyp/adenoma. *Am J Surg Pathol*. 2012;36:1030–1035.

Ueyama H, Yao T, Nakashima Y, et al. Gastric adenocarcinoma of fundic gland type (chief cell predominant type): proposal for a new entity of gastric adenocarcinoma. *Am J Surg Pathol*. 2010;34:609–619.

Adenocarcinoma

Blot WJ, Devesa SS, Kneller RW, et al. Rising incidence of adenocarcinoma of the esophagus and gastric cardia. *JAMA*. 1991;265:1287–1289.

Bunt AM, Hermans J, Smit VT, et al. Surgical /pathologic-stage migration confounds comparisons of gastric cancer survival rates between Japan and Western countries. *J Clin Oncol*. 1995;13:19–25.

Campoli PM, Ejima FH, Cardoso DM, et al. Metastatic cancer to the stomach. *Gastric Cancer*. 2006;9:19–25.

Cunningham SC, Kamangar F, Kim MP, et al. Survival after gastric adenocarcinoma resection: eighteen year experience at a single institution. *J Gastrointest Surg*. 2005;9:718–725.

Dhingra S, Wang H. Nonneoplastic signet-ring cell change in gastrointestinal and biliary tracts: a pitfall for overdiagnosis. *Ann Diagn Pathol*. 2011;15:490–496,.

Eckardt VF, Giessler W, Kanzler G, et al. Clinical and morphological characteristics of early gastric cancer: a case-control study. *Gastroenterol*. 1990;98:708–714.

Esaki Y, Hirayama R, Hirokawa K. A comparison of patterns of metastasis in gastric cancer by histologic type and age. *Cancer*. 1990;65:2086–2090.

Goseki N, Takizawa T, Koike M. Differences in the mode of the extension of gastric cancer classified by histological type: new histological classification of gastric carcinoma. *Gut*. 1991;33:606–612.

Green LK. Hematogenous metastases to the stomach: a review of 67 cases. *Cancer*. 1990;65:1596–1600.

Huang KH, Want RF, Yang MH, et al. Advanced gastric cancer patients with lymphoid stroma have better survival than those without. *J Surg Oncol*. 2013;107:523–528.

Hughes C, Greywoode G, Chetty R. Gastric pseudo-signet ring cells: a potential diagnostic pitfall. *Virchows Arch*. 2011;459:347–349.

Hundahl SA, Phillips JL, Menck HR. The National Cancer Data Base Report on poor survival of U.S. gastric carcinoma patients treated with gastrectomy: Fifth Edition American Joint Committee on Cancer staging, proximal disease, and the "different disease" hypothesis. *Cancer*. 2000;88:921–932.

Ishikura H, Kirimoto K, Shamoto M, et al.: Hepatoid adenocarcinomas of the stomach: an analysis of seven cases. *Cancer*. 1986;58:119–126.

Lauren P. The two histological main types of gastric carcinoma: diffuse and so-called intestinal-type carcinoma-an attempt at a histo-clinical classification. *Acta Pathol Microbiol Scand.* 1965;64:31–49.

Lee SJ, Sohn TS, Lee J, et al. Adjuvant chemoradiation with 5-fluoro-uracil/leucovorin versus S-1 in gastric cancer patients following D2 lymph node dissection surgery: a feasibility study. *Anticancer Res.* 2014;34:6585–6591.

Maehara Y, Orita H, Okuyama T, et al. Predictors of lymph node metastasis in early gastric cancer. *Br J Surg.* 1992;79:245–247.

Meng XM, Zhou Y, Dang T, et al. Magnifying chromoendoscopy combined with immunohistochemical staining for early diagnosis of gastric cancer. *World J Gastroenterol.* 2013;19:404–410.

Mezhir JJ, Gonen M, Ammori JB, et al. Treatment and outcome of patients with gastric remnant cancer after resection for peptic ulcer disease. *Ann Surg Oncol.* 2011;18:670–676.

Mori M, Iwashita A, Enjoji M. Adenosquamous carcinoma of the stomach: a clinicopathologic analysis of 28 cases. *Cancer.* 1986;57:333–339.

Motoyama T, Aizawa K, Watanabe H, et al. α-Fetoprotein producing gastric carcinomas: a comparative study of three different subtypes. *Acta Pathol Jpn.* 1993;43:654–661.

Noda M, Kodama T, Atsumi M, et al. Possibilities and limitations of endoscopic resection for early gastric cancer. *Endoscopy.* 1997;29:361–365.

O'Connell FP, Wang HH, Odze RD, et al. Utility of immunohistochemistry in distinguishing primary adenocarcinomas from metastatic breast carcinomas in the gastrointestinal tract. *Arch Pathol Lab Med.* 2005;129:338–347.

Oda I, Kondo H, Yamao T, et al. Metastatic tumors to the stomach: analysis of 54 patients diagnosed at endoscopy and 347 autopsy cases. *Endoscopy.* 2001;33:507–510.

Okabayashi T, Gotoda T, Kondo H, et al. Early carcinoma of the gastric cardia in Japan: is it different from that in the West? *Cancer.* 2000;89:2555–2559.

Osada M, Aishima S, Hirahashi M, et al. Combination of hepatocellular markers is useful for prognostication in gastric hepatoid adenocarcinoma. *Hum Pathol.* 2014;45:1243–1250.

Saigo PE, Brigati DJ, Sternberg SS, et al. Primary gastric choriocarcinoma: an immunohistological study. *Am J Surg Pathol.* 1981;5:333–342.

Suan ZX, Ueyama T, Yao T, Tsuneyoshi M. Time trends of early gastric carcinoma. A clinicopathologic analysis of 2846 cases. *Cancer.* 1993;72:2889–2894.

Tamura W, Fukami N. Early gastric cancer and dysplasia. *Gastrointestinal Endoscopy Clin N Amer.* 2013;23:77–94.

Wang HH, Wu MS, Shun Ct, et al. Lymphoepithelioma-like carcinoma of the stomach: a subset of gastric carcinoma with distinct clinicopathological features and high prevalence of Epstein-Barr infection. *Hepatogastroenterology.* 1999;46:1214–1219.

Wang K, Weinrach D, Lal A, et al. Signet-ring cell change versus signet-ring cell carcinoma: a comparative analysis. *Am J Surg Pathol.* 2003;27:1429–1433.

Yakirevich E, Resnick MB. Pathology of gastric cancer and its precursor lesions. *Gastroenterol Clin North Am.* 2013;42:261–284.

Yasuda K, Adachi y, Shiraishi N, et al. Papillary adenocarcinoma of the stomach. *Gastric Cancer.* 2000;3:33–38.

Yasuda K, Shiraishi N, Suematsu T, et al. Rate of detection of lymph node metastasis is correlated with the depth of submucosal invasion in early stage gastric carcinoma. *Cancer.* 1999;85:2119–2123.

Ye MF, Tao F, Liu F, Sun AJ. Hepatoid adenocarcinoma of the stomach: a report of three cases. *World J Gastroenterol.* 2013;19:4437–4492.

Hereditary Diffuse Gastric Cancer

Fitzgerald RC, Hardwick R, Huntsman D, et al. Hereditary diffuse gastric cancer: updated consensus guidelines for clinical management and directions for future research. *J Med Genet.* 2010; 47:436–444.

Gayther SA, Gorringe KL, Ramus SJ, et al. Identification of germ-line E-cadherin mutations in gastric cancer families of European origin. *Cancer Res.* 1998;58:4086–4089.

Hebbard PC, Macmillan A, Huntsman D, et al. Prophylactic total gastrectomy (PTG) for hereditary diffuse gastric cancer (HDGC): the Newfoundland experience with 23 patients. *Ann Surg Oncol.* 2009;16:1890–1895.

Kaurah P, MacMillan A, Boyd N, et al. Founder and recurrent CDH1 mutations in families with hereditary diffuse gastric cancer. *JAMA.* 2007; 297:2360.

Oliveira C, Moreira H, Seruca R, et al. Role of pathology in the identification of hereditary diffuse gastric cancer: report of a Portuguese family. *Virchows Arch.* 2005;446:181–184.

Pharoah PD, Guilford P, Caldas C, International Gastric Cancer Linkage Consortium. Incidence of gastric cancer and breast cancer in CDH1 (E-cadherin) mutation carriers from hereditary diffuse gastric cancer families. *Gastroenterology.* 2001;121:1348–1353.

Neuroendocrine Neoplasms (See Also Chapter 3)

Bordi C, Yu JY, Baggi MT, et al. Gastric carcinoids and their precursor lesions. A histologic and immunohistochemical study of 23 cases. *Cancer.* 1991;67(3):663–672.

Bordi C. Gastric carcinoids: an immunohistochemical and clinicopathologic study of 104 patients. *Cancer.* 1995;75(1):129–130.

Bordi C. Neuroendocrine pathology of the stomach: the Parma contribution. *Endocr Pathol.* 2014;25:171–180.

Ishida M, Sekine S, Fukagawa T, et al. Neuroendocrine carcinoma of the stomach: morphologic and immunohistochemical characteristics and prognosis. *Am J Surg Pathol.* 2013;37:949–959.

La Rosa S, Inzani F, Vanoli A, et al. Histologic characterization and improved prognostic evaluation of 209 gastric neuroendocrine neoplasms. *Hum Pathol.* 2011;42(10):1373–1384.

Rindi G, Bordi C, Rappel S, et al. Gastric carcinoids and neuroendocrine carcinomas: pathogenesis, pathology, and behavior. *World J Surg.* 1996;20(2):168–172.

Thomas RM, Baybick JH, Elsayed AM, Sobin LH. Gastric carcinoids. An immunohistochemical and clinicopathologic study of 104 patients. *Cancer.* 1994;73(8):2053–2058.

Yao JC, Hassan M, Phan A, et al. One hundred years after "carcinoid:" epidemiology of and prognostic factors for neuroendocrine tumors in 35,825 cases in the United States. *J Clin Oncol.* 2008;26:3063–3072.

Mesenchymal Neoplasms (See Also Chapter 5)

Doyle LA, Nelson D, Heinrich MC, et al. Loss of succinate dehydrogenase subunit B (SDHB) expression is limited to a distinctive subset of gastric wild-type gastrointestinal stromal tumors: a comprehensive genotype-phenotype correlation study. *Histopathol.* 2012;61:801–809.

Kang G, Park HJ, Kim JY, et al. Glomus tumor of the stomach: a clinicopathologic analysis of 10 cases and review of the literature. *Gut Liver.* 2012;6:52–57.

Lasota J, Dansonka-Mieszkowska A, Sobin LH, Miettinen M. A great majority of GISTs with PDGFRA mutations represent gastric tumors of low or no malignant potential. *Lab Invest.* 2004;84:874–883.

Liu TC, Lin MT, Montgomery EA, Singhi AD. Inflammatory fibroid polyps of the gastrointestinal tract: spectrum of clinical, morphologic, and immunohistochemistry features. *Am J Surg Pathol.* 2013;37(4):586–592.

Miettinen M, Makhlouf HR, Sobin LH, Lasota J. Plexiform fibromyxoma: a distinctive benign gastric antral neoplasm not to be confused with a myxoid GIST. *Am J Surg Pathol.* 2009;33:1624–1632.

Miettinen M, Sobin LH, Lasota J, et al. Gastrointestinal stromal tumors of the stomach. A clinicopathologic, immunohistochemical, and molecular genetic study of 1765 cases with long term follow up. *Am J Surg Pathol.* 2005;29:52–68.

Miettinen M, Want ZF, Sarloma-Rikala M, et al. Succinate dehydrogenase-deficient GISTs: a clinicopathologic, immunohistochemical, and molecular genetic study of 66 gastric GISTs with predilection to young age. *Am J Surg Pathol.* 2011;35:1712–1721.

Ozolek JA, Sasatomi E, Swalsky PA, et al. Inflammatory fibroid polyps of the gastrointestinal tract: clinical, pathologic, and molecular characteristics. *Appl Immunohistochem Mol Morphol.*
2004;12:59–66.

Takahashi Y, Shimizu S, Ishida T, et al. Plexiform angiomyx-
oid myofibroblastic tumor of the stomach. *Am J Surg Pathol.*
2007;31:724–728.

Voltaggio L, Murray R, Lasota J, Miettinen M. Gastric schwannoma: a
clinicopathologic study of 51 cases and critical review of the literature. *Hum Pathol.* 2012;43:650–659.

Hematolymphoid Neoplasms

Burke JS. Lymphoproliferative disorders of the gastrointestinal tract: a
review and pragmatic guide to diagnosis. *Arch Pathol Lab Med.*
2011;135:1283–1297.

Fischbach W. Gastric MALT lymphoma – update on diagnosis and treatment. *Best Pract Res Clin Gastroenterol.* 2014;28:1069–1077.

Kuo SH, Yeh KH, Wu MS, et al. Helicobacter pylori eradication therapy
is effective in the treatment of early-stage H. pylori-positive gastric
diffuse large B-cell lymphomas. *Blood.* 2012;119:4838–4844.

O'Malley DP, Goldstein NS, Banks PM. The recognition and classification of lymphoproliferative disorders of the gut. *Hum Pathol.*
2014;45:899–916.

Owens SR, Smith LB. Molecular aspects of H. pylori-related
MALT lymphoma. *Patholog Res Int.* 2011;2011:193149. doi:
10.4061/2011/193149

Sehn LH, Gascoyne RD. Diffuse large B-cell lymphoma: optimizing outcome in the context of clinical and biologic heterogeneity.
Blood. 2015;125:22–32.

Smith LB, Owens SR. Gastrointestinal lymphomas: entities and mimics.
Arch Pathol Lab Med. 2012;136:865–870.

9

Neoplasms of the Small Intestine

WEI CHEN, SCOTT R. OWENS, AND WENDY L. FRANKEL

INTRODUCTION

The small intestine represents 75% of the length and greater than 90% of the surface area of the gastrointestinal (GI) tract. Despite its length, large surface area, and higher rate of cellular turnover, primary small intestinal tumors are rare, estimated at 40 to 60 times less common than colonic neoplasms, and account for only 3% of GI neoplasms overall. Rapid transit time of the luminal liquid content, lower bacterial load, and detoxification effects of mucosal enzymes are all believed to contribute to decreased production of and/or exposure to carcinogens. The abundant immunoglobulin A (IgA) and lymphoid tissue in the small bowel also enhances immunosurveillance for tumor.

There are four major histologic categories of primary small intestinal malignancies: adenocarcinomas, neuroendocrine tumors (NETs), mesenchymal tumors, and lymphomas (Table 9.1). Epidemiologic studies have shown an increased incidence of all types between 1985 and 2005, with a more than four-fold increase in the incidence of NETs. In fact, in the year 2000, NETs surpassed adenocarcinoma as the most common type of primary small intestinal tumor reported to the National Cancer Data Base. The World Health Organization (WHO) 2010 classification of small intestinal tumors is shown in Table 9.2.

INFLAMMATORY AND NON-NEOPLASTIC LESIONS

Inflammatory lesions can present as polypoid masses, and thus lead to endoscopic biopsies or polypectomies. Several inflammatory and non-neoplastic entities enter into the differential diagnosis of dysplasia and malignancy in the small bowel, and thus will be briefly discussed here.

Peptic duodenitis often appears nodular or erythematous at endoscopy; common histologic findings include reactive epithelial changes, gastric surface cell metaplasia, and increased chronic (and sometimes acute) inflammation in the lamina propria (Figure 9.1A–C). Reactive epithelium with foveolar metaplasia in nodular peptic duodenitis can at times mimic dysplasia. Although many duodenal adenomas do have gastric surface cell metaplasia, adenomas are more likely to be sharply delineated from adjacent normal mucosa than reactive lesions (Figure 9.2A–B). Brunner gland hyperplasia is another common lesion that often presents as a polypoid mass (Figure 9.3A–B).

In the small bowel, gastric heterotopias most commonly occur in the duodenal bulb and in Meckel's diverticulum. These congenital rests are benign, non-neoplastic lesions composed of ectopic gastric mucosa containing both foveolar epithelium and oxyntic glands (Figure 9.4A–B). Heterotopic gastric tissue should be distinguished from foveolar cell metaplasia of the duodenal mucosa, which is typically secondary to peptic injury, Crohn disease, or *Helicobacter pylori* infection.

Pancreatic heterotopia (Figure 9.5A–B) occurs most often in the distal stomach and proximal small bowel, and is also common in Meckel's diverticulum. Heterotopic pancreas can be either mucosal or mural, with the latter often causing more significant clinical symptoms such as abdominal pain, stricture, intussusception, or bleeding. One-third of pancreatic heterotopia cases contain pancreatic islets, in addition to lobules of pancreatic acini and ductules.

Inflammatory pseudopolyps can be sporadic, or associated with inflammatory bowel disease, and may mimic a neoplastic process endoscopically. Histologic examination reveals polypoid granulation tissue with inflammation, edema, and fibrosis, and there may be florid reactive epithelial changes (Figure 9.6).

TABLE 9.1   Clinicopathologic Characteristics of Primary Small Intestinal Malignancies

	Neuroendocrine Tumor	Adenocarcinoma	Lymphoma	Mesenchymal Tumor
Relative Incidence (%)	37.3	36.9	17.3	8.4
Age (median, years)	66	67	66	64
Gender (male: female)	1.1:1	1.1:1	1.4:1	1.1:1
Size (median, cm)	1.6	4.0	NA	7.5
Most common site	Jejunum	Duodenum	Any site	Any site

Source: Data adapted from Bilimoria et al. Small bowel cancer in the United States: changes in epidemiology, treatment, and survival over the last 20 years. *Ann Surg.* 2009;249:63–71.

TABLE 9.2   WHO 2010 Classification of Tumors of the Small Intestine

Epithelial Tumors
  Premalignant Lesions
   Adenoma
    Tubular
    Villous
    Tubulovillous
   Dysplasia (intraepithelial neoplasia)
    Low grade
    High grade
  Hamartomas
   Juvenile polyp
   Peutz–Jeghers polyp
  Carcinoma
   Adenocarcinoma
    Mucinous adenocarcinoma (>50% mucinous)
    Signet ring cell carcinoma (>50% signet ring cells)
   Adenosquamous carcinoma
   Medullary carcinoma
   Squamous cell carcinoma
   Undifferentiated carcinoma
  Neuroendocrine Neoplasms
   Neuroendocrine tumor (NET)
    NET G1 (carcinoid)
    NET G2
   Neuroendocrine carcinoma (NEC)
    Large cell NEC
    Small cell NEC
   Mixed adenoneuroendocrine carcinoma (MANEC)
   Enterochromaffin (EC) cell, serotonin-producing NET
   Gangliocytic paraganglioma
   Gastrinoma
   L cell, glucagon-like peptide-producing and PP/PYY-producing NETs
   Somatostatin-producing NET
Mesenchymal Tumors
  Leiomyoma
  Lipoma
  Angiosarcoma
  Gastrointestinal stromal tumor
  Kaposi sarcoma
  Leiomyosarcoma
Lymphomas
Secondary Tumors

Source: Data adapted from Bosman F, Carneiro F, Hruban R, et al (Eds.) Chapter 6, Tumours of the small intestine. In *World Health Organization classification of tumours of the digestive system.* 4th ed. Lyon, France:IARC Press; 2010.

HAMARTOMATOUS POLYPS

Several types of hamartomatous polyps occur in the small bowel; these are also discussed in detail in Chapter 6. Peutz–Jeghers polyps can occur sporadically or as part of Peutz–Jeghers syndrome (PJS). PJS is an inherited syndrome characterized by a germline mutation of the tumor suppressor gene *STK11/LKB1*. The polyps preferentially affect the small intestine (most frequently the jejunum, followed by the ileum and duodenum), and patients typically have mucocutaneous melanocytic pigmentation. When compared to the general population, PJS patients have a very high relative risk (RR = 520) for the development of small intestinal adenocarcinoma. Histologically, Peutz–Jeghers polyps show papillary architecture with arborizing bundles of smooth muscle that separate the epithelial components into lobules (Figure 9.7A–B). Dysplasia may occur within these polyps (Figure 9.7C–D), and misplacement of both non-neoplastic and dysplastic epithelium is common in pedunculated polyps. Displacement of dysplastic epithelium may mimic invasive cancer, but the identification of smooth muscle bundles around the displaced epithelium, as opposed to a stromal desmoplastic reaction, can help distinguish misplaced glands from invasive adenocarcinoma (Figure 9.7E).

Juvenile polyps may also be either sporadic or syndromic. Sporadic juvenile polyps are restricted to the colorectum, and have no associated cancer risk. Juvenile polyposis syndrome (JPS) is characterized by a germline mutation in the *SMAD4* or *BMPR1A* gene, and multiple juvenile polyps in the GI tract. These polyps are most commonly found in the colorectum, but can be found throughout the upper and lower GI tract as well. JPS patients have a 68% risk of developing colorectal cancer by 60 years of age, with a mean age at diagnosis of 35 years. There is also increased risk for small intestinal, gastric, and possibly pancreatic cancers. Histologically, juvenile polyps show cystically dilated glands embedded in abundant loose, edematous and inflamed stroma (Figure 9.8A–B). Surface ulceration and mucin extravasation from ruptured cysts may be present as well. Syndromic juvenile polyps may give rise to foci of dysplasia (Figure 9.8C–D) and carcinoma, but these findings are very uncommon in sporadic juvenile polyps.

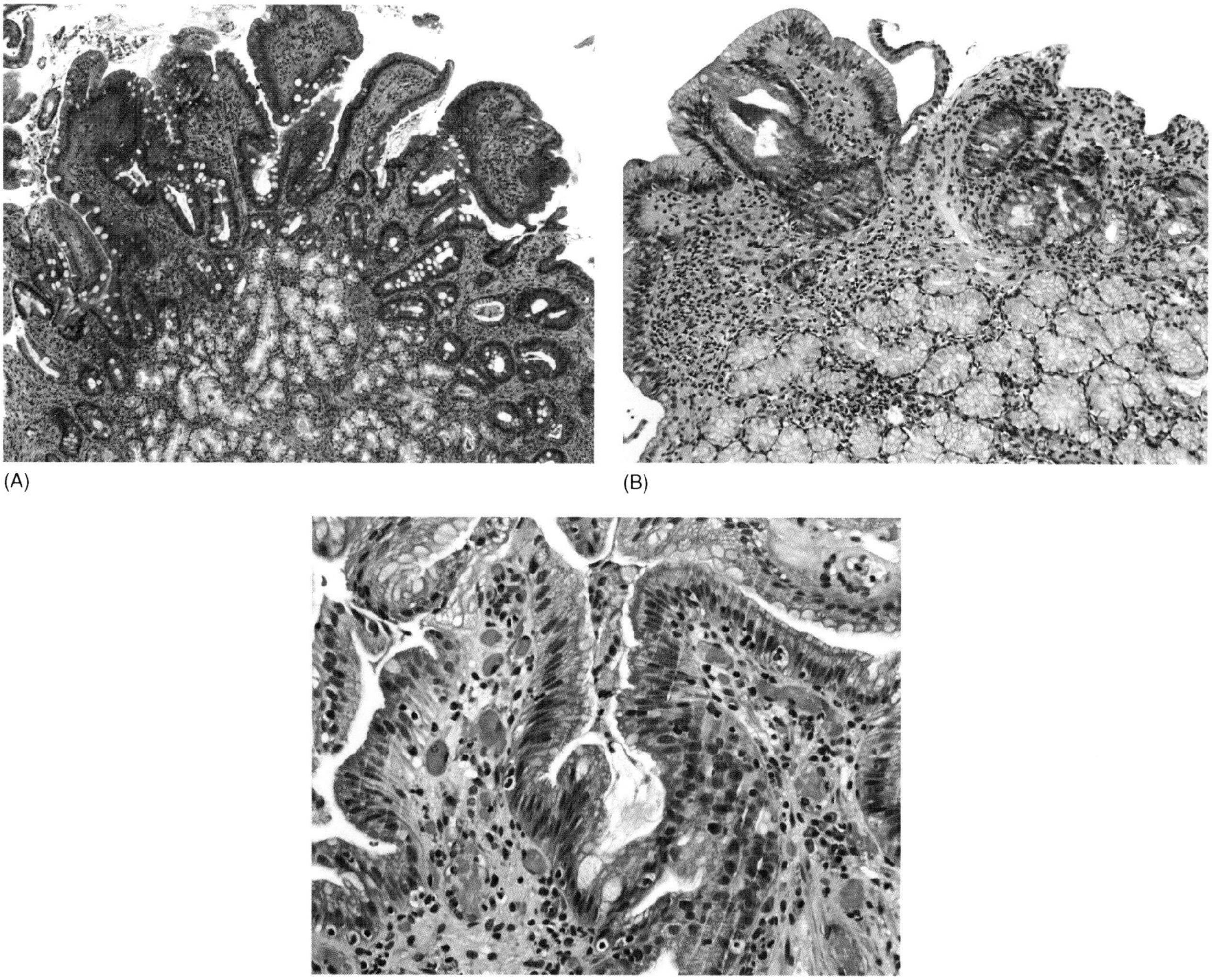

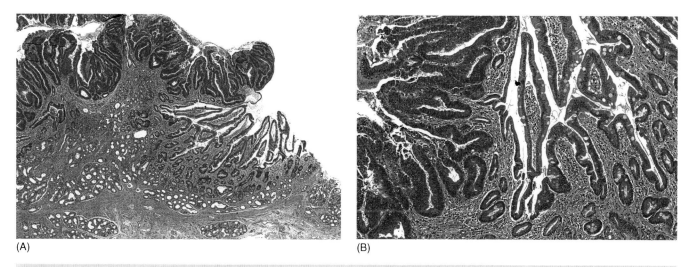

(A)

(B)

(C)

FIGURE 9.1 Nodular peptic duodenitis features Brunner gland hyperplasia, surface gastric metaplasia, acute and chronic inflammation, and reactive epithelial changes (A–B). Reactive surface gastric cell metaplasia may occasionally mimic dysplasia, but the well-developed apical mucin is a clue that this is a reactive, metaplastic change rather than dysplasia (C).

(A)

(B)

FIGURE 9.2 Small bowel adenomas are typically sharply demarcated from the surrounding mucosa, unlike reactive epithelial changes. The adenomatous epithelium on the left abruptly transitions to normal mucosa on the right (A–B).

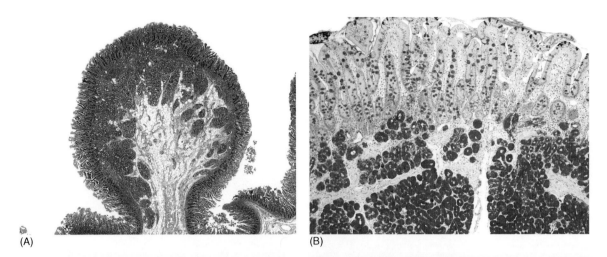

(A)

(B)

FIGURE 9.3 Brunner gland hyperplasia can form a polypoid mass in the duodenum (A). Alcian blue/periodic acid–Schiff stain (B) highlights the goblet cells in the epithelium (blue) and Brunner glands in the submucosa and deep mucosa (magenta).

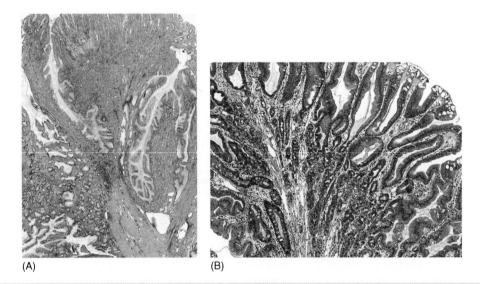

(A)

(B)

FIGURE 9.4 Heterotopic gastric tissue in the small bowel occasionally forms polypoid masses (A). At higher power, the heterotopic tissue is composed of parietal and chief cells (B) admixed with the small bowel mucosa.

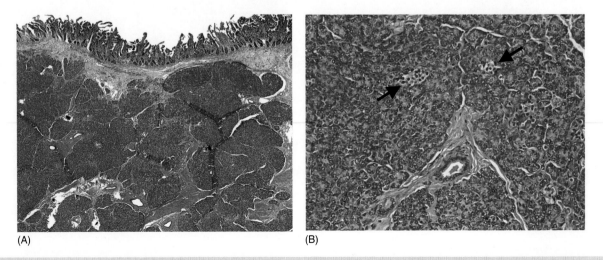

(A)

(B)

FIGURE 9.5 Heterotopic pancreas in the submucosa of the small intestine is composed of a variable mixture of benign pancreatic acini, islets, and ductules (A–B, arrows denoting small islets).

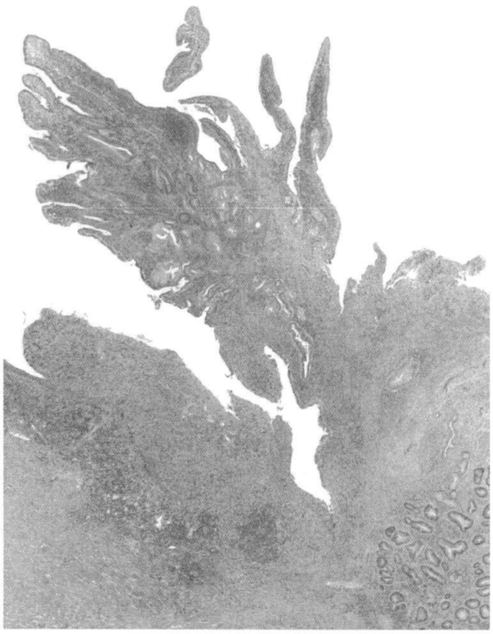

ADENOMATOUS POLYPS

Small intestinal adenomas are polypoid growths of dysplastic epithelium that are most often (80%) found near the ampulla/papilla of Vater or in the second portion of the duodenum. They may be incidental findings, or they can cause clinical signs and symptoms including GI bleeding, abdominal pain, intussusception, or jaundice, particularly if located at the ampulla. Treatment options for small bowel adenomas include endoscopic polypectomy for pedunculated polyps, endoscopic mucosal or surgical resection for large sessile lesions, and Whipple surgery for large periampullary lesions.

Most small intestinal adenomas resemble colonic adenomas both macroscopically and microscopically. One unique feature of small intestinal adenomas is that many of them show gastric surface cell metaplasia, creating the illusion of surface maturation and thus mimicking a reactive process (Figure 9.9A). Small bowel adenomas tend to have a more villous or tubulovillous pattern (Figure 9.9B–C), as compared to the predominantly tubular pattern seen in colonic adenomas. Goblet cells are prevalent in small bowel adenomas as well, and occasional Paneth cells and endocrine cells may also be seen. As with colonic adenomas, dysplasia in small bowel adenomas is classified

FIGURE 9.6   An ileal inflammatory pseudopolyp from a patient with Crohn disease, showing a polypoid projection of disordered mucosa protruding above the surrounding ulcerated mucosa.

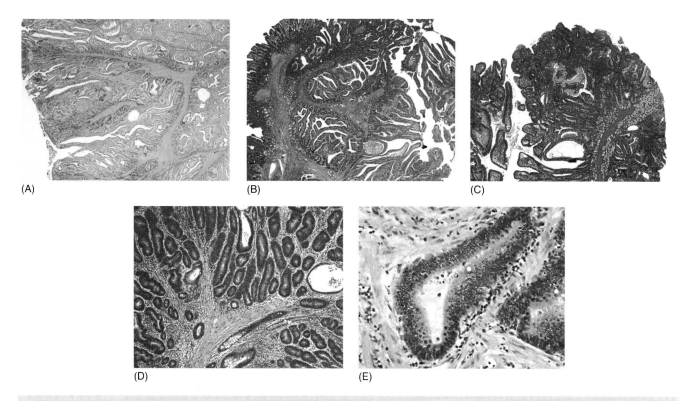

(A)   (B)   (C)

(D)   (E)

FIGURE 9.7   A Peutz–Jeghers polyp of the duodenum features lobules of glandular epithelium separated by complex, arborizing bundles of smooth muscle (A–B). Peutz–Jeghers polyps may contain foci of dysplasia, as in this example with low-grade dysplasia at the surface (C). Note the arborizing muscle fibers that surround the dysplastic glands (D). Epithelial misplacement may pose a diagnostic problem in Peutz–Jeghers polyps, as noted here where dysplastic glands are misplaced within the bundles of smooth muscle in the stalk, mimicking invasive cancer (E). However, muscle bundles surround both the dysplastic glands and the nondysplastic glands, and there is no desmoplasia (B–E, courtesy of Dr. Samir Kahwash).

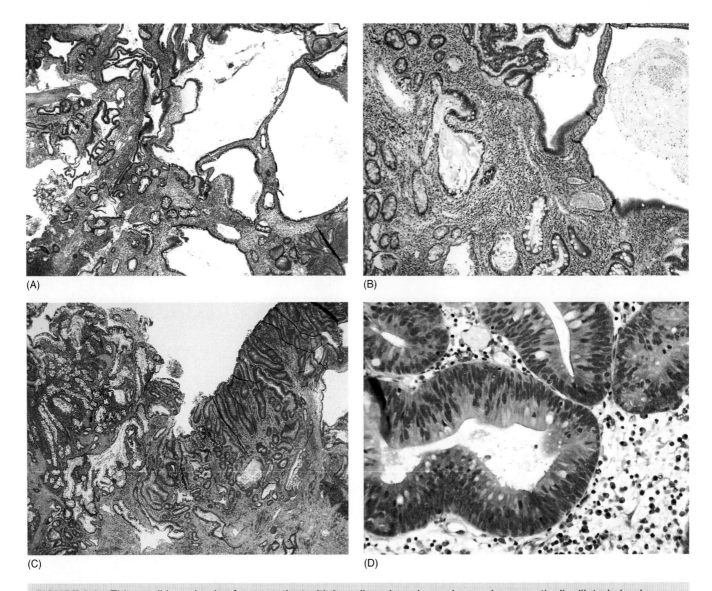

FIGURE 9.8 This small bowel polyp from a patient with juvenile polyposis syndrome shows cystically dilated glands embedded in abundant loose, edematous, and inflamed stroma (A–B). Some glands are filled with mucin and inflammatory debris. Dysplasia can be seen in syndromic juvenile polyps (C–D). In (C), notice the demarcation between the non-dysplastic (left) and dysplastic (right) areas.

as either low or high grade. The risk of progression to adenocarcinomas in adenomas (Figure 9.9D–F) increases with increasing polyp size, with the presence of high-grade dysplasia, and with increasing percentage of villous architecture in the polyp.

Several hereditary cancer syndromes are associated with small bowel adenomas, most notably familial adenomatous polyposis (FAP) and Lynch syndrome (see also Chapter 6). FAP is an autosomal dominant disorder caused by a germline mutation of the adenomatous polyposis coli (*APC*) gene on chromosome 5q21. The lifetime risk for FAP patients to develop duodenal adenomas and small bowel adenocarcinoma is estimated at nearly 100% and 5%, respectively. Periampullary adenomas appear to have a high risk of malignant transformation.

Patients with Lynch syndrome have a 4% lifetime risk of developing small bowel adenocarcinoma, which is 100 times greater than the risk in the general population. MUTYH-associated polyposis is associated with an increased risk for the development of duodenal adenomas and adenocarcinomas as well.

ADENOCARCINOMA

Epidemiology

Primary small bowel adenocarcinoma is rare, with only approximately 3,000 cases diagnosed per year. This is a 50-fold lower incidence than colorectal adenocarcinoma,

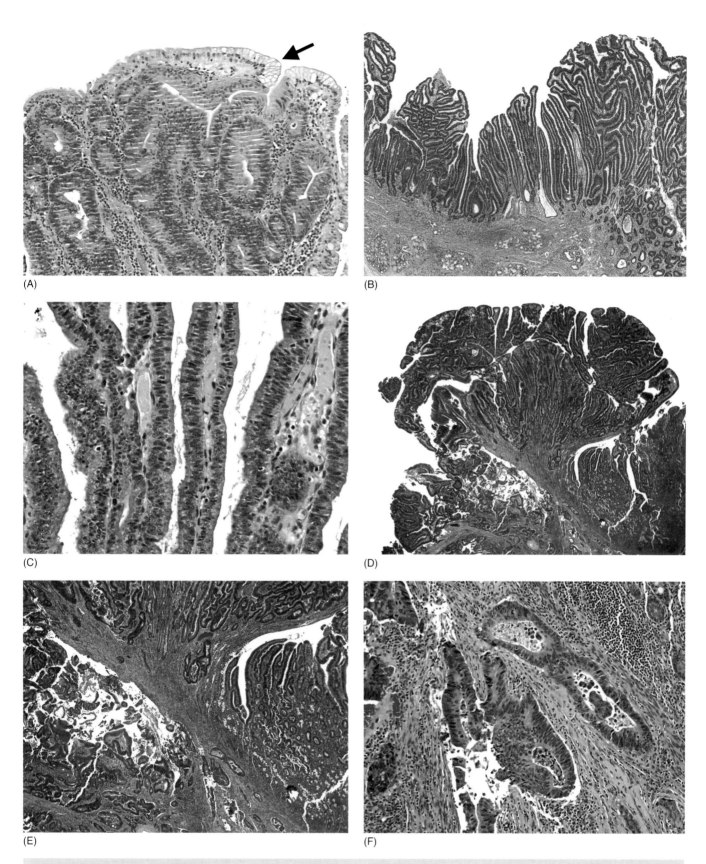

FIGURE 9.9 Small bowel adenomas are in some cases similar to their colonic counterparts (A), but often have a more prominent villous component (B–C). Note the gastric surface cell metaplasia in this duodenal adenoma as well (A, arrow). This jejunal adenoma has a focus of invasive adenocarcinoma in the stalk (D–E). Higher power shows infiltrating irregular glands with associated desmoplasia (F).

despite the fact that the small intestine represents 75% of the length and 90% of the surface area of the alimentary tract.

The mechanisms of carcinogenesis are less well-defined in the small intestine than in the large intestine. The adenoma–adenocarcinoma sequence is assumed to be similar, however, and 80% of duodenal adenocarcinomas have an associated adenomatous component. Patients with polyposis syndromes, such as FAP, Lynch syndrome, PJS, JPS, and PTEN hamartoma tumor syndrome (PHTS), have increased risk of small bowel malignancies. Chronic inflammation is another major risk factor associated with the development of small bowel adenocarcinoma, as demonstrated by the increased incidence of small intestinal adenocarcinoma in patients with Crohn disease, celiac disease, and ileostomies. Other risk factors for small bowel adenocarcinoma include cigarette smoking, alcohol consumption, and toxin exposure to 7,12-dimethylbenz-anthracene (DMBA) and benzopyrene. A summary of diseases associated with the development of small bowel adenocarcinoma is given in Table 9.3.

Small bowel adenocarcinoma occasionally arises in the background of restorative proctocolectomy with ileal pouch. When the small bowel mucosa in ileal pouches adapts to its role as a reservoir, the mucosa often undergoes villous atrophy, and pouchitis may develop. Dysplasia and adenocarcinoma can occur in this background of chronic inflammation, but this is a very rare occurrence.

Additionally, adenocarcinomas rarely arise in heterotopic tissues in the small bowel, such as heterotopic pancreas and Meckel's diverticulum.

Clinical and Prognostic Features

The most common location for sporadic primary small bowel adenocarcinomas is in the duodenum (55%, especially at the ampulla of Vater), followed by jejunum (30%) and ileum (15%). In contrast, adenocarcinomas arising in the setting of celiac disease and Crohn disease preferentially occur in the jejunum and distal ileum, respectively, likely corresponding to the site of the most significant chronic mucosal injury.

The diagnosis of small bowel adenocarcinoma is often made at a more advanced stage (28% and 32% at stages III and IV, respectively) than colorectal cancer (27% and 20% at stages III and IV, respectively), most likely due to the relative inaccessibility of some parts of the small bowel, nonspecific presenting symptoms, and low index of clinical suspicion. In a large population-based comparison of adenocarcinomas of small and large intestine, small bowel adenocarcinoma patients were younger, presented at a higher stage and with a higher histological tumor grade, and had a worse outcome than those with colorectal adenocarcinoma (Table 9.4).

Overall, the prognosis for small bowel adenocarcinomas is poor, with a 5-year relative survival of less than

TABLE 9.3   Diseases Associated With Small Intestinal Adenocarcinoma

	FAP	Lynch Syndrome	Peutz–Jeghers Syndrome	Crohn Disease	Celiac Disease
Molecular alterations	*APC* (5q21)	Mismatch repair genes	*STK11/LKB1* (19p13.3)	NA	NA
Premalignant lesions	Adenomas	Adenomas	Hamartomas with dysplasia and adenomas	Epithelial dysplasia associated with chronic inflammation	Epithelial dysplasia associated with chronic inflammation
Location of polyps	Colon, duodenum/periampulla, jejunum, and ileum	Colon, duodenum, jejunum, ileum	Small intestine, stomach, colon	Ileum	Jejunum
Risk for developing small intestinal adenocarcinoma	Lifetime risk 3%–5%	Relative risk >100 Lifetime risk 2%–8%	13% by age 65 years	Relative risk 33.2	Relative risk 60–80
Recommendations for small bowel surveillance	Gastro-duodenal endoscopy every 1–5 years depending on polyp location and burden	No established guidelines	Upper endoscopy or video capsule endoscopy every 2–3 years from 18 years of age	No established guidelines	No established guidelines

Abbreviation: FAP, familial adenomatous polyposis.
Source: Data from Arber and Moshkowitz. Small bowel polyposis syndromes. *Curr Gastroenterol Rep.* 2011;13:435–441; Canavan et al. Meta-analysis: colorectal and small bowel cancer risk in patients with Crohn's disease. *Aliment Pharmacol Ther.* 2006;23:1097–1104; Jass. Colorectal polyposes: from phenotype to diagnosis. *Pathol Res Pract.* 2008;204:431–447; Koornstra. Small bowel endoscopy in familial adenomatous polyposis and Lynch syndrome. *Best Pract Res Clin Gastroenterol.* 2012;26:359–368; Pan. Epidemiology of cancer of the small intestine. *World J Gastrointest Oncol.* 2011;3:33–42; Rampertab et al. Small bowel neoplasia in coeliac disease. *Gut.* 2003;52:1211–1214.

TABLE 9.4 Comparison of Small and Large Bowel Adenocarcinomas

	Small Bowel Adenocarcinoma	Large Bowel Adenocarcinoma
Age	Younger	Older
Gender	54% Male	49% Male
Race	16% Black	10% Black
Age-standardized incidence rate	Decreased (−1.24%/year)	Increased (+1.47%/year)
High-grade tumor	33%	21%
Stage IV at presentation	32%	20%
Five-year cancer-specific survival (among patients with ≥ 8 lymph nodes assessed)	Stage I: 13% worse	Better
	Stage II: 15.9% worse	Better
	Stage III: 18.5% worse	Better
	Stage IV: No difference	No difference
Molecular alterations	7%–13%	60%–68%
APC mutation	47%	73%
18q-	40%–60%	40%–60%
KRAS mutation	18%–35% (67%–73% in Celiac-related small bowel adenocarcinoma)	15%
Microsatellite Instability		

Source: Data adapted from Overman et al. A population-based comparison of adenocarcinoma of the large and small intestine: insights into a rare disease. *Ann Surg Oncol.* 2012;19:1439–1445; Raghav and Overman 2013. Small bowel adenocarcinomas—existing evidence and evolving paradigms. *Nat Rev Clin Oncol.* 2013;10:534–544.

30%. Other small bowel neoplasms, such as NETs and lymphomas, generally have a better prognosis than adenocarcinoma. Surgical resection is the treatment of choice for small bowel adenocarcinoma. The role of adjuvant therapy remains unclear, and mucin-producing adenocarcinomas are typically resistant to radiation therapy.

Macroscopic and Microscopic Features

Macroscopically, most small bowel adenocarcinomas are annular constricting tumors, but they may also present as flat, polypoid, or ulcerative lesions. Duodenal carcinomas are usually more circumscribed and polypoid, due to frequent association with an adenomatous component. Microscopically, small bowel adenocarcinomas resemble their counterparts in the colorectum (Figure 9.10A–D). Small bowel adenocarcinomas associated with Crohn disease resemble sporadic adenocarcinomas as well, but are more likely to have poorly differentiated or mucinous features.

Rare subtypes of small bowel carcinoma include adenosquamous carcinoma (Figure 9.10E–F), medullary carcinoma, mixed adenocarcinoma/neuroendocrine carcinoma (NEC), tumors with tripartite differentiation (glandular, squamous, and neuroendocrine components), and small cell NECs.

Ancillary Studies

Forty-three percent of small bowel adenocarcinomas are CK7-/CK20+, as opposed to 82% of colorectal adenocarcinomas. Twenty-eight percent are CK7-/CK20- (as compared to 10% in the colon), followed by CK7+/CK20+

(15%, vs. colon 8%), and CK7+/CK20- (13%, vs. colon <1%). CDX2 may be expressed, but less frequently than in the colon. Tumors arising at the ampulla of Vater may show either intestinal or pancreaticobiliary-type morphology as well as immunophenotype; the intestinal type is associated with a better prognosis.

Not surprisingly, small and large bowel adenocarcinomas share some similar molecular alterations, such as 18q loss (less common in the small bowel than colon), *TP53* overexpression, and activating mutations in *KRAS*. Small bowel adenocarcinomas demonstrate similar rates of microsatellite instability (15 to 20%) and CpG island methylator phenotype (27%) to those seen in colorectal cancer. However, celiac-disease-related small bowel adenocarcinomas show higher rates of MSI (67%–73%) due to promoter methylation of *MLH1*. Given the comparable rates of MSI in small and large bowel adenocarcinomas, we suggest incorporating the results of mismatch repair protein immunostains or MSI testing on primary small bowel adenocarcinomas into surgical pathology reports.

Interestingly, *APC* mutation occurs at a much lower rate in small bowel adenocarcinoma (7%–13%) than in tumors of the large bowel (60%–68%), which may partially explain the lower number of adenomas and consequently fewer adenocarcinomas observed in the small bowel.

Diagnostic Challenges

Adenomas with high-grade dysplasia can be difficult to differentiate from invasive adenocarcinoma, particularly

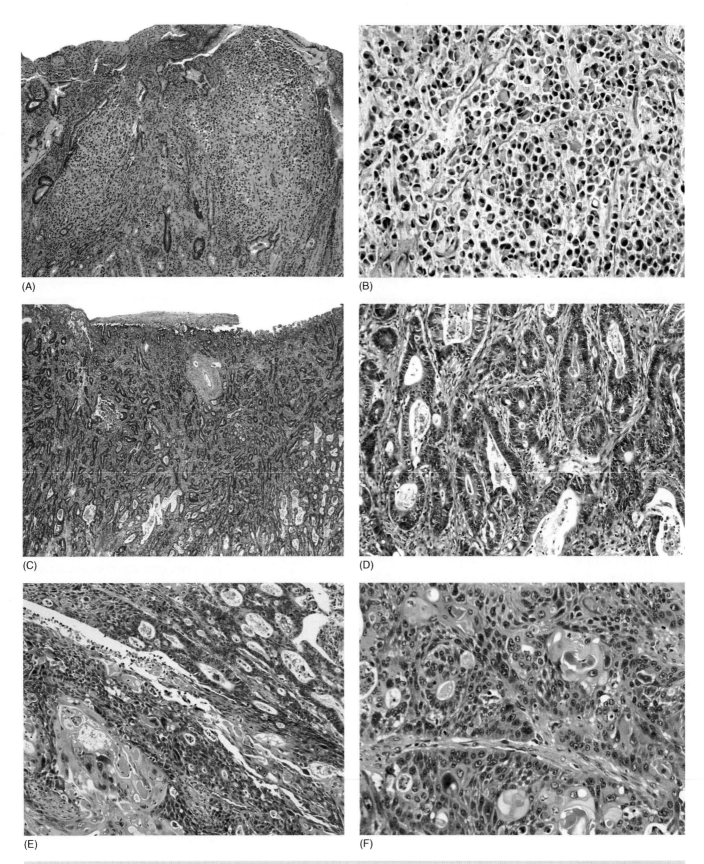

FIGURE 9.10 This case of primary duodenal signet ring cell adenocarcinoma is composed of infiltrating dyscohesive cells with eccentric, crescent-shaped, hyperchromatic nuclei displaced by cytoplasmic mucin (A–B). This ileal adenocarcinoma arising in the context of Crohn disease shows infiltrating small, irregular malignant glands with overlying ulceration (C–D). An ileal adenosquamous carcinoma shows neoplastic glands admixed with malignant squamoid cells with keratin formation (E–F).

in small biopsies, in specimens obtained from around the ampulla due to the complex architecture in this location, or in adenomas with prolapse change/misplaced epithelium. Stromal desmoplasia and the presence of more severe atypia in the putative invasive component than in the surface adenomatous epithelium can be helpful in making the diagnosis of invasion (Figure 9.11A–D). Pancreatic adenocarcinomas in the ampullary/periampullary area can also mimic small bowel adenocarcinoma, as these tumors may extend outwards from the ampulla and grow along the basement membrane of the small bowel epithelium, thus simulating a small bowel adenocarcinoma arising from an adenoma.

Several benign conditions can mimic small bowel adenocarcinoma, including endometriosis (most commonly in the ileum) and as previously discussed in the section on non-neoplastic lesions, ectopic pancreas (more common in proximal than distal small intestine). The presence of endometrial glands (especially the ciliated epithelium associated with tubal metaplasia), hypercellular endometrial stroma, and hemosiderin supports the diagnosis of endometriosis. Positive staining with estrogen receptor (ER), PAX8, and CD10 and negative CDX2 are helpful in confirming the diagnosis of endometriosis as well. Ectopic pancreas may also be misinterpreted as adenocarcinoma, particularly on frozen section evaluation when only pancreatic ducts are present (Figure 9.12A–B). The lobulated architecture and lack of cytologic atypia help to support a diagnosis of ectopic pancreas rather than adenocarcinoma.

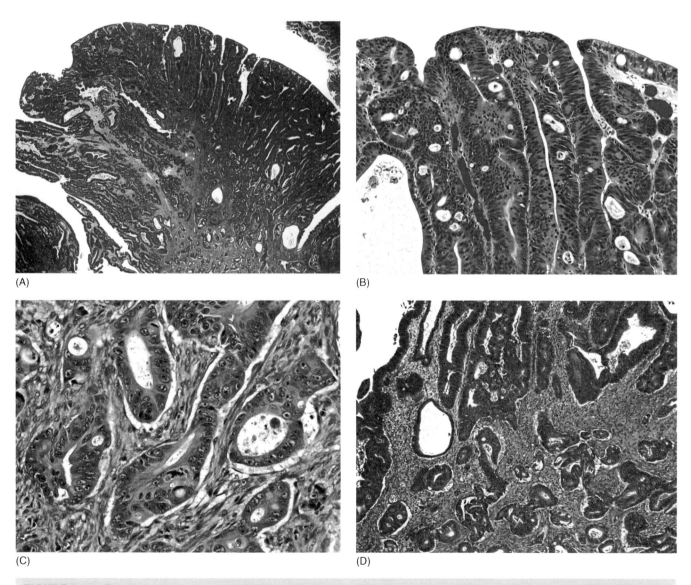

(A)

(B)

(C)

(D)

FIGURE 9.11 This low-power photomicrograph shows invasive adenocarcinoma arising from the base of a jejunal tubulovillous adenoma with high-grade dysplasia (A). When compared to the adenomatous epithelium at the surface (B), the invasive glands demonstrate more severe atypia with vesicular nuclei, open chromatin, prominent nucleoli, and single cell necrosis (C). There is also prominent desmoplasia around the invasive component (D).

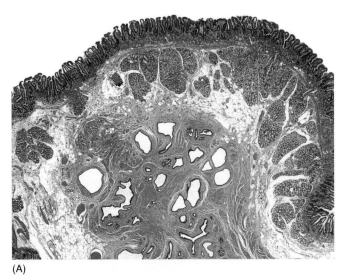
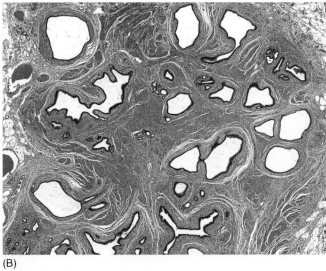

(A)

(B)

FIGURE 9.12 Ectopic pancreas may contain only ducts, without accompanying acini and islets, mimicking invasive adenocarcinoma in the duodenal submucosa (A–B). However, there is retained lobular architecture surrounding smooth muscle, and a lack of cytological atypia.

Grading and Staging

The current grading and staging criteria for small bowel adenocarcinomas are based on *AJCC/UICC TNM*, seventh edition. Grading of small bowel adenocarcinoma is similar to that of colorectal cancer, and is summarized in brief as follows:

- Gx: grade cannot be assessed
- G1: well-differentiated
- G2: moderately differentiated
- G3: poorly differentiated
- G4: small cell carcinoma and undifferentiated carcinoma

By convention, signet ring cell carcinoma is grade 3. Most small bowel adenocarcinomas are moderately (53%) or well differentiated (23%). Overall, 21% are classified as poorly differentiated, and 2% as undifferentiated carcinomas. Grade does not appear to be a strong predictor of outcome.

Staging criteria for small intestinal adenocarcinoma are listed as follows:

- pT1: tumor invades lamina propria or submucosa
- pT2: tumor invades muscularis propria
- pT3: tumor invades through the muscularis propria into the subserosa or into the nonperitonealized perimuscular tissue (mesentery or retroperitoneum) with extension 2 cm or less
- pT4: tumor penetrates visceral peritoneum (serosa) or invades other organs or structures (including other loops of small intestine, mesentery, or retroperitoneum greater than 2 cm, and abdominal wall by way of serosa; for duodenum only, invasion of pancreas or bile duct)

Metastases in one to three regional nodes are classified as pN1, and metastases to four or more nodes are classified as pN2. pM1 indicates distant metastasis. Notably, due to the rich network of lymphatic vessels in the small bowel lamina propria, carcinomas invading the lamina propria of small bowel are staged as pT1a, whereas similar lesions are staged as in situ disease (pTis) in the colon.

NEUROENDOCRINE NEOPLASMS

Epidemiology and Clinicopathologic Features

The majority of GI well-differentiated NETs arise in the small intestine (45%), followed by rectum (20%), appendix (16%), colon (11%), and stomach (7%). Small bowel NETs occur most frequently in the ileum (specifically within 60 cm of the ileocecal valve), followed by duodenum (especially in the first and the second parts), and then jejunum.

The types of small bowel NET parallel the progenitor cell types in the foregut and midgut, and different NETs characteristically present with distinct clinical symptoms. Midgut NETs, including jejunal and ileal tumors, are enterochromaffin (EC) cell tumors, which produce serotonin and other vasoactive substances. When liver metastases are present, they cause classic carcinoid syndrome (flushing and diarrhea) and frequent fibrous endocardial thickening on the right side of the heart. Twenty percent of these tumors are multifocal, and they are not associated with hereditary tumor syndromes. Foregut NETs, including duodenum and proximal jejunum, comprise gastrin-secreting G-cell tumors, somatostatin-producing D-cell tumors, and rarely EC-cell tumors. One third of gastrinomas are associated with Zollinger–Ellison syndrome (hypergastrinemia, gastric hypersecretion, and refractory peptic-ulcer disease). Gastrinomas are also associated with multiple endocrine neoplasia type 1 (MEN1) syndrome. Small (less than 1.0 cm) nonfunctional gastrinomas are often associated with chronic *H. pylori* gastritis and long-term proton pump inhibitor use. In contrast to pancreatic somatostatin-producing NETs, duodenal somatostatinomas are not associated with "somatostatinoma syndrome" (diabetes mellitus, cholelithiasis, and steatorrhea). However, duodenal somatostatinomas are associated with MEN1, neurofibromatosis type 1 (NF1), and von Hippel–Lindau syndrome (VHL). Notably, L-cell, glucagon-like peptide-producing, and pancreatic peptide/peptide YY-producing NETs are much less common in the small bowel (foregut and midgut) than the hindgut (left colon and rectum). NETs are discussed in greater detail in Chapter 3.

Many small bowel NETs are found incidentally, and are asymptomatic at presentation due to hepatic metabolism of vasoactive amines, absence of hormone secretion altogether, and/or small size. Among symptomatic patients, 40% present with vague and nonspecific abdominal pain, secondary to intussusception, mass effect of the tumor, or mesenteric ischemia due to tumor-associated fibrosis. Intermittent bowel obstruction occurs in 25% of small intestinal NET, and duodenal/periampullary NET may also produce biliary obstruction.

Small bowel NETs have a propensity to metastasize to the liver, mesentery, and peritoneum. The metastatic risk of small bowel NET increases when tumors are greater than 2.0 cm, when the muscularis propria is involved, and with increased mitotic activity. The prognosis for small bowel well-differentiated NET is worse than for those arising in the stomach or rectum. Treatment modalities include surgery, somatostatin analogues (if the tumor expresses somatostatin receptors), and chemoradiation. The latter has limited utility in treating well-differentiated NET.

Molecular Features

Molecular features of foregut NETs include frequent abnormalities of the *MEN1* gene, which is absent in midgut (ileal) NETs. Ileal NETs often show mutations in the *APC* gene and upregulation of the *HOXC6* gene. In addition, several growth factors, such as transforming growth factor (TGF), insulin-like growth factor (IGF), and fibroblast growth factor (FGF), play important roles in the stromal fibrosis/desmoplasia seen in EC-cell NETs.

Macroscopic and Microscopic Features

Macroscopically, small bowel NETs can be solitary or multiple (25%–40% cases). They are characteristically

gray in the fresh state, and turn yellow following formalin fixation (Figure 9.13A–B). The overlying mucosa may be intact or ulcerated. In general, the tumor size is small (less than 2 cm), and even smaller in functioning/hormone secreting NETs (eg, gastrinomas are typically less than 0.8 cm, and somatostatinomas average 1.8 cm). In some cases, deep infiltration into the muscular wall, peritoneum, or mesentery is present, which can lead to obstruction, adhesion, and volvulus.

A detailed description of the histologic features of NETs is given in Chapter 3. Briefly, low-grade NET contains uniform round smooth nuclei with stippled chromatin and inconspicuous nucleoli (Figure 9.13C–E). Tumor cells may be arranged in various patterns, including nested/insular, trabecular, glandular/pseudoglandular, or solid. NETs are typically very vascular, with frequent perineural and vascular invasion even in well-differentiated tumors. Well-differentiated small bowel NETs are positive for neuroendocrine markers (synaptophysin, chromogranin, and CD56) and cytokeratin (CK) AE1/3, and negative for mucin, TTF1, and S100. Poorly differentiated small bowel NECs are uncommon, but similar to other poorly differentiated NETs in that they can stain for TTF1 and show weak to absent expression of chromogranin and CK AE1/3.

Gangliocytic paraganglioma is a rare nonfunctional, triphasic tumor that primarily occurs in the second portion of duodenum, and occasionally in the pylorus and jejunum. This tumor is generally regarded as benign, with rare reports of regional lymph node metastases. Macroscopically, gangliocytic paraganglioma is a small submucosal mass that frequently has an ulcerated mucosal surface. It is composed of variable proportions of spindle cells, epithelioid cells, and ganglion-like cells (Figure 9.14A–D). The spindle cells resemble proliferating neural processes and Schwann cells; the epithelioid cells are arranged in an "endocrine" pattern that forms nests or trabeculae; and the ganglion-like cells are large cells with round nuclei and distinct nucleoli. Immunohistochemically, the spindle cell component is positive for S100; the epithelioid component stains for synaptophysin, chromogranin, and occasionally CK AE1/3 (50%); and the ganglion cells express synaptophysin. The major differential diagnosis on hematoxylin and eosin (H&E) evaluation includes GISTs (which are positive for KIT), well-differentiated NETs, and ganglioneuromas. Identification of all three cell components helps to distinguish gangliocytic paraganglioma from the other entities in the differential diagnosis.

Diagnostic Challenges

Somatostatinomas may show a purely glandular pattern that can be confused with conventional adenocarcinomas. Immunohistochemical stains for neuroendocrine markers are useful in such cases. It is also important to

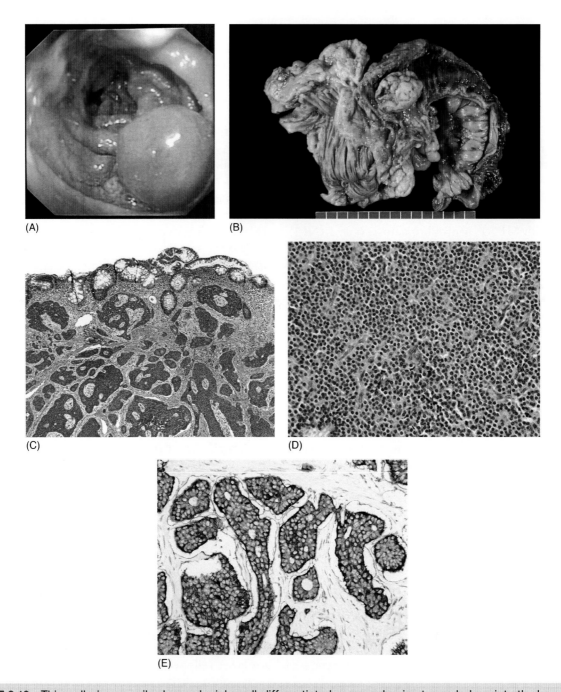

FIGURE 9.13 This well-circumscribed, round, pink, well-differentiated neuroendocrine tumor bulges into the lumen of the duodenum (A, courtesy Dr. Whit Knapple). Neuroendocrine tumors characteristically turn yellow after formalin fixation (B). An example of the typical nested or organoid growth pattern of a well-differentiated NET (C) composed of uniform round nuclei with stippled chromatin and inconspicuous nucleoli (D). Diffuse strong synaptophysin staining is typical (E).

recognize that some NETs produce mucin or have spindle cell components, and the majority of NETs will show CK expression. Some well-differentiated NETs that are arranged in sheets may mimic lymphoma, but lymphomas express CD45, rather than epithelial and neuroendocrine markers.

Grading and Staging

Grading of small bowel NET is performed similarly to other NETs, which is based on mitotic rate and Ki-67 proliferative index (WHO 2010 criteria). This is discussed in detail in Chapter 3. Accurate grading is difficult on small biopsies, given the limited sample, and should be performed

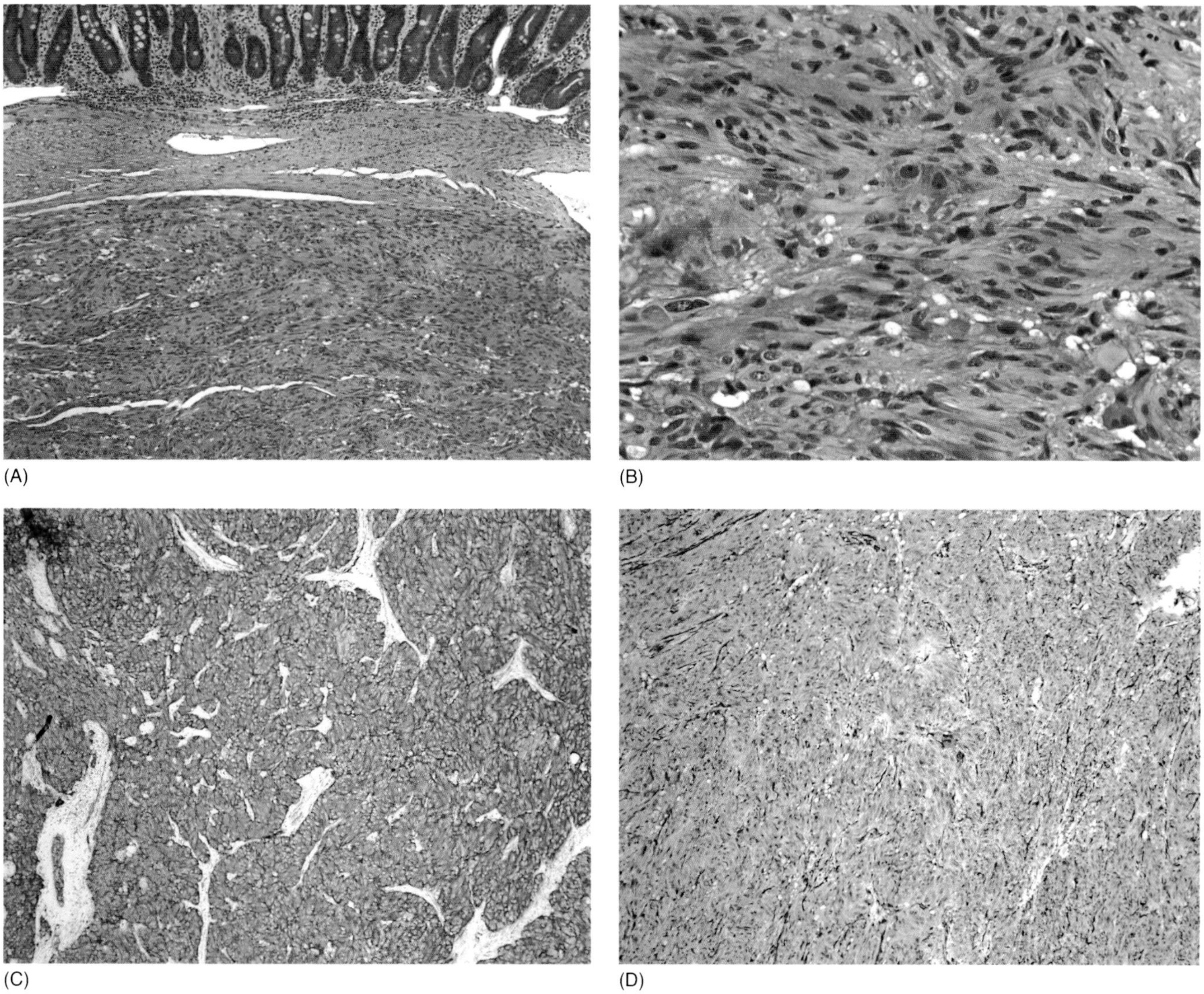

FIGURE 9.14 Duodenal gangliocytic paragangliomas are typically well-circumscribed tumors located in the submucosa (A). They are composed of a mixture of epithelioid cells, spindle cells, and ganglion cells (B). These lesions strongly and diffusely express neuroendocrine markers such as chromogranin and synaptophysin (C), and S100 highlights the sustentacular network (D).

on resection specimens if available. Quantification should be performed at the "hot spot" within the tumor where mitotic activity is the highest. If the mitotic rate and proliferative index suggest different grades, the higher grade is assigned. Of note, cytologic atypia in G1 tumors has no effect on clinical behavior. G2 tumors may show punctate necrosis, although necrosis is not considered a grading criterion in abdominal NETs.

The current grading and staging criteria for small bowel NETs are based on AJCC/UICC TNM, seventh edition. The cancer staging protocol for small bowel adenocarcinoma is used for small bowel neuroendocrine carcinomas (G3) and tumors with mixed glandular/

neuroendocrine differentiation (MANEC), while a unique staging protocol applies to low- and intermediate-grade (G1 and G2) NETs. Since the current staging system is fairly new and remains controversial, it is important for the pathologist to include all important elements in the report, including the diagnosis, site of tumor/metastasis, grade, stage, mitotic rate, proliferation rate, and results of immunohistochemical staining. Table 9.5 summarizes the differences between the staging criteria for small bowel NET and adenocarcinomas/NEC. Notably, if the size of an NET exceeds 1 cm, the tumor is staged as pT2 even if it is confined to the submucosa and does not invade the muscularis propria.

TABLE 9.5 Comparison of Staging Criteria for Small Bowel Adenocarcinoma and Small Bowel Neuroendocrine Tumor

	Small Bowel Adenocarcinoma and Poorly Differentiated Neuroendocrine Carcinoma	Small Bowel Well-Differentiated Neuroendocrine Tumor
pT1	Tumor invades lamina propria or submucosa	Tumor invades lamina propria or submucosa *and* tumor size ≤1 cm
pT2	Tumor invades muscularis propria	Tumor invades muscularis propria *or* tumor size >1 cm
pT3	Tumor invades through the muscularis propria into the subserosa *or* into the nonperitonealized perimuscular tissue (mesentery or retroperitoneum) with extension ≤2 cm	Tumor invades through the muscularis propria into subserosal tissue without penetration of overlying serosa (jejunal or ileal tumors) *or* invades pancreas or retroperitoneum (ampullary or duodenal tumors) or into nonperitonealized tissues
pT4	Tumor penetrates visceral peritoneum (serosa) or directly invades other organs or structures (including other loops of small intestine, mesentery, or retroperitoneum >2 cm, and abdominal wall by way of serosa; for duodenum only, invasion of pancreas or bile duct)	Tumor penetrates visceral peritoneum (serosa) or invades other organs
pN1	Metastases in one to three regional lymph nodes	Metastases in regional lymph nodes
pN2	Metastases in four or more regional lymph nodes	–
pM1	Distant metastasis	Distant metastasis

MESENCHYMAL TUMORS

Mesenchymal tumors are discussed in detail in Chapter 5, thus the focus of this chapter is on the mesenchymal neoplasms that are most common in or unique to the small bowel.

Gastrointestinal Stromal Tumors (GISTs)

GISTs are mesenchymal tumors that arise from the interstitial cells of Cajal. The small bowel is the second most common location for GIST, preceded by the stomach (which accounts for 60% of GIST). The jejunum and ileum are the most commonly affected segments, followed by duodenum. When compared with gastric GISTs, small intestinal GISTs (Figure 9.15A) are more likely to present with acute complications, such as intestinal obstruction and tumor rupture. Histologically, small intestinal GISTs are typically spindle cell tumors (Figure 9.15B–C), like their counterparts in other regions of the GI tract. However, a few histologic features are specific to small bowel GISTs. Approximately half of small bowel GISTs contain microscopically distinctive, extracellular collagen globules known as "skeinoid fibers," which are associated with a lower grade and favorable outcome (Figure 9.15D). In addition, nuclear palisading is less commonly seen in small intestinal tumors when compared to gastric and colorectal GISTs. Focal nuclear pleomorphism is more common in small intestinal GISTs from patients with NF1.

GISTs typically have strong and diffuse KIT and DOG1 positivity (Figure 9.15E–F). Reactivity for other markers, including smooth muscle actin, S100, and CD34, is variable. On a molecular level, *KIT*-activating mutations are common in small intestinal GISTs, and duplication of AY502-503 in *KIT* exon 9 is virtually specific for small intestinal (vs. gastric) GISTs (see Chapter 5 for further discussion of immunohistochemical and molecular aspects of GIST).

Small intestinal GISTs are more likely to be malignant than gastric GISTS (40%–50% of small bowel tumors vs. 20%–25% of gastric GIST). The risk assessment for primary GIST is based on tumor size, location, and mitotic activity. The major differential diagnosis includes other spindle cell mesenchymal tumors, such as leiomyoma, schwannoma, and inflammatory fibroid polyp. This is also discussed in detail in Chapter 5.

Smooth Muscle Tumors

Leiomyomas are much less common in the small bowel than in the esophagus or large intestine. These tumors can arise either in association with the muscularis mucosae or with the muscularis propria (Figure 9.16A). The cells are cytologically bland, arranged in perpendicularly oriented fascicles, and have bright eosinophilic cytoplasm and blunt-ended nuclei (Figure 9.16B). Rare cases may show nuclear atypia, but lack mitotic activity. Leiomyomas are immunoreactive with markers such as smooth muscle actin, smooth muscle myosin heavy chain (Figure 9.16C), myosin, desmin, and caldesmon, but are typically negative for DOG1 and KIT. Leiomyosarcomas are extremely rare in the GI tract. They usually arise in the muscularis propria, and show marked cytologic atypia, significant mitotic activity, and necrosis. Similar to leiomyomas, leiomyosarcomas are actin and desmin positive, and KIT negative.

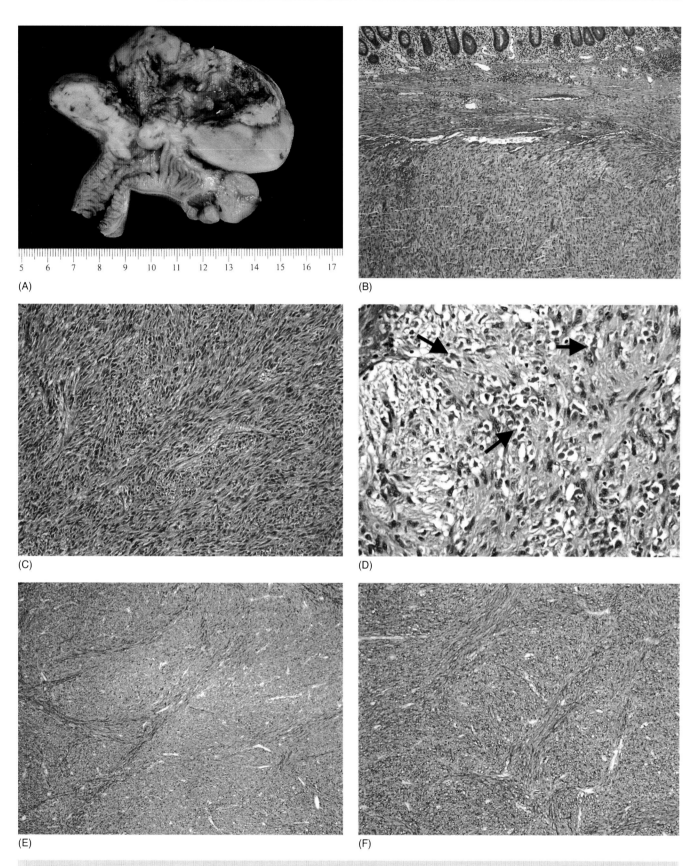

FIGURE 9.15 This gross photograph shows a large gastrointestinal stromal tumor (GIST) arising in the wall of the small bowel and bulging outward (A). The cut surface shows hemorrhage and degenerative changes. The cellular tumor is composed of fascicles of spindle cells (B–C). Skeinoid fibers can also be seen in small bowel GIST (D, arrows). GISTs diffusely express DOG1 (E) and KIT (F).

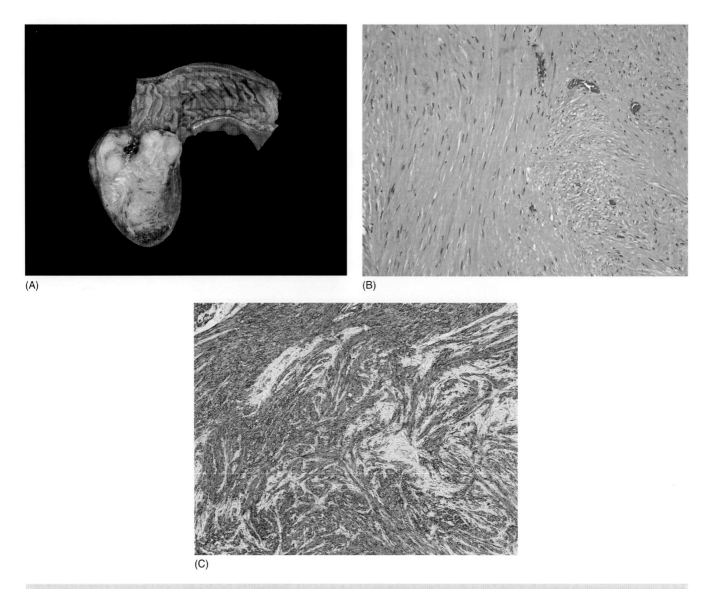

FIGURE 9.16 This gross photograph shows a leiomyoma arising from the wall of the small bowel (A). It has a tan–white, firm, whorled cut surface. At low power, the tumor is composed of cytologically bland spindle cells with elongated nuclei and eosinophilic cytoplasm, with low to medium cellularity (B). Leiomyomas show diffuse strong reactivity to smooth muscle myosin heavy chain (C).

Fibroblastic Tumors

Inflammatory fibroid polyps are benign polypoid submucosal neoplasms; the ileum is the second most common site in the GI tract, after the gastric antrum. These lesions can present as an obstructive mass and may cause intussusception. Histologically, inflammatory fibroid polyps are composed of loose fibromyxoid stroma containing spindle cells, inflammatory cells (particularly eosinophils, plasma cells, and mast cells), and prominent vessels that may have surrounding concentric fibrosis (Figure 9.17A–D). The tumor cells are positive for CD34 and smooth muscle actin, and negative for KIT and DOG1.

Mesenteric fibromatosis (desmoid tumor) (Figure 9.18A–B) originates in the mesentery, but may form a fibrotic mass involving the intestinal wall. This process is a clonal fibroblastic and myofibroblastic proliferation that is associated with *CTNNB1* or *APC* mutations. Mesenteric fibromatosis usually expresses nuclear β-catenin (Figure 9.18C) and estrogen receptor. Fibromatosis is associated with FAP (Gardner syndrome).

Lipomatous Lesions

Lipomatous hypertrophy of the ileocecal valve is characterized by a circumferential deposition of fat in the submucosa of the ileocecal valve. Submucosal deposition of small amounts of mature fat is common throughout the GI tract; however, the prominent fat deposition at the ileocecal valve may result in an elevated mucosal protrusion into the lumen that produces a mass, resulting in occasional mucosal ulceration or even partial

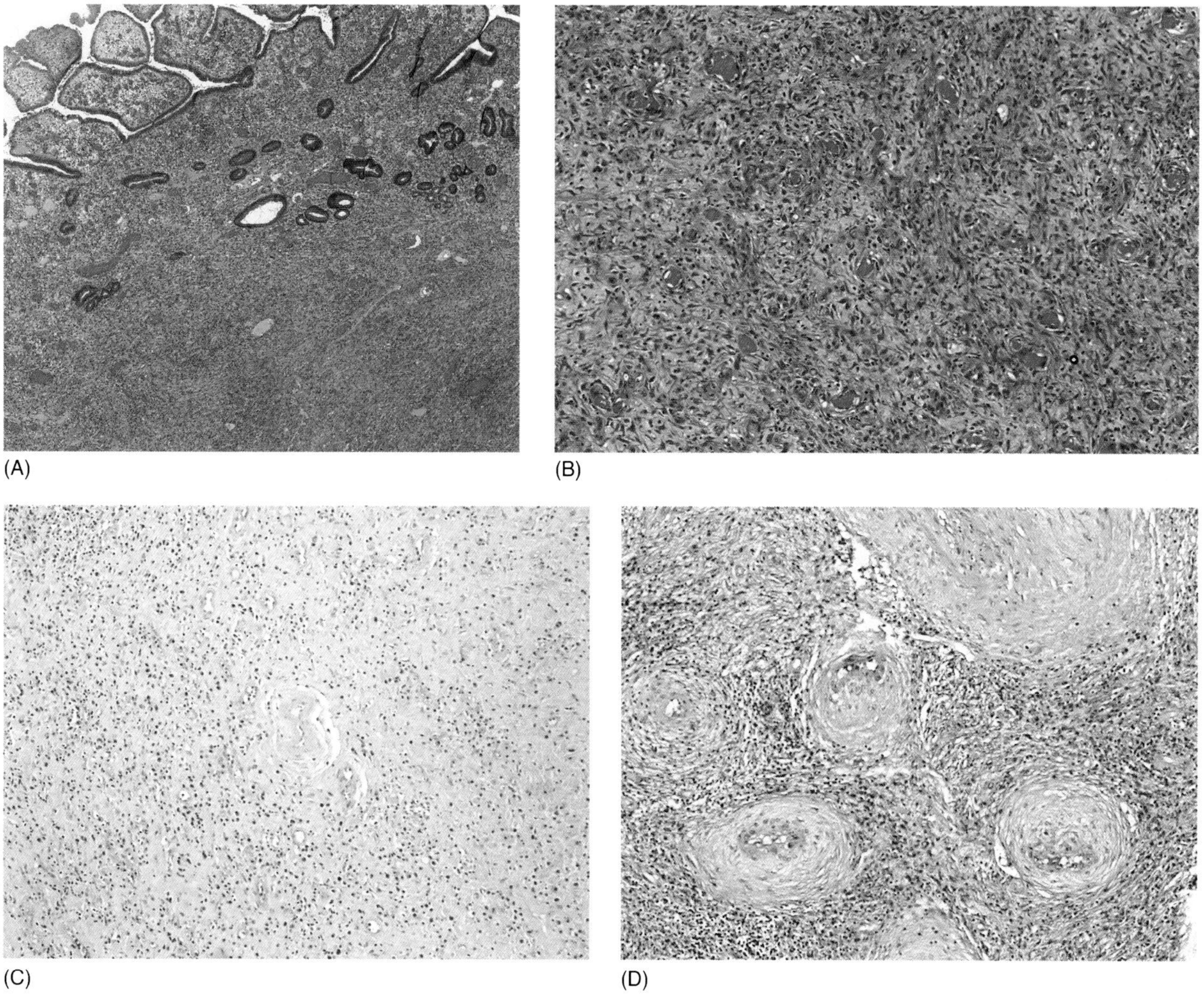

FIGURE 9.17 Inflammatory fibroid polyps are submucosal lesions composed of spindle cells within a loose fibromyxoid stroma (A–B). Higher power reveals cytologically bland spindle cells in a background of myxoid stroma with inflammatory cells including prominent eosinophils, lymphocytes, and plasma cells (C). Vessels are prominent, often surrounded by concentric collagen deposition (D).

obstruction. The etiology of this process is unclear. Lipomas can be seen in other locations in the small bowel as well (Figure 9.19), but are more commonly located in the right colon.

Vascular Tumors

Hemangiomas and lymphangiomas are relatively common mesenchymal lesions throughout the GI tract, and resemble their counterparts elsewhere. Microscopically, multiple cystically dilated spaces are lined by a single layer of flattened endothelium. Hemangiomas generally contain blood, whereas lymphangiomas contain proteinaceous material (Figure 9.20A–B). In addition, lymphangiomas frequently contain lymphoid aggregates. Immunostains can be helpful in this distinction: D2-40 is more frequently positive in lymphangiomas (Figure 9.20C), whereas CD31 and CD34 are more frequently positive in hemangiomas.

Kaposi sarcoma may occur in the GI tract of HIV patients with severe immunosuppression. The duodenum is more commonly involved by Kaposi sarcoma than the jejunum or ileum. Histologically, the tumor is composed of submucosal spindle cell proliferation, forming slit-like vascular channels containing red blood cells (Figure 9.20D–E). Extravasated red blood cells are frequently seen. The tumor cells are positive for CD31 (Figure 9.20F), HHV-8 (Figure 9.20G), CD34, and Factor VIII. Angiosarcoma of the small intestine is rare, and most often occurs in older patients who were previously treated with radiation therapy for uterine or urinary bladder cancer. The tumors are composed of pleomorphic spindle cells or epithelioid cells that form primitive vascular channels (Figure 9.20H–I). The tumor cells are positive for CD31, but show more variable expression for CD34 or Factor VIII. One caveat is that epithelioid variants may show keratin positivity, and mimic a carcinoma.

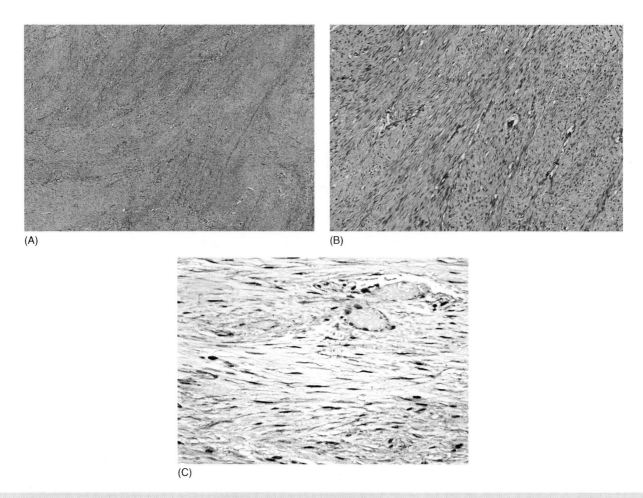

FIGURE 9.18 Mesenteric fibromatosis (desmoid tumor) is composed of intersecting fascicles of bland spindle cells (A). The nuclei have smooth chromatin and inconspicuous nucleoli (B). There is diffuse nuclear expression of β-catenin (C).

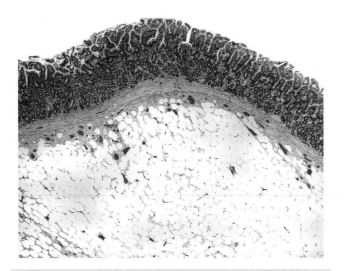

FIGURE 9.19 This lipoma of the small bowel consists of a well-circumscribed submucosal mass composed of mature adipocytes that are relatively uniform in size, and lack cytologic atypia.

Gastrointestinal Clear Cell Sarcoma

GI clear cell sarcoma is a rare tumor with a characteristic t(2;22)(q32;q12) chromosome translocation leading to *EWSR1–CREB1* fusion. This tumor is more commonly found in the small intestine than the stomach and colon. It often presents as a mural mass in young adults, with frequent metastases to mesenteric lymph nodes and liver. The tumor cells are rounded to mildly spindled (Figure 9.21A–B) and can contain multinucleated osteoclast-like giant cells. The tumors share morphologic similarity with peripheral clear cell sarcoma and cutaneous malignant melanoma, and likewise they express S100. However, unlike the other two entities, GI clear cell sarcomas do not express HMB-45 and melan-A. A recent ultrastructural examination demonstrates primitive neuroectodermal differentiation in the tumor cells; therefore, a new designation of malignant GI neuroectodermal tumor has been proposed for this tumor type.

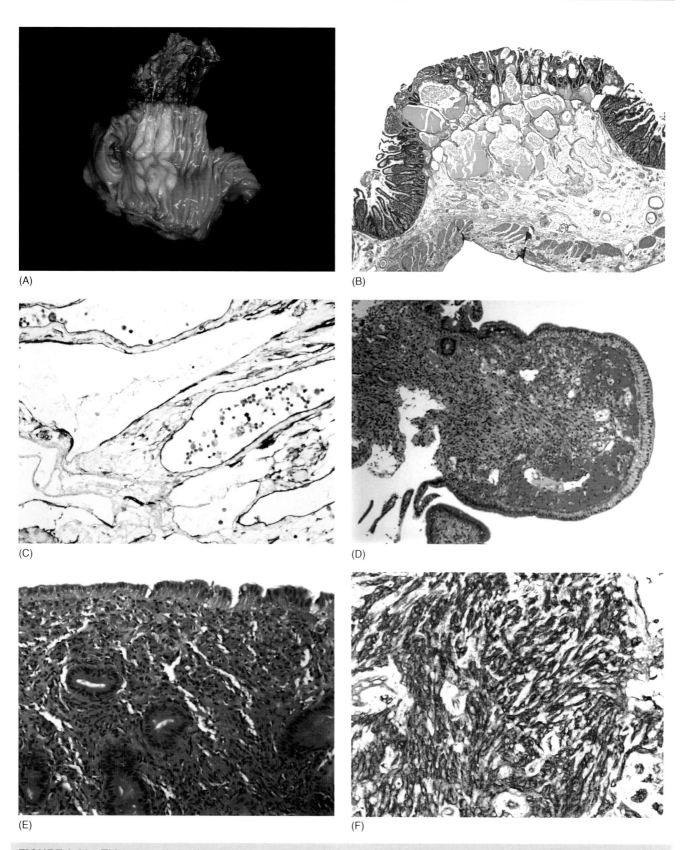

FIGURE 9.20 This gross photo demonstrates a circumscribed, lobulated mucosal lesion containing milky white lymph, typical of lymphangioma (A). The lesion is centered in the submucosa, but the dilated, lymph-filled spaces extend into the mucosa (B). Multiple cystically dilated, endothelial-lined spaces are filled with thin pink amorphous material. D2-40 highlights the endothelial cells of the lymphatic channels (C). Kaposi sarcoma consists of a proliferation of spindle cells, forming slit-like vascular channels with red blood cells and extravasated red cells (D–E). (*continued*)

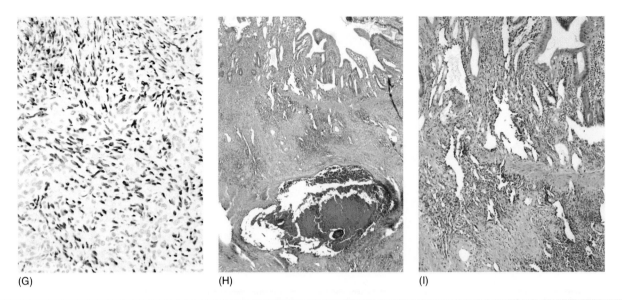

(G)   (H)   (I)

FIGURE 9.20 (*continued*) The tumor expresses CD31 (F) and HHV-8 (G). Angiosarcomas are composed of spindled or epithelioid cells that form primitive vascular channels (H–I). This example extends entirely through the wall of the small bowel.

HEMATOLYMPHOID TUMORS

Overview

Any of the lymphomas described in this text can involve the small bowel, but several types have a propensity for occurring at this site, and thus will be discussed in detail in this chapter. As in the rest of the GI tract, B cell lymphomas are most common, but two unique T cell lymphomas also involve the small intestine. For additional information on a general approach to lymphoma diagnosis in the GI tract, see Chapter 4.

Enteropathy-Associated T Cell Lymphoma (EATL)

This T cell lymphoma has historically been associated with underlying gluten-sensitive enteropathy (celiac disease),

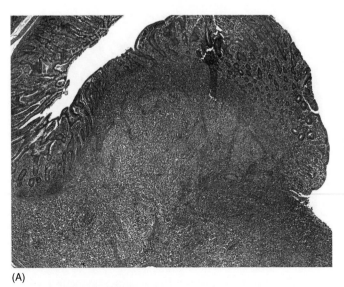

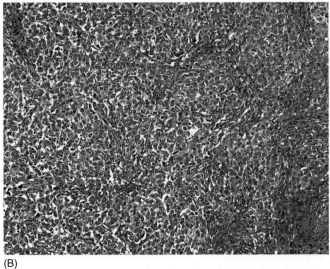

(A)   (B)

FIGURE 9.21 This gastrointestinal clear cell sarcoma from a 30-year-old woman shows sheets of epithelioid cells arranged in a vaguely nested pattern in the submucosa of the small bowel (A). The tumor cells show focal clearing of cytoplasm, small nucleoli, and scattered mitoses (B, courtesy of Dr. Paul Wakely Jr.).

though more recently a subtype has been identified that most often occurs outside the clinical setting, termed "Type II EATL." A small number of patients who develop EATL have a history of celiac disease diagnosed in childhood, but more commonly the diagnosis occurs in adulthood or is made concurrently with the diagnosis of lymphoma. It occurs most commonly in the jejunum, where there is overlap with what has in the past been termed "ulcerative jejunitis." In this era of molecular clonality analysis, it has been demonstrated that patients with celiac disease who become refractory to a gluten-free diet, and subsequently progress to EATL, can harbor identical T cell clones in their intestinal mucosa both before and after the development of lymphoma. In addition, the same clonal T cells can be found in other locations throughout the GI tract. This finding suggests a spectrum of neoplastic disease in these patients.

EATL causes ulcerating masses that infiltrate transmurally (Figure 9.22A). This may lead to perforation, which may be the presenting sign of disease, even in patients who have not been previously diagnosed with celiac disease. "Classical" (or Type I) EATL accounts for the majority of cases, and is usually associated with the celiac-disease-related HLA DQ2 or DQ8 haplotypes. It consists of variably pleomorphic, intermediate- or large-sized cells with prominent nucleoli that most commonly express CD3 and CD7 (Figure 9.22B–C). They classically lose expression of the pan-T cell marker CD5, and are CD4-negative. CD8 is most often negative but may be expressed, and the neoplastic cells have other evidence of a cytotoxic phenotype, including expression of cytotoxic granule-associated proteins including TIA-1 and granzyme B. CD56 is negative and the cells express the $\alpha\beta$ T cell receptor. Frequently, the neoplastic T cells express CD30, which may lead to confusion with other CD30-positive T cell lymphomas such as anaplastic large cell lymphoma (particularly when the cells are markedly pleomorphic). Other morphologic signs of celiac disease, from an isolated increase in intraepithelial lymphocytes to fully developed celiac-type changes with mucosal flattening, may be present in the intact mucosa elsewhere in the intestine (Figure 9.22D).

In contrast, the monomorphic (Type II) variant is composed of monotonous, small- to intermediate-sized cells with inconspicuous nucleoli and less cytoplasm (Figure 9.22E). The immunophenotype differs from the classic form, with most cases expressing CD8 (approximately 80%) and CD56 (greater than 90%), along with CD3 and CD7. CD5 is negative, and this variant may express either the $\alpha\beta$ or $\gamma\delta$ T cell receptor. These differences, along with the lack of close association with celiac disease and the HLA DQ2 and DQ8 haplotypes, have led some to question whether this disease should truly be regarded as a variant of EATL or as a separate disease.

In either form, EATL has a very aggressive course and a poor prognosis, particularly in the setting of intestinal perforation. This is due to the inherent characteristics of the lymphoma and, often in the case of classic/Type I disease, to the underlying effects of celiac disease. Median survivals are measured in months.

Extranodal NK/T Cell Lymphoma (ENKTL), Nasal Type

This relatively rare lymphoma is important to consider in the differential diagnosis of EATL in the small bowel. While it is uncommon and usually found in the sinonasal tract, as implied by its name, the most frequent extranasal site of involvement by ENKTL is the GI tract. Like Type II EATL, the lymphoma cells of ENKTL usually express CD56, although they are usually negative for both CD4 and CD8. Surface CD3 is also negative, although cytoplasmic CD3ε can be found, depending on the specific anti-CD3 antibody used for immunohistochemistry (or flow cytometry). Cytotoxic molecules including TIA-1 and granzyme B are also expressed. ENKTL is essentially invariably related to Epstein–Barr virus (EBV), which can be demonstrated by in situ hybridization EBV-encoded ribonucleic acid (EBER) studies.

The cells of ENKTL have variable morphology, ranging from small lymphocytes to large and anaplastic cells. When it involves mucosa, including that of the GI tract, ulceration is a frequent feature. An angiocentric and angiodestructive pattern of infiltration is quite characteristic, with lymphoma cells overrunning and destroying the walls of mural blood vessels, which can lead to extensive tissue necrosis (Figure 9.23).

Follicular Lymphoma (FL)

This mature B cell lymphoma occurs throughout the GI tract, both as a primary tumor and as secondary involvement by a neoplasm centered elsewhere, such as in retroperitoneal lymph nodes. It is discussed here because there is also a primary form that appears to be unique to the small intestine (often the duodenum), which, while morphologically and immunophenotypically indistinguishable from other forms of FL, is believed to have a very good prognosis with conservative therapy. Nonetheless, it must be distinguished from systemic cases of FL by full staging procedures including bone marrow biopsy.

FL is composed of B lymphocytes with the characteristic features of follicle center (or germinal center) cells, and most often has a nodular or follicular pattern (Figure 9.24A). The neoplastic cells have variable morphology, some with small, cleaved nuclei and scant cytoplasm characteristic of follicular "centrocytes," and others that are large with open chromatin and more abundant cytoplasm characteristic of "centroblasts" (Figure 9.24B). FL is graded, based on the proportion of centroblast-like cells, into three grades that have prognostic significance.

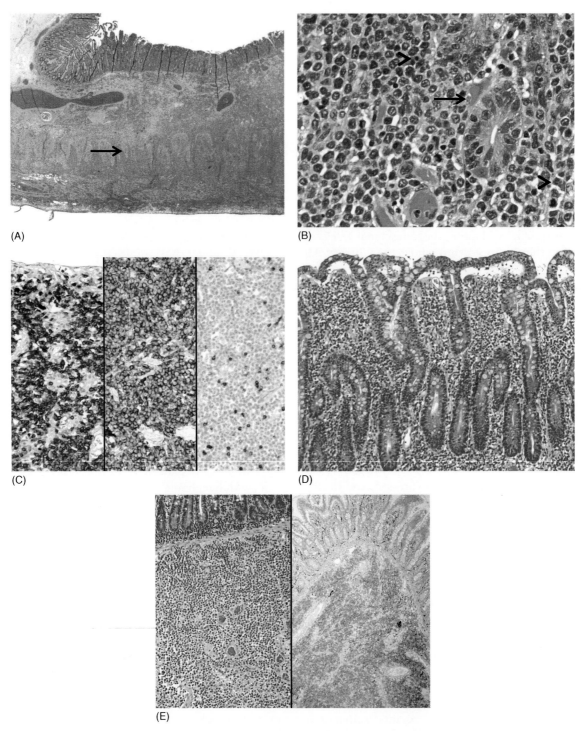

FIGURE 9.22 Enteropathy-associated T cell lymphoma (EATL) arising in the small intestine and infiltrating transmurally (A). The lymphoma involves the mucosa, penetrates the fibers of the muscularis propria (arrow), and involves the subserosa. The cells of classical EATL are intermediate to large, with pleomorphic nuclei and occasional prominent nucleoli (B). Endothelial cells of admixed blood vessels (arrow) are a convenient internal standard for large nuclear size. Note the presence of scattered eosinophils (arrowhead). Immunohistochemically (C), most cases are positive for the pan-T cell markers CD3 (left panel) and CD7 (center panel). CD5 (right panel) is usually negative. The positive-staining cells are scattered non-neoplastic T cells. A careful examination of the mucosa of uninvolved small intestine will very often reveal the presence of sprue-type changes indicating underlying celiac disease, particularly in classic (non-Type II) EATL. In this panel (D), the mucosa is flattened, with numerous intraepithelial lymphocytes on the surface and crypt epithelium. There is also a prominent lamina propria lymphoplasmacytic infiltrate. Studies have shown that the intraepithelial lymphocytes even in areas away from the lymphoma can be clonal. The so-called Type II EATL (E) is less often associated with underlying celiac disease and tends to be composed of monotonous, small- or intermediate-sized cells (left panel) that often express CD56 (right panel). Note the relatively intact villous architecture of the overlying mucosa in the right panel.

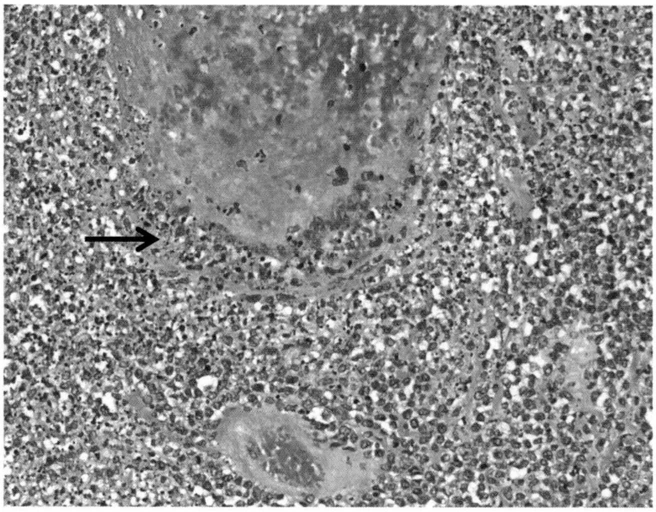

FIGURE 9.23 Extranodal NK/T cell lymphoma, nasal type. This rare lymphoma occurs in the head and neck, but the GI tract is the most commonly involved extranasal site. Histologically, it bears a resemblance to EATL (especially the classic type), with relatively large and pleomorphic cells. It is essentially always related to underlying Epstein–Barr virus and has a distinctive, angiocentric and angiodestructive infiltration pattern. Here, lymphoma cells invade and disrupt the wall of a medium-sized vessel (arrow).

Grade 3 is further subdivided into grades 3A and 3B (see Table 9.6). Current practice is to combine grades 1 and 2 into an effective "low-grade" category, reported as "follicular lymphoma, grade 1–2." As with other B cell lymphomas, the appearance of a significant (reported as greater than 25% by some authorities) diffuse large cell component should be regarded and reported as diffuse large B cell lymphoma (DLBCL) with a precursor FL in the background (Figure 9.24C).

The characteristic nodular/follicular pattern, along with the monotonous appearance of the lymphoma cells making up these nodules, makes it possible to essentially render a definite diagnosis even on routine H&E stained sections in classic cases. Nonetheless, a typical immunohistochemical panel shows that the lymphoma cells express pan-B cell markers including CD20 and CD79a, as well as the markers of follicle center cell differentiation CD10 and BCL-6. As noted in Chapter 4, the diagnosis of FL and, in particular, its separation from a reactive follicular hyperplasia that can accompany many conditions, is greatly aided by the use of a BCL-2 immunohistochemical stain (Figure 9.24D). While many B cell lymphomas, along with numerous normal hematolymphoid cells, express this protein, it is negative in reactive, non-neoplastic germinal centers. In contrast, the vast majority of FL, including nearly all low-grade (grades 1–2) tumors, are BCL-2 positive. Thus, a follicular proliferation that is

CD10 and/or BCL-6 positive that also expresses BCL-2 is diagnostic of FL.

The unique "primary intestinal" FL mentioned earlier is morphologically identical to other forms, but is localized to the small intestine, very often the duodenum. It is more common in young or middle-aged patients, often women, and can appear as a polyp or polyps endoscopically (Figure 9.24E). There is evidence that patients with this form of the disease have a very good prognosis with endoscopic "excision" of the polyp alone. The only way to be certain of the primary intestinal form of the disease, however, is to perform full clinical staging to rule out systemic involvement. Systemic FL is relentlessly progressive and incurable, with a significantly worse prognosis than the localized small intestinal form.

Burkitt Lymphoma (BL)

BL occurs in endemic and sporadic forms, as well as in an immunodeficiency-related variety. The classic de novo presentation of the sporadic form of this rare B cell lymphoma is in the ileocecal region, where it can create large masses that grow at a seemingly impossible rate. In the area of the ileocecal valve, this can lead to dramatic clinical presentations that include rapid-onset obstruction and perforation (Figure 9.25A). Most patients are relatively young, although immunodeficiency-associated cases, many of which are related to underlying HIV infection, occur in older patients. EBV infection is a fairly frequent association with BL, especially in the endemic form, but also in sporadic and immunodeficiency-associated cases. The endemic form is limited to equatorial Africa and New Guinea and will not be discussed further.

The cells of BL are intermediate in size with round, monotonous nuclei and one or more relatively inconspicuous nucleoli (Figure 9.25B). In touch or aspirate preparations, perinuclear cytoplasmic vacuoles may be seen, but these are not usually apparent in formalin-fixed tissue preparations. A characteristic "starry sky" pattern reflects the extremely rapid proliferative rate, with numerous tingible-body macrophages interspersed with the monotonous lymphoma cells (Figure 9.25C). This proliferative rate can be confirmed using Ki-67 immunohistochemistry, which will reveal near-100% labeling in the lymphoma cells (Figure 9.25D). The neoplastic cells are CD20-positive B cells and have a germinal center phenotype, expressing BCL-6 and CD10. Unlike many other B cell lymphomas, BL is usually BCL-2 negative, a finding that helps distinguish it from the diffuse form of FL. The diagnosis can be confirmed with molecular studies for translocations involving the *MYC* gene on chromosome 8, which are almost invariably present. By far, the most common of these is t(8;14), which brings together *MYC* and the *IGH* gene, but t(2;8) and t(8;22) are also found, involving the genes for kappa and lambda light chains, respectively.

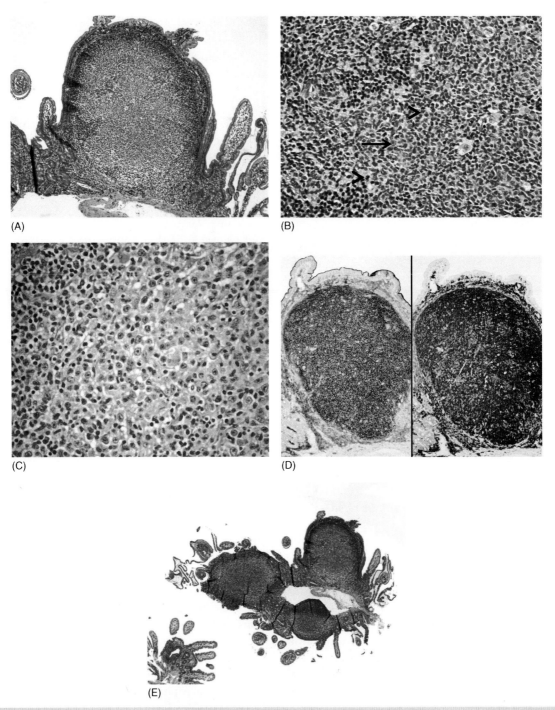

FIGURE 9.24 Follicular lymphoma involving the small intestine. Here, a nodular lymphoid aggregate with a follicular architecture expands the enteric mucosa (A). At high magnification (B), the infiltrate of follicular lymphoma contains a mixture of small cells with irregular nuclear contours (centrocytes) and larger cells with more vesicular nuclei and prominent nucleoli (centroblasts; arrow). The centrocytes often have a nuclear indentation or cleft ("cleaved" nuclei; arrowhead), which is best seen by changing the plane of focus slightly under the microscope. This low-grade case has a preponderance of centrocytes. Cases with sheets of large and pleomorphic cells that do not have a follicular pattern, such as this case (C), should be diagnosed as diffuse large B cell lymphoma (DLBCL). If other areas of the lymphoma have a recognizable precursor follicular lymphoma, this should be mentioned in the diagnosis, as the DLBCL is potentially curable, but the underlying follicular lymphoma may be relatively resistant to therapy. The neoplastic follicles in follicular lymphoma (D) are CD10 positive (left panel), indicating their follicle center cell phenotype. BCL-6 is also positive. Note the CD10 staining of the brush border on the luminal side of the epithelium as well. In addition, BCL-2 is positive in the neoplastic follicles (right panel), a useful feature in distinguishing follicular lymphoma (positive) from reactive follicular hyperplasia (negative). This duodenal follicular lymphoma (E) had a polypoid endoscopic appearance, which is reflected in the low-power histological appearance as well. In this case, the lymphoma was found only in the small intestine, making it a case of so-called "primary intestinal" follicular lymphoma.

TABLE 9.6 Grading Scheme for Follicular Lymphoma

Lymphoma Grade	Features	
1	0–5 centroblasts/HPF	Low grade
2	6–15 centroblasts/HPF	
3A	>15 centroblasts/HPF with centrocytes	High grade
3B	>15 centroblasts/HPF without centrocytes (ie, all centroblasts in follicular structures)	

Abbreviation: HPF = high-power field (40x objective). Counts are made by counting 10 HPF (when available) and dividing by 10.

As introduced in Chapter 4 and further discussed in Chapter 8, in association with DLBCL, a recently recognized subset of B cell lymphoma has been found to harbor genetic abnormalities *MYC*, as well as *BCL2* and/or *BCL6*. These so-called "double-hit" lymphomas are currently included in the nebulous category of "B cell lymphoma, unclassifiable, with features intermediate between diffuse large B cell lymphoma and Burkitt lymphoma" in the most recent (2008) WHO classification. These lymphomas may be categorized differently in subsequent WHO classifications but, for now, it is thought that their recognition and separation from BL and DLBCL has prognostic, and

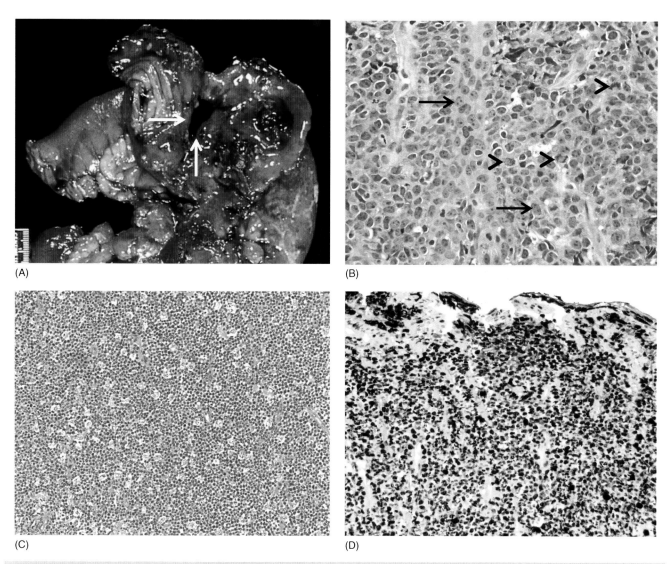

(A)

(B)

(C)

(D)

FIGURE 9.25 Burkitt lymphoma can cause clinically impressive changes, including large masses that grow at a seemingly impossible rate, and which can result in perforation (arrows) as in this case (A). Histologically, Burkitt lymphoma is composed of intermediate-sized lymphocytes that are quite monomorphic (B), with fine nuclear chromatin and, often, several inconspicuous nucleoli (arrows). The lymphoma has a brisk proliferative rate, as evidenced by several mitotic figures in this single field (arrowheads). The rapid proliferation of Burkitt lymphoma is also reflected in the so-called "starry sky" appearance at low magnification (C). The lighter colored "stars" in the monotonous field of lymphoma cells are tingible-body macrophages, which contain nuclear and cellular debris. The final confirmation of Burkitt lymphoma's impressive proliferative ability is a Ki-67 immunostain (D), which usually reveals a proliferative rate (as indicated by positive nuclear staining) of nearly 100%.

potentially therapeutic, significance, especially in younger patients. Double-hit lymphoma can strongly resemble BL, with a high proliferative rate (though usually not 100%) and a germinal center cell immunophenotype. It may be either BCL-2 positive or negative, and molecular assays for the genetic abnormalities described earlier in this paragraph are the only way to confirm the diagnosis at this point.

BL is a very clinically aggressive neoplasm. While this behavior leads to impressive and life-threatening clinical presentations, it also means that BL is potentially curable when subjected to appropriate therapy. Depending on patient age, long-term survival rates range from 70% to 90% when intensive chemotherapy is employed.

METASTASES TO THE SMALL BOWEL

Metastases to the small intestine are 2.5 times more common than primary small bowel carcinomas in large autopsy studies. The most common metastatic tumors to the small intestine include tumors from the skin (particularly melanoma), breast, ovary, lung, and pancreas.

Metastatic tumors typically present as intestinal wall thickening with submucosal spread, but may present as mucosal polyps or nodules (Figure 9.26A–C). In the latter situation, it can be challenging to distinguish metastatic from primary carcinomas, due to both morphologic overlap and to mucosal spread of some metastatic tumors, which mimics in situ growth and suggests an adenomatous precursor lesion. Because of this propensity for mucosal spread, the finding of an apparent precursor lesion and growth along a basement membrane cannot be reliably used to distinguish primary from metastatic lesions in the small bowel. This is especially problematic in cases of metastases from other sites in the GI or pancreaticobiliary tract, (Figure 9.27A–B) or gynecologic adenocarcinomas.

In most cases, the history and radiographic findings are sufficient to determine the site of origin in potentially metastatic cases. It can be extremely helpful to review the primary tumor if it is available for comparison. In difficult cases, immunohistochemical stains can be used to help determine the site of origin. An initial panel of CK7, CK20, and CDX2 is helpful in ascertaining the site of origin. Additional commonly used markers include TTF1

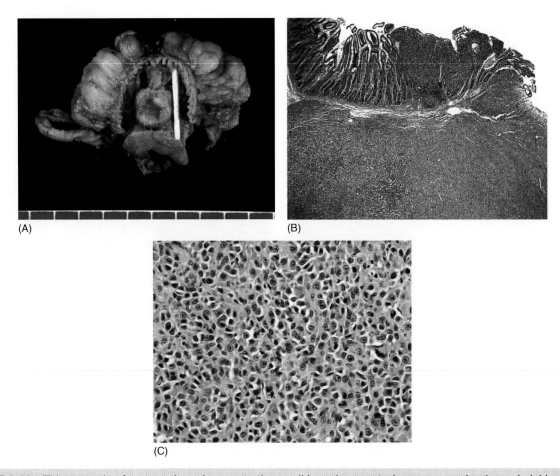

(A)

(B)

(C)

FIGURE 9.26 This example of metastatic melanoma to the small bowel presented as a mucosal polyp, mimicking a primary tumor (A). Another example of metastatic melanoma to the small bowel demonstrates a growth pattern centered in the submucosa, which extends into the surface epithelium (B). The tumor cells are dyscohesive with a plasmacytoid appearance and prominent nucleoli (C), typical of melanoma.

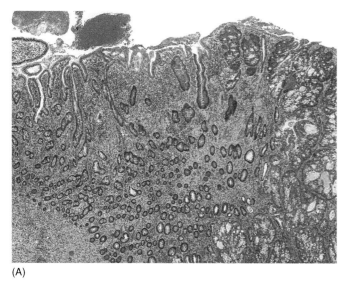
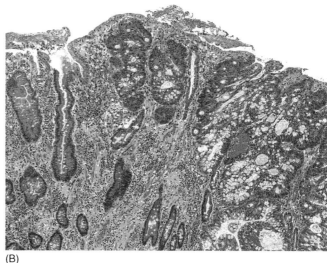

(A)   (B)

FIGURE 9.27   Intramucosal involvement of small intestine by a metastatic adenocarcinoma of the appendix (A). The metastatic tumor glands inconspicuously merge with the small intestinal epithelium at the surface (B) mimicking the in situ component of a small intestinal primary.

(lung, thyroid), ER/PR (breast, Müllerian), PAX8 (kidney, Müllerian, thyroid), p53 and WT1 (serous carcinoma with the latter also expressed by mesothelioma), napsin A (lung or papillary renal cell carcinoma), and prostate-specific antigen (prostate). Attention to the extent and intensity of the immunoreactivity is sometimes helpful in appreciating the subtle differences in those tumors with morphologic and frequent immunophenotypic similarities. As always, immunohistochemical stains are most useful when used in panels with attention to the clinical findings.

SELECTED REFERENCES

General

Ashley SW, Wells SA. Tumors of the small intestine. *Semin Oncol* 1988;15:116–128.

Bellizzi AM. Immunohistochemistry in gastroenterohepatopancreatobiliary epithelial neoplasia: Practical application, pitfalls, and emerging markers. *Surg Pathol Clin.* 2013;6:567–609.

Bosman F, Carneiro F, Hruban R, et al (Eds.). Tumours of the small intestine. In *World Health Organization Classification of Tumours of the Digestive System.* 4th ed. Lyon, France: IARC Press; 2010:chap 6.

Darling RC and Welch CE. Tumors of the small intestine. *N Engl J Med.* 1959;260:397–408.

Dye CE, Gaffney RR, Dykes TM, et al. Endoscopic and radiographic evaluation of the small bowel in 2012. *Am J Med.* 2012;125:1228. e1–1228.e12

Piscaglia AC, Campanale M, Gasbarrini G. Small bowel nonendocrine neoplasms: current concepts and novel perspectives. *Eur Rev Med Pharmacol Sci.* 2010;14:320–326.

Rampertab SD, Forde KA, Green PH. Small bowel neoplasia in coeliac disease. *Gut.* 2003;52:1211–1214.

Schottenfeld D, Beebe-Dimmer JL, Vigneau FD. The epidemiology and pathogenesis of neoplasia in the small intestine. *Ann Epidemiol.* 2009;19:58–69.

Siegel R, Naishadham D, Jemal A. Cancer statistics. *CA Cancer J Clin.* 2013;63:11–30.

Umar A, Boland R, Terdiman JP, et al. Revised Bethesda guidelines for hereditary nonpolyposis colorectal cancer (Lynch syndrome) and microsatellite instability. *J Nat Cancer Inst.* 2004;96:261–268.

van Ree K, Thurley P, Singh R, et al. The imaging features of small bowel tumours. *J Gastrointest Cancer.* 2012;43:405–412.

Reactive/Benign Lesions

Chen ZM, Scudiere JR, Abraham SC, et al. Pyloric gland adenoma: an entity distinct from gastric foveolar type adenoma. *Am J Surg Pathol.* 2009; 33:186–193.

Genta RM, Kinsey RS, Singhal A, et al. Gastric foveolar metaplasia and gastric heterotopia in the duodenum: no evidence of an etiologic role for Helicobacter pylori. *Hum Pathol.* 2012;41:1593–1600

Lambert MP, Heller DS, Bethel C. Extensive gastric heterotopia of the small intestine resulting in massive gastrointestinal bleeding, bowel perforation, and death: report of a case and review of the literature. *Pedatr Dev Pathol.* 2000;3:277–280.

Limaiem F, Haddad I, Marsaoui L, et al. Pancreatic heterotopia of the small intestine: two case reports. *Pathologica.* 2013;105:18–20.

Uppal K, Tubbs RS, Matusz P, et al. Meckel's diverticulum: a review. *Clin Anat.* 2011;24:416–422.

Hamartomatous Polyp Syndromes

Adolph VR and Bernabe K. Polyps in Children. *Clin Colon Rectal Surg.* 2008;21:280–285.

Arber N and Moshkowitz M. Small bowel polyposis syndromes. *Curr Gastroenterol Rep.* 2011;13:435–441.

McGarrity TJ and Amos C. Peutz-Jeghers syndrome: clinicopathology and molecular alterations. *Cell Mol Life Sci.* 2006;63: 2135–2144.

Adenomatous Polyps

Genta RM, Feagins LA. Advanced precancerous lesions in the small bowel mucosa. *Best Pract Res Clin Gastroenterol.* 2013;27:225–233.

Jass JR. Colorectal polyposes: from phenotype to diagnosis. *Pathol Res Pract.* 2008;204:431–447.

Kadmon M, Tandara A, Herfarth C. Duodenal adenomatosis in familial adenomatous polyposis coli. A review of the literature and results from the Heidelberg Polyposis Register. *Int J Colorectal Dis.* 2001; 16:63–75

Koornstra JJ. Small bowel endoscopy in familial adenomatous polyposis and Lynch syndrome. *Best Pract Res Clin Gastroenterol.* 2012;26:359–368.

Martin JA and Haber GB. Ampullary adenoma: clinical manifestations, diagnosis, and treatment. *Gastrointest Endosc Clin N Am.* 2003;13:649–669

Adenocarcinoma

Benhammane H, El M'rabet FZ, Idrissi Serhouchni K, et al. Small bowel adenocarcinoma complicating coeliac disease: a report of three cases and the literature review. *Case Rep Oncol Med.* 2012;2012:935183.

Bilimoria KY, Bentrem DJ, Wayne JD, et al. Small bowel cancer in the United States: changes in epidemiology, treatment, and survival over the last 20 years. *Ann Surg.* 2009;249:63–71.

Canavan C, Abrams KR, Mayberry J. Meta-analysis: colorectal and small bowel cancer risk in patients with Crohn's disease. *Aliment Pharmacol Ther.* 2006;23:1097–1104.

Chang HK, Yu E, Kim J, et al. Adenocarcinoma of the small intestine: a multi-institutional study of 197 surgically resected cases. *Hum Pathol.* 2010;41:1087–1096.

Diosdado B, Buffart TE, Watkins R, et al. High-resolution array comparative genomic hybridization in sporadic and celiac disease-related small bowel adenocarcinomas. *Clin Cancer Res.* 2010;16:1391–401.

Edge SB, Byrd DR, Compton CC, Fritz AG, Greene FL, Trotti A eds. *AJCC cancer staging manual.* New York, NY: Springer; 2010.

Fu T, Pappou EP, Guzzetta AA, et al. CpG island methylator phenotype-positive tumors in the absence of MLH1 methylation constitute a distinct subset of duodenal adenocarcinomas and are associated with poor prognosis. *Clin Cancer Res.* 2012;18:4743–4752.

Goodman MT, Matsuno RK, Shvetsov YB. Racial and ethnic variation in the incidence of small-bowel cancer subtypes in the United States, 1995-2008. *Dis Colon Rectum.* 2013;56:441–448.

Green PH, Rampertab SD. Small bowel carcinoma and coeliac disease. *Gut.* 2004; 53:774.

Haan JC, Buffart TE, Eijk PP, et al. Small bowel adenocarcinoma copy number profiles are more closely related to colorectal than to gastric cancers. *Ann Oncol.* 2012;23:367–374.

Neely D, Ong J, Patterson J, et al. Small intestinal adenocarcinoma: rarely considered, often missed? *Postgrad Med J.* 2013;89: 197–201.

Nilubol N, Scherl E, Bub DS, et al. Mucosal dysplasia in ileal pelvic pouches after restorative proctocolectomy. *Dis Colon Rectum.* 2007;50:825–831.

Overman MJ, Hu CY, Kopetz S, et al. A population-based comparison of adenocarcinoma of the large and small intestine: insights into a rare disease. *Ann Surg Oncol.* 2012;19:1439–1445.

Overman MJ, Hu CY, Wolff RA, et al. Prognostic value of lymph node evaluation in small bowel adenocarcinoma: analysis of the surveillance, epidemiology, and end results database. *Cancer.* 2010;116:5374–5382.

Overman MJ. Rare but real. Management of Small Bowel Adenocarcinoma. *Am Soc Clin Oncol Educ Book.* 2013:189–193.

Pan SY and Morrison H. Epidemiology of cancer of the small intestine. *World J Gastrointest Oncol.* 2011;3:33–42.

Planck M, Ericson K, Piotrowska Z, et al. Microsatellite instability and expression of MLH1 and MSH2 in carcinomas of the small intestine. *Cancer.* 2003;97:1551–1557.

Potter DD, Murray JA, Donohue JH, et al. The role of defective mismatch repair in small bowel adenocarcinoma in celiac disease. *Cancer Res.* 2004;64:7073–7077.

Raghav K, Overman MJ. Small bowel adenocarcinomas—existing evidence and evolving paradigms. *Nat Rev Clin Oncol.* 2013;10:534–544.

Richir M, Songun I, Wientjes C, et al. Small Bowel Adenocarcinoma in a Patient with Coeliac Disease: Case Report and Review of the Literature. *Case Rep Gastroenterol.* 2010;4:416–420.

Zouhairi ME, Venner A, Charabaty A, et al. Small bowel adenocarcinoma. *Curr Treat Options Oncol.* 2008;9:388–399.

Neuroendocrine Tumors

Klimstra DS. Pathology reporting of neuroendocrine tumors: essential elements for accurate diagnosis, classification, and staging. *Semin Oncol.* 2013;40:23–36.

Maggard MA, O'Connell JB, Ko CY. Updated population-based review of carcinoid tumors. *Ann Surg.* 2004;240:117–122.

Soga J, Tazawa K. Pathologic analysis of carcinoids. Histologic reevaluation of 62 cases. *Cancer.* 1971;28:990–998.

Soga J. Carcinoids of the small intestine: a statistical evaluation of 1102 cases collected from the literature. *J Exp Clin Cancer Res.* 1997;16:353–363

Strosberg J. Neuroendocrine tumours of the small intestine. *Best Pract Res Clin Gastroenterol.* 2012;26:755–773.

Yang Z, Tang LH, Klimstra DS. Gastroenteropancreatic neuroendocrine neoplasms: historical context and current issues. *Semin Diagn Pathol.* 2013;30:186–196.

Yantiss RK, Odze RD, Farraye FA, et al. Solitary versus multiple carcinoid tumors of the ileum: a clinical and pathologic review of 69 cases. *Am J Surg Pathol.* 2003;27:811–817.

Yao JC, Hassan M, Phan A, et al. One hundred years after "carcinoid": epidemiology of and prognostic factors for neuroendocrine tumors in 35,825 cases in the United States. *J Clin Oncol.* 2008;26:3063–3072.

Mesenchymal Tumors

Akbulut S. Intussusception due to inflammatory fibroid polyp: a case report and comprehensive literature review. *World J Gastroenterol.* 2012; 18:5745–5752

Al Ali J, Ko HH, Owen D, et al. Epithelioid angiosarcoma of the small bowel. *Gastrointest Endosc* 2006; 64:1018–1021

Arora M, Goldberg EM. Kaposi sarcoma involving the gastrointestinal tract. *Gastroenterol Hepatol (NY)* 2010; 6:459–462

Boyle L, Lack EE. Solitary cavernous hemangioma of small intestine. Case report and literature review. *Arch Pathol Lab Med.* 1993; 117:939–941

Cabaud PG and Harris LT. Lipomatosis of the Ileocecal Valve. *Ann Surg.* 1959;150:1092–1098.

Chang CW, Wang TE, Chang WH, et al. Unusual presentation of desmoid tumor in the small intestine: a case report. *Med Oncol.* 2011;28:159–162

Chatterjee C, Khan D, U De. A rare presentation of gastrointestinal stromal tumors as a small bowel perforation: A single institution based clinical experience of three cases. *J Dr. NTR Univ. Health Sci.* 2013;2:118–121

Corless CL. Gastrointestinal stromal tumors: what do we know now? *Mod Pathol.* 2014;Suppl 1: S1–S16

Miettinen M, Lasota J. Gastrointestinal stromal tumors: review on morphology, molecular pathology, prognosis, and differential diagnosis. *Arch Pathol Lab Med.* 2006;130:1466–1478.

Morris-Stiff G, Falk GA, EL-Hayek K, et al. Jejunal cavernous lymphangioma. *BJM Case Rep.* 2011; pii:bcr0320114022

Ni Q, Shang D, Peng H, et al. Primary angiosarcoma of the small intestine with metastasis to the liver: a case report and review of the literature. *World J Surg Oncol.* 2013; 11:242

Pahwa M, Girotra M, Rautela A, et al. Periampullary leiomyosarcoma presenting with cutaneous metastases: a rare entity. *South Med J.* 2010;103:1190–1191

Rampone B, Pedrazzani C, Marrelli D, et al. Updates on abdominal desmoid tumors. *World J Gastroenterol.* 2007;13:5985–5988

Regula J, Wronska E, Pachlewski J. Vascular lesions of the gastrointestinal tract. *Best Pract Res Clin Gastroenterol.* 2008; 22: 313–328

Stockman DL, Miettinen M, Suster S, et al. Malignant gastrointestinal neuroectodermal tumor: clinicopathologic, immunohistochemical, ultrastructural, and molecular analysis of 16 cases with a reappraisal of clear cell sarcoma-like tumors of the gastrointestinal tract. *Am J Surg Pathol.* 2012;36:857–868

Suryawanshi KH, Patil TB, Damle RP, et al. Gastrointestinal stromal tumour of small intestine presenting as a mesenteric mass. *J Clin Diagn Res.* 2014;8:FD14–FD16

Wysocki AP, Taylor G, Windsor JA. Inflammatory fibroid polyps of the duodenum: a review of the literature. *Dig Surg.* 2007; 24:162–168

Hematolymphoid Neoplasms

Burke JS. Lymphoproliferative disorders of the gastrointestinal tract: a review and pragmatic guide to diagnosis. *Arch Pathol Lab Med.* 2011;135:1283–1297.

Damaj G, Verkarre V, Delmer A, et al. Primary follicular lymphoma of the gastrointestinal tract: a study of 25 cases and a literature review. *Ann Oncol.* 2003;14:623–629.

Hawkes EA, Wotherspoon A, Cunningham D. Diagnosis and management of rare gastrointestinal lymphomas. *Leuk Lymphoma.* 2012;53:2341–2350.

O'Malley DP, Goldstein NS, Banks PM. The recognition and classification of lymphoproliferative disorders of the gut. *Hum Pathol.* 2014;45:899–916.

Smith LB, Owens SR. Gastrointestinal lymphomas: entities and mimics. *Arch Pathol Lab Med.* 2012;136:865–870.

Swerdlow SH, Jaffe ES, Brousset P, et al. Cytotoxic T-cell and NK-cell lymphomas: current questions and controversies. *Am J Surg Pathol.* 2014;38:e60–e71.

Metastases

Disibio G, French SW. Metastatic patterns of cancers: results from a large autopsy study. *Arch Pathol Lab Med.* 2008;132:931–939.

Estrella JS, Wu TT, Rashid A, et al. Mucosal colonization by metastatic carcinoma in the gastrointestinal tract: a potential mimic of primary neoplasia. *Am J Surg Pathol.* 2011;35:563–572.

Hess KR, Varadhachary GR, Taylor SH, et al. Metastatic patterns in adenocarcinoma. *Cancer.* 2006;106:1624–1633.

Lianos GD, Messinis T, Doumos R, et al. A patient presenting with acute abdomen due to metastatic small bowel melanoma: a case report. *J Med Case Rep.* 2013; 7:216.

Newton RC, Penney N, Nind N, et al. Small bowel malignant melanoma presenting as a perforated jejunal diverticulum: a case report and literature review. *Gastroenterol Rep (Oxf).* 2014; pii:gou058. [Epub ahead of print]

Sundersingh S, Majhi U, Chandrasekar SK, et al. Metastatic malignant melanoma of the small bowel-report of two cases. *J Gastrointest Cancer.* 2012;43:332–335.

10

Neoplasms of the Appendix

RHONDA K. YANTISS

INTRODUCTION

Most appendiceal neoplasms are incidentally detected in appendectomy or colectomy specimens obtained for other indications. Slightly more than 50% of tumors are neuroendocrine tumors (NETs), most of which share biochemical properties with similar lesions of the distal small intestine. The majority of the remaining non-neuroendocrine appendiceal tumors are mucinous in nature, whereas nonmucinous neoplasms, including serrated lesions, villous adenomas, and nonmucinous adenocarcinomas, are relatively less common.

Mucinous neoplasms are usually limited to the mucosa (ie, adenomas), but they may invade the appendiceal wall or disseminate in the peritoneal cavity, resulting in substantial disease-related morbidity and mortality despite the relatively bland appearance of neoplastic epithelium. The discordance between the histologic features and biologic behavior among mucinous tumors, and the infrequent nature of nonmucinous lesions, has generated considerable confusion regarding their nomenclature and classification.

NEUROENDOCRINE TUMORS OF THE APPENDIX

Overview

Neuroendocrine tumors (NETs) are identified in less than 1% of patients undergoing appendectomy, and are more common among adults. Patients tend to be slightly younger than those with other NETs of the gastrointestinal tract, and lesions show a slight female predominance. It is likely that these features reflect the frequency of appendectomy procedures among young patients and women undergoing gynecologic surgery.

Enterochromaffin (EC) Cell Neuroendocrine Tumors

As mentioned in Chapter 3, the majority of appendiceal NETs are composed of serotonin-producing enterochromaffin (EC) cells, similar to jejunoileal tumors. Previously, these tumors have been known as "classic" carcinoid tumors. These tumors show a predilection for the distal appendiceal tip, where they form solitary yellow nodules (Figure 10.1A–B). They are unencapsulated, well-circumscribed aggregates of tightly packed nests and acini (Figure 10.2A–B), the latter of which harbor luminal material that is positive for periodic acid–Schiff stain, but do not contain mucin. Tumor cells contain abundant faintly eosinophilic or clear cytoplasm and are both argentaffin and argyrophil positive. Some tumor cells contain brightly eosinophilic cytoplasmic granules. The nuclei are typically round with a stippled chromatin pattern likened to "salt and pepper." Nucleoli tend to be small, but conspicuous, and mitotic figures are infrequent. Occasional tumors display degenerative-type nuclear atypia with hyperchromasia and multinucleation, which has no bearing on their biologic behavior. EC cells show strong immunopositivity for chromogranin A, synaptophysin, and serotonin. Most (70%) of these NETs are smaller than 1 cm in diameter and show a very low Ki-67 proliferation index (less than 1%).

Enteroglucagon (L) Cell Endocrine Tumors

Approximately 10% to 20% of appendiceal NETs are composed of enteroglucagon (L) cells. These tumors are small (2–3 mm) nodules composed of trabeculae and cords of cytologically bland tumor cells. Some tumors display a predominantly acinar, or tubular, growth pattern with inspissated mucin; hence their previous classification as tubular

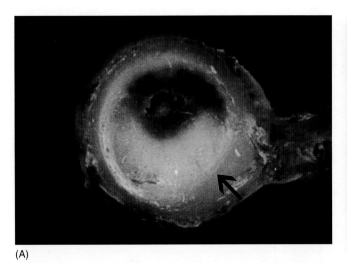

(A)

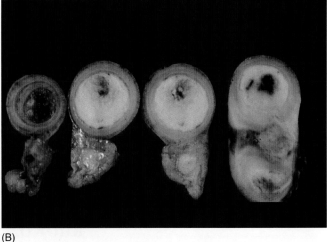

(B)

FIGURE 10.1 This appendiceal neuroendocrine (carcinoid) tumor forms a yellow nodule in the distal appendix. The tumor obliterates the muscularis propria (arrow) (A, courtesy of Dr. Henry Appelman). This appendix cut in cross section illustrates the firm, yellow appearance of the carcinoid tumor on the cut section. The tumor infiltrates the mesoappendix (B, courtesy of Dr. George Gray).

NETs or tubular carcinoids (Figure 10.2C–D). Lesions with either a trabecular or tubular appearance harbor enteroglucagons, glucagon-like peptides, pancreatic polypeptide, and peptide YY. Small red basophilic neuroendocrine granules may be visible. The tumor cells are argyrophilic and show immunopositivity for chromogranin B, glucagon, and carcinoembryonic antigen (CEA) but do not stain for chromogranin A. The Ki-67 proliferation index is usually very low. Because of the infiltrative growth pattern and the lack of chromogranin A expression, tubular carcinoids may be mistaken for metastatic carcinoma.

Pathologic Reporting of Appendiceal Endocrine Tumors

Appendiceal neuroendocrine neoplasms are now included in the *American Joint Committee on Cancer Staging Manual* and, thus, should be graded and staged in accordance with the Tumor Nodes Metastases (TNM) staging system. Grading is determined based on a combination of mitotic activity and immunolabeling with Ki-67, as discussed in Chapter 3, and thus Ki-67 staining should be performed in all cases. Other important criteria, such as the status of the resection margin, presence of lymphovascular invasion, and involvement of mesoappendiceal soft tissues, should also be included in surgical pathology reports.

Biologic Behavior and Management

Appendiceal NETs usually behave in a benign fashion, especially if they are small. Indeed, less than 1% of tumors spanning less than 2 cm metastasize. Those that do behave aggressively first spread to regional lymph nodes followed by the liver, similar to NETs of other organs in the gastrointestinal tract. Tumors that metastasize to the liver or produce bulky peritoneal disease may produce the carcinoid syndrome. Management decisions are largely based on tumor size. Small lesions (up to 1 cm in diameter) are adequately treated with appendectomy alone, provided the resection margin is negative. Right colectomy with lymph node dissection is generally limited to tumors larger than 2 cm or those with vascular invasion since these tumors have a greater likelihood of regional lymph node involvement. Management of tumors ranging from 1 to 2 cm in diameter is somewhat controversial. Completely resected tumors may be treated with appendectomy and clinical follow-up. Features suggestive of aggressive behavior (eg, invasion of the mesoappendix, vascular invasion, mitotic activity, and high Ki-67 labeling) may prompt right colectomy and lymph node dissection, although the added benefit of extensive surgery in these patients has not been clearly documented in the literature.

MUCINOUS NEOPLASMS OF THE APPENDIX AND PERITONEUM

Overview

The low-grade features of appendiceal mucinous neoplasms and confusing, descriptive terminology used to classify them have led to several misconceptions regarding their biologic potential. Older reports described appendiceal adenomas that metastasized to the abdomen,

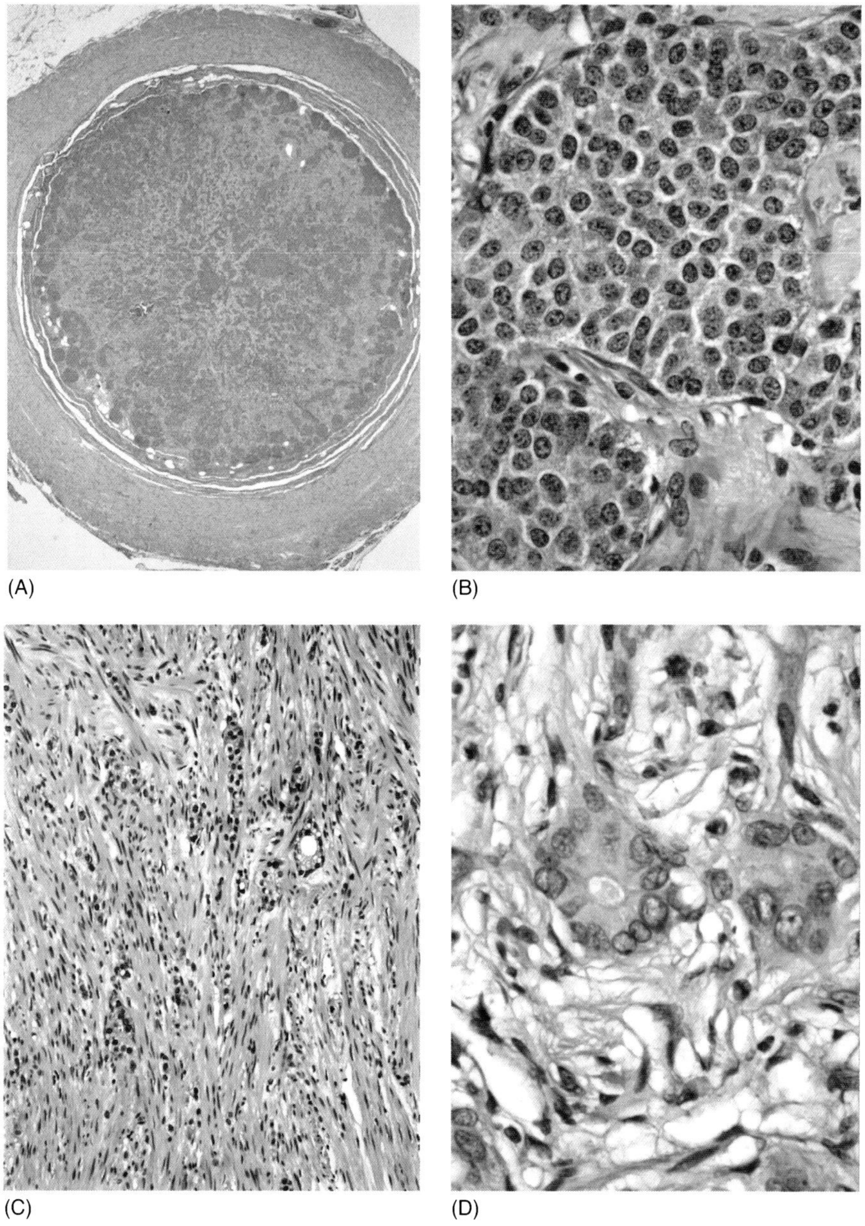

FIGURE 10.2   This classic neuroendocrine tumor forms a nodule in the distal appendix, obliterating the lumen and expanding the submucosa. The tumor consists of cellular nests enmeshed in collagenous stroma (A). Lesional cells contain abundant, faintly eosinophilic cytoplasm and round nuclei with stippled chromatin and small nuclei (B). In contrast to classic tumors, hindgut neuroendocrine tumors contain cords and clusters of cells in a fibroblast-rich, cellular stroma (C). Some of these lesions contain small acinar structures and tubules. Lesional cells are polarized around a central lumen. The nuclei have smooth contours and small nucleoli (D).

producing clinical findings of pseudomyxoma peritonei, which resulted in their historical classification as tumors of uncertain malignant potential or adenomucinosis. However, it is now clear that mucinous tumors confined to the appendiceal mucosa are generally benign with no biologic risk, whereas those with peritoneal mucin deposits pursue an indolent but relentless course and thus many authors classify these tumors as well-differentiated mucinous carcinomas for treatment and staging purposes. Criteria for classification of appendiceal mucinous

tumors that have not yet seeded the peritoneum, but extend into the appendiceal wall or show mucin on the serosal surface, remain poorly defined and somewhat controversial.

Mucinous Adenoma and Mucinous Cystadenoma

Some appendiceal adenomas do not produce any gross abnormalities, whereas others cause localized or fusiform appendiceal dilatation (Figure 10.3A–C). Although these lesions have been termed mucinous cystadenomas in the past, they are now mostly considered to be adenomas. By definition, mucinous adenomas are confined to the appendiceal mucosa and, with rare exception, do not display mucin on the serosal surface (Figure 10.3D). Some authors require the presence of intact muscularis mucosae to make a diagnosis of adenoma, and consider atrophy and fibrosis of the mucosa and muscularis mucosae to be evidence of low-grade appendiceal mucinous neoplasms (LAMNs; Figure 10.3E). Adenomas generally lack complex architectural features. They frequently contain flat or undulating epithelium, but villous projections are present in many cases. The crypts have straight luminal edges similar to those of the non-neoplastic appendix. Some lesions contain crypts with a serrated appearance near the lumen.

Most adenomas display low-grade cytologic atypia characterized by nuclear hyperchromasia and pseudostratification with rare mitotic figures. High-grade dysplasia is uncommon, and is characterized by architectural abnormalities, including cribriform and micropapillary growth, as well as nuclear pleomorphism with loss of cell polarity and readily identifiable mitotic figures. Appendiceal mucinous adenomas are cured by appendectomy regardless of the degree of dysplasia. However, some authors have proposed that adenoma at the surgical resection margin warrants concern for recurrent disease or metastasis, and consider such tumors to have uncertain malignant potential or low risk for recurrence. Submission of the entire appendix is recommended in cases of mucinous adenoma, in order to exclude the possibility of extra-appendiceal epithelium and/or mucin.

Low-Grade Appendiceal Mucinous Neoplasm

Low-grade appendiceal mucinous neoplasm (LAMN) is a term applied to appendiceal mucinous tumors that show features portending increased risk of peritoneal dissemination. They may appear grossly unremarkable or produce a cystically dilated appendix filled with tenacious mucin, resembling a mucinous (cyst)adenoma (Figure 10.4A–C). Grossly visible mucin on the serosal surface is an important finding and, if present, should be submitted entirely for histologic evaluation to document the presence, or absence, of extra-appendiceal neoplastic epithelium. Appendices that are encased in mucin, or essentially replaced by mucinous neoplasia, are highly likely to represent mucinous adenocarcinomas associated with peritoneal tumor deposits.

The histologic features of LAMNs are poorly defined. Some authors use this terminology to describe lesions limited to the luminal epithelium of the appendix that show mucosal alterations, such as atrophy or fibrosis of the mucosa and muscularis mucosae with hyalinization or calcification (Figure 10.4D). This term has also been used to

denote lesions confined to the mucosa that show neoplastic mucinous epithelium with a villous, undulating, or flat appearance at the luminal surface (Figure 10.5A). Others, including the World Health Organization, use the term "low-grade appendiceal mucinous neoplasm" to describe cases that show mucin and/or epithelium that shows a broad "pushing" front, rather than an infiltrative pattern of invasion (Figure 10.5B–D), as well as those that display low-grade malignant mucinous epithelium in the peritoneum (ie, pseudomyxoma peritonei). Opponents of the latter argue that although application of this terminology to such a broad spectrum of lesions, ranging from those that are clearly benign to those that behave in a malignant fashion, makes classification easier, its clinical utility is limited.

In our practice, we use the term "low-grade appendiceal mucinous neoplasm" to describe situations in which there is uncertainty regarding biologic risk, namely those cases containing mucin pools (but no neoplastic epithelium) that transgress the muscularis mucosae and extend into the appendiceal wall or onto the serosal surface, but are confined to the right lower quadrant. We classify lesions entirely confined to the mucosa as mucinous adenomas, and those with peritoneal tumor deposits as low-grade mucinous adenocarcinomas. In our experience, the overwhelming majority of appendiceal mucinous tumors are amenable to this classification scheme, which allows one to clearly convey information to the clinicians regarding biologic risk. However, as mentioned in the previous section, accurate classification depends on adequate gross evaluation and sectioning as well as careful histologic examination.

Mucinous neoplasms that transgress the muscularis mucosae and show high-grade cytology are classified as high-grade mucinous adenocarcinomas, regardless of growth pattern, and should never be considered in the spectrum of LAMN. High-grade lesions infrequently produce the clinical appearance of pseudomyxoma peritonei and are less likely to respond to cytoreductive surgery and chemotherapy. Of note, both low- and high-grade tumors that extend beyond the muscularis mucosae are staged as adenocarcinomas in the seventh edition of the *American Joint Committee on Cancer (AJCC) Staging Manual*. In other words, cases classified as either LAMN or well-differentiated mucinous carcinoma are similarly staged in the TNM system.

Mucinous tumors associated with acellular mucin confined to the right lower quadrant have an extremely low risk of progression to pseudomyxoma peritonei, whereas one-third of patients with *any amount of neoplastic epithelium* outside the appendix develop peritoneal dissemination that can result in the death of the patient. For this reason, low-grade appendiceal mucinous neoplasms with periappendiceal mucin should be submitted entirely for histologic evaluation, in order to exclude the presence of extra-appendiceal neoplastic epithelium. Management of patients with extra-appendiceal mucin limited to the periappendiceal region is controversial. They should undergo

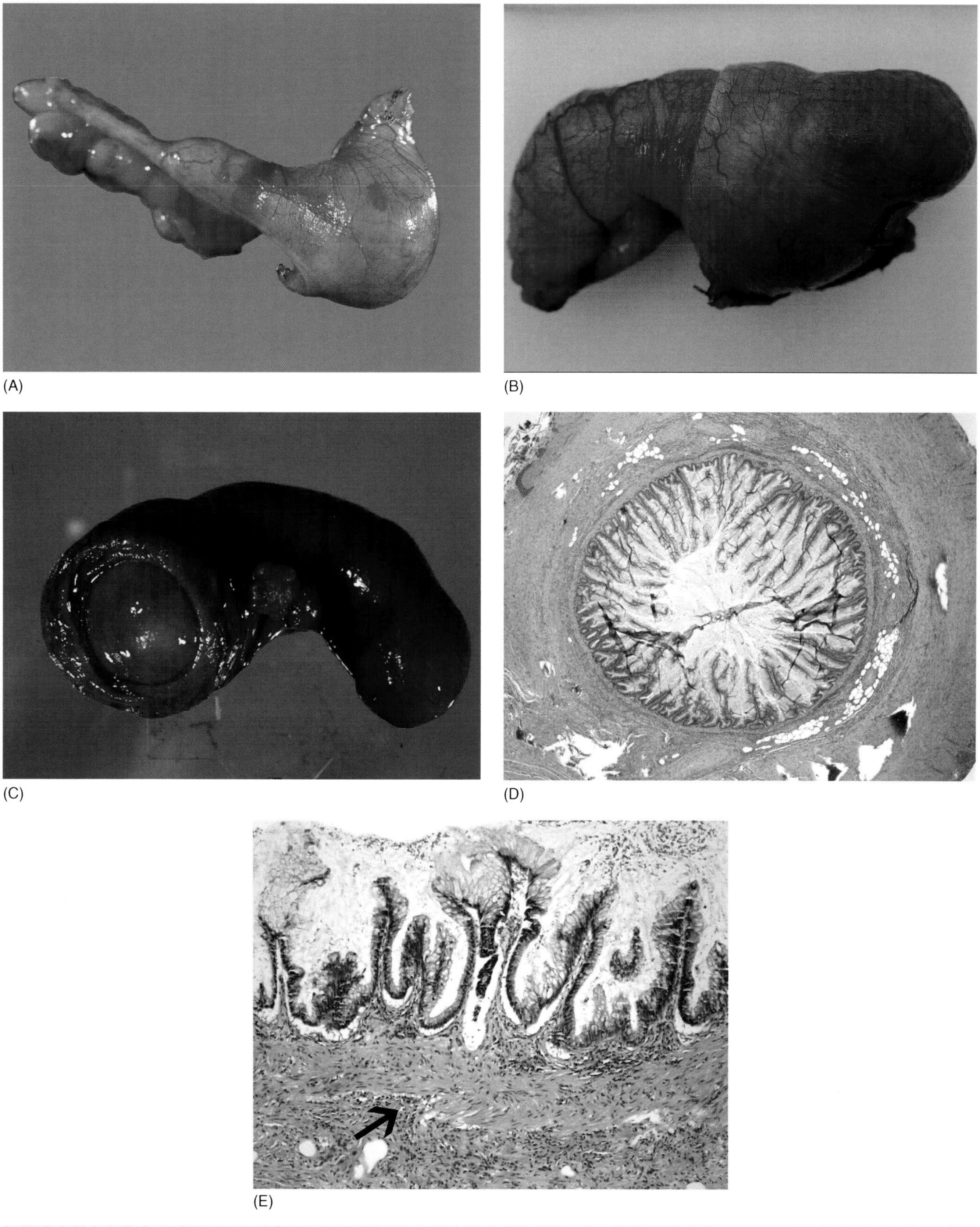

(A)

(B)

(C)

(D)

(E)

FIGURE 10.3 Mucinous cystadenomas cause localized (A) or fusiform (B–C) dilatation of the appendix (C, courtesy of Dr. George Gray). This adenoma has circumferential villous architecture and is surrounded by an intact muscularis mucosae (D). Higher magnification reveals diminished lamina propria and lymphoid tissue overlying the muscularis mucosae (arrow). The submucosa is slightly cellular and fibrotic (E).

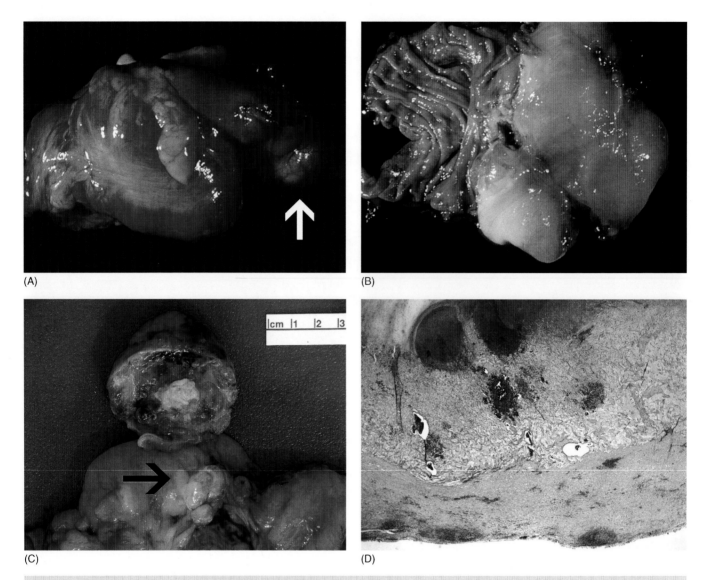

FIGURE 10.4 A low-grade appendiceal mucinous neoplasm distends the appendix (arrow), but is not associated with extra-appendiceal mucin (A). Opening the appendix of the same case reveals copious amounts of tenacious mucin (B). Cross sections through another mucinous tumor reveal distention of the appendix by thick mucinous secretions (C). Although one may consider a diagnosis of either mucinous (cyst)adenoma or low-grade mucinous neoplasm based on these features, careful examination of the pericolic fat reveals mucinous nodules in the colonic mesentery (arrow), and additional biopsies from the peritoneum reveal disseminated disease. Thus, this lesion is best classified as a low-grade mucinous adenocarcinoma. Sections through the wall of a low-grade appendiceal neoplasm demonstrate extensive denudation of the surface epithelium with pools of dissecting mucin in the wall. The muscularis propria is largely effaced and replaced by fibrosis with lymphoid aggregates (D).

radiographic surveillance to evaluate for development of mucinous ascites, but there are no data to support cytoreductive surgery with intraperitoneal chemotherapy as a preventive measure, and right colectomy offers no survival benefit over appendectomy alone.

Mucinous Adenocarcinoma and Pseudomyxoma Peritonei

Pseudomyxoma peritonei is a descriptive term denoting mucin accumulation in the peritoneal cavity. Most cases develop secondary to the spread of low-grade mucinous tumors of the appendix, although rare cases are associated with origins from other sites (eg, ovary). Mucin accumulates in dependent areas, including the greater omentum, under the right hemidiaphragm, behind the liver, and left abdominal gutter and pelvis (Figure 10.6A). Patients are usually older adults, and women are reportedly affected more frequently than men, although this difference may reflect a reporting bias in relatively small series of patients presenting to gynecologic oncologists with ovarian involvement.

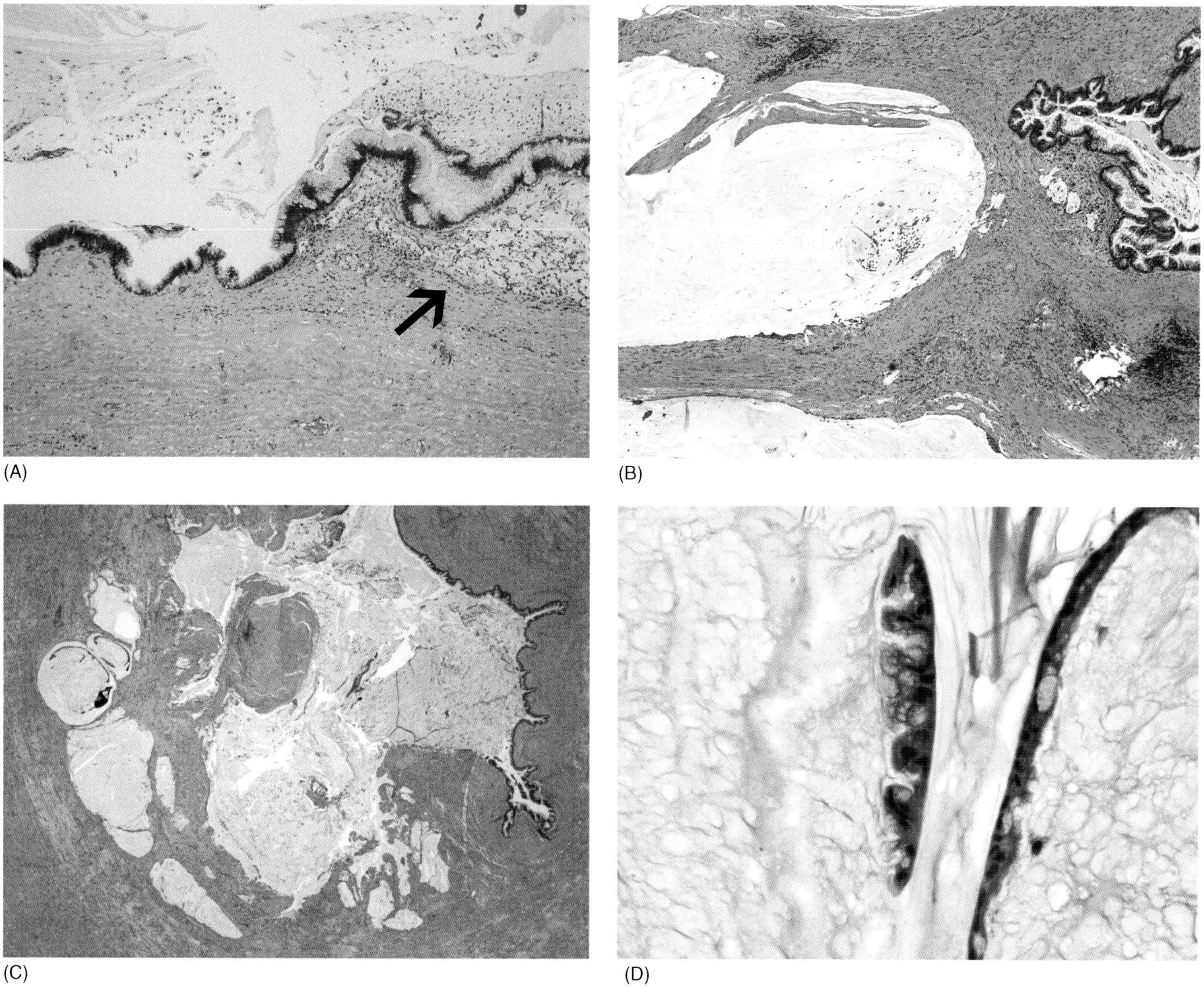

FIGURE 10.5 This low-grade appendiceal mucinous neoplasm is lined by undulating epithelium that rests on fibrotic connective tissue without an apparent lamina propria or muscularis mucosae. Dissecting mucin is present subjacent to the epithelium (arrow), which shows low-grade cytologic features (A). Another mucinous neoplasm is associated with large mucin pools in the appendiceal wall (B). This same mucinous tumor also displays round mucin pools confined to the appendiceal wall (C). The pools contain strips of low-grade epithelium that warrant a diagnosis of at least low-grade appendiceal mucinous neoplasm, although the AJCC classifies this type of lesion as a carcinoma for staging purposes (D).

Peritoneal tumor deposits are morphologically similar to the primary appendiceal tumor in most cases. Low-grade lesions consist of mucin pools containing scant strips of mucinous epithelium with mild cytologic atypia and a paucity of mitotic activity (Figure 10.6B–C). The background tissue is abnormal, frequently showing hyalinized bands of collagen and reactive fibrosis around mucin pools.

Although distinguishing criteria between low- and high-grade neoplasms are not well-defined, tumors that show more abundant epithelium in mucin pools or destructive tissue invasion with infiltrative tumor cells should be classified as high-grade mucinous carcinomas (Figure 10.6D–F).

High-grade features also include solid cell clusters that display nuclear enlargement and hyperchromasia, single cell necrosis and mitotic activity (Figure 10.6F). Single infiltrating signet ring cells are believed to be a poor prognostic factor and, if present, should be specifically mentioned. Peritoneal deposits that show high-grade features with a desmoplastic tissue response (Figure 10.6E) and lymph node metastases only rarely represent metastases arising from low-grade mucinous appendiceal tumors, although progression from low-grade to high-grade cytologic atypia does occur in patients who develop multiple tumor recurrences or those who fail treatment. Indeed, the presence of high-grade epithelial atypia in peritoneal deposits should

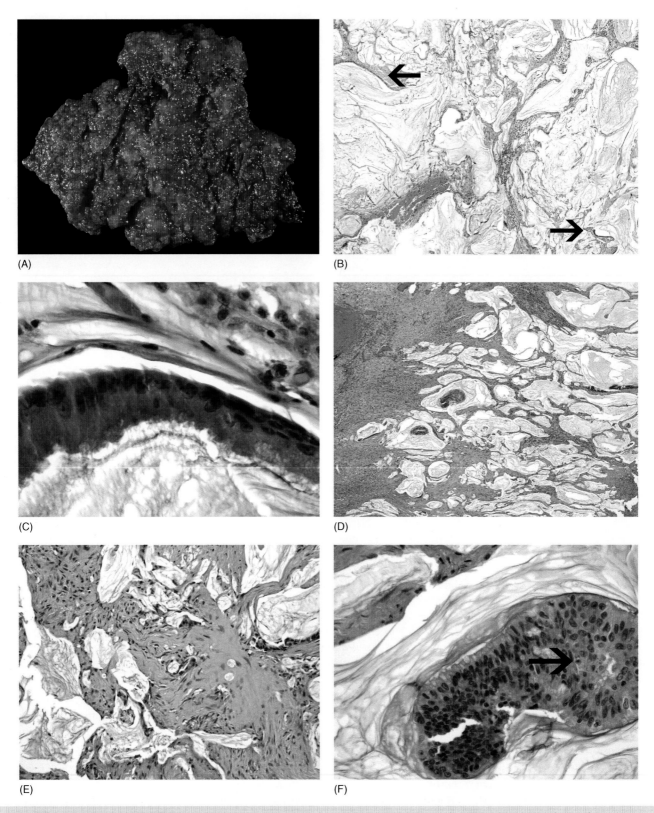

FIGURE 10.6 Low-grade appendiceal mucinous adenocarcinomas spread to the peritoneal cavity in the form of mucinous ascites (ie, pseudomyxoma peritonei). They have a tendency to spare the bowel surfaces early in the course of disease, but commonly affect the omentum, producing confluent mucinous nodules (A). Although the criteria used to distinguish between low- and high-grade neoplasms are not well-defined, low-grade lesions should contain rare strips of epithelium (arrow) in otherwise paucicellular mucin pools (B). Lesional cells are polarized with abundant cytoplasm and small nuclei, without appreciable mitotic activity (C). Tumors that show more abundant epithelium in mucin pools (D) or destructive tissue invasion with infiltrative tumor cells and glands (E) are best classified as mucinous carcinomas. High-grade features include solid cell clusters that display nuclear enlargement and hyperchromasia, single cell necrosis (arrow), and mitotic activity (F).

lead one to suspect a nonappendiceal origin, such as the small bowel, colon, or pancreas. Alternatively, such lesions may represent peritoneal metastases from nonmucinous appendiceal carcinomas.

Most patients with peritoneal mucinous adenocarcinoma develop multiple tumor recurrences that require several interventions and lead to extensive adhesions that prohibit further abdominal therapy. The natural history of the disease is dictated by tumor grade and pathologic stage. Patients with low-grade mucinous adenocarcinoma in the peritoneum have 5- and 10-year survival rates of 75% and 68%, compared to approximately 55% and 13%, respectively, for high-grade carcinomas. Aggressive modern therapeutic approaches include a combination of surgery and intra-abdominal chemotherapy. Surgical peritonectomy with resection of multiple organs (eg, omentum, spleen, gallbladder, some, or all of the affected stomach, colon, and small bowel, uterus, ovaries, and fallopian tubes) is aimed at complete tumor cytoreduction. Chemotherapy is in the form of hyperthermic intra-operative intraperitoneal chemotherapy (HIPEC) supplemented by additional cycles of early postoperative intraperitoneal chemotherapy (EPIC). Five-year survival rates of 86% are achievable among low-grade tumors that are treated with cytoreductive surgery and chemotherapy compared to 50% for high-grade tumors. Complete cytoreduction improves survival compared to cases in which gross residual disease is left behind following surgery.

Ancillary Studies

Appendiceal mucinous neoplasms and pseudomyxoma peritonei usually show immunoexpression of cytokeratin (CK)20, CDX2, and MUC2, and up to 40% coexpress CK7. Appendiceal adenomas and mucinous adenocarcinomas show *KRAS* mutations in approximately 50% of cases, but do not harbor abnormalities in *BRAF*, *APC*, or *DCC*, or show microsatellite instability. Carcinomas may also have loss of heterozygosity or chromosome 18q mutations affecting *DPC4*, a tumor suppressor gene.

Differential Diagnosis of Appendiceal Mucinous Neoplasms

Several lesions that have no biologic risk can cause diagnostic confusion with appendiceal mucinous neoplasms. Some appendices contain mucosal hyperplasia that can be misinterpreted as a neoplasm, particularly when associated with other findings, such as mucus retention or diverticula. Non-neoplastic hyperplasia contains a mixed population of mucin-containing columnar epithelial cells without cytologic atypia or appreciable mitotic activity. Diverticula represent herniations of mucosa through the muscularis propria and are best appreciated at low magnification (Figure 10.7A–D). They may be solitary or multiple and occur in association with mucinous adenomas or in non-neoplastic appendices.

Diverticula are frequently encountered in association with mucinous adenomas, potentially reflecting increased intraluminal pressures resulting from inspissated mucin. When they occur in association with mucinous adenomas, diverticula can be confused with the "pushing front" of a low-grade appendiceal neoplasm, particularly if they are colonized by neoplastic epithelium. Features suggesting a diverticulum, rather than a LAMN, include the presence of non-neoplastic epithelial cells and/or lamina propria in the appendiceal wall or subserosa, continuity of mural epithelium with that lining the lumen, and an intact, normal-appearing muscularis propria. Denuded diverticula may appear as solitary mucin pools associated with lamina propria elements and variable inflammatory changes.

Appendiceal mucinous adenomas may be associated with rupture and extrusion of mucin onto the serosal surface, in which case a diagnosis of LAMN may be considered. Ruptured adenomas generally show a single focus of transmural extra-appendiceal mucin associated with attenuation of the appendiceal wall, striking inflammation and organizing granulation tissue at the serosal surface, and an absence of neoplastic epithelium on the serosa or in the appendiceal wall deep to the muscularis mucosae. Multifocal or extensive transgression of the muscularis mucosae by mucin pools, copious amounts of mucin on the serosal surface, mucin beyond the right lower quadrant, and extra-appendiceal neoplastic epithelium should be considered evidence of a LAMN at a minimum, and some would classify such a lesion as low-grade mucinous adenocarcinoma. Cases classified as "ruptured" adenomas should be submitted entirely for histologic evaluation and designated with a comment implying a low risk of recurrent disease and a need for clinical follow-up as appropriate.

NONMUCINOUS APPENDICEAL NEOPLASMS

Overview

Nonmucinous adenomas of the appendix generally resemble their colonic counterparts in that they display tubular, villous, or serrated crypt architecture. Most are asymptomatic and, thus, reporting bias in the literature is heavily skewed toward appendectomy specimens removed for symptoms of appendicitis and colectomy specimens obtained for unrelated reasons. Invasive nonmucinous adenocarcinomas of the appendix are not well described, but generally arise in association with serrated neoplasms and goblet cell carcinoid tumors. Nonmucinous adenocarcinomas involving the proximal appendix often represent extension of a colonic tumor into the appendix.

Colonic-Type Adenomas of the Appendix

Colonic-type adenomas of the appendix are uncommon, and lesions involving the proximal appendix likely

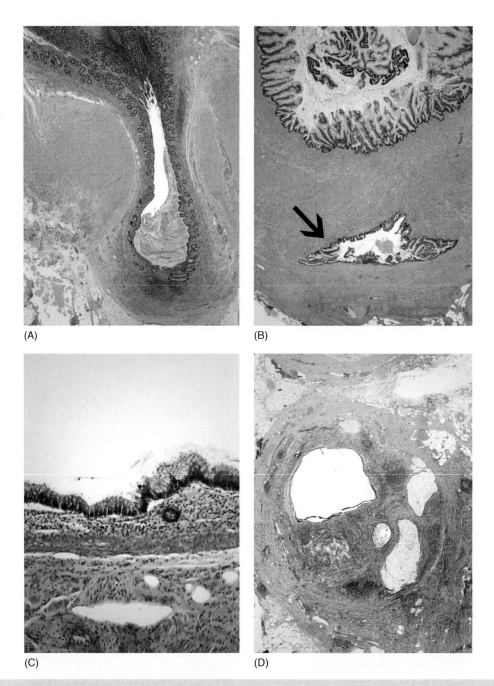

FIGURE 10.7 The differential diagnosis of appendiceal mucinous neoplasia includes appendiceal diverticulosis either with, or without, an associated mucinous neoplasm. Diverticula represent herniations of mucosa and submucosa through the muscularis propria. The diagnosis is straightforward when diverticula contain non-neoplastic epithelium (A), but can be challenging when diverticula are colonized by mucinous neoplasia (arrow) that simulates the appearance of a low-grade appendiceal mucinous neoplasm (B). The presence of a lamina propria investing the epithelium of this diverticulum is a helpful feature indicating that this is a cystadenoma rather than a LAMN (C). Some diverticula rupture and are associated with inflammatory changes, including fibrosis, mucin pools, and lymphoid aggregates (D). Although one may be concerned that such findings reflect a mucinous neoplasm, the luminal epithelium of this case was essentially normal.

represent extension of colonic adenomas into the appendiceal orifice. They are also encountered in appendices removed with colectomy specimens from patients with familial adenomatous polyposis. Colonic-type adenomas do not circumferentially involve the appendiceal mucosa, but form polypoid projections that are sharply demarcated from adjacent normal-appearing mucosa. They contain crowded, tubular crypts lined by dysplastic epithelial cells with elongated, hyperchromatic nuclei, similar to tubular and villous adenomas of the colon (Figure 10.8).

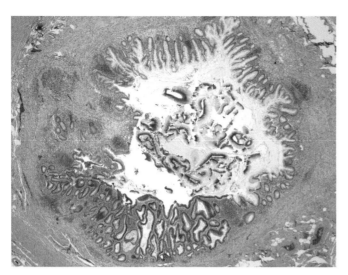

FIGURE 10.8 This colonic-type adenoma forms a sessile plaque in the appendix of this patient with familial adenomatous polyposis. The lesion is sharply demarcated from the adjacent mucosa and contains crowded, variably dilated crypts lined by low-grade dysplastic epithelium.

Serrated Lesions of the Appendix

Serrated appendiceal neoplasms show a spectrum of histologic features paralleling those of serrated colorectal polyps. Hyperplastic polyps are sessile nodules that do not involve the entire luminal circumference. They are reminiscent of "microvesicular" hyperplastic polyps of the colorectum and contain a dual population of goblet cells and nongoblet columnar cells with microvesicles of cytoplasmic mucin. Sessile serrated polyps (also termed sessile serrated adenoma) circumferentially involve the mucosa and contain elongated crypts with a serrated appearance (Figure 10.9A). Similar to colonic lesions, those of the appendix contain dilated crypts that display lateral branching or budding and mild cytologic atypia (Figure 10.9B).

Dysplastic serrated polyps of the appendix resemble their colonic counterparts with conventional cytologic dysplasia, and are much less common than appendiceal hyperplastic polyps and sessile serrated adenomas without conventional dysplasia. Some contain crypts lined by cells with abundant eosinophilic cytoplasm and pencillate nuclei (Figure 10.9C), resembling traditional serrated adenomas of the left colon. Nuclei have smooth contours and small nucleoli and mitotic figures are infrequent. The cytologic dysplasia in appendiceal sessile serrated polyps is often focal, and can display a tubular, villous, or serrated appearance. Some dysplastic serrated polyps contain crypts that architecturally resemble those of a sessile serrated polyp, but are lined by dysplastic epithelium, often with high-grade cytologic features (Figure 10.9D).

Non-dysplastic serrated polyps of the appendix show strong immunopositivity for MUC6 and asymmetric Ki-67 labeling of crypt epithelial cells, similar to colorectal serrated polyps. They also display decreased staining for DNA repair proteins in the superficial epithelium, reflecting its nonproliferative nature, but staining is preserved at the crypt bases and the lesions are mismatch proficient by polymerase chain reaction (PCR). Mutually exclusive *BRAF* and *KRAS* mutations are detected in approximately 50% and 20% of appendiceal sessile serrated polyps, respectively, whereas *BRAF* mutations are far more common and *KRAS* mutations are less frequent among similar-appearing colonic polyps.

Serrated polyps may precede the development of invasive adenocarcinomas. Most of these adenocarcinomas are asymptomatic until they penetrate the visceral peritoneum and cause abdominal pain, so they tend to be locally advanced at the time of diagnosis. Adenocarcinomas associated with serrated lesions show a destructive growth pattern with infiltrative glands that may have a tubular or serrated appearance. Some tumors contain abundant extracellular mucin, but they are typically more cellular and show high-grade cytologic features and desmoplasia beyond the spectrum of changes seen in appendiceal mucinous neoplasms that cause pseudomyxoma peritonei. Distinction from the latter is important, as nonmucinous carcinomas of the appendix pursue an aggressive clinical course and are unlikely to respond to cytoreductive surgery and heated intraperitoneal chemotherapy.

Goblet Cell Carcinoid Tumor

Most goblet cell carcinoid tumors (also known as crypt cell carcinomas, among other names) are incidentally discovered in patients with symptoms suggesting acute appendicitis, and the diagnosis is rarely suspected at the time of surgery. Goblet cell carcinoid tumors are virtually unique to the vermiform appendix and show features of both neuroendocrine and epithelial differentiation. Unlike classic carcinoid tumors, goblet cell carcinoid tumors occur anywhere in the appendix but are more common in the midportion, producing an ill-defined mural thickening that is difficult to identify at the time of gross examination (Figure 10.10A). Aggregates of tumor cells resembling abortive colonic crypts permeate the deep mucosa. Cells infiltrate the appendiceal wall in nests, cords, and clusters arranged circumferentially around the lumen. The tumor cells are usually associated with a densely collagenous stroma (Figure 10.10B). Tumor cells are distended with large cytoplasmic mucin vacuoles that compress the nuclei (Figure 10.10C). Mitotic activity is generally inconspicuous and Ki-67 immunolabeling indices are low (less than 2%). Goblet cell carcinoid tumors show divergent differentiation with patchy immunopositivity for neuroendocrine markers and strong, diffuse mucicarmine positivity.

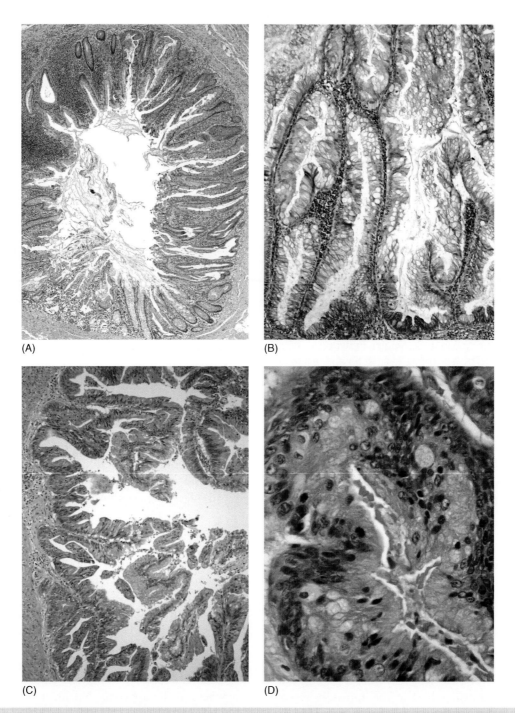

FIGURE 10.9 Serrated appendiceal lesions share morphologic features with their colonic counterparts. Sessile serrated polyps circumferentially surround the appendiceal lumen (A) and contain elongated crypts that show dilatation and branching in the deep mucosa (B). Some serrated polyps with conventional cytologic dysplasia contain serrated crypts lined by cells with enlarged, hyperchromatic nuclei and abundant eosinophilic cytoplasm, similar to those of a (traditional) serrated adenoma (C). They may show high-grade cytologic features with increased mitotic activity and apoptotic debris (D).

At least 50% of goblet cell carcinoid tumors contain areas of adenocarcinoma, which have been called "adenocarcinoma ex goblet cell carcinoid." Approximately half of these cases cause symptoms related to an abdominal mass, which may reflect the enlarged appendix, or metastases to other organs, such as the ovary. The carcinomatous components may display signet ring cell morphology, although mucinous, intestinal, and poorly differentiated areas are also encountered (Figure 10.10D–F). Features suggestive of carcinoma include nuclear atypia, the presence of single infiltrating cells, loss of mucin production, and increased Ki-67 immunolabeling. Cases in which goblet cell carcinoid tumors are identified in initial sections should be submitted entirely to exclude the possibility of

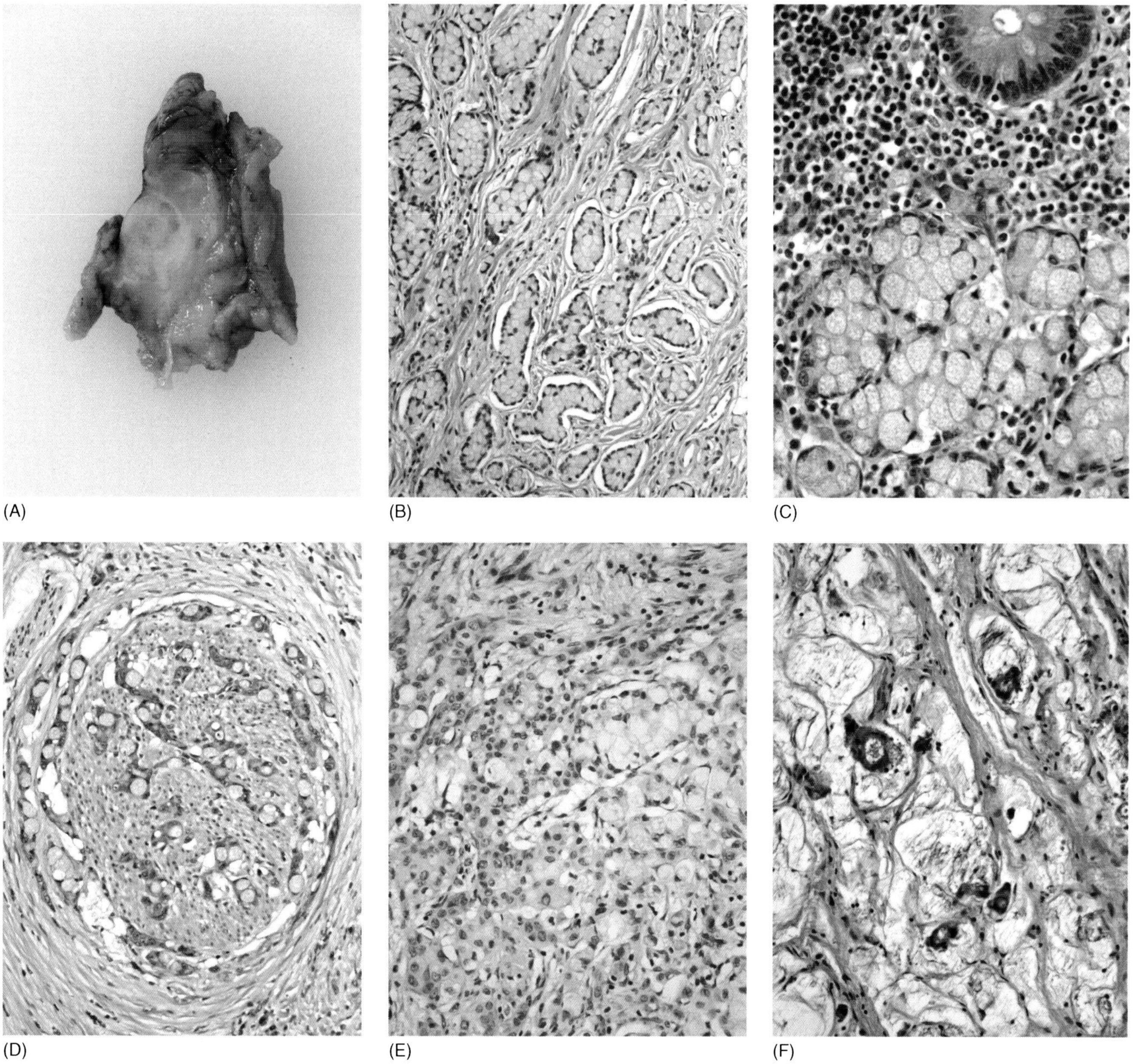

FIGURE 10.10 This goblet cell carcinoid tumor shows subtle features on gross examination. The muscularis propria is obliterated by a tumor in the mid-appendix that infiltrates periappendiceal fat (A). The tumor consists of nests of goblet cells embedded in densely collagenous stroma that lacks the cellularity seen in typical desmoplasia (B). Goblet cell carcinoid tumors are cytologically bland and contain crescentic nuclei with minimal mitotic activity. This lesion expands the deep mucosa (C). This adenocarcinoma ex goblet cell carcinoid contains poorly formed nests of goblet cells and single infiltrating signet ring cells. Perineural invasion is present (D). Another adenocarcinoma ex goblet cell carcinoid contains nests of goblet cells and sheets of poorly differentiated malignant cells (E). Adenocarcinomas associated with goblet cell carcinoid tumors may also display mucinous differentiation, as in this case, where small, round pools of extracellular mucin contain nests and tubules of malignant cells (F).

concomitant carcinoma. Carcinomas derived from goblet cell carcinoid tumors do not show alterations affecting β-catenin, *KRAS*, *DPC4*, or *TP53* typical of malignancies of the lower gastrointestinal tract.

Most goblet cell carcinoid tumors deeply invade the appendiceal wall to penetrate the serosa, and frequently metastasize to regional lymph nodes, peritoneum, and ovaries. Both the World Health Organization and American Joint Commission on Cancer classify and stage goblet cell carcinoid tumors as adenocarcinomas. Management of goblet cell carcinoid tumors is not standardized, although appendectomy alone is unlikely to be adequate therapy owing to their high metastatic potential. Surgical management generally consists of right colectomy with lymph node staging. Extra-appendiceal tumor deposits are more likely to contain carcinomatous elements, in which case the natural history is dictated by the tumor grade and stage.

SUMMARY AND CONCLUSIONS

Appendiceal tumors are uncommon lesions that show unique clinicopathologic features. Most neuroendocrine tumors are small, incidentally discovered tumors of the distal appendix that are adequately managed by appendectomy alone, whereas larger tumors may require more extensive surgery with lymph node dissection due to increased metastatic potential. These tumors should be assessed for grade and stage using Ki-67 immunohistochemistry and criteria enumerated in the *AJCC Cancer Staging Manual*, 7th Edition. Appendiceal mucinous neoplasms are also subject to new grading and staging criteria aimed at predicting biologic behavior. Tumors confined to the mucosa are classified as adenomas and cured by appendectomy alone, whereas those that extend into the appendiceal wall or periappendiceal soft tissue may spread to the peritoneal cavity and, thus, should be classified as LAMNs or mucinous adenocarcinoma in order to imply biologic risk. Mucinous tumor deposits in the peritoneum (ie, pseudomyxoma peritonei) may respond to cytoreductive surgery in combination with intraperitoneal chemotherapy, particularly if they contain low-grade neoplastic epithelium. Most nonmucinous carcinomas of the appendix are derived from serrated appendiceal neoplasms and goblet cell carcinoid tumors. They share some morphologic and molecular features with their colonic counterparts, including frequent *BRAF* or *KRAS* mutations. Goblet cell carcinoid tumors frequently behave in a more aggressive fashion than classic neuroendocrine tumors and may give rise to high-grade carcinomas that behave in a stage dependent fashion. For this reason, they are classified as adenocarcinomas, rather than neuroendocrine tumors.

SELECTED REFERENCES

General

Appendix. In: Edge, S, Byrd, D, Compton, CC, Fritz, A, Green, F, Trotti, A, eds. *AJCC Cancer Staging Manual.* 7th ed. New York: Springer; 2009:133–141.

Carr NJ, Sobin LH. Tumors of the appendix. In: Bosman FT, Carneir F, Hruban RH, Theise ND, eds. *WHO Classification of Tumours of the Digestive System.* 4th ed. Lyon: International Agency for Research on Cancer (IARC); 2010:122–125.

Neuroendocrine Tumors

Burke AP, Sobin LH, Federspiel BH, Shekitka KM. Appendiceal carcinoids: correlation of histology and immunohistochemistry. *Mod Pathol.* 1989;2(6):630–637.

Carr NJ, Sobin LH. Neuroendocrine tumors of the appendix. *Semin Diagn Pathol.* 2004;21(2):108–119.

Hemminki K, Li X. Incidence trends and risk factors of carcinoid tumors: a nationwide epidemiologic study from Sweden. *Cancer.* 2001;92(8):2204–2210.

In't Hof KH, van der Wal HC, Kazemier G, Lange JF. Carcinoid tumour of the appendix: an analysis of 1,485 consecutive emergency appendectomies. *J Gastrointest Surg.* 2008;12(8):1436–1438.

Komminoth P, Arnold R, Capella C, et al. Neuroendocrine Neoplasms of the Appendix. In: Bosman FT, Carneiro F, Hruban RH, Theise ND, eds. *WHO Classification of Tumours of the Digestive System.* 4th ed. Lyon: International Agency for Research on Cancer; 2010:126–128.

Matsukuma KE, Montgomery EA. Tubular carcinoids of the appendix: the CK7/CK20 immunophenotype can be a diagnostic pitfall. *J Clin Pathol.* 2012;65(7):666–668.

Murray SE, Lloyd RV, Sippel RS, Chen H, Oltmann SC. Postoperative surveillance of small appendiceal carcinoid tumors. *Am J Surg.* 2014;207(3):342–345.

Plockinger U, Couvelard A, Falconi M, et al. Consensus guidelines for the management of patients with digestive neuroendocrine tumours: well-differentiated tumour/carcinoma of the appendix and goblet cell carcinoma. *Neuroendocrinology.* 2008;87(1):20–30.

Williams GT. Endocrine tumours of the gastrointestinal tract-selected topics. *Histopathology.* 2007;50(1):30–41.

Mucinous Tumors

Bradley RF, Stewart JH 4th, Russell GB, Levine EA, Geisinger KR. Pseudomyxoma peritonei of appendiceal origin: a clinicopathologic analysis of 101 patients uniformly treated at a single institution, with literature review. *Am J Surg Pathol.* 2006;30(5):551–559.

Chua TC, Al-Zahrani A, Saxena A, et al. Secondary cytoreduction and perioperative intraperitoneal chemotherapy after initial debulking of pseudomyxoma peritonei: a study of timing and the impact of malignant dedifferentiation. *J Am Coll Surg.* 2010;211(4):526–535.

Davison JM, Hartman DA, Singhi AD, et al. Loss of SMAD4 protein expression is associated with high tumor grade and poor prognosis in disseminated appendiceal mucinous neoplasms. *Am J Surg Pathol.* 2014;38(5):583–592.

Elias D, Gilly F, Quenet F, et al. Pseudomyxoma peritonei: a French multicentric study of 301 patients treated with cytoreductive surgery and intraperitoneal chemotherapy. *Eur J Surg Oncol.* 2010;36(5):456–462.

Fish R, Selvasekar C, Crichton P, et al. Risk-reducing laparoscopic cytoreductive surgery and hyperthermic intraperitoneal chemotherapy for low-grade appendiceal mucinous neoplasm: early outcomes and technique. *Surg Endosc.* 2014;28(1):341–345.

Foster JM, Gupta PK, Carreau JH, et al. Right hemicolectomy is not routinely indicated in pseudomyxoma peritonei. *Am Surg.* 2012;78(2):171–177.

Gonzalez-Moreno S, Sugarbaker PH. Right hemicolectomy does not confer a survival advantage in patients with mucinous carcinoma of the appendix and peritoneal seeding. *Br J Surg.* 2004;91(3):304–311.

Jarvinen P, Jarvinen HJ, Lepisto A. Survival of patients with pseudomyxoma peritonei treated by serial debulking. *Col Dis.* 2010;12(9):868–872.

Kabbani W, Houlihan PS, Luthra R, et al. Mucinous and nonmucinous appendiceal adenocarcinomas: different clinicopathological features but similar genetic alterations. *Mod Pathol.* 2002;15(6):599–605.

Lamps LW, Gray GF Jr, Dilday BR, Washington MK. The coexistence of low-grade mucinous neoplasms of the appendix and appendiceal diverticula: a possible role in the pathogenesis of pseudomyxoma peritonei. *Mod Pathol.* 2000;13(5):495–501.

Miner TJ, Shia J, Jaques DP, et al. Long-term survival following treatment of pseudomyxoma peritonei: an analysis of surgical therapy. *Ann Surg.* 2005;241(2):300–308.

Misdraji J, Burgart LJ, Lauwers GY. Defective mismatch repair in the pathogenesis of low-grade appendiceal mucinous neoplasms and adenocarcinomas. *Mod Pathol.* 2004;17(12):1447–1454.

Misdraji J, Yantiss RK, Graeme-Cook FM, et al. Appendiceal mucinous neoplasms: a clinicopathologic analysis of 107 cases. *Am J Surg Pathol.* 2003;27(8):1089–1103.

Pai RK, Beck AH, Norton JA, Longacre TA. Appendiceal mucinous neoplasms: clinicopathologic study of 116 cases with analysis of factors predicting recurrence. *Am J Surg Pathol.* 2009;33(10):1425–1439.

Ronnett BM, Yan H, Kurman RJ, et al. Patients with pseudomyxoma peritonei associated with disseminated peritoneal adenomucinosis have a significantly more favorable prognosis than patients with peritoneal mucinous carcinomatosis. *Cancer.* 2001;92:85–91.

Ronnett BM, Zahn CM, Kurman RJ, et al. Disseminated peritoneal adenomucinosis and peritoneal mucinous carcinomatosis. A clinicopathologic analysis of 109 cases with emphasis on distinguishing pathologic features, site of origin, prognosis, and relationship to "pseudomyxoma peritonei." *Am J Surg Pathol.* 1995;19(12):1390–1408.

Schomas DA, Miller RC, Donohue JH, et al. Intraperitoneal treatment for peritoneal mucinous carcinomatosis of appendiceal origin after operative management: long-term follow-up of the Mayo Clinic experience. *Ann Surg.* 2009;249(4):588–595.

Smeenk RM, van Velthuysen ML, Verwaal VJ, Zoetmulder FA. Appendiceal neoplasms and pseudomyxoma peritonei: a population based study. *Eur J Surg Oncol.* 2008;34(2):196–201.

Smeenk RM, Verwaal VJ, Antonini N, Zoetmulder FA. Survival analysis of pseudomyxoma peritonei patients treated by cytoreductive surgery and hyperthermic intraperitoneal chemotherapy. *Ann Surg.* 2007;245(1):104–109.

Yantiss RK, Shia J, Klimstra DS, et al. Prognostic significance of localized extra-appendiceal mucin deposition in appendiceal mucinous neoplasms. *Am J Surg Pathol.* 2009;33:248–255.

Youssef H, Newman C, Chandrakumaran K, et al. Operative findings, early complications, and long-term survival in 456 patients with pseudomyxoma peritonei syndrome of appendiceal origin. *Dis Col Rect.* 2011;54(3):293–299.

Zauber P, Berman E, Marotta S, Sabbath-Solitare M, Bishop T. Ki-ras gene mutations are invariably present in low-grade mucinous tumors of the vermiform appendix. *Scand J Gastroenterol.* 2011;46(7–8):869–874.

Nonmucinous Tumors

Alsaad KO, Serra S, Schmitt A, Perren A, Chetty R. Cytokeratins 7 and 20 immunoexpression profile in goblet cell and classical carcinoids of appendix. *Endocr Pathol.* 2007;18(1):16–22.

Bellizzi AM, Rock J, Marsh WL, Frankel WL. Serrated lesions of the appendix: a morphologic and immunohistochemical appraisal. *Am J Clin Pathol.* 2010;133(4):623–632.

Burke AP, Sobin LH, Federspiel BH, Shekitka KM, Helwig EB. Goblet cell carcinoids and related tumors of the vermiform appendix. *Am J Clin Pathol.* 1990;94(1):27–35.

Butler JA, Houshiar A, Lin F, Wilson SE. Goblet cell carcinoid of the appendix. *Am J Surg.* 1994;168(6):685–687.

Carr NJ, McCarthy WF, Sobin LH. Epithelial noncarcinoid tumors and tumor-like lesions of the appendix. A clinicopathologic study of 184 patients with a multivariate analysis of prognostic factors. *Cancer.* 1995;75(3):757–768.

Cortina R, McCormick J, Kolm P, Perry RR. Management and prognosis of adenocarcinoma of the appendix. *Dis Colon Rectum.* 1995;38(8):848–852.

Gui X, Qin L, Gao ZH, Falck V, Harpaz N. Goblet cell carcinoids at extraappendiceal locations of gastrointestinal tract: an underrecognized diagnostic pitfall. *J Surg Onc.* 2011;103(8):790–795.

Holt N, Gronbaek H. Goblet cell carcinoids of the appendix. *Scientific World Journal.* 2013;2013:543696.

Maru D, Wu TT, Canada A, et al. Loss of chromosome 18q and DPC4 (Smad4) mutations in appendiceal adenocarcinomas. *Oncogene.* 2004;23(3):859–864.

Moran B, Baratti D, Yan TD, Kusamura S, Deraco M. Consensus statement on the loco-regional treatment of appendiceal mucinous neoplasms with peritoneal dissemination (pseudomyxoma peritonei). *J Surg Onc.* 2008;98(4):277–282.

Pai RK, Hartman DJ, Gonzalo DH, et al. Serrated lesions of the appendix frequently harbor KRAS mutations and not BRAF mutations indicating a distinctly different serrated neoplastic pathway in the appendix. *Hum Pathol.* 2014;45(2):227–235.

Palanivelu C, Rangarajan M, Annapoorni S, et al. Laparoscopic right hemicolectomy for goblet-cell carcinoid of the appendix: report of a rare case and literature survey. *J Laparoendosc Adv Surg Tech A.* 2008;18(3):417–421.

Renshaw AA, Kish R, Gould EW. Sessile serrated adenoma is associated with acute appendicitis in patients 30 years or older. *Am J Clin Pathol.* 2006;126(6):875–877.

Rubio CA. Serrated adenomas of the appendix. *J Clin Pathol.* 2004;57(9):946–949.

Stancu M, Wu TT, Wallace C, et al. Genetic alterations in goblet cell carcinoids of the vermiform appendix and comparison with gastrointestinal carcinoid tumors. *Mod Pathol.* 2003;16(12):1189–1198.

Sugarbaker PH, Chang D. Results of treatment of 385 patients with peritoneal surface spread of appendiceal malignancy. *Ann Surg Onc.* 1999;6(8):727–731.

Sugarbaker PH, Jablonski KA. Prognostic features of 51 colorectal and 130 appendiceal cancer patients with peritoneal carcinomatosis treated by cytoreductive surgery and intraperitoneal chemotherapy. *Ann Surg.* 1995;221(2):124–132.

Tang LH, Shia J, Soslow RA, et al. Pathologic classification and clinical behavior of the spectrum of goblet cell carcinoid tumors of the appendix. *Am J Surg Pathol.* 2008;32(10):1429–1443.

van Eeden S, Offerhaus GJ, Hart AA, et al. Goblet cell carcinoid of the appendix: a specific type of carcinoma. *Histopathology.* 2007;51(6):763–773.

Yajima N, Wada R, Yamagishi S, et al. Immunohistochemical expressions of cytokeratins, mucin core proteins, p53, and neuroendocrine cell markers in epithelial neoplasm of appendix. *Hum Pathol.* 2005;36(11):1217–1225.

Yantiss RK, Panczykowski A, Misdraji J, et al. A comprehensive study of nondysplastic and dysplastic serrated polyps of the vermiform appendix. *Am J Surg Pathol.* 2007;31(11):1742–1753.

Younes M, Katikaneni PR, Lechago J. Association between mucosal hyperplasia of the appendix and adenocarcinoma of the colon. *Histopathology.* 1995;26(1):33–37.

11

Neoplasms of the Colon

BENJAMIN J. SWANSON, SCOTT R. OWENS, AND WENDY L. FRANKEL

INTRODUCTION

Adenocarcinoma is the most common malignancy arising in the colorectum, and colorectal adenocarcinoma (CRC) is the third most common malignancy overall in the United States. It is estimated that approximately 133,000 people will be diagnosed with CRC in 2015, and about 50,000 people will die of the disease. Furthermore, 1.4 million new cases of CRC were diagnosed worldwide in 2012, with approximately 694,000 deaths. Although a wide variety of other benign and malignant tumors are seen in the colon, they are much less common; often these lesions present as polyps that are found on screening colonoscopy.

Similar to the small bowel, there are four major categories of primary colorectal malignancies: adenocarcinoma, neuroendocrine tumors (NETs), mesenchymal tumors, and lymphomas (Table 11.1). The World Health Organization (WHO) 2010 classification for colorectal tumors is shown in Table 11.2.

INFLAMMATORY AND NON-NEOPLASTIC LESIONS

Inflammatory lesions in the colon often present as polyps, which are then endoscopically biopsied or removed. Many colonic inflammatory lesions are considered to be within the spectrum of mucosal prolapse and related conditions, including solitary rectal ulcer syndrome, diverticular polyps, colitis cystica profunda, inflammatory cap polyps, and inflammatory cloacogenic polyps. All are believed to be caused by traction and twisting of the mucosa from peristalsis-induced trauma, with torsion of blood vessels and ischemic damage to the mucosa. The polyps included in the spectrum of mucosal prolapse-associated lesions all

have some degree of overlapping morphologic findings, and are discussed here because they may occasionally enter into the differential diagnosis with adenomas and CRC.

Patients with mucosal prolapse are often symptomatic, with melena and rectal bleeding among the most common complaints. These lesions may present as polyps, ulcers, or masses, or a combination of those lesions. Histologic features include perpendicular fibromuscular hyperplasia and splaying and disorganization of the muscularis mucosae/lamina propria interface; proliferating, dilated, and thrombosed blood vessels in the lamina propria; mucosal erosion and ulceration with an overlying acute inflammatory exudate with abundant fibrin; reactive epithelial changes such as crypt hyperplasia and serration; and diamond or triangular-shaped crypts (Figure 11.1A–C).

Diverticular polyps (also known as polypoid prolapsing mucosal folds) are similar lesions that develop in association with diverticular disease. Early in their development, these polyps may contain congested blood vessels, hemorrhage and hemosiderin deposition (Figure 11.2A–C), which may impart a red–brown discoloration macroscopically. Older polyps show histologic findings similar to other mucosal prolapse polyps, including fibromuscular hyperplasia and reactive epithelial changes.

Inflammatory cap polyposis is also considered within the spectrum of prolapse polyps. They are usually found in the rectosigmoid colon, but occasionally involve the entire colon. Inflammatory cap polyposis appears in two clinical settings: patients (usually women) with prolapse-type symptoms who have solitary or a few lesions confined to the rectum, and patients with more extensive disease who do not have a history of constipation. The most striking feature is a "cap" of fibrinopurulent exudate (Figure 11.3)

TABLE 11.1 Clinicopathologic Characteristics of Primary Colorectal Malignancies

	Adenocarcinoma	Neuroendocrine Tumor/Carcinoma	B Cell Lymphoma	Malignant Mesenchymal Tumor
Relative Incidence (%)	90%–95%	0.4%	0.2%–0.4%	Extremely rare
Age (median, years)	72	Colon 66 Rectum 56	50–70	Variable
Gender (male:female)	Colon 1.2:1 Rectum 1.5:1	Colon 0.66:1 Rectum 1.02:1	2:1	Variable
Most common site(s)	Sigmoid, rectum	Rectum, cecum, sigmoid	Cecum	Variable

Source: Data adapted from *WHO Classification of Tumours of the Digestive System* (2010).

TABLE 11.2 WHO 2010 Classification of Tumors of the Colon

Epithelial Tumors
 Hamartomas
  Juvenile polyp
  Peutz–Jeghers polyp
  Cowden-associated polyp (PTEN hamartomatous syndrome)
 Premalignant Lesions
  Adenoma
   Tubular
   Villous
   Tubulovillous
  Dysplasia (intraepithelial neoplasia)
   Low grade
   High grade
  Serrated Lesions
   Hyperplastic polyp
   Sessile serrated adenoma/polyp
   Traditional serrated adenoma
 Carcinoma
  Adenocarcinoma
   Cribriform comedo-type adenocarcinoma
   Medullary carcinoma
   Micropapillary carcinoma
   Mucinous adenocarcinoma
   Serrated adenocarcinoma
   Signet ring cell carcinoma
  Adenosquamous carcinoma
  Spindle cell carcinoma
  Squamous cell carcinoma
  Undifferentiated carcinoma
 Neuroendocrine Neoplasms
  Neuroendocrine tumor (NET)
   NET G1 (carcinoid)
   NET G2
  Neuroendocrine carcinoma (NEC)
   Large cell NEC
   Small cell NEC
  Mixed adenoneuroendocrine carcinoma (MANEC)
  EC cell, serotonin-producing NET
  L cell, glucagon-like peptide-producing, and PP/PYY-producing NET
Mesenchymal Tumors
 Leiomyoma
 Lipoma
 Angiosarcoma
 Gastrointestinal stromal tumor
 Kaposi sarcoma
 Leiomyosarcoma
Lymphomas
Secondary Tumors

Source: Data adapted from *WHO Classification of Tumours of the Digestive System*, 4th Edition, 2010.

overlying an eroded or ulcerated surface, often with prominent granulation tissue. Crypt hyperplasia and fibromuscular change of the lamina propria are variably present.

Colitis cystica profunda most commonly occurs as a solitary lesion in the rectum, but can be found anywhere in the colon, often in association with inflammatory bowel disease, ostomy sites, or other conditions that feature mucosal ulceration and repair. These lesions often regress after the underlying mechanism of traumatic injury is removed. Histologically, colitis cystica profunda features misplaced, cystically dilated, mucin-filled crypts lined by intestinal epithelium, which are present within the submucosa and even the muscularis propria in rare cases (Figure 11.4A–B). The misplaced crypts are lobular in arrangement and are surrounded by lamina propria; there are often associated hemosiderin-laden macrophages as well. The epithelium in the misplaced crypts is not neoplastic. The main differential diagnosis is colorectal adenocarcinoma, both clinically and histologically. Invasive adenocarcinoma, however, features neoplastic epithelium (with much more significant atypia than the surface epithelium), irregular or angulated glands, and associated desmoplastic stroma. The glands in colitis cystica profunda, in contrast, are not angulated, and are surrounded by lamina propria; desmoplasia is absent. If there is any cytologic atypia in the context of colitis cystica profunda, it should be similar in degree to that seen in the overlying surface epithelium.

Inflammatory cloacogenic polyps are prolapse-type polyps that typically present as a single polypoid mass in the anterior wall of the anorectum. Histologically, due to the anatomic location, these lesions may have colorectal columnar mucosa in addition to anal stratified squamous epithelium, or a combination of both. The most striking feature of this polyp is the villiform morphology of the surface epithelium (Figure 11.5). Similar to other prolapse-type polyps, there may be stromal hyalinization, which is most prominent at the base of the polyp, as well as elastin deposition, which is unique to this type of polyp. Due to the villous growth pattern, these may mimic a villous adenoma at low power. However, inflammatory cloacogenic polyps lack cytologic dysplasia.

Inflammatory myoglandular polyps are rare, usually solitary, and primarily found in the distal colon. Many

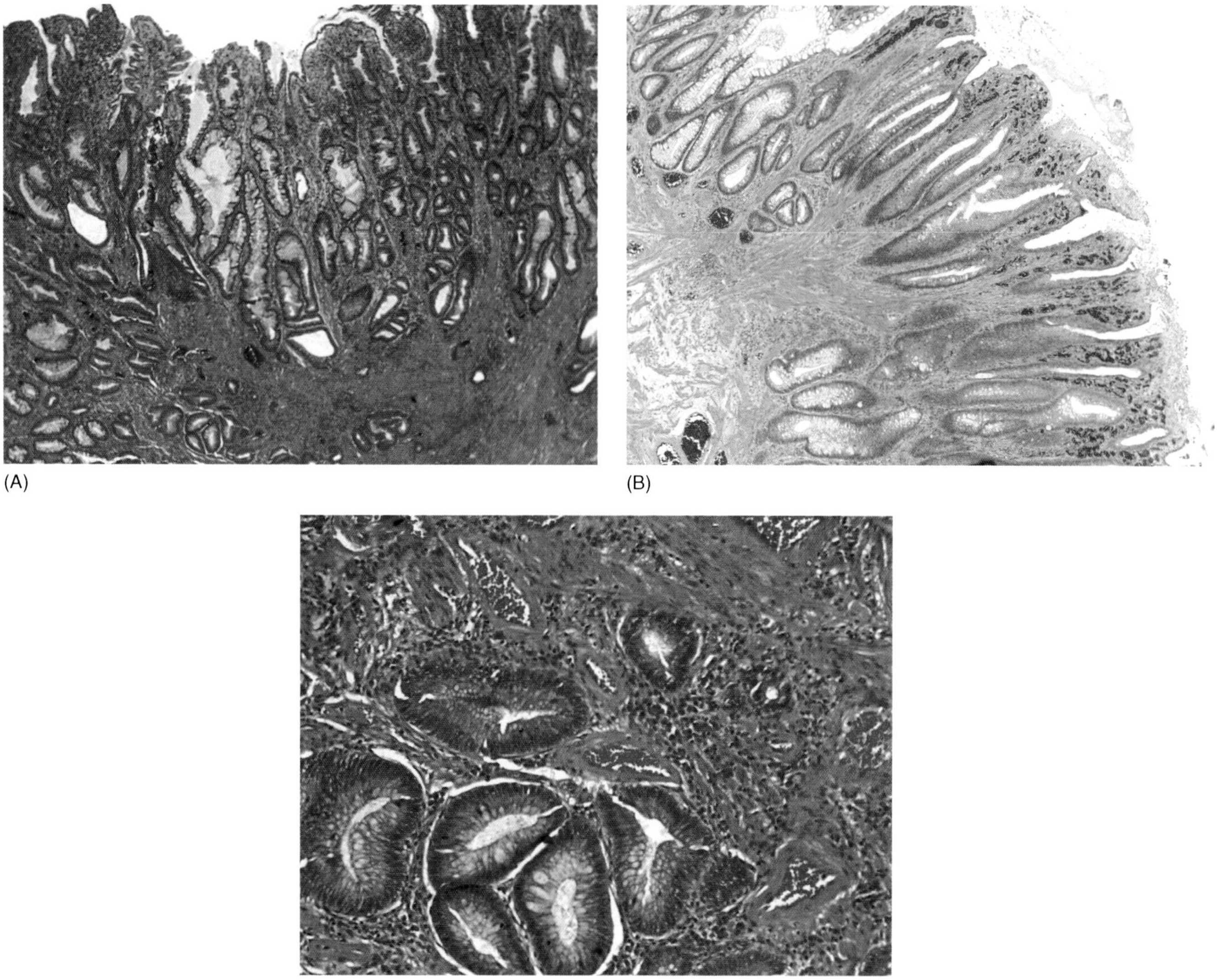

(A)

(B)

(C)

FIGURE 11.1 A low-power view of a prolapse polyp shows reactive epithelial changes such as crypt hyperplasia and serration (A). Disorganization of the muscularis mucosae/lamina propria interface and perpendicular fibromuscular hyperplasia are common (B), as are proliferating, dilated, and sometimes thrombosed blood vessels in the lamina propria and mucosal erosion and ulceration. Diamond- or triangular-shaped crypts are often seen at the base of prolapse polyps (C).

consider these to be within the spectrum of colonic mucosal prolapse polyps because of the significant histologic overlap. However, inflammatory myoglandular polyps often lack the well-formed granulation tissue cap seen in inflammatory cap polyps, the villous architecture of inflammatory cloacogenic polyps, and the misplaced epithelium of colitis cystica profunda; in addition, they are not necessarily associated with diverticular disease or inflammatory bowel disease. For these reasons, other authorities believe these polyps could represent hamartomas. Myoglandular polyps have a radially arranged network of muscularis mucosae that may closely resemble Peutz–Jeghers-type polyps; however, in contrast to Peutz–Jeghers polyps, the surface epithelium is often eroded or ulcerated, with an associated fibrinopurulent exudate and reactive epithelial changes (Figure 11.6). Glands are typically hyperplastic and/or cystically dilated, and there is often hemosiderin deposition in the lamina propria. An older age at presentation favors inflammatory myoglandular polyp over Peutz–Jeghers polyp, and Peutz–Jeghers polyps typically do not have surface erosions, ulcerations, or marked inflammatory epithelial changes.

Although all of the above-mentioned lesions within the spectrum of mucosal prolapse are reactive, it can be challenging to distinguish them from other types of neoplastic polyps and even invasive adenocarcinoma. This may be a

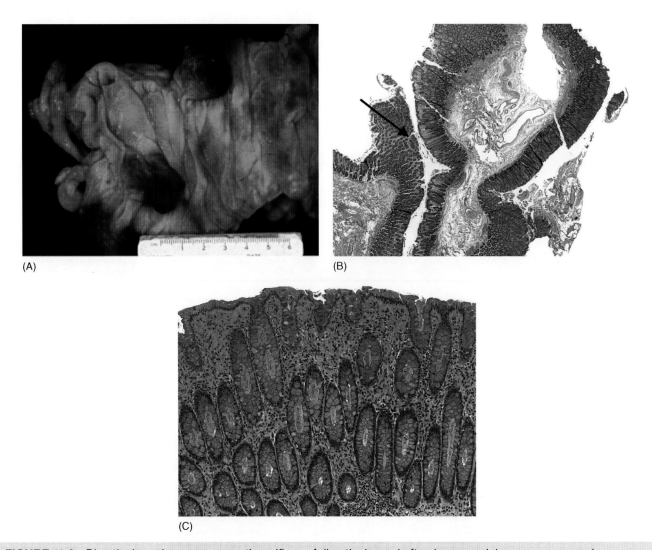

FIGURE 11.2 Diverticular polyps occur near the orifices of diverticula, and often have a red–brown macroscopic appearance due to hemorrhage and hemosiderin deposition (A). This low-power view shows dilated and congested blood vessels in the submucosa; the diverticular orifice is to the left (B, arrow). In early diverticular polyps, prominent mucosal hemorrhage and hemosiderin deposition are present (C).

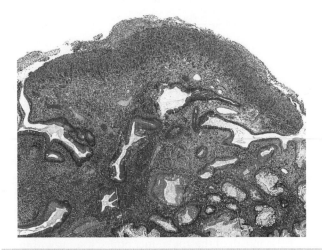

FIGURE 11.3 Inflammatory cap polyps feature a prominent "cap" of fibrinopurulent exudate overlying an ulcerated surface, with marked capillary proliferation.

particular problem during intraoperative frozen section evaluation, when the splaying and fibromuscular hyperplasia with entrapped glands mimic invasive adenocarcinoma.

Inflammatory polyps (or pseudopolyps) are another common inflammatory lesion of the colon. These polyps occur as a result of regeneration and repair secondary to mucosal injury, and are present in numerous contexts, including inflammatory bowel disease, ischemic colitis, and infectious colitis. The histologic features of these polyps are related to the regenerative biology of the mucosa, and include variable amounts of surface ulceration, granulation tissue, crypt distortion, and neutrophilic inflammation that may extend into the crypts (Figure 11.7). The epithelium may exhibit marked atypia due to regenerative and reactive changes, which can be concerning for dysplasia. Maturation at the mucosal surface, as well as the presence of surrounding inflammation and ulceration, helps distinguish reactive changes from true dysplasia.

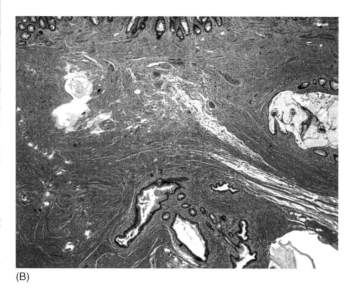

(A)   (B)

FIGURE 11.4 Colitis cystica profunda consists of misplaced mucosal elements, including markedly dilated crypts filled with mucin (A). The misplaced epithelium has a lobular configuration, and is surrounded by lamina propria (B). The misplaced epithelium is not dysplastic, and resembles the overlying surface epithelium, helping to distinguish it from invasive adenocarcinoma.

HAMARTOMATOUS POLYPS

Several types of hamartomatous polyps are seen in the gastrointestinal tract; these are discussed in detail in Chapter 6. Features pertinent to the colon are briefly mentioned here.

Juvenile polyps (Figure 11.8A–C) may occur sporadically or as part of juvenile polyposis syndrome (JPS). Sporadic juvenile polyps are the most common colorectal polyp in children 10 years of age and younger. Patients with JPS have mutations or deletions in the *SMAD4/ DPC4* or *BMPR1A* genes. JPS patients have a 68% risk

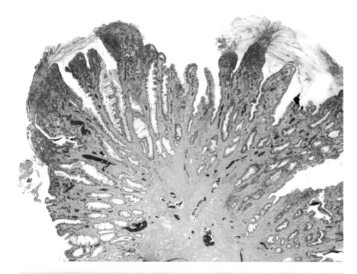

FIGURE 11.5 The most striking feature of inflammatory cloacogenic polyps, which are included in the spectrum of prolapse polyps, is the villiform morphology of the surface epithelium. Similar to other prolapse polyps, there may be stromal hyalinization, perpendicular fibromuscular hyperplasia, and proliferation of capillaries in the lamina propria. Photograph, courtesy of Dr. Rhonda Yantiss.

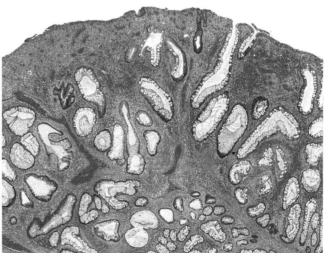

FIGURE 11.6 Myoglandular polyps contain well-developed smooth muscle surrounding lobules of benign epithelium, which may resemble Peutz–Jeghers-type polyps. The surface epithelium is often eroded or ulcerated, with an associated fibrinopurulent exudate and reactive epithelial changes.

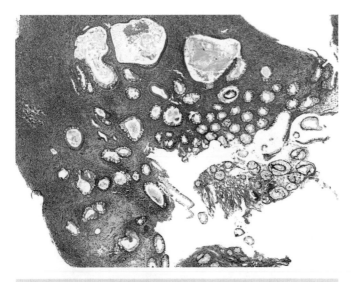

FIGURE 11.7 Inflammatory polyps (also known as inflammatory pseudopolyps) feature inflamed polypoid colonic mucosa with surface ulceration, prominent granulation tissue, and crypt distortion.

of developing colorectal cancer by 60 years of age, with a mean age at diagnosis of 35 years; there is also increased risk of small intestinal, gastric, and possibly pancreatic cancer. Syndromic juvenile polyps may also give rise to foci of dysplasia and carcinoma, but these findings are very uncommon in sporadic juvenile polyps, and, if identified, should prompt consideration of JPS.

Peutz–Jeghers polyps (Figure 11.9) typically occur in patients with Peutz–Jeghers syndrome (PJS), an autosomal dominant disorder caused by mutation to the gene *STK11*; they rarely occur sporadically. PJS polyps can be found in the stomach, small intestine, and large intestine, and may give rise to dysplasia and carcinoma. Care must be taken not to misdiagnose herniated/misplaced epithelium as invasive adenocarcinoma, particularly if the displaced epithelium is dysplastic.

PTEN hamartoma syndrome is an autosomal dominant syndrome that encompasses several syndromes that were previously thought to be distinct, including Cowden syndrome, Bannayan–Ruvalcaba–Riley syndrome, and Lhermitte–Duclos disease, among others. All of these disorders have mutations in the tumor suppressor *PTEN* (phosphatase and tensin homolog) on chromosome 10. These patients have hamartomatous gastrointestinal tract polyps as well as a variety of extra-intestinal manifestations, and an increased risk of malignancy at various sites including breast, thyroid, and the colon. Patients with this syndrome may also have hyperplastic, inflammatory, adenomatous, and ganglioneuromatous polyps in the colon. The hamartomatous polyps in PTEN hamartoma syndrome are not believed to have neoplastic potential.

Cronkhite–Canada syndrome is an idiopathic gastroenterocolopathy affecting older adults (see also Chapter 8). Patients with this disease have diffuse polyposis of the gastrointestinal tract that spares the esophagus, as well as extraintestinal manifestations. The natural history of the disease is variable, but mortality is high. Histologically, the polyps in Cronkhite–Canada syndrome resemble

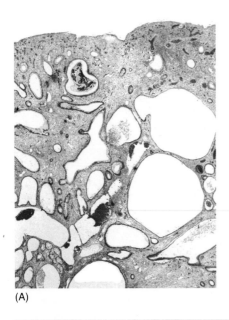
(A)

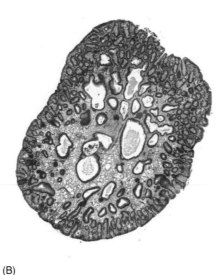
(B)

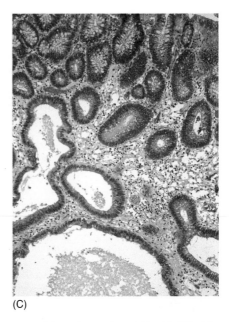
(C)

FIGURE 11.8 Juvenile polyps are composed of markedly dilated glands containing inspissated mucin and inflammatory cells, with associated stromal expansion by edema and inflammation (A). This juvenile polyp from a JPS patient shows extensive low-grade dysplasia (B–C). Note that the presence of cystically dilated glands is still detectable.

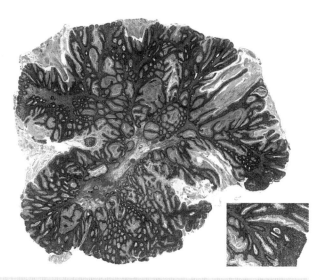

FIGURE 11.9 Peutz–Jeghers polyps have a distinct arborizing architecture featuring lobules of benign colonic epithelium surrounded by prominent bundles of smooth muscle. The epithelium resembles normal colonic epithelium, with abundant goblet cells (inset).

other hamartomatous polyps, but Cronkhite–Canada can usually be distinguished based on the clinical presentation and the fact that the intervening mucosa shows similar changes to the hamartomatous polyps.

ADENOMATOUS AND SERRATED POLYPS

Conventional (Intestinal-Type) Adenomas

Conventional (intestinal-type) adenomas of the colorectum are extremely common, as illustrated by the fact that up to 16% of patients in the sixth decade of life have at least one adenoma identified on screening colonoscopy. The incidence of conventional adenomas increases with age as well. These adenomas can be classified based on the degree of villous architecture as well as the degree of dysplasia. Adenomas with less than 25% villous architecture are considered tubular adenomas; adenomas with greater than 75% villous architecture are considered villous adenomas; and adenomas with 25% to 75% villous formation are classified as tubulovillous adenomas. Despite these definitions, there is high interobserver variability in the quantification of the villous component in adenomatous polyps, even among pathologists with interest/experience in gastrointestinal pathology. Furthermore, the definition of "villous" is not particularly well established either. Some authorities have defined a villus, in this context, as a villiform structure that is two times higher than the surrounding colonic mucosa. However, this definition is arbitrary and not supported by studies that evaluate the prognostic significance of this morphologic definition. Likewise, the

criterion of a minimum amount of 25% villous architecture for classification as a tubulovillous adenoma is also arbitrary. Due to poor reproducibility and lack of strict definitions, some have questioned the clinical utility of reporting the presence or absence of a villous component, but the supposed significance of a villous component is firmly embedded in the clinical literature.

Conventional adenomas of the colon, by definition, contain at least low-grade dysplastic epithelium. Histologically, low-grade dysplasia features pseudostratified, hyperchromatic, pencillate nuclei (Figure 11.10A–G). Prominent large nucleoli are not typically present, and nuclear polarity is maintained with the nuclei predominately restricted to the basal portion of the cells. Mitotic figures and apoptotic bodies are frequently seen. The glands do not form confluent sheets, cribriforming architecture, or complex budding. The dysplastic changes typically involve the surface epithelium.

Metaplastic changes can also be found in conventional adenomas (Figure 11.10D–G). Squamoid metaplasia is very common, affecting 0.44% of colon adenomas. Histologically, the metaplastic component is composed of monotonous nests of cells that do not have significant nuclear pleomorphism, mitoses, or necrosis. These nests of cells are often found at the base of the adenoma, and rarely have stroma surrounding them that mimics desmoplasia. The epithelial cells stain for squamous markers, and are sometimes immunoreactive for neuroendocrine markers. For these reasons, it was recently proposed that squamous metaplasia is related or equivalent to an adenoma with a focus of microscopic carcinoid tumor. Salaria et al. demonstrated that both the adenomatous component as well as the microcarcinoid component are positive for nuclear β-catenin, suggesting that the two components were derived from a common progenitor via the adenomatous polyposis coli (APC)/Wnt signaling pathway. It remains controversial whether this represents true metaplasia or an alternative differentiation of a stem cell. The main differential diagnosis for this entity is an invasive, poorly differentiated carcinoma arising from an adenoma. Close examination of the low-grade cytologic features of the squamous metaplasia, as well as the lobular architecture, helps distinguish this entity from invasive carcinoma.

The second most common type of metaplasia found in conventional adenomas, (reportedly 0.20%) is Paneth cell metaplasia. This metaplasia is usually not diagnostically challenging and should not suggest a diagnosis of inflammatory bowel disease (IBD) even if seen in the left colon or rectum. The Paneth cells contain apically located eosinophilic granules and are similar to those seen normally in the small bowel and right colon. Other rare metaplasias arising in conventional adenomas include clear cell, osseous, gastric, and melanocytic metaplasia.

High-grade dysplasia is characterized by high-grade nuclear features and/or high-grade architectural features.

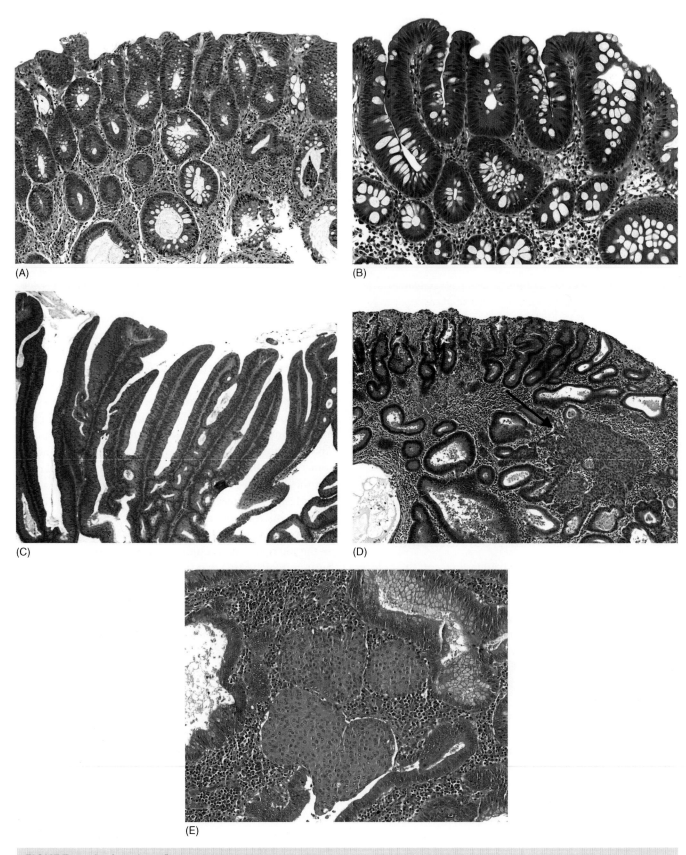

(A)

(B)

(C)

(D)

(E)

FIGURE 11.10 (*continued*)

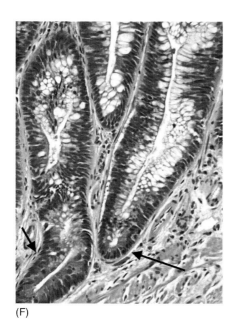
(F)

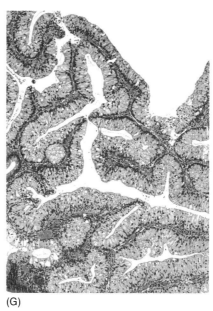
(G)

FIGURE 11.10 Low-grade adenomatous epithelium in colon polyps is typically composed of cigar-shaped, pseudostratified hyperchromatic nuclei that reach the epithelial surface (A–B). Goblet cells are often decreased. Adenomas with villous architecture have long villi covered by dysplastic epithelium (C). Squamous metaplasia is common in tubular adenomas, which some classify as foci of microcarcinoid based on the immunophenotype (D [arrow], E). Paneth cell metaplasia is common in tubular adenomas (F, arrow). Clear cell change can also be seen in tubular adenomas; this has no clinical significance (G; courtesy Dr. Shawn Kinsey).

The nuclei show pleomorphism as well as an increased nuclear:cytoplasmic ratio (Figure 11.11A–C). The nucleoli may be large with interspersed areas of clear chromatin. Nuclear polarity is typically lost, and bizarre mitotic figures may be seen. Architectural findings include cribriformed glands, confluent sheets of dysplastic cells, and complex budding. Most pathologists consider carcinoma in situ to be within the spectrum of high-grade dysplasia; furthermore, most discourage the use of the term carcinoma in situ because it is not believed to have the potential to metastasize, and may lead to confusion and possible overtreatment.

The concept of "advanced" adenomas has arisen in the clinical literature to describe those adenomas that require closer follow-up than typical conventional intestinal-type adenomas. Advanced adenomas are characterized by at least one of the following features: high-grade dysplasia, a villous component, or size greater than 1.0 cm. Similar to the debate regarding the reproducibility and definitional criteria of villous components in adenomatous polyps, there are similar challenges to reporting high-grade dysplasia in adenomatous polyps. There is poor interobserver agreement, even among pathologists with interest/experience in gastrointestinal pathology, regarding the designation of high-grade dysplasia, particularly in small (< 1 cm) adenomatous polyps. In addition, some pathologists believe that the

size of the polyp is more important than the other less reproducible features of an advanced adenoma, and thus they prefer not to mention villous architecture or high-grade dysplasia. This opinion, together with concern about overly aggressive therapy for lesions that do not have metastatic potential, has led some pathologists to refrain from using any other morphologic descriptors for conventional adenomas (villous, tubular, or high-grade dysplasia). Other pathologists continue to use these descriptors at the request of their colleagues in gastroenterology and surgery.

Treatment and Surveillance Guidelines

The current recommendation for screening is to begin at age 50 for average-risk individuals, with complete removal of any adenomas. The endoscopic follow-up for adenomatous polyps depends on the number, size, and histologic characteristics of the polyp. A patient with a small (< 1 cm) tubular adenoma usually has a follow-up colonoscopy in 5 to 10 years, as the risk of neoplasia developing in a patient with a small tubular adenoma in the Veterans Affairs (VA) cooperative study was less than 1% after 5 years. If a patient has greater than three tubular adenomas, the surveillance interval may be decreased to 3 years; in addition, the typical endoscopic follow-up interval for an advanced adenoma is 3 years (rather than 5–10 years).

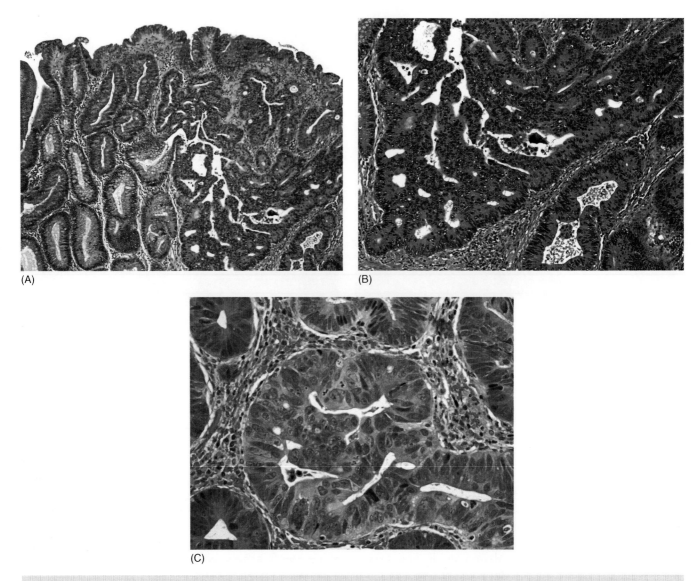

FIGURE 11.11 High-grade dysplasia typically shows both architectural complexity (such as cribriform gland architecture, A–B) and high grade cytologic changes including prominent nucleoli and loss of nuclear polarity (C).

The risk of developing neoplasia in a polyp of any size with high-grade dysplasia, according to the VA cohort study, is 11% after 5 years.

Diagnostic Challenges

Florid reactive epithelial changes can mimic conventional adenomas, particularly when the reactive epithelium features nuclear hyperchromasia and stratification, increased or atypical mitotic figures, and mucin depletion. However, reactive/reparative epithelium typically shows maturation toward the luminal surface, as opposed to conventional adenomas, which show nuclear hyperchromasia, pseudostratification, and mitoses that extend to the mucosal surface. When the reactive epithelium is associated with an erosion or ulcer bed, the identification of granulation tissue and abundant acute inflammation helps in the distinction from dysplasia. Close examination of the adjacent mucosa may also help to identify the epithelial changes as reactive, particularly if they are adjacent to an ulcer or an area of ischemia (Figure 11.12A–B). Finally, true dysplasia is usually very well demarcated from the surrounding mucosa, whereas reactive changes tend to be less sharply delineated.

The distinction between sporadic adenomatous polyps and IBD-related polypoid or adenoma-like dysplasia (also known as dysplasia-associated lesion or mass [DALM]) can be extremely challenging. Patients with both ulcerative colitis and Crohn's disease are at increased risk for both dysplasia and eventual progression to carcinoma. Dysplasia in IBD can present as a flat, elevated but indistinct lesion, or a discrete polypoid lesion, and can contain either low- or high-grade dysplasia.

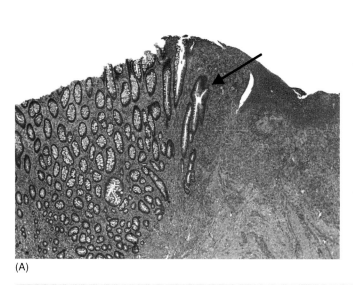
(A)

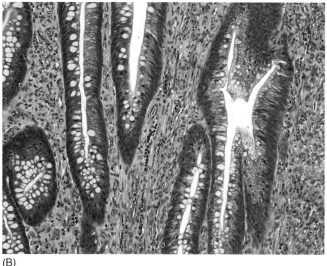
(B)

FIGURE 11.12 Reactive/regenerative epithelium near an ulcer (A, arrow; and B) shows nuclear hyperchromasia and stratification that mimics dysplasia. Note the gradual, indistinct transition to clearly benign crypts more distant to the ulcer (A).

Histologically, it has been reported in the literature that polypoid dysplasia in IBD may contain more inflammation and chronic mucosal injury than that seen in sporadic adenomas (Figure 11.13A–B). Sporadic adenomas also tend to have adenomatous glands that populate the entire polyp, whereas polypoid dysplasia in IBD may show a combination of adenomatous and nonadenomatous crypts. However, these observations cannot be used as definite criteria, as there is considerable morphologic overlap between sporadic adenomas in IBD and polypoid

dysplasia arising from the background of IBD. The most useful histologic finding in these cases often results from endoscopic sampling of the mucosa adjacent to the polypoid lesion. In IBD, the mucosa adjacent to the polypoid dysplasia tends to show histologic features of IBD, whereas these features should be absent in the case of a sporadic adenoma. Although it has been proposed that polypoid dysplasia in IBD shows stronger expression of p53 and less frequent nuclear β-catenin labeling, most practicing pathologists do not routinely use these

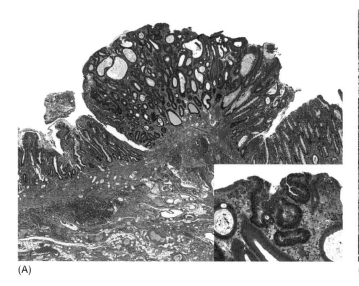
(A)

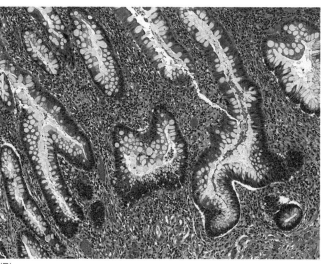
(B)

FIGURE 11.13 This focus of dysplasia in a case of inflammatory bowel disease forms a distinct polyp that is elevated above the surrounding mucosa (A; high power view shown in inset). The surrounding mucosa shows chronic minimally active colitis with crypt distortion and increased basal lymphoplasmacytosis, consistent with the history of chronic idiopathic inflammatory bowel disease (B).

immunostains to distinguish between these lesions. The distinction between a sporadic adenoma and polypoid low grade dysplasia in the setting of IBD may have little clinical importance, because polypectomy appears to be the adequate treatment in either case. The most important endoscopic question is whether the dysplasia is polypoid or not. If it is polypoid, polypectomy may be sufficient treatment, whereas a flat or indistinct elevated area of dysplasia is more concerning and may require additional treatment in the setting of IBD.

Serrated Polyps

Serrated polyps are common overall, comprising up to 15% to 45% of all colorectal polyps. The diagnostic classification of serrated polyps has undergone significant change in the past two decades. The unifying histologic feature of these polyps is sawtooth or serrated architecture that is thought to occur due to alterations in both apoptosis and senescence of crypt epithelial cells. Although historically the majority of serrated polyps were classified as hyperplastic polyps, it was observed that some cases of CRC appeared to arise in the context of certain serrated polyps, particularly those that were large and right-sided. Based on distinct morphologic, genetic, and clinical findings, the WHO now classifies serrated polyps as follows: hyperplastic polyp, sessile serrated adenoma/polyp (SSA/P), and traditional serrated adenoma (TSA) (see Table 11.3).

Hyperplastic polyps are the most common type of serrated polyp, representing 75% to 90% of serrated lesions. Endoscopically, hyperplastic polyps tend to be small (less than 5 mm), flat, pale, smooth, and located in the left colon. These polyps have essentially no malignant potential. Histologically, hyperplastic polyps are characterized by straight crypts that narrow at the base, with serration limited to the upper half of the crypts (Figure 11.14A–E). The basement membrane beneath the surface may be thickened. In comparison to SSA/Ps the crypt bases are not T- or L-shaped, nor are they dilated. The nuclei of hyperplastic

polyps are basally oriented with no significant hyperchromasia, pseudostratification, nor abundant apoptotic bodies. Neuroendocrine cells and mitotic figures may be present, but they are typically confined to the crypt bases. The proliferative zone, which can be highlighted by Ki-67 immunohistochemistry, is expanded but limited to the basal half of the crypt. Hyperplastic polyps can be morphologically subdivided into three types (microvesicular, goblet-cell-rich, and mucin-poor), but it is not currently necessary to distinguish between them in clinical practice.

SSA/P is a relatively recently described polyp that has distinct histologic and biologic features as compared to hyperplastic polyps. These polyps are common, comprising 10% to 20% of serrated polyps. Prior to their relatively recent description, SSA/Ps were thought to be within the spectrum of hyperplastic polyps, but it is now recognized that SSA/Ps are precursor lesions to CRC via the serrated pathway.

SSA/Ps typically are flat and sessile endoscopically (Figure 11.15A–J), with indistinct borders and a mucin cap. These polyps are usually greater than 5 mm in size, and often resemble a prominent colonic mucosal fold; SSA/Ps are more common in the right colon than the left. The defining histologic features of SSA/Ps are architectural, rather than cytologic. The most distinct architectural changes are identified at the base of the crypts, which show abnormal branching and dilatation that can resemble a "T," "L," "boot," or fish mouth shape (Figure 11.15E–F). The current minimum criteria for SSA/P consists of a single dilated crypt with convincing architectural distortion. In comparison to hyperplastic polyps, the serration of the glands in SSA/Ps extends to the base of the crypts, and is not confined to the upper half of the gland. Mature gastric foveolar cells and goblet cells may also be found at the base of the crypts, which is known as "reverse maturation." An inverted growth pattern can occur when there is herniation of crypts through the muscularis mucosae. Conventional cytologic dysplasia is not present in SSA/Ps although it may develop (see subsequent paragraphs).

TABLE 11.3   Clinical, Endoscopic, and Molecular Features of Colorectal Serrated Polyps

World Health Organization Classification	Prevalence	Shape and Endoscopic Appearance	Most Common Colorectal Site	Malignant Potential	Molecular Features
HP	Very common	Sessile/flat, smooth, and pale	Distal	Minimal to none	*KRAS* or *BRAF* mutation
SSA/P	Common	Sessile/flat mucous cap	Proximal		
No dysplasia				Present	*BRAF* mutation and CIMP
Dysplastic				Significant	*MLH1* promoter hypermethylation
TSA	Rare	Sessile or pedunculated	Distal	Present	*KRAS* mutation *BRAF* mutation or CIMP

Source: Modified from Lieberman DA, Rex DK, Winawer SJ, et al. Guidelines for colonoscopy surveillance after screening and polypectomy: a consensus update by the US Multi-Society Task Force on Colorectal Cancer. *Gastroenterology.* 2012;143:844–857.

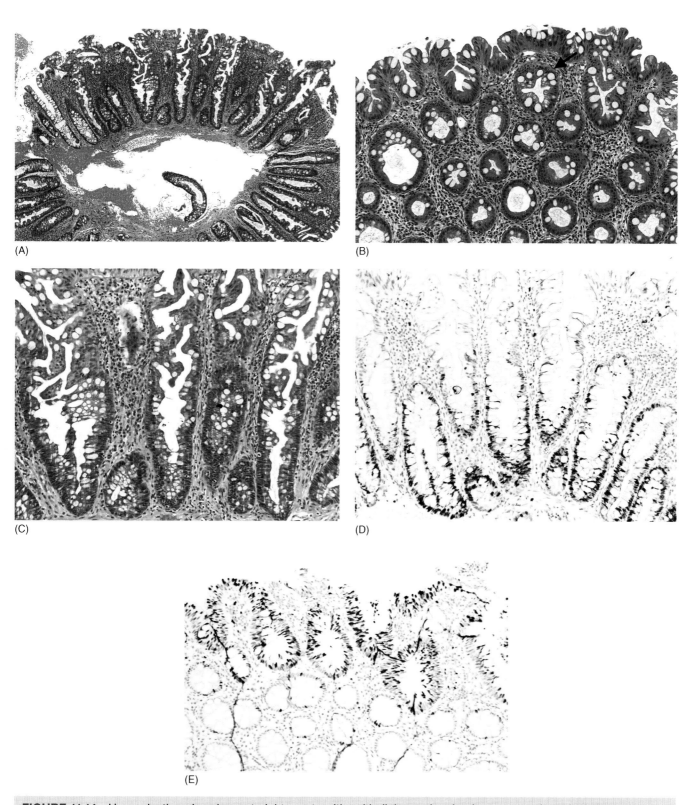

FIGURE 11.14 Hyperplastic polyps have straight crypts with epithelial serration that is most prominent in the upper half of the glands (A). A tangential section of the crypts shows a star-shaped configuration (B, arrow). The nuclei are basally oriented with no significant hyperchromasia, pseudostratification, or prominent apoptotic bodies. The basal zone of the crypts is narrow, without branching (C). A Ki-67 immunostain demonstrates that the proliferation zone of a hyperplastic polyp is confined to the basal crypts (D). This is in contrast to a tubular adenoma, in which the proliferation zone extends all the way up to the surface (E).

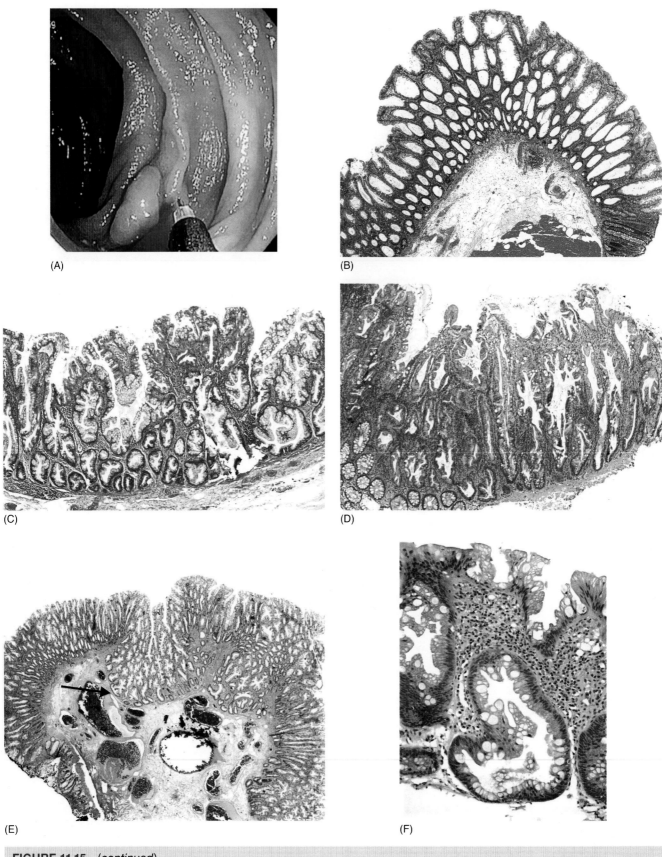

(A)

(B)

(C)

(D)

(E)

(F)

FIGURE 11.15   (*continued*)

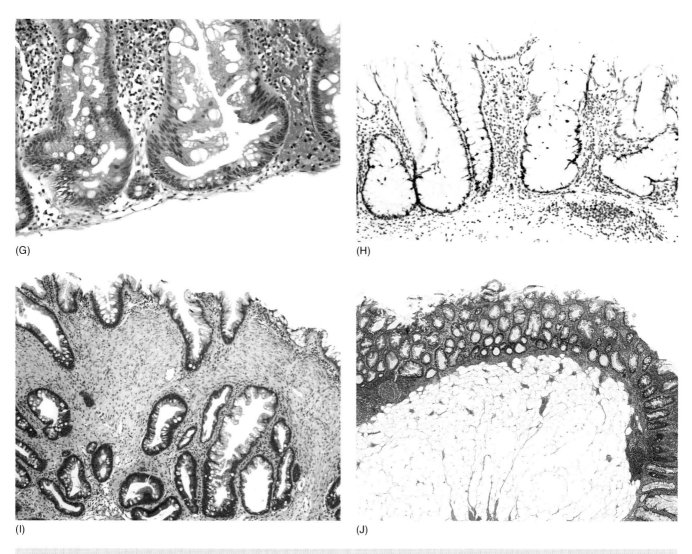

(G)

(H)

(I)

(J)

FIGURE 11.15   Sessile serrated adenomas are flat and sessile, with indistinct borders (A, courtesy Dr. Rhonda Yantiss). Sessile serrated adenomas demonstrate prominently dilated crypts (B) as well as serrations that involve the entire length of the crypt (C–D). T- and L-shaped crypts are present at the base of the lesion (E [arrow], F). The base of SSA/P also contains mature goblet cells and foveolar-type cells, a feature known as "reverse maturation" (G). A Ki-67 immunostain demonstrates that the proliferation zone is at the sides of the crypts and extends to the upper region of the crypts, unlike tubular adenomas (See Figure 11.14E) (H). Sessile serrated adenomas can have associated perineurioma-like stroma (I), as well as underlying lipomatous change (J).

SSA/Ps have an atypical proliferative area that can be highlighted using Ki-67 immunostaining; staining can be found in an irregular and asymmetric pattern anywhere from the base to the surface of the crypts. In addition, mitotic figures are "upwardly displaced" and located above the base of the crypts, in contrast to the location of mitotic figures in hyperplastic polyps. This helps explain, in part, why the crypts may proliferate in a horizontal configuration leading to T- and L-shaped crypts.

Some SSA/Ps contain mesenchymal changes including perineuriomatous change (Figure 11.15I). Both the SSA/P and perineuriomatous areas have been reported to show *BRAF* mutations. In addition, SSA/Ps have been associated with lipoma-like adipose tissue in the submucosa

(Figure 11.15J). It remains unclear if this represents an association between an SSA/P and a typical lipoma, or is a type of change induced in the mesenchymal tissue by the epithelium.

SSA/Ps that develop cytologic dysplasia (Figure 11.16A–D) similar to that seen in conventional adenomatous polyps are termed "SSA/P with cytologic dysplasia." Previously, these were often classified as mixed serrated/adenomatous polyps, or mixed hyperplastic/adenomatous polyps. They are now thought to represent molecular progression in SSA/Ps, and are clinically significant as they may progress to carcinoma more rapidly than conventional adenomas or SSA/P due to the additional molecular "hit." Histologically, these lesions have

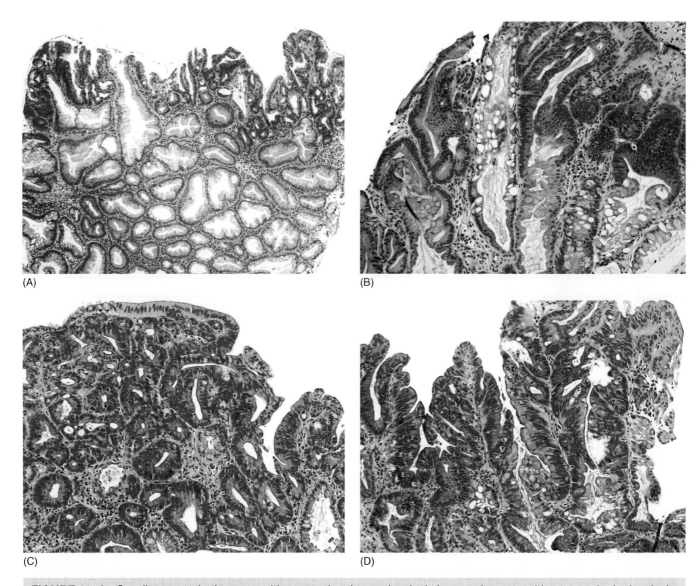

FIGURE 11.16 Sessile serrated adenomas with conventional-type dysplasia have a sharp transition to cytologic dysplasia that reaches the epithelial surface (A–B). The cytologic dysplasia is similar to conventional adenomas with elongated, hyperchromatic nuclei and pseudostratification. This sessile serrated adenoma with progression to high-grade dysplasia shows cribriform architecture (C) with residual serrated architecture in the background. The serrated form of epithelial dysplasia features prominent serration with dysplastic cells containing eosinophilic cytoplasm, more similar to a traditional serrated adenoma (D).

areas characteristic of SSA/P, with an abrupt transition to conventional-type cytologic dysplasia (adenomatous change). The cytologic dysplasia is usually low grade, but high-grade conventional-type dysplasia can be seen as well. A "serrated" form of cytologic dysplasia has also been described, featuring more cuboidal cells with open chromatin, similar to TSA.

TSAs are rare (1%–2% of serrated polyps), and almost exclusively located in the distal colorectum. Endoscopically, they may be pedunculated or sessile. Histologically, these polyps show a villous or tubulovillous architecture and surface cytologic dysplasia (typically low grade) (Figure 11.17A–C). The tall and columnar

cells have basally or centrally located nuclei with striking eosinophilic cytoplasm; given these features, these are often referred to as "eosinophilic pencillate cells." Unlike conventional adenomas, mitotic figures are rare. In addition, they show ectopic crypt buds in the villi that are oriented perpendicular to the long axis of the villi, and do not connect to the muscularis mucosae. This is in contrast to hyperplastic polyps and SSA/Ps in which the crypts are anchored to the muscularis mucosae. These ectopic crypts are the location of the proliferation zone and are one of the most characteristic histologic features of TSA; however, they are reportedly only seen in approximately one-third of cases.

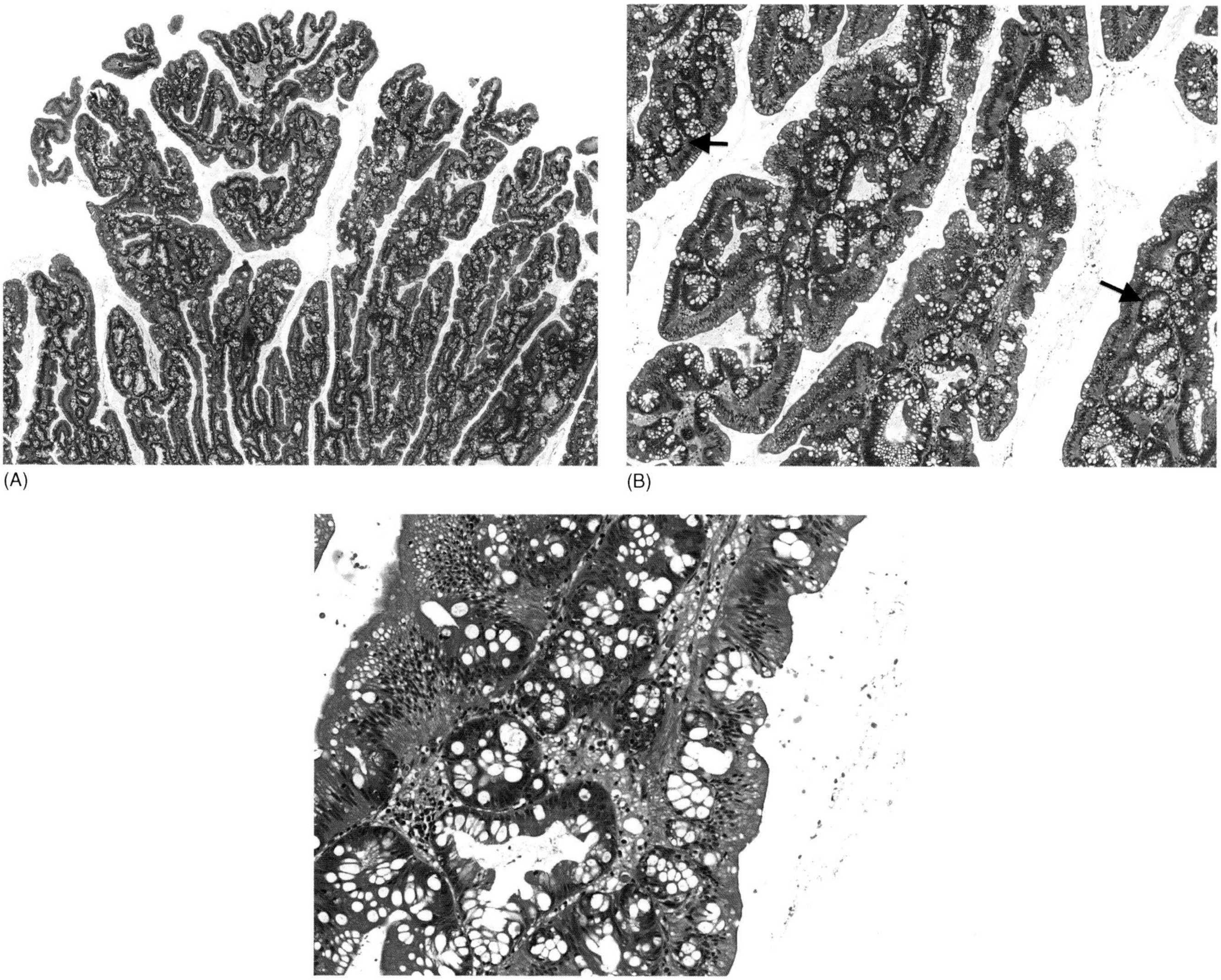

FIGURE 11.17 Traditional serrated adenomas have a complex villiform growth pattern at low power (A). Numerous ectopic crypts (B, arrows and C) are present along the sides of the villi. TSAs typically display low-grade cytologic dysplasia at the surface, with tall columnar epithelium with striking eosinophilic cytoplasm.

Serrated polyposis syndrome is an ill-defined and probably underrecognized disorder characterized by multiple serrated polyps throughout the colorectum, with an associated increased risk of CRC. The polyps can be hyperplastic polyps, SSA/Ps TSAs, or a combination thereof. The genetic features of serrated polyposis syndrome are not well understood. Compared to other syndromes with a predisposition to CRC, this syndrome is unusual in that it primarily affects older adults (although there is a wide age range).

The criteria for diagnosing serrated polyposis syndrome consist of at least one of the following:

- At least five serrated polyps proximal to the sigmoid colon, two of which are greater than 10 mm.
- Any number of serrated polyps proximal to the sigmoid colon in an individual who has a first-degree relative with serrated polyposis syndrome.

- Greater than 20 serrated polyps of any size found anywhere in the colon.

Based on molecular analysis, there are likely two subtypes of this syndrome, with overlapping features. The first subgroup corresponds to the first criterion listed above (at least five serrated polyps, at least two greater than 10 mm). These polyps can be large hyperplastic polyps, SSA/P or SSA/P with dysplasia. These polyps commonly have molecular alterations including CpG island methylator phenotype (CIMP) and *BRAF* mutation; *KRAS* mutations are less common. The second subtype corresponds to the third criterion listed above (greater than 20 polyps of any size). The polyps in this subtype are often hyperplastic polyps, and frequently have mutations in *KRAS*. This subtype has a lower overall risk of CRC.

Molecular Alterations in Serrated Polyps

KRAS mutations are more characteristically present in goblet-cell-rich hyperplastic polyps, while *BRAF* mutations are associated with microvesicular hyperplastic polyps, and some authors believe that a subset of microvesicular hyperplastic polyps may progress to SSA/Ps. SSA/Ps are thought to develop through *BRAF* mutations and CpG island methylation. If CpG island methylation of the *MLH1* promoter region occurs, the SSA/Ps may progress to dysplasia and possibly subsequent adenocarcinoma. The promoter hypermethylation causes downregulation of gene transcription with resultant decrease/loss of MLH1 protein expression; thus, MLH1 immunostaining may be lost in areas of cytologic dysplasia. This molecular alteration in the serrated pathway leads to microsatellite instability and possibly to an accelerated path to adenocarcinoma when additional molecular events occur. In fact, serrated precursor lesions are sometimes seen at the edge of sporadic microsatellite unstable adenocarcinomas. TSAs can have *KRAS* or *BRAF* mutations or a CIMP.

Treatment and Surveillance Guidelines

These guidelines are dictated by the risk of progression to malignancy. Most patients with hyperplastic polyps detected at initial colonoscopy should undergo repeat surveillance after 10 years. More than four hyperplastic polyps at the time of endoscopy, and/or any hyperplastic polyp greater than 5 mm, may warrant follow-up at 5 years. SSA/Ps are followed with repeat endoscopy every 5 years, similar to conventional-type adenomas, and should be completely removed if possible. When there are greater than three SSA/Ps at endoscopy or one SSA/P is greater than 10 mm, the current guidelines recommend follow-up at 3 years, similar to follow-up recommendations for conventional adenomas with high-risk features. SSA/Ps with dysplasia should be completely removed and patients should undergo surveillance in 1 year. Patients with serrated polyposis syndrome should undergo surveillance every 1 to 3 years. These guidelines are summarized in Table 11.4.

Diagnostic Challenges

The most common diagnostic dilemma is distinguishing between an SSA/P and another type of serrated polyp, usually a hyperplastic polyp. Attention to the lack of dilatation, serration, and complex shapes at the base of the crypts typically helps support the diagnosis of hyperplastic polyp rather than SSA/P. Poor orientation or tissue fragmentation, however, may preclude a definite distinction between the two. If the distinction cannot be made due to tissue fragmentation, lack of orientation, or the fact that a small biopsy of a large lesion is received for evaluation, a diagnosis of "serrated polyp" can be rendered with an explanatory comment. Correlation with the macroscopic size and location of the polyp can also be very helpful. A similar issue can arise when multiple fragments of serrated polyp are submitted, and some of them contain conventional-type cytologic dysplasia, as it may be difficult to ascertain whether the tissue fragments represent SSA/P and a separate conventional adenoma, or an SSA/P with conventional dysplasia (progression). The identification of both the SSA/P area and conventional dysplastic portion in the same tissue fragment can help confirm this as progression within the SSA/P. Furthermore, correlation with the macroscopic findings (ie, whether one or two lesions were sampled) can be very useful.

TABLE 11.4 Recommended Surveillance Intervals After Endoscopic Resection of Polyps

Histology	Size	Number	Location	Interval in Years
Hyperplastic polyp (HP)	<10 mm	Any number	Rectosigmoid	10
HP	≤5 mm	≤3	Proximal sigmoid	10
HP	Any size	≥4	Proximal sigmoid	5
HP	>5 mm	≥1	Proximal sigmoid	5
SSA/P or TSA	<10 mm	<3	Any site in colon	5
SSA/P or TSA	≥10 mm	1	Any site in colon	3
SSA/P or TSA	<10 mm	≥3	Any site in colon	3
SSA/P	≥10 mm	≥2	Any site in colon	1–3
SSA/P w/dysplasia	Any size	Any number		1–3
TA	< 10 mm	1–2	Any site in colon	5–10
TA	<10 mm	3–10	Any site in colon	3
TA, TVA, VA	Any size	>10	Any site in colon	<3
TA	≥10 mm	Any number	Any site in colon	3
VA or TVA	Any size	Any number	Any site in colon	3
Adenoma with high-grade dysplasia (HGD)	Any size	Any number	Any site in colon	3
Serrated polyposis syndrome	Any size	Any number	Any site in colon	1

Source: Modified from Rex DK, Ahnen DJ, Baron JA, et al. Serrated lesions of the colorectum: review and recommendations from an expert panel. *Am J Gastroenterol. 2012*;107:1315–1329; Lieberman DA, Rex DK, Winawer SJ, et al. Guidelines for colonoscopy surveillance after screening and polypectomy: a consensus update by the US Multi-Society Task Force on Colorectal Cancer. *Gastroenterology*. 2012;143:844–857.

TSA can also be in the differential diagnosis with SSA/P although this is a less common dilemma. The villous architecture, together with the low-grade surface dysplasia and ectopic crypts, should help support the diagnosis of TSA. If a right-sided polyp has features suggestive of a TSA, the possibility of an SSA/P with progression and dysplasia should be considered. The most common polyp in the differential diagnosis of a TSA is tubulovillous adenoma. Tubulovillous adenomas typically show more significant dysplasia than that seen in TSAs, and do not contain ectopic crypts.

Other entities in the differential diagnosis of SSA/P are prolapse and inflammatory-type polyps. These polyps can contain elongation and serration of crypts that mimic SSA/P (Figure 11.18A–C). Features favoring prolapse/inflammatory-type polyps include inflammation, fibromuscular hyperplasia of the lamina propria, triangular or diamond-shaped crypts, and location in the distal colon or rectum. Features favoring SSA/P include location in the proximal colon and irregular T-shaped or fish-mouth-shaped crypts. Additionally, SSA/P typically lack prominent inflammation, ulceration, granulation tissue, and fibromuscular proliferation in the stroma.

COLORECTAL ADENOCARCINOMA

Epidemiology

CRC is the third most common malignancy in both women and men, although men are more commonly affected. There is a great degree of geographical variation in the incidence of CRC, with industrialized nations having a much higher incidence than developing countries due to

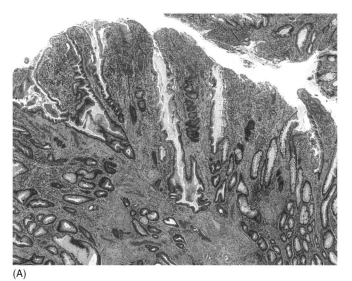

(A)

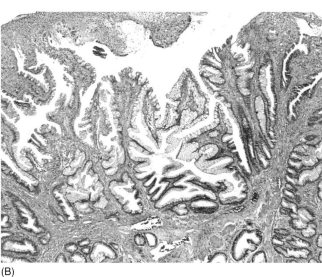

(B)

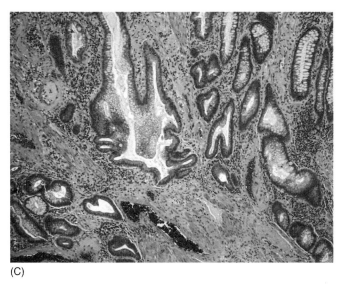

(C)

FIGURE 11.18 Prolapse polyps may contain irregularly shaped hyperplastic crypts that mimic SSA/Ps; however, the perpendicular fibromuscular stroma and inflammatory changes of prolapse polyps help to distinguish the two (A–C).

differences in diet as well as genetic alterations. Likewise, survival varies with geography, due to differences in the availability of screening colonoscopy and the variation in the quality of medical care among different countries.

Both genetic and environmental factors influence the risk of development of CRC. Genetic polyposis syndromes (see also Chapter 6) have a strong penetrance, but account for only a minority of cases (approximately 5%). Some cases of CRC appear to be familial, but no known genetic mutation is detectable. Chronic idiopathic inflammatory bowel disease, which has a strong genetic component, is also a risk factor for CRC, particularly in the context of long-standing disease. Table 11.5 summarizes diseases associated with increased risk of CRC.

One of the greatest risk factors for the development of CRC is advanced age. Additional risk factors include a prior history of CRC, an adenomatous polyp greater than 1.0 cm, a first-degree relative with a history of CRC (family history), African American ethnicity, smoking, alcohol consumption, diabetes mellitus, physical inactivity, obesity, previous uretero-sigmoidectomy, and a history of abdominal irradiation. Conversely, environmental factors that are protective against CRC include diets rich in fibers and vegetables, physical activity, nonsteroidal anti-inflammatory drugs, and folate, among others.

Clinical Features

Patients who present with CRC often have vague generalized complaints such as weight loss or fever. Symptoms often include changes in bowel habits, stool size, and hematochezia. Left-sided CRCs are more likely than right-sided CRCs to present with a change in bowel habits and hematochezia, due to the smaller lumen of the bowel on the left side. Rectal cancer can present with pain and tenesmus as well as pencil-thin stools. Alternatively, right-sided CRCs are more likely to present with anemia rather than obstruction or change in bowel habits. Laboratory findings can include iron deficiency anemia, elevated serum carcinoembryonic antigen, and, rarely, *Streptococcus bovis* bacteremia.

Macroscopic and Microscopic Features

Colorectal cancer can have several different growth patterns macroscopically, including polypoid/exophytic, ulcerating, and endophytic lesions. When CRC grows circumferentially around the lumen of the large bowel, it is described as annular. Rarely, CRC has a diffuse growth pattern with indistinct borders, similar to linitis plastica of the stomach.

Histologically, about 85% of CRC are intestinal-type adenocarcinomas, with the remaining 15% comprising various subtypes that will be discussed in the subsequent paragraphs. Similar to the remainder of the gastrointestinal tract, CRC is usually composed of malignant glands (Figure 11.19A–E). The glands may be incompletely formed and have central dirty or comedo-type necrosis. The nuclei often have vesicular chromatin with prominent nucleoli. The glands are often angulated and surrounded by a fibroinflammatory stromal response.

The most common immunohistochemical profile of colorectal carcinoma is cytokeratin (CK)20 positive, CDX2 positive, and CK7 negative. However, not all CRCs show this immunoprofile (see also Chapter 13). CK20 positivity is more common in well-differentiated tumors than poorly differentiated ones. CK7 positivity, when present, is often patchy, and is more commonly found in the rectum where approximately 25% of rectal adenocarcinomas express of CK7. CDX2 expression is present in about 70% of CRC, and is more common in well- and moderately differentiated tumors compared to poorly differentiated tumors. Microsatellite unstable tumors are more commonly negative for CK20 and CDX2, and medullary carcinoma is negative for CDX2 in approximately 85% of cases. Signet ring cell carcinoma expresses CK7 in up to 33% of cases.

The histologic classification of CRC from the WHO is summarized in Table 11.2. When a subtype of CRC is present but the percentage fails to meet the WHO diagnostic criteria for classification as that subtype, the minor component(s) may be listed in the report along with the diagnosis of conventional adenocarcinoma (eg, poorly differentiated adenocarcinoma with mucinous and signet ring cell components).

Mucinous adenocarcinoma of the colorectum is diagnosed when greater than 50% of the tumor is composed of mucin pools, with tumor cells floating within the mucin (Figure 11.20A–B). The floating epithelium commonly appears as detached strips, and there may be a minor component of signet ring cells. This subtype of CRC is relatively common, accounting for 10% of all CRC. Mucinous adenocarcinoma is more common in microsatellite unstable tumors and younger patients. The prognostic significance of this subtype has been disputed, but it appears that mucinous adenocarcinomas associated with microsatellite instability have a more favorable course than those that are microsatellite stable. Of note, the term "mucinous adenocarcinoma" should not be used to describe the extracellular mucin pools found after neoadjuvant chemoradiation in rectal cancer.

Signet ring cell carcinomas are the third most common subtype of CRC, accounting for approximately 1% of CRC. Designation as a signet ring cell carcinoma requires that greater than 50% of the tumor be composed of signet ring cells. Signet ring cells, characterized by a nucleus that is eccentrically displaced by a mucin vacuole (Figure 11.21A–B), are typically dyscohesive with an infiltrating

TABLE 11.5 Diseases Associated With Colorectal Adenocarcinoma

	Familial Adenomatous Polyposis (FAP)	Lynch Syndrome	Peutz-Jehgers Syndrome	Cowden Syndrome	MUTYH-Associated Polyposis	Juvenile Polyposis Syndrome	Ulcerative Colitis	Crohn disease
Inheritance mode	Autosomal Dominant	Autosomal Dominant	Autosomal Dominant	Autosomal Dominant	Autosomal Recessive	Autosomal Dominant	Partial contribution/penetrance of multiple genes	Partial contribution/penetrance of multiple genes
Molecular alterations	APC (5q21-q22)	MLH1 (3p21-p23), MSH2 or MSH6 (2p21), PMS2 (7p22)	STK11/LKB1 (19p13.3)	PTEN (10q23)	MUTYH (former MYH) (1p34.1)	SMAD4/DPC4 (18q21.1) or BMPR1A/ALK3 (10q22.3)	Variable	Variable
Premalignant lesions	Adenomas	Adenomas	Hamartomas with dysplasia	Hamartomas with dysplasia	Adenomas	Juvenile polyp with dysplasia	Dysplasia	Dysplasia
Polyp number	100s-1,000s	Varies	Varies	Varies	5-100s	3-200	Varies	Varies
Location of polyps within the GI tract	Colorectum (especially left colon), small intestine	Colorectum (especially right colon), small intestine	Small intestine, stomach, colorectum	Stomach, small intestine, colorectum	Colorectum, small intestine, stomach	Colorectum, small intestine, stomach	Colorectum	Colorectum
Lifetime risk for developing colorectal adenocarcinoma	100%, mean age 35-40	10-53%	39%	Little or no risk	93-fold increased risk	39%, Relative risk 34	30% risk by age 30 in patients with pancolitis before age 15 years	Relative risk 2.9% at 10 years following diagnosis
Recommendations for surveillance	Lower & upper endoscopy every 1-5 years depending on polyp location and burden	Colonoscopy every 1-2 years from age 20-25 years or 10 years prior to the earliest age of colon cancer diagnosis in the family (whichever comes first)	Lower & upper endoscopy every 2-3 years from age 18 years	Baseline colonoscopy at age 35 years then every 5 to 10 years or more frequently if symptomatic or polyps are noted	Biannual lower & upper endoscopy from age 25-30 years	Lower & upper endoscopy annually from age 15 years	Variable	Variable

Source: Data from Arber and Moshkowitz, *Curr Gastroenterol Rep.* 2011;13:435-41; Canavan et al, *Aliment Pharmacol Ther.* 2006;23:1097-104; Jass, *Pathol Res Pract.* 2008;204:431-47; Koornstra, *Best Pract Res Clin Gastroenterol.* 2012;26:359-68; Pan, *World J Gastrointest Oncol.* 2011;3:33-42; Rampertab et al, *Gut.* 2003;52:1211-4; Adapted from *WHO classification of tumours of the digestive system,* 4th edition, 2010.

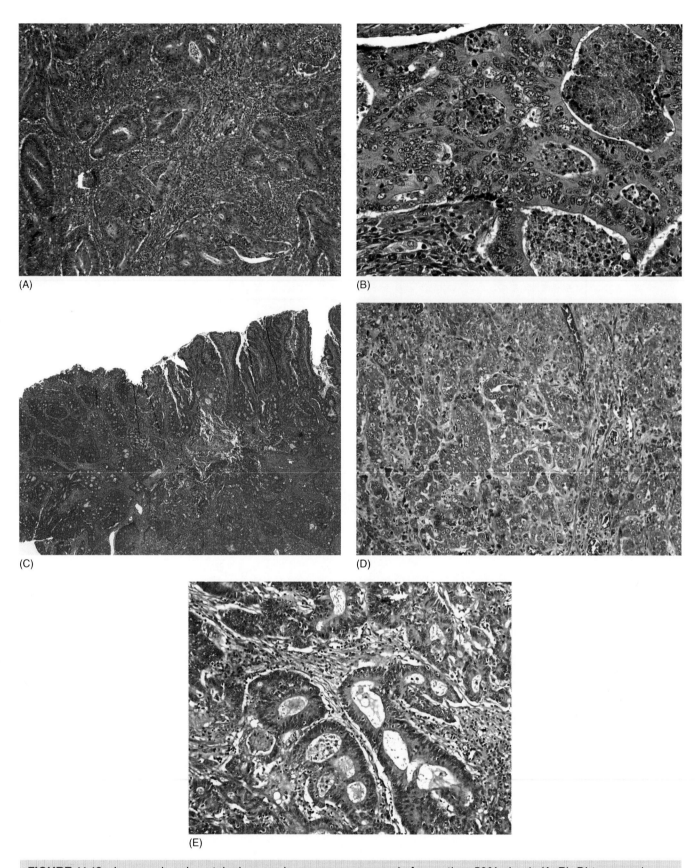

FIGURE 11.19 Low-grade colorectal adenocarcinomas are composed of more than 50% glands (A–B). Dirty necrosis is a common feature. Poorly differentiated adenocarcinomas (high grade) have predominately solid and cribriform growth patterns with only focal gland formation, and high-grade nuclear features (C–D). Tumors with numerous intratumoral lymphocytes should raise the possibility of MSI and Lynch Syndrome (E).

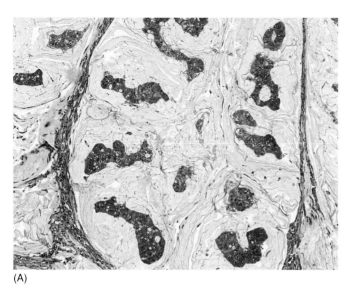
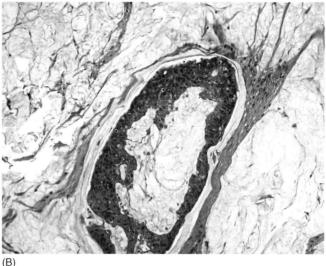

(A)   (B)

FIGURE 11.20 Mucinous adenocarcinomas feature lakes of dissecting mucin containing floating strips of malignant epithelium (A–B). The epithelium typically has low-grade cytologic features (B).

growth pattern. Signet ring cell tumors are usually aggressive and are considered by convention to be poorly differentiated. This subtype has also been associated with microsatellite unstable CRC.

Medullary carcinoma is a unique subtype of CRC that is strongly associated with MSI. Microscopically, these tumors are composed of uniform cells that may have a round or polygonal shape, with eosinophilic cytoplasm and a characteristic lymphocytic infiltrate (Figure 11.22A–B). The tumor cells may form nests and cords, and therefore, may mimic NETs. However, medullary carcinomas are

negative for neuroendocrine markers. Medullary carcinomas may not express CK20 or CDX2, and occasionally express CK7 in contrast to the typical immunoprofile of CRC. Despite the aggressive appearance of medullary carcinoma, this tumor has a more favorable prognosis, as do other tumors associated with MSI.

There are several rare subtypes of CRC. Pure squamous cell carcinomas are composed of invasive nests of cells with variable keratin formation. Primary squamous cell carcinoma of the colorectum is a diagnosis of exclusion, as proximal extension of an anal tumor, metastatic disease, and

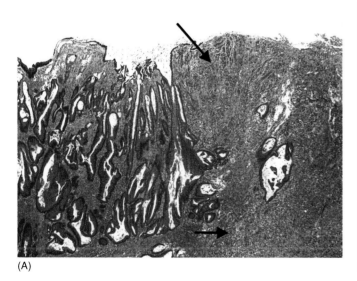
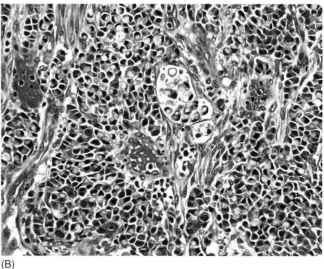

(A)   (B)

FIGURE 11.21 Areas of signet ring cell adenocarcinoma (arrows) can occur along with a component of conventional intestinal-type adenocarcinoma (A). The signet ring cells are dyscohesive, have an eccentrically placed nucleus, and intracytoplasmic vacuoles that contain mucin (B).

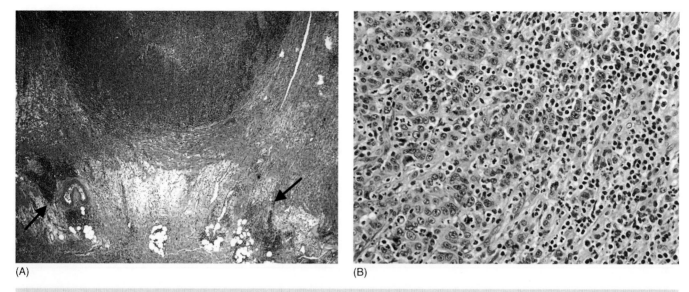

(A)   (B)

FIGURE 11.22   This medullary carcinoma has an associated lymphocytic Crohn-like reaction at the periphery (arrows), typical of microsatellite unstable tumors (A). This tumor is composed of sheets of polygonal, monotonous cells with an intratumoral inflammatory infiltrate composed mainly of lymphocytes (B).

squamous cell carcinoma arising from a fistula tract must all be excluded. These tumors tend to have a very poor prognosis. Clear cell adenocarcinoma of the colon is composed of polygonal cells arranged in nests (Figure 11.23A–B). The cytoplasm of the tumor cells is optically clear to eosinophilic. There is often a conventional adenocarcinoma component and/or a tubular adenoma adjacent to this tumor, which, along with immunohistochemistry (CK20+ and CDX2+, negative for PAX8 and PAX2) helps to distinguish it from metastatic clear cell carcinoma of the kidney.

Other rare variants include sarcomatoid carcinoma, which is a biphasic tumor composed of both carcinomatous and sarcomatous components; choriocarcinoma, which usually demonstrates foci of conventional CRC as well as areas of both cytotrophoblasts and syncytiotrophoblasts; and adenosquamous carcinoma, which shows areas of both squamous cell carcinoma and adenocarcinoma and may be associated with hypercalcemia and elevated levels of Parathyroid hormone (PTH)-related protein.

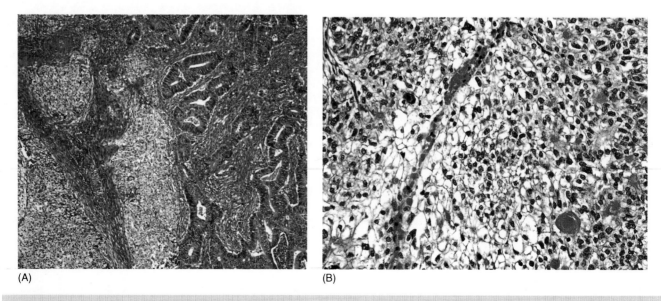

(A)   (B)

FIGURE 11.23   Clear cell carcinoma is a rare subtype of colorectal carcinoma that can occur in association with conventional intestinal-type adenocarcinoma (A). The cell borders are well-defined and contain clear cytoplasm (B).

Adenocarcinoma presenting in a polyp may lead to unique diagnostic challenges. A malignant polyp is defined as one that harbors adenocarcinoma extending beyond the muscularis mucosae into the submucosa of the polyp. Carcinoma confined to a polypectomy specimen represents a unique circumstance in which the biopsy specimen may be both diagnostic and curative. Depending on the microscopic findings in the specimen, patients may not need to undergo further surgical treatment for their carcinoma.

Malignant polyps that are pedunculated can often be safely managed by endoscopic resection, provided pathologists are able to evaluate specific histologic features. It is helpful for the polyp to be removed as a single piece with a clearly defined stalk margin, whereas one may not be able to evaluate the margin status of fragmented specimens. Patients whose margin status is uncertain may need to undergo further resection, although sometimes rebiopsy of the polypectomy site may prove sufficient if the rebiopsy is negative. In contrast, the extent of invasive carcinoma in sessile polyps may be difficult to appreciate, and endoscopic resection may not be adequate.

Once the diagnosis of invasive adenocarcinoma is made in a polypectomy specimen, there are three critical morphologic features that must be assessed and reported: margin status, tumor grade, and lymphovascular invasion. An increased risk of adverse outcome has been associated with tumor present less than 1 to 2 mm from the cauterized margin. The presence of lymphovascular invasion is another histologic feature that is unfavorable. Retraction artifact around malignant glands can mimic lymphovascular invasion, so if there is any doubt about the presence of lymphovascular invasion, immunostains such as D2-40 or CD31 may be helpful. Finally, the presence of any high-grade (poorly differentiated) component of invasive carcinoma is considered a risk factor for disease recurrence or regional lymph node metastases. Thus, the presence of any poorly differentiated component in a malignant polyp should be noted in the pathology report. Other histologic features that some authors have found to correlate with adverse prognosis include the depth of submucosal invasion and tumor budding. Although these features have not been incorporated into patient management guidelines yet, future studies may warrant their inclusion.

Diagnostic Challenges

One major pitfall in the diagnosis of invasive adenocarcinoma is misplaced adenomatous epithelium, also known as pseudoinvasion, particularly in pedunculated adenomas of the distal colorectum. The primary mechanism for pseudoinvasion is thought to be traumatic mechanical forces that push mucosa into the submucosa, similar to colitis cystica profunda.

Microscopic features favoring invasive adenocarcinoma include a prominent desmoplastic response, infiltrating small angulated glands or single cells, and architectural complexity including a cribriform growth pattern and/or solid sheets of cells (Figure 11.24A–B). Furthermore, in true invasion, the malignant epithelium tends to be of a higher grade in the invasive component than in the overlying adenoma. Invasive adenocarcinomas also typically lack associated hemorrhage and hemosiderin-laden macrophages seen in cases of misplaced adenomatous epithelium. If mucin pools are present in cases of invasive adenocarcinoma, they characteristically have irregular dissecting borders and contain malignant cells.

Histologic features that favor misplaced epithelium include the presence of lamina propria around the misplaced glands, hemorrhage, hemosiderin-laden macrophages, and rounded glands in an orderly arrangement (Figure 11.24C–E). Misplaced epithelium does not have associated desmoplasia, and does not contain angulated glands. Misplaced epithelium can sometimes contain high-grade dysplasia and even architectural complexity. However, the degree of cytologic atypia should be similar to the dysplasia in the surface adenomatous epithelium. Benign mucin pools in the submucosa have round edges and do not contain epithelial cells, although low-grade epithelium at the peripheries of mucin pools may be present. In addition, the epithelium associated with the benign mucin pools should be similar in grade to the mucosa in the overlying associated polyp.

Another diagnostic challenge in the diagnosis of CRC is the distinction from endometriosis, particularly when endometriosis involves the wall of the colon. Endometriosis/endosalpingiosis occurs in women of reproductive age, who often present with infertility, hematochezia (sometimes coinciding with menstruation), or abdominal pain. Endoscopically, endometriosis may present as a polyp or mass, or may be found incidentally. Endometriosis may be found in the serosa, muscularis propria, submucosa, or lamina propria. It is histologically composed of benign haphazardly arranged columnar glands reminiscent of endometrium (Figure 11.25A–C). The columnar epithelium may appear hyperchromatic, but does not contain goblet cells. Endometrial stroma may be present, which can vary in morphology depending on the menstrual cycle. Features favoring endometriosis include identification of endometrial stroma, benign nuclear features, a lack of "dirty" necrosis (seen in CRCs), and hemosiderin deposition. The endometrial epithelium is positive for CK7 and PAX8, while negative for CK20 and CDX2, in contrast to typical CRC. In addition, the endometrial stroma may be decidualized and expresses CD10, ER, and PR. Rarely, Müllerian tumors may develop from endometriosis in the colon.

Endosalpingiosis is thought to be due to metaplasia of the peritoneal mesothelial surface into an epithelial type that resembles fallopian tube epithelium. It is usually an incidental finding. Because it is due to metaplasia of mesothelial cells, it is commonly found on the peritoneal

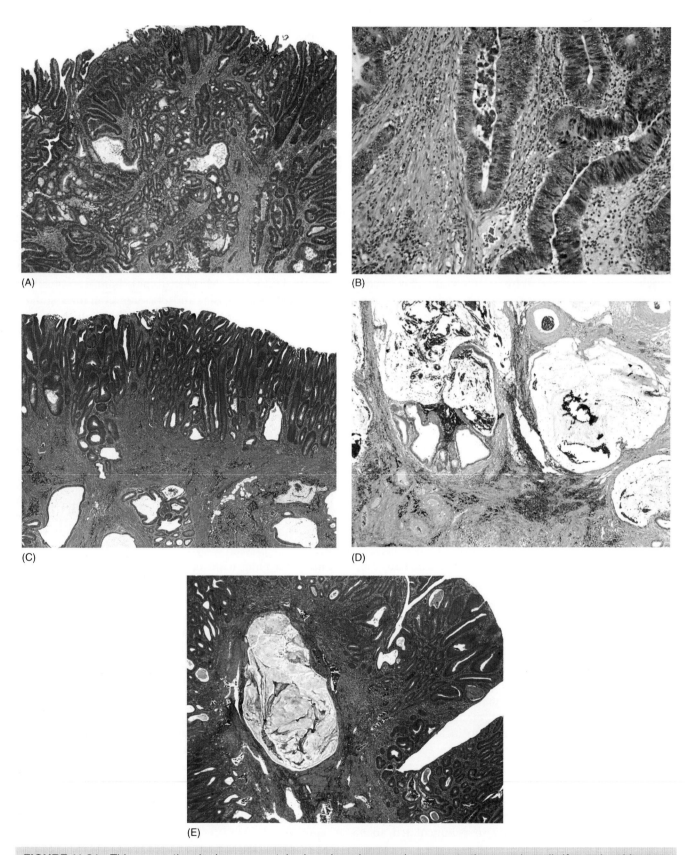

FIGURE 11.24 This conventional adenoma contains invasive adenocarcinoma; note the complex cribriformed architecture (A). A surrounding desmoplastic reaction and high grade nuclear features are readily apparent (B). This adenoma contains misplaced epithelium deep to the surface; the degree of dysplasia in the misplaced epithelium is similar to that seen at the surface (C). Other features favoring misplaced glands over invasive adenocarcinoma include surrounding lamina propria and hemosiderin-laden macrophages (D). The mucin beneath the surface of an adenoma with prolapse-type changes shows rounded edges that do not dissect tissue (E).

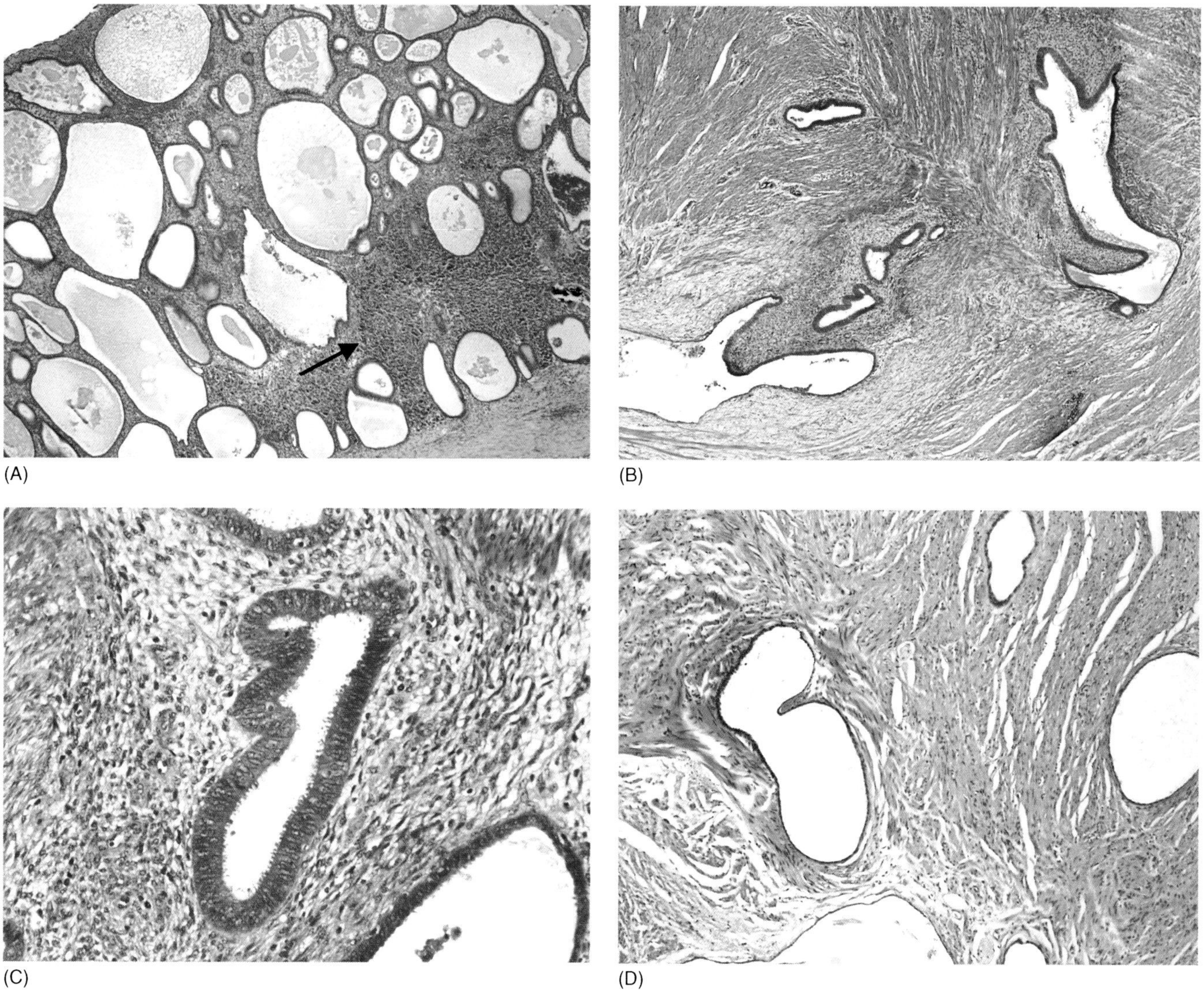

FIGURE 11.25 Endometriosis of the bowel may mimic invasive adenocarcinoma, and may even form a mass (A). However, the columnar epithelium lacks goblet cells, and there is associated endometrial stroma, hemosiderin-laden macrophages, and hemorrhage (A, arrow, and B). High-grade nuclear features should be absent as well, although nuclei may be enlarged and hyperchromatic (C). Endosalpingiosis is commonly found on the peritoneal surface of the bowel, and may also mimic adenocarcinoma (D). Histologically, the epithelium is very low grade, and there is no associated desmoplastic reaction to the glands.

surface (Figure 11.25D). Histologically, endosalpingiosis is composed of tubular-type epithelium that is ciliated, and endometrial-type stroma is not present. The distinction of endosalpingiosis from CRC is usually more straightforward than endometriosis, but if the diagnosis is not considered it can be missed. Features favoring endosalpingiosis include primarily peritoneal location, low-grade cytologic features, and ciliation.

Grading and Staging

CRCs are graded and staged according to the seventh edition of AJCC TNM, which was released in 2009 and contains many changes and clarifications from previous editions. Fortunately, many of the pathologic parameters are relatively straightforward, but some of the staging parameters remain challenging and/or controversial and require additional explanation. These include the concept of intramucosal adenocarcinoma, the identification of invasion through the muscularis propria and into pericolonic/perirectal soft tissues (T3), proper classification of serosal involvement (T4a) or adhesions to adjacent organs (T4b), evaluation of total mesorectal excision (TME), assessment of acellular mucin pools after neoadjuvant chemoradiation, tumor regression grade, tumor budding, and the definition of tumor deposits and N1c.

Similar to other adenocarcinomas, CRCs have traditionally been graded as well, moderately, and poorly differentiated; the justification for this is that the degree of differentiation is an independent predictor of outcome. Due to interobserver variability in the distinction/interpretation of well-differentiated from moderately differentiated tumors, however, a two-tiered system is currently used. Tumors are categorized as either low grade (well- and moderately differentiated) or high-grade (poorly differentiated). Tumors exhibiting less than 50% gland formation are classified as high grade when assessing the entire area of the tumor.

According to the American Joint Committee on Cancer (AJCC), seventh edition, carcinoma in situ and tumors for which invasion is restricted to the lamina propria are staged as carcinoma in situ (Tis), whereas tumors that invade the submucosa are staged as T1. Once a tumor has invaded the muscularis propria, it is staged as T2. Invasion of the pericolorectal soft tissues beyond the muscularis propria is considered T3. When a tumor is present at the visceral peritoneal surface, it is staged as T4a. Finally, invasion or adherence of adjacent organs is considered T4b. In most circumstances, analysis of the depth of invasion is straightforward. However, certain scenarios can present diagnostic challenges that can lead to inconsistent or incorrect staging; these are discussed in the immediately following sections.

Tis and T1

As mentioned in the previous paragraph, most pathologists consider carcinoma in situ to be within the spectrum of high-grade dysplasia in the colon, and the use of this term is discouraged because this lesion is not believed to have the potential to metastasize. In the AJCC, seventh edition, however, the term carcinoma in situ (Tis) is included, and (unlike most other organs) the definition includes tumors that are restricted to the glandular basement membrane as well as tumors that invade the lamina propria (sometimes called intramucosal carcinoma). The logic for this classification of Tis rather than T1 for intramucosal carcinoma in the colon arose from studies by Fenoglio et al. that demonstrated the absence of lymphatics in the lamina propria of the large bowel. It was therefore hypothesized that carcinoma that only invaded the lamina propria, but not the submucosa, did not have the ability to metastasize. Whether or not the lamina propria of the bowel contains lymphatics remains controversial, but most authorities believe that colorectal tumors confined to the lamina propria have minimal, if any, chance of metastasis. Although the classification of Tis exists for the colorectum in the AJCC scheme, many authorities discourage the use of this term.

T3

The identification of invasion through the muscularis propria and into pericolonic soft tissue (pT3) can be challenging when invasion by the leading edge of tumor is obscured by a fibrotic reaction to the tumor, which makes it difficult to determine where the muscularis propria ends and the pericolonic adipose tissue begins. This can be particularly challenging if invasion into the pericolonic soft tissue is focal. It has been proposed that the loss of muscle fibers between glands of tumor at the invasive front should be classified as pT3, but long-term studies are necessary to determine if these "minimal" pT3 cases behave similarly to those that are unequivocally classified as pT3. Taking additional sections of the area in question may also be helpful in getting a better look at the interface between the muscular wall and the pericolonic soft tissue.

T4a

Once a tumor has invaded beyond the muscularis propria and into the pericolorectal soft tissues, determination of whether the serosal surface is involved is of vital importance. A tumor is classified as pT4a when it is present at the visceral peritoneal surface or the tumor has perforated the bowel wall (Figure 11.26A–B). Assessment of serosal involvement is important because it may indicate the need for systemic adjuvant chemotherapy, even in those patients with stage II (lymph node negative) cancers (most of whom would not receive adjuvant chemotherapy unless there are high-risk features such as inadequate evaluation of the lymph nodes, T4 pathologic stage, lymphovascular invasion, bowel perforation, or poorly differentiated tumor).

One important study regarding the importance of serosal surface involvement was conducted by Shepherd et al., in an analysis of 412 colon cancers in which local peritoneal involvement (LPI) was carefully assessed. Tumors that had spread beyond the muscularis propria were classified into four groups: tumors cells well clear of the peritoneal surface (LPI1), tumor cells close to but not at the serosal surface with an associated mesothelial inflammatory and/or mesothelial hyperplastic reaction (LPI2), tumor cells present at the serosal surface with an inflammatory reaction, mesothelial hyperplasia, or "ulceration" (LPI3), and free floating tumor cells in the peritoneum with evidence of adjacent "ulceration" (LPI4). LPI groups correlated with overall survival, predicted intraperitoneal recurrence, and were a stronger independent prognostic indicator than the extent of local spread and lymph node involvement.

Controversy remains, however, in cases where tumor cells are close (less than 1 mm) to the serosal surface with circumstantial evidence of serosal involvement such as hemorrhage, ulceration, and/or a mesothelial reaction (Figure 11.26C). Colorectal tumors less than 1 mm from the serosal surface with a fibroinflammatory tissue

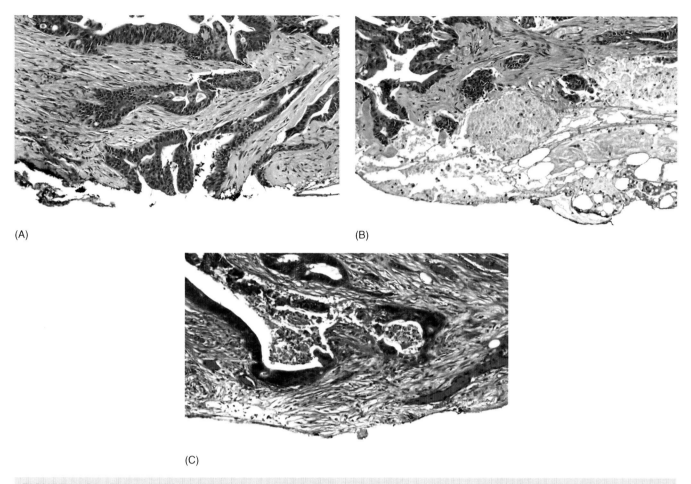

(A)

(B)

(C)

FIGURE 11.26 This case of colorectal carcinoma shows malignant glands present at the inked serosal surface and is staged as T4a (A). A different case shows necrosis extending from the tumor to the serosal surface; this would be considered T4a as well (B). This case shows tumor that is less than 1.0 mm from the serosal surface, with a fibrous reaction (C); staging as T3 versus T4a is controversial. Many would stage as T3 with a comment in the report.

reaction have been shown to have positive serosal scrape cytology and outcome more similar to T4 tumors, thus suggesting peritoneal involvement. In cases where serosal involvement is considered, it is often helpful to get deeper levels and take additional samples of the serosal surface. Tumor cells may involve natural clefts of the serosal surface, and these areas should be carefully assessed and considered T4a if involved by tumor. Since identification of mesothelial cells can be challenging, some have advocated the use of CK7 or calretinin to identify mesothelial cells, but this has not proven to be useful due to the lack of mesothelial cells lining the serosal surface in many cases.

Other authors have suggested that invasion of the subserosal elastic lamina can be used as a surrogate marker for serosal invasion. In the colon, the subserosal elastic lamina is found near the peritoneal surface (Figure 11.27A–D), and thus the hypothesis is that tumors that have invaded through this subserosal elastic lamina are more likely to gain access to the serosal surface and behave more aggressively. However, there are several

challenges in the interpretation and reporting of elastic lamina invasion. The elastic lamina is not easily identifiable in all colon cancer cases, notably the right colon. In addition, the subserosal elastic lamina often does not form a contiguous line. In our own practice, we have found that most cases do not show continuous staining and some do not stain at all. Currently, it remains unclear how to report tumor invasion of the elastic lamina and how this should affect staging, and studies examining the behavior of tumors that show penetration of the elastic lamina, but not the visceral peritoneum, have shown mixed results. Therefore, reporting of elastic lamina invasion is not recommended, nor is routine use of the elastic stain to help stage or predict outcome.

A common misunderstanding in staging rectal tumors is the belief they cannot invade the serosal surface. Proximal rectal tumors at or above the peritoneal reflection *do* have a serosal surface, and tumor involvement of this surface would be classified as T4a. In addition, the anterior serosa extends more distally than the posterior

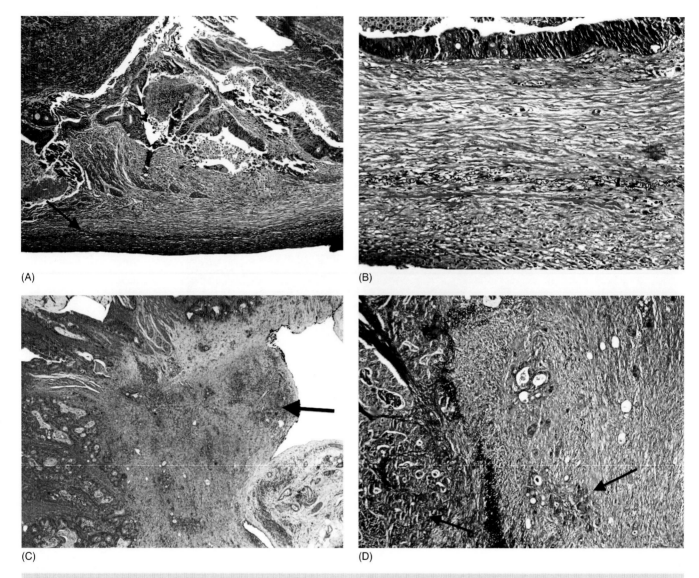

(A)

(B)

(C)

(D)

FIGURE 11.27 This elastic stain image shows an intact elastic lamina (A, arrow) without invasion by tumor (A–B, high power). Note that the elastic lamina forms a nearly continuous line that is black on elastic stain. Another case shows tumor cells very close to the serosal surface (C, arrow). When this area of tumor was stained for elastin, carcinoma is present on both the mucosal and serosal sides of the elastic lamina (D, arrows), suggesting that the tumor may have gained access to the serosal surface.

serosa in the rectum. Rectal tumors distal to the peritoneal reflection *do not* have a serosal surface, however. Therefore, a case with tumor cells present at the peripheral edge/surface of a distal rectal specimen would be classified as a positive radial margin but not serosal involvement.

Invasion of Adjacent Organs (T4b)

Invasion of adjacent organs, which is classified as T4b, is usually straightforward. Adhesions between the resected colorectum and adjacent organs should be staged as T4b when tumor cells are present within the adhesion, or directly invading adjacent organs. In other words, one need not identify carcinoma in an adjacent organ to assign a stage pT4b; tumor in the adhesion alone is adequate.

Previous data suggested that tumors with serosal involvement behave worse than those with invasion of adjacent organs. Therefore, the previous edition of AJCC (sixth edition) classified serosal involvement as T4b and involvement of adjacent organs as T4a. More recent data (Surveillance, Epidemiology, and End Results [SEER]) demonstrated that invasion of adjacent organs behaves worse than serosal involvement, which resulted in the current classification in the AJCC, seventh edition.

Radial (Circumferential) Margin and Mesenteric Margin

There is a great deal of confusion inherent in the definitions of the radial (circumferential) margin and the mesenteric margin. It is important to remember, as well, that these definitions differ according to site in the colorectum. A radial (circumferential) margin is surgically created by dissection of soft tissue. Thus, peritonealized surfaces (eg, the cecum) are *not* considered to be circumferential (radial) margins because they are not a surgically created plane. Therefore, in a segment of colon encased by peritoneum, only the surgically created mesenteric margin is equivalent to the radial margin. The remaining peritonealized surface is not a margin. The ascending and descending colons lack posterior serosalized surfaces; thus this area is considered the circumferential/radial margin. Very few pathologists (<10%) actually document the status of the posterior radial margins of ascending and descending colon cancers. Fortunately, available data suggest that this margin is likely of limited practical importance; tumors that involve this margin are generally of advanced with regional lymph node or distant metastases.

In the distal portion of the rectum not encased in peritoneum, the entire circumference of the bowel is considered a radial margin. The more proximal rectum does contain a peritonealized surface and, therefore, could be staged as T4a when involved by tumor, while the distal rectum would be staged as T3 with a positive radial margin. The radial margin is considered positive if the tumor is 1 mm or less from the nonperitonealized surface. Furthermore, if the tumor is present within a lymph node 1 mm or less from the nonperitonealized surface, this is also considered a positive radial margin. A positive radial margin is predictive of both local recurrence and death in rectal carcinomas.

Total Mesorectal Excision

Rectal cancers that lie below the peritoneal reflection are often removed by a surgical procedure known as total mesorectal excision (TME). This procedure is now considered the standard of care for low rectal cancers. The adequacy of the resection, is a strong independent predictor of local recurrence of the tumor and is noted to be complete, nearly complete or incomplete depending on the appearance of the mesorectal envelope (Figure 11.28). An incomplete mesorectum may be a surrogate marker for the local biologic aggressiveness of the tumor, or may be due to technical difficulties during the procedure.

Mesorectal resection specimens should be assessed grossly in the fresh state, and the entire mesorectal surface should be carefully examined; the worst appearing area should be used to score the specimen (Figure 11.28A–E). The mesorectum is considered complete when it is bulky with a smooth surface or only minor surface irregularities. There should not be any defect greater than 5 mm in depth, and there should not be coning (ie, tapering of the distal aspect of the specimen). The mesorectum is considered nearly complete when there is moderate bulk to the mesorectum and only mild surface irregularities with

none extending to the muscularis propria. One should not be able to visualize the muscularis propria in a nearly complete specimen. The mesorectum is considered incomplete when there is little bulk to the mesorectum, and/or defects are present in the mesorectum that clearly communicate with the muscularis propria. Assessment of completeness can be particularly challenging in abdominoperineal resection specimens, because the area in which the distal rectum crosses the levator muscles appears tapered, and this can be misinterpreted as distal coning. Robotically performed resections are becoming more common as well, and these types of specimens can also present challenges if the specimen is damaged during robotic removal. Controversy exists as to whether robotic procedures are superior to, equivalent, or inferior to open resections; however, experienced surgeons are able to perform robotic TME with complete preservation of the mesorectum.

Lymph Node Assessment

All lymph nodes that are identified during gross evaluation of a colectomy should be submitted for histologic evaluation. In the vast majority of cases, standard gross examination is sufficient to identify lymph nodes. Fat clearing agents can help identify lymph nodes when standard grossing fails to yield sufficient numbers of lymph nodes. These agents are composed of formalin, ethanol, and acetic acid, and make lymph nodes appear firm and white after fixation. However, routine use of fat clearing agents is not considered the standard of care and is not required for adequate lymph node dissection.

The typical minimum number of lymph nodes for adequate assessment of CRC ranges from 12 (College of American Pathologists [CAP]) or 10 to 14 (AJCC, seventh edition). It is important to note that when less than the minimal number of lymph nodes is identified, the designation Nx should not be used, but the tumor should be staged according to the number of nodes that are involved. It is well known that rectal tumors treated with neoadjuvant chemoradiation tend to have fewer lymph nodes identified, and lymphoid tissue may decrease with age as well. Therefore, there is no suggested minimum number of lymph nodes for rectal cancers treated with neoadjuvant chemoradiation, but as many as possible should be identified.

The definition, nomenclature, and role of tumor nodules or deposits in staging CRC have evolved with recent iterations of the AJCC. The fifth edition AJCC (1997) defined tumor deposits as foci of tumor measuring less than 3 mm without residual lymph node architecture. In the sixth edition AJCC (2002), the contour, rather than the size, of the tumor focus was used to distinguish totally replaced lymph nodes (rounded) from tumor deposits (irregular contour), and the latter were then coded as V1 (microscopic venous invasion) or V2 (grossly evident disease), depending on microscopic/gross findings. Tumor

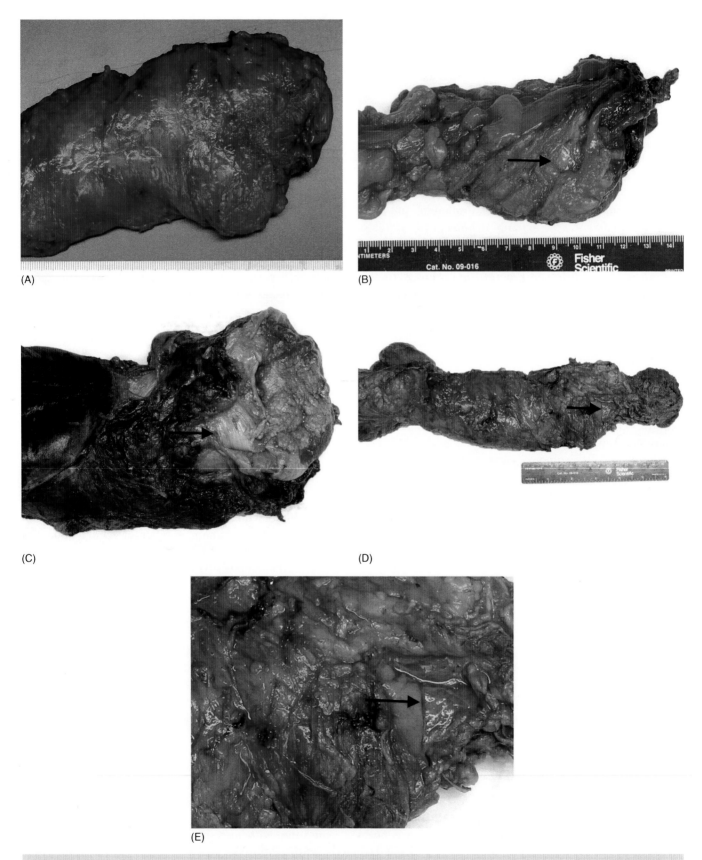

FIGURE 11.28 This example of a *complete* total mesorectal excision shows a bulky surface with no significant surface defects (A). A *nearly complete* total mesorectal excision has moderate bulk, with a small defect that does not extend to the muscularis propria (B, arrow). Incomplete total mesorectal excisions have defects (arrow) that extend to the muscularis propria (C–E). The narrow distal portion of the excision at the right of the specimen (D, abdominoperineal resection) should not be considered coning, and is due to the normal anatomical resection at the levators.

nodules helped define the T stage in both the AJCC, fifth and sixth editions, and were considered a discontinuous extension of the primary tumor; the T stage was therefore upstaged when necessary. In contrast, tumor deposits do not count toward the T stage in the AJCC, seventh edition.

Pericolonic tumor deposits are currently defined in the AJCC 7th edition as "discrete foci of tumor found in the pericolic or perirectal fat or in adjacent mesentery (mesocolic fat) away from the leading edge of the tumor and showing no evidence of residual lymph node tissue." This definition relies on the pathologist's interpretation of what constitutes residual lymph node tissue, and in some cases this is subjective. Interobserver variability exists when defining tumor deposits, even among pathologists with an interest/expertise in gastrointestinal pathology.

In challenging cases, helpful features in distinguishing lymph nodes from tumor deposits include round shape, peripheral lymphocyte rim, peripheral lymphoid follicles, possible subcapsular sinus, residual lymph node present in surrounding fibroadipose tissue, and a thick capsule (Figure 11.29A–C). When a tumor deposit is present within a discernible blood vessel, this should be recorded as lymphovascular invasion rather than a tumor deposit. Table 11.6 shows the evolution of tumor deposit definitions from AJCC, 5th, 6th, and 7th editions.

The AJCC 7th edition also created a new category termed N1c for cases in which there are tumor deposits present, but no positive lymph nodes. The letter "c" was chosen since it was the next alphabetic option after N1a and N1b. N1c does not, by definition, indicate a worse

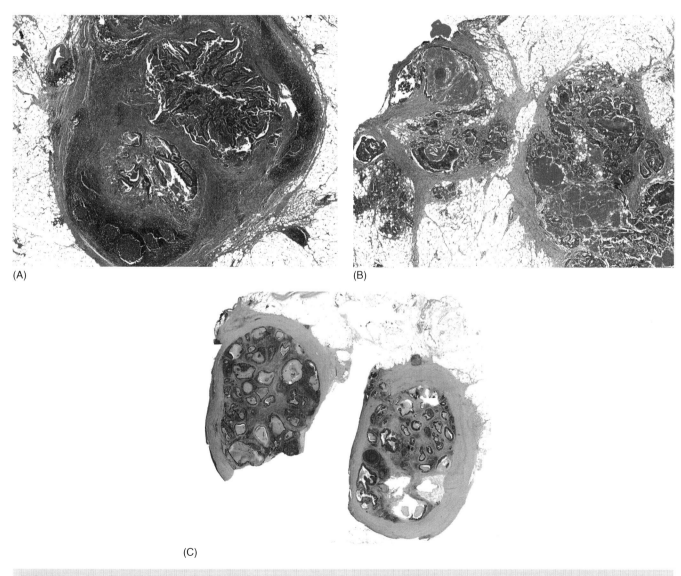

(A)

(B)

(C)

FIGURE 11.29   This photomicrograph shows an obvious lymph node containing metastatic adenocarcinoma; the residual peripheral lymphoid tissue is easily seen (A). This image shows focus of tumor with irregular borders and no definite residual lymph node architecture; this would be classified as a tumor deposit (B). This focus of metastatic carcinoma has a round shape and a thick capsule, which many would classify as a positive lymph node rather than a tumor deposit even though there is no residual lymph node tissue (C).

TABLE 11.6 Evolution of Colorectal Carcinoma Tumor Deposits With Recent Editions of the American Joint Committee on Cancer Staging Manual

AJCC Edition	Tumor Deposit Size Criteria	Tumor Deposit Shape Criteria	Other Definitional Criteria	Effect on T Stage	Effect on N Stage
Fifth	Less than 3 mm	No	No residual lymph node architecture	Considered discontinuous tumor extension, upstage when needed	None
Sixth	No	Irregular shape	No residual lymph node architecture	Considered discontinuous tumor extension, upstage when needed	None
Seventh	No	No	No residual lymph node architecture	None	N1c category used when no other lymph node metastasis is present

prognosis than N1a and N1b. In cases in which there are both lymph nodes and tumor deposits involved, N should be classified only by the number of positive lymph nodes (ie, N1a, N1b, N2a, N2b) and it is not appropriate to use the N1c classification in this circumstance. Tumor deposits do not count toward the total lymph node count, but the number of tumor deposits should be recorded independently of the lymph node count per CAP protocol.

Selected Stage-Independent Issues

The term lymphovascular invasion was created due to the difficulty in distinguishing tumor invasion of small lymphatic spaces from invasion of postcapillary venules. Regardless, the presence of lymphovascular invasion is an independent predictor of outcome in patients lacking metastatic lymph node disease, and may influence the use of systemic therapy in certain circumstances. Morphologically, lymphovascular invasion is identified as tumor cells within flat endothelial-lined spaces (Figure 11.30A). It is usually readily apparent on hematoxylin and eosin (H&E) stained sections, although the use of antibodies such as D2-40, CD31, or elastin may be helpful in cases where vessels and lymphatic spaces are difficult to identify with certainty. The presence of perineural invasion should also be dutifully sought in resection specimens, as it is an independent prognostic factor as well (Figure 11.30B).

Tumor budding is a more recently described feature of colorectal carcinoma that may be associated with aggressive behavior. It is believed to represent a type of epithelial-to-mesenchymal transition, indicating that tumor cells have gained migratory capability, including loss of cell

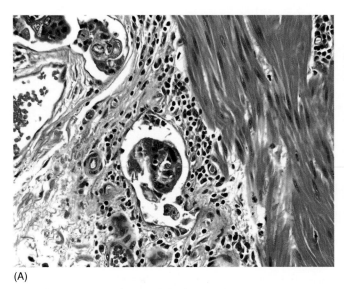

(A)

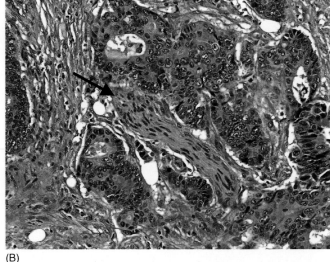

(B)

FIGURE 11.30 This example of lymphovascular invasion shows tumor cells present within endothelial-lined spaces (A). Perineural invasion consists of tumor cells within the perineurium of the nerve (B, arrow).

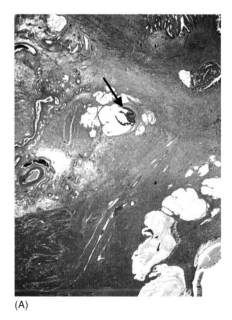

FIGURE 11.31 Tumor budding consists of groups of five cells or less at the invasive front of the tumor.

adhesion and loss of cell polarity. This gain of migratory capability and loss of cell adhesion is believed to be one of the first biologic steps toward metastasis. Histologically, tumor budding is identified at the invasive front of the tumor, and consists of groups of up to five cells (cords or aggregates) (Figure 11.31) that "bud" or invade away from the invasive front. There are several scoring systems that have been developed for assessing the amount of tumor budding in any given case, but a standardized scoring system has not been agreed upon.

Assessment of tumor budding may be most useful in cases where treatment could be affected, such as when carcinoma is confined to a polyp and additional resection is being considered, or in stage II colorectal cancers (lymph node negative), where a decision regarding adjuvant chemotherapy could be affected by the amount of tumor budding. To date, however, tumor budding is not routinely reported in either polypectomies or resections for CRC. Furthermore, although tumor budding has been independently associated with poor outcome and lymph node metastasis, large prospective studies assessing the long-term prognostic utility of this histologic parameter are still lacking.

Neoadjuvant Chemoradiation

The standard of care for locally advanced rectal cancers (tumors that are T3 or T4 and/or lymph node positive) is neoadjuvant chemoradiation followed by resection. Common histologic findings described after neoadjuvant chemotherapy include acellular mucin pools, fibrosis, necrosis, hemosiderin deposition, foamy macrophages, and calcification. Acellular mucin pools can be found in the wall of the rectum as well as in lymph nodes (Figure 11.32A–B). Although it is presumed that these pools once contained viable tumor cells, residual acellular mucin after neoadjuvant therapy pools is not used in staging, and only viable tumor cells within mucin pools count toward both T and N stages. Deeper levels of blocks may be of help in this scenario. Although the finding of acellular mucin pools is not used in staging, it is nonetheless useful to mention the presence of these pools and their location within the surgical pathology report.

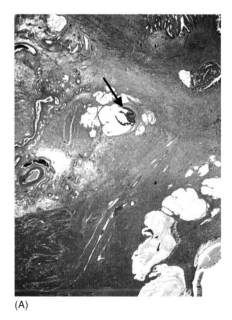
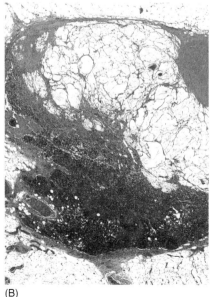

(A)   (B)

FIGURE 11.32 After neoadjuvant chemotherapy, this tumor has acellular mucin pools present in the muscularis propria, but the only viable tumor cells are present in the submucosa (arrow), and thus it is classified as ypT1 (A). This lymph node shows acellular mucin pools with no residual tumor cells (B).

The tumor's response to the chemoradiation is measured as the tumor regression grade (Figure 11.33A–D). Different classification schemes exist to evaluate the tumor regression grade; AJCC 7th edition uses a score from 0 to 3. Complete response (score 0) is defined by the absence of viable cancer cells. Moderate response (score 1) is characterized by rare residual single cells or small groups of cancer cells, while minimal response (score 2) includes residual cancer outgrown by fibrosis. Poor response (score 3) is defined by minimal or no tumor kill with extensive residual cancer. Not surprisingly, the grading of response to therapy shows considerable interobserver variability in several studies. The tumor regression grade should be scored in the primary colorectal tumor and not in lymph nodes or other sites harboring metastatic tumor. When these cases are pathologically staged, the prefix "y"

should be used, indicating neoadjuvant therapy. Although the clinical significance of tumor regression grading is not well understood, complete response of a colorectal tumor to neoadjuvant chemotherapy is associated with improved disease-free survival, decreased chance of recurrence, and decreased metastasis. Careful gross sampling of the tumor site should be performed to adequately assess if any viable tumor remains, especially if no visible gross lesion remains.

MOLECULAR GENETICS OF COLORECTAL CANCER

The molecular basis of CRC is one of the best studied among human neoplasms, in large part because adenomas

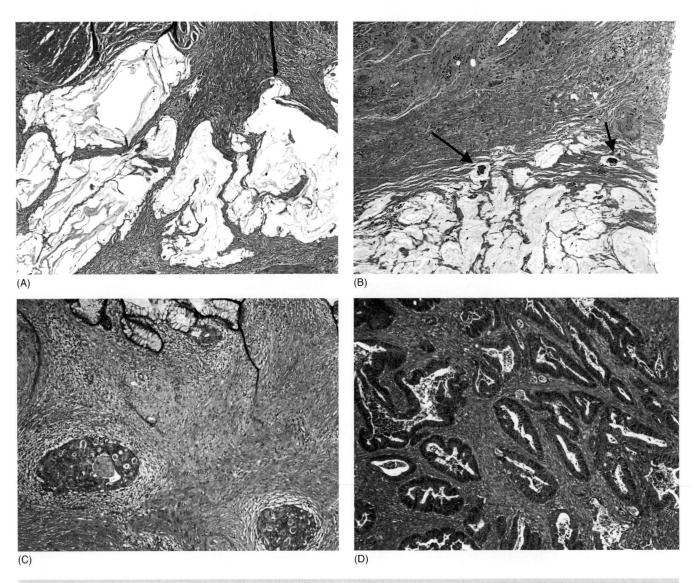

(A)

(B)

(C)

(D)

FIGURE 11.33 Tumor status post neoadjuvant therapy with no identifiable tumor cells, but only acellular mucin pools and fibrosis, is graded as tumor regression grade 0 (A). Tumor regression grade 1 shows rare malignant glands in mucin pools (B, arrows). Tumor regression grade 2 has foci of tumor, but with a greater proportion of fibrosis (C). Tumor regression grade 3 shows no definite tumor response to therapy (D).

are easily accessible via colonoscopy. It has long been known that CRC usually develops from adenomatous polyps, with an interval of approximately 10 to 15 years for the development of invasive carcinoma from an adenoma.

Fearon and Vogelstein expanded on Knudson's two-hit hypothesis model of tumor suppressor genes and proposed a model of colorectal tumorigenesis with four features:

1. CRC has both activating mutations in oncogenes and inactivating mutations in tumor suppressor genes.
2. At least four to five genes must be mutated for CRC to arise.
3. The accumulation of genetic changes, rather than the chronologic order of those changes, determines the biologic behavior of CRC.
4. Tumor suppressor genes with mutational inactivation of only one allele still appear to exert a phenotypic effect on the tumor.

In addition to alterations of genes by mutations, deletions, and insertions, epigenetic mechanisms can influence the expression of genes in CRC. These epigenetic mechanisms include cytosine methylation of DNA, histone modification, and microRNAs, among others.

Currently, three separate but overlapping pathways have been identified for the development of CRC: the chromosomal instability pathway, the CIMP pathway, and the microsatellite instability/mismatch repair pathway. These are discussed and illustrated in detail in Chapters 6, 13, and 14.

NEUROENDOCRINE NEOPLASMS

Epidemiology and Clinicopathologic Features

Well-differentiated neuroendocrine tumors (NETs), formerly known as carcinoid tumors in the tubular gut, are now referred to as NETs in the current WHO 2010 Classification. NETs of the colon and rectum account for 11% and 20% of all gastrointestinal tumors, respectively (see also the detailed discussion in Chapter 3). The most common location for NET in the large bowel is the rectum, followed by the cecum. Most colonic NETs arise sporadically; in contrast to NETs elsewhere in the gastrointestinal tract, there is no association with multiple endocrine neoplasia type 1 syndrome.

Poorly differentiated neuroendocrine neoplasms are now referred to as neuroendocrine carcinomas (NECs) in the WHO 2010 Classification. The term NEC encompasses small cell and large cell neuroendocrine carcinoma (as well as mixed small and large cell carcinomas). NECs can arise anywhere in the colorectum, and are very aggressive tumors regardless of location or morphologic subtype.

Rectal NETs are typically asymptomatic, and are incidentally found at the time of colonoscopy for another reason. They are characteristically small, and tend to behave in a benign fashion with low metastatic potential. Presentation with classic "carcinoid syndrome" symptoms such as diarrhea, cutaneous flushing, bronchospasms, and venous telangiectasia is quite rare among tumors at this site. NETs arising in the ascending and transverse colon are more likely to have metastatic potential, which correlates with size, presence of lymphovascular invasion, grade, and stage.

Most rectal NETs measure less than 1 cm. Macroscopically, these tumors often appear as submucosal nodules (Figure 11.34A–D); larger tumors may produce overlying mucosal ulceration. Right-sided NETs are frequently larger than NETs arising in the distal colon and rectum. Similar to NETs elsewhere in the gastrointestinal tract, these tumors are gray in color when fresh and turn yellow after fixation in formalin. A comprehensive discussion of the histology, immunophenotype, and grading of NET/NEC is found in Chapter 3.

Diagnostic Challenges

The distinction between CRCs and NETs is generally straightforward by routine histology. The acinar pattern of low-grade NETs occasionally mimics a well-differentiated adenocarcinoma, but neuroendocrine markers will confirm the distinction. It is important to remember that MOC31 is not useful in this situation, as it will mark both types of tumors. The solid growth pattern of NETs may occasionally resemble a low-grade lymphoma; this differential can also be resolved with immunohistochemistry. Prostate cancer can sometimes enter into the differential diagnosis for rectal NETs, given the location and low-grade cytologic findings. Immunohistochemistry for prostate markers (PSA and PSAP) as well as neuroendocrine markers help make this distinction. When seen in the liver, the trabecular pattern of NETs may mimic hepatocellular carcinoma. Hepatocellular markers such as HepPar1 do not typically mark NETs, and neuroendocrine markers do not typically stain hepatocellular carcinomas (with the exception of the fibrolamellar variant, which can coexpress synaptophysin and some hepatocellular markers).

Mixed adenoneuroendocrine carcinomas (MANECs) are often a diagnostic consideration in high-grade NECs of the colon and rectum. This distinction is further complicated by the fact that NECs usually arise from colorectal adenomas and adenocarcinomas. The diagnosis of MANEC requires a neuroendocrine component of at least 30%, which should be confirmed by immunohistochemistry. Approximately 40% of CRCs will have at least focal staining with neuroendocrine markers, and this does not fulfill the criteria for MANEC. Staining for neuroendocrine markers is not recommended unless neuroendocrine histologic features are present.

The staging of NETs of the colon and rectum is slightly different than adenocarcinomas from the same location, and Table 11.7 highlights these differences. The staging guidelines for adenocarcinomas of the colon and rectum should be used for NECs as well as MANECs.

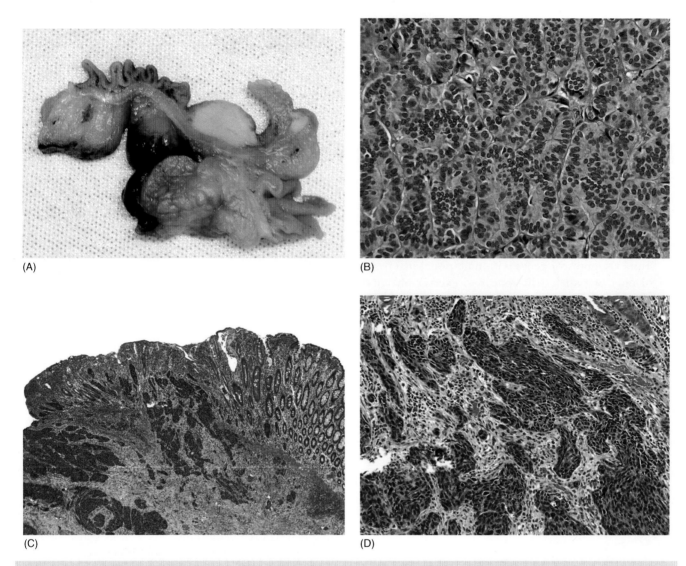

FIGURE 11.34 This well-differentiated neuroendocrine tumor forms a submucosal mass with a yellow cut surface (A). Well-differentiated neuroendocrine tumors are composed of nests and trabeculae of monotonous cells with amphophilic cytoplasm and "salt-and-pepper" chromatin (B). This poorly differentiated neuroendocrine carcinoma shows high-grade cytologic features with nuclear pleomorphism and large nucleoli (C, D).

MESENCHYMAL TUMORS

A detailed discussion of mesenchymal tumors (including gastrointestinal stromal tumor [GIST] and mesenteric fibromatosis) is given in Chapter 5. This section will focus in brief on the most common mesenchymal tumors of the colon and rectum.

Smooth Muscle Tumors

Leiomyomas of the colon most often arise from the muscularis mucosae, and are similar to smooth muscle tumors found elsewhere in the body (Figure 11.35A–B). They often present as polyps in the distal colon, and are usually found incidentally during screening colonoscopy. They are slightly more common in men than women. In

comparison, leiomyomas of the muscularis propria (intramural) and leiomyosarcomas are very rare in this location, and are more likely to present with clinically evident rectal bleeding or obstruction.

Lipomatous Tumors

Lipomas are the most common submucosal mesenchymal polyp in the colorectum; they are rarely seen in the muscularis propria or subserosa as well. They are more often found on the right side of the colon and in older women. Small lipomas (less than 2 cm) are usually asymptomatic, while larger lesions (greater than 2 cm) may present with abdominal pain, bleeding per rectum, or a change in bowel habits. Lipomas are composed of mature adipocytes typically based in the submucosa (Figure 11.36A–B). The

TABLE 11.7 Comparison of Staging Criteria for Colorectal Adenocarcinoma and Colorectal Neuroendocrine Tumor

	Colorectal Adenocarcinoma and Poorly Differentiated Neuroendocrine Carcinoma	Colorectal Well-Differentiated Neuroendocrine Tumor
pTis	Carcinoma in situ, intraepithelial (no invasion of lamina propria) Carcinoma in situ, invasion of lamina propria/muscularis mucosae	—
pT1	Tumor invades submucosa	Tumor invades lamina propria or submucosa and size 2 cm or less
pT1a	—	Tumor size less than 1 cm in greatest dimension
pT1b	—	Tumor size 1 to 2 cm in greatest dimension
pT2	Tumor invades muscularis propria	Same or tumor size >2 cm with invasion of lamina propria or submucosa
pT3	Tumor invades through the muscularis propria into pericolorectal tissues	Same
pT4	—	Tumor invades peritoneum or other organs
pT4a	Tumor penetrates the visceral peritoneum	—
pT4b	Tumor directly invades or is adherent to other organs or structures	—
pN0	No regional lymph node metastasis	Same
pN1		Metastasis in regional lymph nodes
pN1a	Metastasis in one regional lymph node	—
pN1b	Metastasis in two to three regional lymph nodes	—
pN1c	Tumor deposit(s) in the subserosa, or nonperitonealized pericolic or perirectal tissues without regional lymph node metastasis	—
pN2a	Metastasis in four to six regional lymph nodes	—
pN2b	Metastasis in seven or more regional lymph nodes	—
pM1	Distant metastasis	Same
pM1a	Metastasis to single organ or site (eg, liver, lung, ovary, nonregional lymph node)	—
pM1b	Metastasis to more than one organ/site or to the peritoneum	—

mucosa covering the lipoma may be unremarkable, hyperplastic, ulcerated, or atrophic. When mucosal ulceration is present, reactive changes can include fibrosis, increased mitoses, and adipocyte hyperchromasia. Primary liposarcomas of the colorectum occur but are extremely rare.

Neural Lesions

Ganglioneuromas (GNs) (Figure 11.37A) are most often found in the colon as solitary sporadic lesions. These are usually incidental findings on the left side of the colon, measuring less than 1.0 cm. GNs are also found in the context of ganglioneuromatous polyposis, which is associated with Cowden syndrome and NF1, and in the context of diffuse ganglioneuromatosis, which is associated with MEN-2B and NF1. The colon is the second most common site in the tubular GI tract (after esophagus) for granular cell tumors (Figure 11.37B). Schwannoma and Schwann cell hamartoma occur in the colon but are relatively rare.

Perineuriomas (also referred to as benign fibroblastic polyps, Figure 11.37C) are typically single polyps that are found incidentally on screening colonoscopy; there is a slight female predominance. They are often associated with serrated polyps. These lesions are occasionally confused with GISTs or other types of neural polyps.

HEMATOLYMPHOID NEOPLASMS OF THE COLON

The colon can be involved by any of the hematolymphoid neoplasms discussed in earlier chapters. Here, as elsewhere, B cell lymphomas far outnumber T cell lymphomas, and diffuse large B cell lymphoma (DLBCL, discussed in detail in Chapter 8) is the most common primary colonic lymphoma. A few entities, however, can have a fairly characteristic appearance in this location and will be discussed here, including a disease manifestation usually associated with mantle cell lymphoma (MCL) that can mimic inherited polyposis syndromes, the so-called "lymphomatous polyposis"; Langerhans cell histiocytosis (LCH); and systemic mastocytosis (SM), all of which may be encountered in colon biopsies.

Mantle Cell Lymphoma

This lymphoma of small B lymphocytes typically has a deceptively low-grade appearance, but is actually relentless in its progression and more aggressive than many other small B cell lymphomas. It is closely associated with the t(11;14)(q13;q32) translocation, involving the CCND1 (cyclin-D1) gene, which comes under the influence of the promoter for the immunoglobulin heavy chain (IGH) gene. MCL is fairly uncommon, accounting for only a few percentage of non-Hodgkin lymphomas, and tends to occur in middle-aged to older individuals (median age 60 years), with men outnumbering women about two to one. The GI tract is the most common extranodal site of occurrence of MCL, and is involved in about one third of patients with the disease. Common presentations include hepatosplenomegaly, lymphadenopathy, and peripheral blood involvement by circulating lymphoma cells.

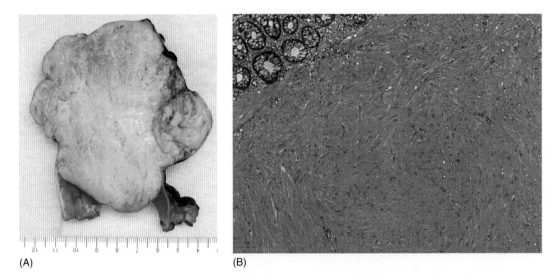

(A)   (B)

FIGURE 11.35   This gross photomicrograph shows a leiomyoma arising from the muscularis propria in the colon (A). The tumor is composed of intersecting fascicles with monomorphic spindle cells without significant nuclear atypia, mitoses, or necrosis (B).

In the colon, MCL is the lymphoma most commonly associated with the clinical presentation of lymphomatous polyposis, although essentially any lymphoma can present with this appearance. This manifestation involves nodular aggregates of MCL that protrude from the mucosa, creating "polyps" that can look essentially identical to those found in inherited polyposis syndromes such as familial adenomatous polyposis. Histologically, these nodular aggregates are composed of collections of small- or medium-sized lymphocytes with scant cytoplasm and dark nuclei that have irregular, often angulated, contours (Figure 11.38). These collections distort the overlying mucosa, protruding into the intestinal lumen. The cells are quite monotonous, but there may be prominent vessels and occasional admixed eosinophilic ("pink") histiocytes.

In addition to the nodular pattern of MCL involvement described in the previous paragraph and in Figure 11.38, this type of lymphoma can have a more diffuse pattern, or may surround reactive germinal centers in an easily overlooked pattern analogous to the normal mantle zones found in other sites of mucosa-associated lymphoid tissue (MALT) such as Peyer's patches. Mercifully, this last pattern is quite rare. In addition to the small cells with angulated nuclei typically encountered, MCL can also be composed of larger cells that resemble lymphoblasts

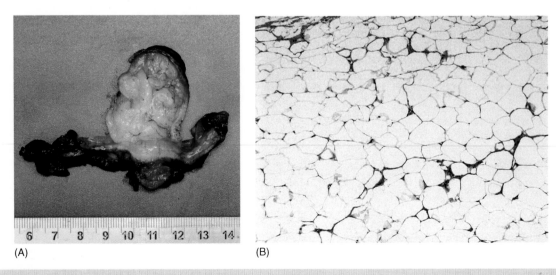

(A)   (B)

FIGURE 11.36   Lipomas often arise in the submucosa, as illustrated here in a gross specimen (A). Lipomas are composed of mature adipocytes without atypia (B).

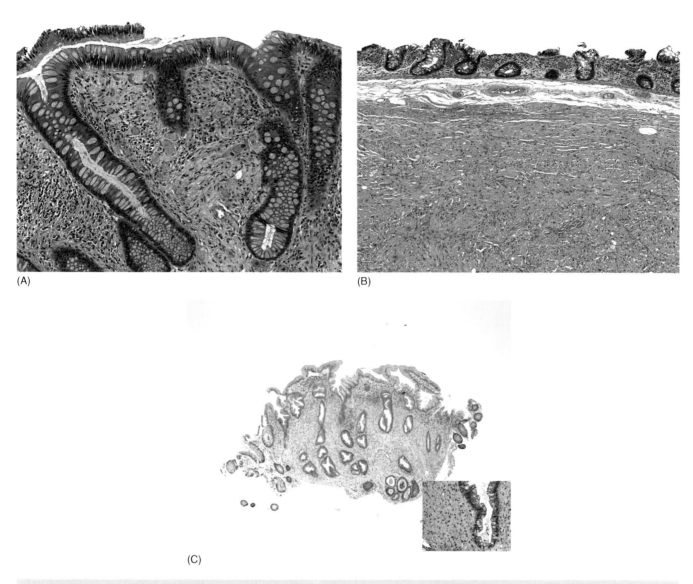

FIGURE 11.37 Ganglioneuromas are composed of a mixture of spindled Schwann cells and ganglion cells (A). This granular cell tumor is well-circumscribed (B) and shows polygonal cell borders with granular eosinophilic cytoplasm. Perineuromas are composed of bland spindle cells restricted to the colonic lamina propria (C, courtesy Dr. Rhonda Yantiss; inset, high power) and are often associated with serrated crypts in hyperplastic polyps or SSA/Ps.

(the "blastoid" variant) or the cells of DLBCL (the "pleomorphic" variant). These variants are associated with a higher proliferative rate and are considered to be clinically important, because they are more aggressive than typical MCL.

Immunophenotypically, MCL consists of CD20-positive B cells that aberrantly coexpress CD5 and, usually, CD43. This pattern is similar to that seen in chronic lymphocytic leukemia/small lymphocytic lymphoma (CLL/SLL). One aid to distinction between the two entities is CD23, which is often positive in CLL/SLL and negative in MCL. FMC7, which is usually assessed by flow cytometry, has the opposite pattern, being most often positive in MCL and negative in CLL/SLL. Rarely, MCL can be CD5-negative, which can lead to diagnostic confusion. Thankfully, almost all cases of MCL express cyclin-D1 in a nuclear pattern and, if the suspicion for MCL is high (eg, in a patient with atypical lymphoid aggregates in colon biopsies who carries the diagnosis already), this may be the only stain needed to make the diagnosis.

The prognosis for MCL is, unfortunately, relatively poor, particularly in cases primarily involving the GI tract. Median survival is in the range of 3 to 5 years. It is important to make the distinction between the aggressive variants (blastoid and pleomorphic) and the other hematolymphoid conditions that they mimic, because DLBCL and lymphoblastic leukemia/lymphoma are often curable with aggressive therapy, while MCL typically is not.

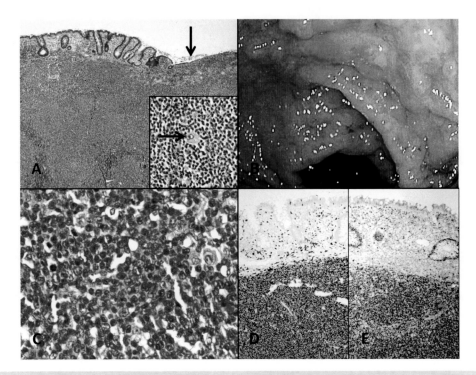

FIGURE 11.38 Mantle cell lymphoma (MCL) often makes nodular or polypoid collections of monotonous lymphocytes that protrude into the lumen of the GI tract (A). In this case of colonic MCL, there is an erosion/ulcer of the overlying mucosa (arrow). At high magnification (A, inset), the malignant cells exhibit an "angulated" contour and there are admixed, epithelioid histiocytes with eosinophilic cytoplasm ("pink histiocytes," arrow). Endoscopically (B), the mucosa often has a nodular or polypoid appearance, and the process may mimic inherited polyposis syndromes (so-called "lymphomatous polyposis"). Some cases (C) have a more pleomorphic cytologic appearance. In such cases, MCL may be confused with diffuse large B cell lymphoma or lymphoblastic lymphoma. A "pink histiocyte" is visible at the right of the panel. MCL is immunohistochemically positive for CD5 (D) and nuclear cyclin-D1 (E).

Systemic Mastocytosis

GI involvement by SM is rare, and occurs as part of more widespread systemic involvement. Symptoms related to GI involvement are usually nonspecific, including diarrhea, abdominal pain, and dyspepsia, and are thought to be secondary to mediator release by the mast cells. According to the most recent WHO classification of hematolymphoid tumors, SM is a clonal myeloproliferative disorder, and is very commonly associated with mutation of the *KIT*

gene, the D816V mutation being the most common. The WHO classification also sets forth diagnostic criteria for the diagnosis of SM (Table 11.8).

GI involvement by SM can be suspected based on endoscopic findings, particularly in a patient already known to have the disease who develops GI symptoms. The mucosa may be nodular, pigmented, or thickened and edematous-appearing. Histologically, SM is characterized by increased numbers of atypical-appearing mast

TABLE 11.8   Diagnostic Criteria for Systemic Mastocytosis

	Major Criterion	**Minor Criteria**
Systemic mastocytosis can be diagnosed with the major and one minor criterion *or* with at least three minor criteria	Multifocal, dense infiltrates of mast cells (≥15 in aggregates) in sections of bone marrow and/or other organs	>25% of mast cells in infiltrates in bone marrow or other extracutaneous organ are spindled or have atypical morphology or, of all mast cells in bone marrow aspirate smears, >25% are immature or atypical Activating point mutation at codon 816 of *KIT* detected in bone marrow, blood, or other extracutaneous organs Expression of CD2 and/or CD25 (in addition to normal mast cell markers) by mast cells in bone marrow, blood, or other extracutaneous organs Serum total tryptase persistently >20 ng/mL (not valid if there is another associated clonal myeloid disorder)

Source: Adapted From WHO *Classification of Tumours of Haematopoietic and Lymphoid Tissues*, 2008.

cells, which very often occur in clusters (Figure 11.39). These cells have ovoid or elongated nuclei and can have a spindled appearance that can make them difficult to recognize for what they are. In addition, neoplastic mast cells often lack the cytoplasmic granules characteristic of their normal counterparts and, when combined with extensive spindled morphology can make them appear like fibroblasts such as may be seen at the site of healing mucosal injury. Immunohistochemically, the neoplastic cells of SM express the typical mast cell antigens KIT and mast cell tryptase, but can aberrantly express CD2 and/or CD25. They may also express CD68, which can lead to their confusion with histiocytes.

Mastocytosis has several forms, and the prognosis is heavily dependent on which type the patient has. Patients with aggressive disease can have a poor prognosis, surviving only a few months. While there is no cure, systemic therapy can be employed for patients with widespread and aggressive forms.

Langerhans Cell Histiocytosis

This rare entity may occasionally make an appearance in the GI tract, and can be seen in colon biopsies. Its etiology has been controversial, but LCH is now thought to be a clonal disorder (based on molecular evidence), and a high proportion of cases have been found to harbor the *BRAF V600E* mutation. This has opened the door to targeted therapy with the BRAF inhibitor vermurafenib. LCH has a variety of other names, including histiocytosis X and eosinophilic granuloma, and it has several forms that include solitary involvement (usually of bone, lymph node, or skin), multifocal involvement of one organ system (usually bones), and multifocal involvement of multiple organ systems (usually skin, bone, and visceral organs). The multifocal, unisystem form has the eponym "Hand–Schüller–Christian disease" and the multifocal, multiorgan form "Letterer–Siwe disease."

Histologically, LCH consists of clusters of Langerhans-like cells, which have ovoid nuclei that often contain a longitudinal groove, giving a so-called "coffee bean" appearance. These cells are immunohistochemically positive for S100 and CD1a (Figure 11.40) and are usually admixed with numerous inflammatory cells, among which eosinophils can be very prominent. Ultrastructurally, the cells contain characteristic inclusions ("Birbeck granules") that have a zipper-like appearance, and which may be dilated at one end like a tennis racket.

The primary importance in recognizing LCH in a GI biopsy is the ability to point the treating physician in the direction of the diagnosis so that additional studies may be performed to look for more widespread involvement.

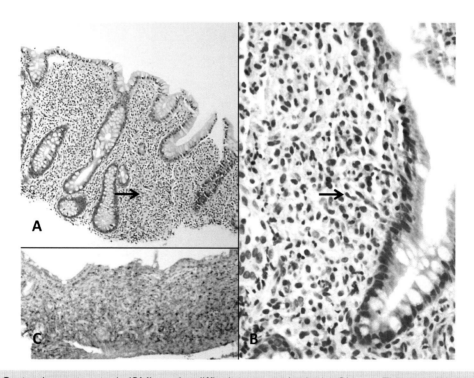

FIGURE 11.39 Systemic mastocytosis (SM) can be difficult to recognize in the GI tract. This case (A) was initially thought to be some type of inflammatory bowel disease before the identification of clusters of unusual-appearing cells (arrow). At high magnification (B), these cells had, in many cases, a spindled appearance (arrow) and there were numerous admixed eosinophils. The cells were immunohistochemically positive for KIT and they had aberrant expression of CD25 (C), establishing the diagnosis of SM.

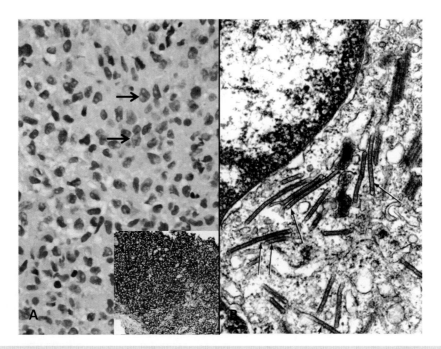

FIGURE 11.40 Langerhans cell histiocytosis (LCH) is a clonal proliferation of cells with the phenotype of Langerhans cells. They typically have ovoid nuclei (A), many of which contain a longitudinal groove (arrows), imparting a coffee-bean-like appearance. The cells of LCH are positive for S100 protein as well as CD1a (inset). While the diagnosis is most often made without the benefit of electron microscopy, ultrastructural studies reveal characteristic cytoplasmic Birbeck granules (B), which have a zipper-like morphology (electron micrograph, courtesy of Bertram Schnitzer, MD).

The prognosis of LCH depends on the extent of involvement, with solitary forms having the best outcome and multifocal, multisystem forms the worst, often requiring systemic therapy. The advent of molecular therapy for cases harboring the *BRAF* mutation seems to promise new hope for treatment.

Rectal Lymphoid Polyps

Occasionally in the rectum (and, rarely, in the more proximal colon), biopsies will sample a polypoid mass of benign lymphoid tissue with prominent lymphoid follicles that usually have well-developed germinal centers (Figure 11.41). These benign lymphoid polyps have been branded with the somewhat evocative name of "rectal tonsils" in the literature, and they can mimic malignant lymphoma, particularly MALT lymphoma (discussed in Chapter 8), which can have reactive germinal centers surrounded by lymphoma cells with a marginal zone phenotype and follicular lymphoma (discussed in Chapter 9), where the follicular structures themselves are neoplastic. In addition to their ability to mimic lymphoma, there are scattered reports in the literature raising the question of whether these lymphoid proliferations may be associated with infectious etiologies such as Epstein–Barr virus or chlamydia.

While the morphology can be striking and these polyps can be as large as a centimeter or more, the differential diagnosis with lymphoma is usually straightforward once a diagnosis of "rectal tonsil" is entertained. Unlike true

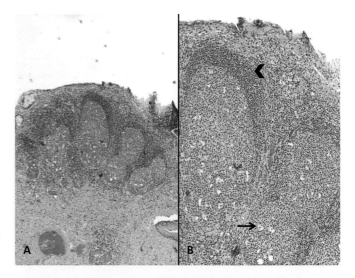

FIGURE 11.41 Rectal lymphoid polyps can have an impressive endoscopic appearance, and can raise the differential diagnosis of lymphoid neoplasia under the microscope. At low magnification (A), a cluster of follicular structures is seen underlying the distal rectal mucosa. While the normal mucosal elements are pushed aside, there is no destructive infiltration of the mucosa. At high magnification (B), the follicular structures have reassuring histologic features, including polarization, with a "dark zone" containing tingible-body macrophages (arrow) oriented away from the lumen, and a well-formed mantle zone (arrowhead) oriented toward the lumen. These benign lymphoid follicles would be negative for BCL-2 expression. Photomicrographs, courtesy of Henry Appelman, MD.

MALT lymphomas, there is no destructive infiltration of the epithelial structures of the mucosa. Well-formed, polarized germinal centers with tingible-body macrophages are common, and these structures are negative for BCL-2 on immunohistochemistry, ruling out follicular lymphoma.

METASTATIC TUMORS TO THE COLON

Although primary colon cancer is common, secondary involvement of the colon by other tumors does occur

and may be an important diagnostic consideration (Figure 11.42A–D). Tumors from the lung, prostate, ovary, uterus, breast, and pancreas can involve the colon, among other primary sites, as well as melanomas.

Müllerian endometrioid adenocarcinomas (Figure 11.42A–B) can be especially difficult to distinguish from well-differentiated CRC. Squamous differentiation is a common feature in Müllerian endometrioid adenocarcinomas but is quite rare in CRC. Furthermore, endometrioid adenocarcinomas tend to have less cytologic atypia and less "dirty" necrosis compared to CRC. Immunohistochemical

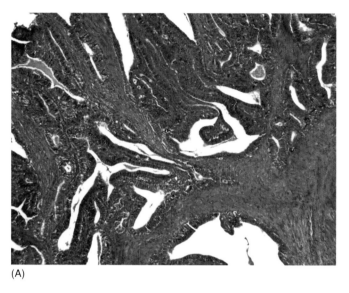

(A)

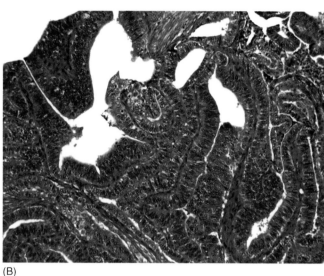

(B)

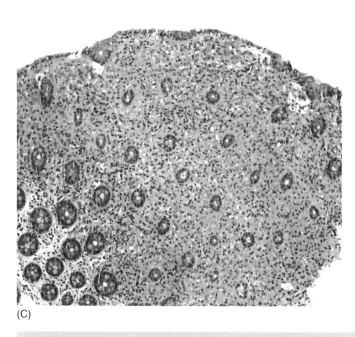

(C)

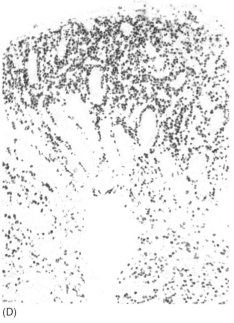

(D)

FIGURE 11.42   This metastatic endometrioid adenocarcinoma to the colon shows crowded and branching glands (A–B) that mimic colorectal adenocarcinoma. It was positive for CK7, PAX8, ER, and PR, and negative for CK20 and CDX2, supporting the diagnosis. This colon biopsy contains an infiltrating poorly differentiated carcinoma with signet ring cells that fills the lamina propria (C); there is no associated adenomatous component. GATA3 immunostain is positive (D), whereas CK20 and CDX2 are negative, consistent with the patient's history of previous breast carcinoma.

stains useful in the distinction include CK20 and CDX2 for colon and CK7, CD10, and PAX8 for Müllerian origin.

Often, there is a known history of an extracolonic tumor and the case is relatively straightforward, but there are several morphologic features that may help suggest a metastatic tumor rather than a primary CRC. Tumors that lack an adenomatous intramucosal component should raise the diagnostic consideration of a metastasis; however, metastatic tumors often overgrow the overlying mucosa and can mimic low- or high-grade dysplasia. Growth based deep in the wall rather than the mucosa, diffuse lymphovascular invasion, pigment (for melanoma), and histology atypical for CRC are all clues indicating metastases from other primary sites.

Immunostains can be extremely useful in the distinction of primary CRC from metastases. The most common immunophenotype for CRC is CK7-/CK20+/CDX2+. However, several caveats exist in the interpretation of these markers. A significant portion (25%) of rectal cancers expresses CK7. Furthermore, up to 13% of rectal tumors are negative for all three markers. A more recently described antibody that is useful for marking the intestine is SATB2, which stains approximately 85% of CRC. SATB2 is highly specific, with only a small percentage (3%–5%) of breast, ovarian, and lung tumors staining positive. Additional immunostains that may be useful to confirm tumors of extracolonic origin include TTF1 (lung), PSA/PSAP/androgen receptor (prostate), PAX8 (ovary, uterus), GATA3/BRST2/mammaglobulin (breast), and SOX10/S100/HMB-45/melan-A (melanoma). As always, immunohistochemical stains are best used in a panel and in conjunction with the history and morphologic findings.

SELECTED REFERENCES

Selected references for Hamartomatous Polyps are included in Chapter 6. Selected references for Neuroendocrine Neoplasms are included in Chapter 3. Additional references for Mesenchymal Neoplasms are included in Chapter 5.

Inflammatory Lesions

Chetty R, Bhathal PS, Slavin JL. Prolapse-induced inflammatory polyps of the colorectum and anal transitional zone. *Histopathology.* 1993;23:63–67.

Chiang JM, Changchien CR, Chen JR. Solitary rectal ulcer syndrome: an endoscopic and histological presentation and literature review. *Int J Colorectal Dis.* 2006;21:348–356.

De Petris G, Leung ST. Pseudoneoplasms of the gastrointestinal tract. *Arch Pathol Lab Med.* 2010;134:378–392.

du Boulay CE, Fairbrother J, Isaacson PG. Mucosal prolapse syndrome—a unifying concept for solitary ulcer syndrome and related disorders. *J Clin Pathol.* 1983;36:1264–1268.

Guest CB, Reznick RK. Colitis cystica profunda. Review of the literature. *Dis Colon Rectum.* 1989;32:983–988.

Huang CC, Frankel WL, Doukides T, et al. Prolapse-related changes are a confounding factor in misdiagnosis of sessile serrated adenomas in the rectum. *Hum Pathol.* 2013;44:480–486.

Kelly JK. Polypoid prolapsing mucosal folds in diverticular disease. *Am J Surg Pathol.* 1991;15:871–878.

Nakamura S, Kino I, Akagi T. Inflammatory myoglandular polyps of the colon and rectum. A clinicopathological study of 32 pedunculated polyps, distinct from other types of polyps. *Am J Surg Pathol.* 1992;16:772–779.

Ng KH, Mathur P, Kumarasinghe MP, et al. Cap polyposis: further experience and review. *Dis Colon Rectum.* 2004;47:1208–1215.

Parfitt JR, Shepherd NA. Polypoid mucosal prolapse complicating low rectal adenomas: beware the inflammatory cloacogenic polyp! *Histopathology.* 2008;53:91–96.

Singh B, Mortensen NJ, Warren BF. Histopathological mimicry in mucosal prolapse. *Histopathology.* 2007;50:97–102.

Conventional Adenoma

Appelman HD. Con: High-grade dysplasia and villous features should not be part of the routine diagnosis of colorectal adenomas. *Am J Gastroenterol.* 2008;103:1329–1331.

Bansal M, Fenoglio CM, Robboy SJ, King DW. Are metaplasias in colorectal adenomas truly metaplasias? *Am J Pathol.* 1984;115:253–265.

Brown LJ, Smeeton NC, Dixon MF. Assessment of dysplasia in colorectal adenomas: an observer variation and morphometric study. *J Clin Pathol.* 1985;38:174–179.

Jensen P, Krogsgaard MR, Christiansen J, et al. Observer variability in the assessment of type and dysplasia of colorectal adenomas, analyzed using kappa statistics. *Dis Colon Rectum.* 1995;38:195–198.

Lasisi F, Mouchli A, Riddell R, et al. Agreement in interpreting villous elements and dysplasia in adenomas less than one centimetre in size. *Dig Liver Dis.* 2013;45:1049–1055.

Levine JS, Ahnen DJ. Clinical practice. Adenomatous polyps of the colon. *N Engl J Med.* 2006;355:2551–2557.

Lieberman DA, Prindiville S, Weiss DG, et al. Risk factors for advanced colonic neoplasia and hyperplastic polyps in asymptomatic individuals. *JAMA.* 2003;290:2959–2967.

Lieberman DA, Weiss DG, Bond JH, et al. Use of colonoscopy to screen asymptomatic adults for colorectal cancer. Veterans Affairs Cooperative Study Group 380. *N Engl J Med.* 2000;343:162–168.

Lin J, Goldblum JR, Bennett AE, et al. Composite intestinal adenoma-microcarcinoid. *Am J Surg Pathol.* 2012;36:292–295.

Mahajan D, Downs-Kelly E, Liu X, et al. Reproducibility of the villous component and high-grade dysplasia in colorectal adenomas <1 cm: implications for endoscopic surveillance. *Am J Surg Pathol.* 2013;37:427–433.

Odze RD. Pathology of dysplasia and cancer in inflammatory bowel disease. *Gastroenterol Clin North Am.* 2006;35:533–552.

Pai RK, Rybicki LA, Goldblum JR, et al. Paneth cells in colonic adenomas: association with male sex and adenoma burden. *Am J Surg Pathol.* 2013;37:98–103.

Rex DK, Goldblum JR. Pro: Villous elements and high-grade dysplasia help guide post-polypectomy colonoscopic surveillance. *Am J Gastroenterol.* 2008;103:1327–1329.

Salaria SN, Abu Alfa AK, Alsaigh NY, et al. Composite intestinal adenoma-microcarcinoid clues to diagnosing an under-recognised mimic of invasive adenocarcinoma. *J Clin Pathol.* 2013;66:302–306.

Terry MB, Neugut AI, Bostick RM, et al. Reliability in the classification of advanced colorectal adenomas. *Cancer Epidemiol Biomarkers Prev.* 2002;11:660–663.

Torres C, Antonioli D, Odze RD. Polypoid dysplasia and adenomas in inflammatory bowel disease: a clinical, pathologic, and follow-up study of 89 polyps from 59 patients. *Am J Surg Pathol.* 1998;22:275–284.

Ullman T, Odze R, Farraye FA. Diagnosis and management of dysplasia in patients with ulcerative colitis and Crohn's disease of the colon. *Inflamm Bowel Dis.* 2009;15:630–638.

Winawer SJ, Zauber AG, Fletcher RH, et al. Guidelines for colonoscopy surveillance after polypectomy: a consensus update by the US Multi-Society Task Force on Colorectal Cancer and the American Cancer Society. *Gastroenterology.* 2006;130:1872–1885.

Serrated Polyps

Aust DE, Baretton GB, Members of the Working Group GI-Pathology of the German Society of Pathology. Serrated polyps of the colon and rectum (hyperplastic polyps, sessile serrated adenomas, traditional serrated adenomas, and mixed polyps)-proposal for diagnostic criteria. *Virchows Arch.* 2010;457:291–297.

Bettington M, Walker N, Clouston A, et al. The serrated pathway to colorectal carcinoma: current concepts and challenges. *Histopathology.* 2013;62:367–386.

Crowder CD, Sweet K, Lehman A, Frankel WL. Serrated polyposis is an underdiagnosed and unclear syndrome: the surgical pathologist has a role in improving detection. *Am J Surg Pathol.* 2012;36:1178–1185.

Dhir M, Yachida S, Van Neste L, et al. Sessile serrated adenomas and classical adenomas: an epigenetic perspective on premalignant neoplastic lesions of the gastrointestinal tract. *Int J Cancer.* 2011;129:1889–1898.

Farris AB, Misdraji J, Srivastava A, et al. Sessile serrated adenoma: challenging discrimination from other serrated colonic polyps. *Am J Surg Pathol.* 2008;32:30–35.

Goldstein NS. Small colonic microsatellite unstable adenocarcinomas and high-grade epithelial dysplasias in sessile serrated adenoma polypectomy specimens: a study of eight cases. *Am J Clin Pathol.* 2006;125:132–145.

Iino H, Jass JR, Simms LA, et al. DNA microsatellite instability in hyperplastic polyps, serrated adenomas, and mixed polyps: a mild mutator pathway for colorectal cancer? *J Clin Pathol.* 1999;52:5–9.

Kalady MF, Jarrar A, Leach B, et al. Defining phenotypes and cancer risk in hyperplastic polyposis syndrome. *Dis Colon Rectum.* 2011;54:164–170.

Kim YH, Kakar S, Cun L, et al. Distinct CpG island methylation profiles and BRAF mutation status in serrated and adenomatous colorectal polyps. *Int J Cancer.* 2008;123:2587–2593.

Leggett B, Whitehall V. Role of the serrated pathway in colorectal cancer pathogenesis. *Gastroenterology.* 2010;138:2088–2100.

Leonard DF, Dozois EJ, Smyrk TC, et al. Endoscopic and surgical management of serrated colonic polyps. *Br J Surg.* 2011;98:1685–1694.

Li D, Jin C, McCulloch C, et al. Association of large serrated polyps with synchronous advanced colorectal neoplasia. *Am J Gastroenterol.* 2009;104:695–702.

Lieberman DA, Rex DK, Winawer SJ, et al. Guidelines for colonoscopy surveillance after screening and polypectomy: a consensus update by the US Multi-Society Task Force on Colorectal Cancer. *Gastroenterology.* 2012;143:844–857.

Limketkai BN, Lam-Himlin D, Arnold MA, Arnold CA. The cutting edge of serrated polyps: a practical guide to approaching and managing serrated colon polyps. *Gastrointest Endosc.* 2013;77:360–375.

Lu FI, van Niekerk dW, Owen D, et al. Longitudinal outcome study of sessile serrated adenomas of the colorectum: an increased risk for subsequent right-sided colorectal carcinoma. *Am J Surg Pathol.* 2010;34:927–934.

Pai RK, Hart J, Noffsinger AE. Sessile serrated adenomas strongly predispose to synchronous serrated polyps in non-syndromic patients. *Histopathology.* 2010;56:581–588.

Pai RK, Mojtahed A, Rouse RV, et al. Histologic and molecular analyses of colonic perineurial-like proliferations in serrated polyps: perineurial-like stromal proliferations are seen in sessile serrated adenomas. *Am J Surg Pathol.* 2011;35:1373–1380.

Patil DT, Shadrach BL, Rybicki LA, et al. Proximal colon cancers and the serrated pathway: a systematic analysis of precursor histology and BRAF mutation status. *Mod Pathol.* 2012;25:1423–1431.

Rex DK, Ahnen DJ, Baron JA, et al. Serrated lesions of the colorectum: review and recommendations from an expert panel. *Am J Gastroenterol.* 2012;107:1315–1329.

Rosty C, Buchanan DD, Walsh MD, et al. Phenotype and polyp landscape in serrated polyposis syndrome: a series of 100 patients from genetics clinics. *Am J Surg Pathol.* 2012;36:876–882.

Rosty C, Hewett DG, Brown IS, et al. Serrated polyps of the large intestine: current understanding of diagnosis, pathogenesis, and clinical management. *J Gastroenterol.* 2013;48:287–302.

Salaria SN, Streppel MM, Lee LA, et al. Sessile serrated adenomas: high-risk lesions? *Hum Pathol.* 2012;43:1808–1814.

Schreiner MA, Weiss DG, Lieberman DA. Proximal and large hyperplastic and nondysplastic serrated polyps detected by colonoscopy are associated with neoplasia. *Gastroenterology.* 2010;139:1497–1502.

Sheridan TB, Fenton H, Lewin MR, et al. Sessile serrated adenomas with low- and high-grade dysplasia and early carcinomas: an immunohistochemical study of serrated lesions "caught in the act." *Am J Clin Pathol.* 2006;126:564–571.

Snover DC, Jass JR, Fenoglio-Preiser C, Batts KP. Serrated polyps of the large intestine: a morphologic and molecular review of an evolving concept. *Am J Clin Pathol.* 2005;124:380–391.

Snover DC. Update on the serrated pathway to colorectal carcinoma. *Hum Pathol.* 2011;42:1–10.

Torlakovic E, Skovlund E, Snover DC, et al. Morphologic reappraisal of serrated colorectal polyps. *Am J Surg Pathol.* 2003;27:65–81.

Torlakovic E, Snover DC. Serrated adenomatous polyposis in humans. *Gastroenterology.* 1996;110:748–755.

Torlakovic EE, Gomez JD, Driman DK, et al. Sessile serrated adenoma (SSA) vs. traditional serrated adenoma (TSA). *Am J Surg Pathol.* 2008;32:21–29.

Colorectal Adenocarcinoma

Abdul-Jalil KI, Sheehan KM, Kehoe J, et al. The prognostic value of tumour regression grade following neoadjuvant chemoradiation therapy for rectal cancer. *Colorectal Dis.* 2014;16:O16–O25.

Allam MF, Lucena RA. Aetiology of sex differences in colorectal cancer. *Eur J Cancer Prev.* 2001;10:299–300.

Arai T, Esaki Y, Sawabe M, et al. Hypermethylation of the hMLH1 promoter with absent hMLH1 expression in medullary-type poorly differentiated colorectal adenocarcinoma in the elderly. *Mod Pathol.* 2004;17:172–179.

Benson AB, Schrag D, Somerfield MR, et al. American Society of Clinical Oncology recommendations on adjuvant chemotherapy for stage II colon cancer. *J Clin Oncol.* 2004;22:3408–3419.

Bond JH. Polyp guideline: diagnosis, treatment, and surveillance for patients with colorectal polyps. Practice Parameters Committee of the American College of Gastroenterology. *Am J Gastroenterol.* 2000;95:3053–3063.

Bruce WR, Giacca A, Medline A. Possible mechanisms relating diet and risk of colon cancer. *Cancer Epidemiol Biomarkers Prev.* 2000;9:1271–1279.

Burt RW. Colon cancer screening. *Gastroenterology.* 2000;119:837–853.

Chang GJ, Rodriguez-Bigas MA, Skibber JM, Moyer VA. Lymph node evaluation and survival after curative resection of colon cancer: systematic review. *J Natl Cancer Inst.* 2007;99:433–441.

Chetty R, Gill P, Govender D, et al. International study group on rectal cancer regression grading: interobserver variability with commonly used regression grading systems. *Hum Pathol.* 2012;43:1917–1923.

Compton C, Fenoglio-Preiser CM, Pettigrew N, Fielding LP. American Joint Committee on Cancer Prognostic Factors Consensus Conference: Colorectal Working Group. *Cancer.* 2000;88:1739–1757.

Connelly JH, Robey-Cafferty SS, Cleary KR. Mucinous carcinomas of the colon and rectum. An analysis of 62 stage B and C lesions. *Arch Pathol Lab Med.* 1991;115:1022–1025.

Cooper HS, Deppisch LM, Gourley WK, et al. Endoscopically removed malignant colorectal polyps: clinicopathologic correlations. *Gastroenterology.* 1995;108:1657–1665.

Cranley JP, Petras RE, Carey WD, et al. When is endoscopic polypectomy adequate therapy for colonic polyps containing invasive carcinoma? *Gastroenterology.* 1986;91:419–427.

de Campos-Lobato LF, Stocchi L, de Sousa JB, et al. Less than 12 nodes in the surgical specimen after total mesorectal excision following neoadjuvant chemoradiation: it means more than you think! *Ann Surg Oncol.* 2013;20:3398–3406.

De Lott LB, Morrison C, Suster S, et al. CDX2 is a useful marker of intestinal-type differentiation: a tissue microarray-based study of 629 tumors from various sites. *Arch Pathol Lab Med.* 2005;129:1100–1105.

Dillman RO, Aaron K, Heinemann FS, McClure SE. Identification of 12 or more lymph nodes in resected colon cancer specimens as an indicator of quality performance. *Cancer.* 2009;115:1840–1848.

Edge S, Byrd DR, Compton cc, et al. Colon and Rectum. *AJCC Cancer Staging Manual.* 7th ed:New York, NY; Springer-Verlag; 2010.

Fenoglio CM, Kaye GI, Lane N. Distribution of human colonic lymphatics in normal, hyperplastic, and adenomatous tissue. Its relationship to metastasis from small carcinomas in pedunculated adenomas, with two case reports. *Gastroenterology.* 1973;64:51–66.

Garfinkel L, Mushinski M. U.S. cancer incidence, mortality and survival: 1973–1996. *Stat Bull Metrop Insur Co.* 1999;80:23–32.

Gleisner AL, Mogal H, Dodson R, et al. Nodal status, number of lymph nodes examined, and lymph node ratio: what defines prognosis after resection of colon adenocarcinoma? *J Am Coll Surg.* 2013;217:1090–1100.

Goldstein NS, Long A, Kuan SF, Hart J. Colon signet ring cell adenocarcinoma: immunohistochemical characterization and comparison with gastric and typical colon adenocarcinomas. *Appl Immunohistochem Mol Morphol.* 2000;8:183–188.

Goldstein NS, Turner JR. Pericolonic tumor deposits in patients with T3N+MO colon adenocarcinomas: markers of reduced disease free survival and intra-abdominal metastases and their implications for TNM classification. *Cancer.* 2000;88:2228–2238.

Goldstein NS. Lymph node recoveries from 2427 pT3 colorectal resection specimens spanning 45 years: recommendations for a minimum number of recovered lymph nodes based on predictive probabilities. *Am J Surg Pathol.* 2002;26:179–189.

Gopal P, Lu P, Ayers GD, et al. Tumor deposits in rectal adenocarcinoma after neoadjuvant chemoradiation are associated with poor prognosis. *Mod Pathol.* 2014;27:1281–1287.

Govindarajan A, Gönen M, Weiser MR, et al. Challenging the feasibility and clinical significance of current guidelines on lymph node examination in rectal cancer in the era of neoadjuvant therapy. *J Clin Oncol.* 2011;29:4568–4573.

Greene FL. Epithelial misplacement in adenomatous polyps of the colon and rectum. *Cancer.* 1974;33:206–217.

Grin A, Messenger DE, Cook M, et al. Peritoneal elastic lamina invasion: limitations in its use as a prognostic marker in stage II colorectal cancer. *Hum Pathol.* 2013;44:2696–2705.

Gunderson LL, Jessup JM, Sargent DJ, et al. Revised tumor and node categorization for rectal cancer based on surveillance, epidemiology, and end results and rectal pooled analysis outcomes. *J Clin Oncol.* 2010;28:256–263.

Hase K, Shatney C, Johnson D, et al. Prognostic value of tumor "budding" in patients with colorectal cancer. *Dis Colon Rectum.* 1993;36:627–635.

Jass JR. Classification of colorectal cancer based on correlation of clinical, morphological and molecular features. *Histopathology.* 2007;50:113–130.

Jass JR. Hereditary Non-Polyposis Colorectal Cancer: the rise and fall of a confusing term. *World J Gastroenterol.* 2006;12:4943–4950.

Jessurun J, Romero-Guadarrama M, Manivel JC. Medullary adenocarcinoma of the colon: clinicopathologic study of 11 cases. *Hum Pathol.* 1999;30:843–848.

Jiang W, Roma AA, Lai K, et al. Endometriosis involving the mucosa of the intestinal tract: a clinicopathologic study of 15 cases. *Mod Pathol.* 2013;26:1270–1278.

Jin M, Roth R, Rock JB, et al. The Impact of Tumor Deposits on Colonic Adenocarcinoma AJCC TNM Staging and Outcome. *Am J Surg Pathol.* 2014;39(1):109–115.

Kakar S, Aksoy S, Burgart LJ, Smyrk TC. Mucinous carcinoma of the colon: correlation of loss of mismatch repair enzymes with clinicopathologic features and survival. *Mod Pathol.* 2004;17:696–700.

Keshava A, Chapuis PH, Chan C, et al. The significance of involvement of a free serosal surface for recurrence and survival following resection of clinicopathological stage B and C rectal cancer. *Colorectal Dis.* 2007;9:609–618.

Kojima M, Nakajima K, Ishii G, et al. Peritoneal elastic laminal invasion of colorectal cancer: the diagnostic utility and clinicopathologic relationship. *Am J Surg Pathol.* 2010;34:1351–1360.

Kojima M, Shimazaki H, Iwaya K, et al. Practical utility and objectivity: does evaluation of peritoneal elastic laminal invasion in colorectal cancer overcome these contrary problems? *Am J Surg Pathol.* 2014;38:144–145.

Kojima M, Yokota M, Saito N, et al. Elastic laminal invasion in colon cancer: diagnostic utility and histological features. *Front Oncol.* 2012;2:179.

Le Voyer TE, Sigurdson ER, Hanlon AL, et al. Colon cancer survival is associated with increasing number of lymph nodes analyzed: a secondary survey of intergroup trial INT-0089. *J Clin Oncol.* 2003;21:2912–2919.

Liang WY, Chang WC, Hsu CY, et al. Retrospective evaluation of elastic stain in the assessment of serosal invasion of pT3N0 colorectal cancers. *Am J Surg Pathol.* 2013;37:1565–1570.

Lipper S, Kahn LB, Ackerman LV. The significance of microscopic invasive cancer in endoscopically removed polyps of the large bowel. A clinicopathologic study of 51 cases. *Cancer.* 1983;52:1691–1699.

Ludeman L, Shepherd NA. Serosal involvement in gastrointestinal cancer: its assessment and significance. *Histopathology.* 2005;47:123–131.

McCluggage WG, Clements WD. Endosalpingiosis of the colon and appendix. *Histopathology.* 2001;39:645–646.

Medani M, Kelly N, Samaha G, et al. An appraisal of lymph node ratio in colon and rectal cancer: not one size fits all. *Int J Colorectal Dis.* 2013;28:1377–1384.

Miller ED, Robb BW, Cummings OW, Johnstone PA. The effects of preoperative chemoradiotherapy on lymph node sampling in rectal cancer. *Dis Colon Rectum.* 2012;55:1002–1007.

Min BS, Kim NK, Ko YT, et al. Clinicopathological features of signet-ring cell carcinoma of the colon and rectum: a case-matched study. *Hepatogastroenterology.* 2009;56:984–988.

Moon SH, Kim DY, Park JW, et al. Can the new American Joint Committee on Cancer staging system predict survival in rectal cancer patients treated with curative surgery following preoperative chemoradiotherapy? *Cancer.* 2012;118:4961–4968.

Morson BC, Whiteway JE, Jones EA, et al. Histopathology and prognosis of malignant colorectal polyps treated by endoscopic polypectomy. *Gut.* 1984;25:437–444.

Moug SJ, Oliphant R, Balsitis M, et al. The lymph node ratio optimises staging in patients with node positive colon cancer with implications for adjuvant chemotherapy. *Int J Colorectal Dis.* 2014;29:599–604.

Muto T, Bussey HJ, Morson BC. Pseudo-carcinomatous invasion in adenomatous polyps of the colon and rectum. *J Clin Pathol.* 1973;26:25–31.

Nagtegaal ID, Quirke P. Colorectal tumour deposits in the mesorectum and pericolon; a critical review. *Histopathology.* 2007;51:141–149.

Panarelli NC, Schreiner AM, Brandt SM, et al. Histologic features and cytologic techniques that aid pathologic stage assessment of colonic adenocarcinoma. *Am J Surg Pathol.* 2013;37:1252–1258.

Parfitt JR, Driman DK. The total mesorectal excision specimen for rectal cancer: a review of its pathological assessment. *J Clin Pathol.* 2007;60:849–855.

Puppa G, Maisonneuve P, Sonzogni A, et al. Pathological assessment of pericolonic tumor deposits in advanced colonic carcinoma: relevance to prognosis and tumor staging. *Mod Pathol.* 2007;20:843–855.

Puppa G, Shepherd NA, Sheahan K, Stewart CJ. Peritoneal elastic lamina invasion in colorectal cancer: the answer to a controversial area of pathology? *Am J Surg Pathol.* 2011;35:465–469.

Puppa G, Sonzogni A, Colombari R, Pelosi G. TNM staging system of colorectal carcinoma: a critical appraisal of challenging issues. *Arch Pathol Lab Med.* 2010;134:837–852.

Puppa G, Ueno H, Kayahara M, et al. Tumor deposits are encountered in advanced colorectal cancer and other adenocarcinomas: an expanded classification with implications for colorectal cancer staging system including a unifying concept of in-transit metastases. *Mod Pathol.* 2009;22:410–415.

Puppa G. Enhanced pathologic analysis for pericolonic tumor deposits: is it worth it? *Am J Clin Pathol.* 2010;134:1019–1021.

Rock JB, Washington MK, Adsay NV, et al. Debating deposits: an interobserver variability study of lymph nodes and pericolonic tumor deposits in colonic adenocarcinoma. *Arch Pathol Lab Med.* 2014;138:636–642.

Rüschoff J, Dietmaier W, Lüttges J, et al. Poorly differentiated colonic adenocarcinoma, medullary type: clinical, phenotypic, and molecular characteristics. *Am J Pathol.* 1997;150:1815–1825.

Ryan R, Gibbons D, Hyland JM, et al. Pathological response following long-course neoadjuvant chemoradiotherapy for locally advanced rectal cancer. *Histopathology.* 2005;47:141–146.

Seitz U, Bohnacker S, Seewald S, et al. Is endoscopic polypectomy an adequate therapy for malignant colorectal adenomas? Presentation of 114 patients and review of the literature. *Dis Colon Rectum.* 2004;47:1789–1797.

Shepherd NA, Baxter KJ, Love SB. Influence of local peritoneal involvement on pelvic recurrence and prognosis in rectal cancer. *J Clin Pathol.* 1995;48:849–855.

Shepherd NA, Baxter KJ, Love SB. The prognostic importance of peritoneal involvement in colonic cancer: a prospective evaluation. *Gastroenterology.* 1997;112:1096–1102.

Shia J, Klimstra DS, Bagci P, et al. TNM staging of colorectal carcinoma: issues and caveats. *Semin Diagn Pathol.* 2012;29:142–153.

Shinto E, Ueno H, Hashiguchi Y, et al. The subserosal elastic lamina: an anatomic landmark for stratifying pT3 colorectal cancer. *Dis Colon Rectum.* 2004;47:467–473.

Snaebjornsson P, Coupe VM, Jonasson L, et al. pT4 stage II and III colon cancers carry the worst prognosis in a nationwide survival analysis. Shepherd's local peritoneal involvement revisited. *Int J Cancer.* 2014;135:467–478.

Soga K, Konishi H, Tatsumi N, et al. Clear cell adenocarcinoma of the colon: a case report and review of literature. *World J Gastroenterol.* 2008;14:1137–1140.

Swamy R. Histopathological reporting of pT4 tumour stage in colorectal carcinomas: dotting the 'i's and crossing the 't's. *J Clin Pathol.* 2010;63:110–115.

Taliano RJ, LeGolvan M, Resnick MB. Immunohistochemistry of colorectal carcinoma: current practice and evolving applications. *Hum Pathol.* 2013;44:151–163.

Ueno H, Hashiguchi Y, Shimazaki H, et al. Peritumoral deposits as an adverse prognostic indicator of colorectal cancer. *Am J Surg.* 2014;207:70–77.

Ueno H, Mochizuki H, Hashiguchi Y, et al. Risk factors for an adverse outcome in early invasive colorectal carcinoma. *Gastroenterology.* 2004;127:385–394.

Ueno H, Mochizuki H, Shirouzu K, et al. Multicenter study for optimal categorization of extramural tumor deposits for colorectal cancer staging. *Ann Surg.* 2012;255:739–746.

Volk EE, Goldblum JR, Petras RE, et al. Management and outcome of patients with invasive carcinoma arising in colorectal polyps. *Gastroenterology.* 1995;109:1801–1807.

Wang HS, Liang WY, Lin TC, et al. Curative resection of T1 colorectal carcinoma: risk of lymph node metastasis and long-term prognosis. *Dis Colon Rectum.* 2005;48:1182–1192.

Washington MK, Berlin J, Branton P, et al. Protocol for the examination of specimens from patients with primary carcinoma of the colon and rectum. *Arch Pathol Lab Med.* 2009;133:1539–1551.

Washington MK, Berlin J, Branton P, et al. Protocol for the examination of specimens from patients with primary carcinoma of the colon and rectum. *Arch Pathol Lab Med.* 2009;133:1539–1551.

Wünsch K, Müller J, Jähnig H, et al. Shape is not associated with the origin of pericolonic tumor deposits. *Am J Clin Pathol.* 2010;133:388–394.

Xie J, Itzkowitz SH. Cancer in inflammatory bowel disease. *World J Gastroenterol.* 2008;14:378–389.

Zhang J, Lv L, Ye Y, et al. Comparison of metastatic lymph node ratio staging system with the 7th AJCC system for colorectal cancer. *J Cancer Res Clin Oncol.* 2013;139:1947–1953.

Mesenchymal Tumors (See Also Chapter 5)

Eslami-Varzaneh F, Washington K, Robert ME, et al. Benign fibroblastic polyps of the colon: a histologic, immunohistochemical, and ultrastructural study. *Am J Surg Pathol.* 2004;28:374–378.

Gibson JA, Hornick JL. Mucosal Schwann cell "hamartoma": clinicopathologic study of 26 neural colorectal polyps distinct from neurofibromas and mucosal neuromas. *Am J Surg Pathol.* 2009;33:781–787.

Groisman GM, Polak-Charcon S. Fibroblastic polyp of the colon and colonic perineurioma: 2 names for a single entity? *Am J Surg Pathol.* 2008;32:1088–1094.

Hancock BJ, Vajcner A. Lipomas of the colon: a clinicopathologic review. *Can J Surg.* 1988;31:178–181.

Hornick JL, Fletcher CD. Soft tissue perineurioma: clinicopathologic analysis of 81 cases including those with atypical histologic features. *Am J Surg Pathol.* 2005;29:845–858.

Mendelsohn G, Diamond MP. Familial ganglioneuromatous polyposis of the large bowel. Report of a family with associated juvenile polyposis. *Am J Surg Pathol.* 1984;8:515–520.

Miettinen M, Furlong M, Sarlomo-Rikala M, et al. Gastrointestinal stromal tumors, intramural leiomyomas, and leiomyosarcomas in the rectum and anus: a clinicopathologic, immunohistochemical, and molecular genetic study of 144 cases. *Am J Surg Pathol.* 2001;25:1121–1133.

Miettinen M, Sarlomo-Rikala M, Sobin LH. Mesenchymal tumors of muscularis mucosae of colon and rectum are benign leiomyomas that should be separated from gastrointestinal stromal tumors—a clinicopathologic and immunohistochemical study of eighty-eight cases. *Mod Pathol.* 2001;14:950–956.

Miettinen M, Shekitka KM, Sobin LH. Schwannomas in the colon and rectum: a clinicopathologic and immunohistochemical study of 20 cases. *Am J Surg Pathol.* 2001;25:846–855.

Rogy MA, Mirza D, Berlakovich G, et al. Submucous large-bowel lipomas—presentation and management. An 18-year study. *Eur J Surg.* 1991;157:51–55.

Shekitka KM, Sobin LH. Ganglioneuromas of the gastrointestinal tract. Relation to Von Recklinghausen disease and other multiple tumor syndromes. *Am J Surg Pathol.* 1994;18:250–257.

Singhi AD, Montgomery EA. Colorectal granular cell tumor: a clinicopathologic study of 26 cases. *Am J Surg Pathol.* 2010;34:1186–1192.

Hematolymphoid Tumors

Behdad A, Owens SR. Langerhans cell histiocytosis involving the gastrointestinal tract. *Arch Pathol Lab Med.* 2014;138:1350–1352.

Behdad A, Owens SR. Systemic mastocytosis involving the gastrointestinal tract: case report and review. *Arch Pathol Lab Med.* 2013;137:1220–1223.

Burke JS. Lymphoproliferative disorders of the gastrointestinal tract: a review and pragmatic guide to diagnosis. *Arch Pathol Lab Med.* 2011;135:1284–1297.

Cramer SF, Romansky S, Hulbert B, et al. The rectal tonsil: a reaction to chlamydial infection? *Am J Surg Pathol.* 2009;33:483–485.

Detlefsen S, Fagerberg CR, Ousager LB, et al. Histiocytic disorders of the gastrointestinal tract. *Hum Pathol.* 2013;44:683–696.

Doyle LA, Hornick JL. Pathology of extramedullary mastocytosis. *Immunol Allergy Clin North Am.* 2014;34:323–339.

Doyle LA, Sepehr GJ, Hamilton MJ, et al. A clinicopathologic study of 24 cases of systemic mastocytosis involving the gastrointestinal tract and assessment of mucosal mast cell density in irritable bowel syndrome and asymptomatic patients. *Am J Surg Pathol.* 2014;38:832–843.

Farris AB, Lauwers GY, Ferry JA, Zukerberg LR. The rectal tonsil: a reactive lymphoid proliferation that may mimic lymphoma. *Am J Surg Pathol.* 2008;32:1075–1079.

Foukas PG, de Leval L. Recent advances in intestinal lymphomas. *Histopathology.* 2015;66:112–136.

Hashimoto Y, Omura H, Tanaka T, et al. CD5-negative mantle cell lymphoma resembling extranodal marginal zone lymphoma of mucosa-associated lymphoid tissue: a case report. *J Clin Exp Hematop.* 2012;52:185–191.

Hawkes EA, Wotherspoon A, Cunningham D. Diagnosis and management of rare gastrointestinal lymphomas. *Leuk Lymphoma.* 2012;53:2341–2350.

Kojima M, Itoh H, Motegi A, et al. Localized lymphoid hyperplasia of the rectum resembling polypoid mucosa-associated lymphoid tissue lymphoma: a report of three cases. *Pathol Res Pract.* 2005;201:757–761.

O'Malley DP, Goldstein NS, Banks PM. The recognition and classification of lymphoproliferative disorders of the gut. *Hum Pathol.* 2014;45:899–916.

Skarbnik AP, Goy AH. Mantle cell lymphoma: state of the art. *Clin Adv Hematol Oncol.* 2015;13:44–55.

Metastatic Tumors

Disibio G, French SW. Metastatic patterns of cancers: results from a large autopsy study. *Arch Pathol Lab Med.* 2008;132:931–939.

Estrella JS, Wu TT, Rashid A, Abraham SC. Mucosal colonization by metastatic carcinoma in the gastrointestinal tract: a potential mimic of primary neoplasia. *Am J Surg Pathol.* 2011;35:563–572.

Magnusson K, de Wit M, Brennan DJ, et al. SATB2 in combination with cytokeratin 20 identifies over 95% of all colorectal carcinomas. *Am J Surg Pathol.* 2011;35:937–948.

Samo S, Sherid M, Husein H, et al. Metastatic malignant melanoma to the colon: a case report and review of the literature. *J Gastrointest Cancer.* 2014;45:221–224.

Yang Q, Wang H, Cho HY, et al. Carcinoma of müllerian origin presenting as colorectal cancer: a clinicopathologic study of 13 Cases. *Ann Diagn Pathol.* 2011;15:12–18.

12

Neoplasms of the Anus

SCOTT R. OWENS

INTRODUCTION

The anus/anal canal is the site of a handful of diseases that pathologists encounter relatively infrequently. Nonetheless, it is an important site of disease in that its anatomically restricted space leaves little room for mass-forming processes to grow before causing relatively significant symptoms. In addition, the anal region is subject to squamous dysplasias and neoplasms that are identical to their counterparts in the genitalia. Finally, the meeting of several different tissue types (columnar rectal mucosa, anal glands, squamous mucosa, and skin) leads to a number of unique disease entities that can affect this small anatomic location.

The anal canal develops from a mixture of endoderm, comprising the upper two thirds of the canal, and ectoderm, comprising the lower third. The division between these epithelial origins is the dentate line, which is normally the dividing line between rectal mucosa above and squamous mucosa below. At the junction between these epithelial types, there is usually a hybrid "transitional" mucosa that appears histologically as a mixture of stratified squamoid cells and more columnar mucus-producing cells (Figure 12.1). In some specimens from this region, the transitional mucosa can be difficult to find, because it can be very focal and/or overgrown by more distal squamous epithelium secondary to prolapse changes (Figure 12.2). Anal glands (or ducts) are lined by similar transitional-type epithelium, and secrete into the canal near the dentate line (Figure 12.3A–B).

The complex anatomy and histology of this small region of the gastrointestinal (GI) tract can give rise to several different types of malignancy, any of which may be biopsied and encountered by the diagnostic pathologist. Most common are squamous dysplasias and carcinomas, which are pathophysiologically related to squamous conditions elsewhere in the anogenital region, and which are frequently the result of infection by human papillomavirus (HPV). The classification of squamous dysplasia has evolved to match that in the male and female genitalia, adopting the "squamous intraepithelial lesion" terminology that will be discussed in the Squamous Dysplasia section. Less common lesions include adenocarcinomas arising from the anal gland/duct epithelium, which must be distinguished from adenocarcinomas that arise from the distal rectum and involve the anus by distal extension. The anus can be involved by extramammary Paget disease, either primary (similar to the vulva) or associated with underlying colorectal neoplasia, and it can be the site of primary melanoma. Finally, tumors of the perianal skin, such as basal cell carcinoma, can appear as anal lesions, and can present a diagnostic challenge in their separation from squamous carcinomas with a "basaloid" histologic appearance.

BENIGN CONDITIONS AND TUMOR MIMICS

Several conditions can result in tumor- or mass-like lesions in the anal canal, and are worth discussing in the differential diagnosis of anal malignancies. Perhaps the most clinically ominous-appearing of these are the inflammatory masses that can result from prolapse of the rectal mucosa just above the anal canal (also known as "inflammatory cloacogenic polyp;" see also Chapter 11). Other masses and nodules in and around the anus can be caused by hemorrhoids and fibroepithelial "tags."

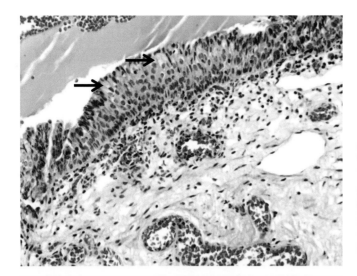

FIGURE 12.1 The anal transition zone contains a "hybrid" epithelium, with stratified squamous-like cells that are admixed with mucus-producing cells (arrows). This type of epithelium occupies the zone between the anal squamous mucosa below and the colonic mucosa above, and is variable in length from person to person.

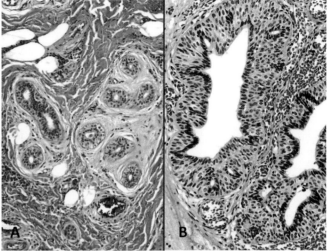

FIGURE 12.3 The anal glands have a variable appearance, and can be found in the subepithelial tissues surrounding the anal canal in the region of the dentate line. They can have an adnexal-like appearance (A), or appear larger and more duct-like (B). They are lined by epithelium with similar characteristics to that of the anal transition zone.

Hemorrhoids

These dilated submucosal vessels, part of the arteriovenous complex of the anal region, often arise in the same clinical setting(s) as mucosal prolapse, including conditions and

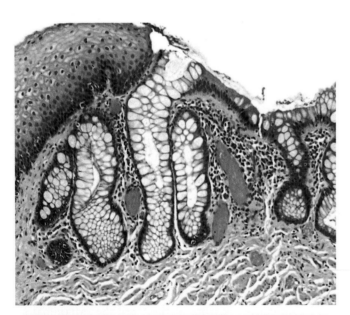

FIGURE 12.2 In some cases, the transition zone is difficult or impossible to find, often because of overgrowth of squamous epithelium secondary to prolapse. In this photomicrograph, the colonic mucosa on the right directly abuts the anal squamous mucosa on the left, without the characteristic transitional epithelium. There is even some overgrowth of squamous cells superficial to colonic crypts.

situations leading to increased intra-abdominal pressure such as pregnancy, ascites, prolonged sitting, and straining at stool. Their incidence is difficult to ascertain, but they are thought to affect at least 5% of the population. They can affect the mucosa/submucosa proximal (internal hemorrhoids) or distal (external hemorrhoids) to the dentate line. The venous plexuses that give rise to these dilated vessels are referred to as the superior and inferior hemorrhoidal plexuses, reflecting how often this condition occurs. Grossly, hemorrhoids are not usually a diagnostic challenge and are mentioned in many endoscopic reports, typically occurring in the left and right posterolateral and right anterior anus. Histologically, they are characterized by dilated submucosal vessels, often containing thrombi in varying states of organization (Figure 12.4A–B). The overlying squamous epithelium frequently has prolapse-related hyperparakeratosis as well.

While hemorrhoids are typically innocuous, other diseases that will be discussed in detail later may complicate them, and it is important to keep these things in mind when grossing and when addressing yet another seemingly uninspiring "hemorrhoid" under the microscope. First, anything that appears as a mass in the anal canal, including carcinomas and melanomas, can mimic a hemorrhoid and may be excised for that clinical indication, appearing unexpectedly when the tissue is examined histologically. In addition, squamous dysplasias, usually related to HPV, can complicate bona fide hemorrhoids (Figure 12.5). This can range from low-grade condylomatous lesions to carcinomas in situ, and is perhaps more easily overlooked than invasive carcinoma or melanoma because the other typical

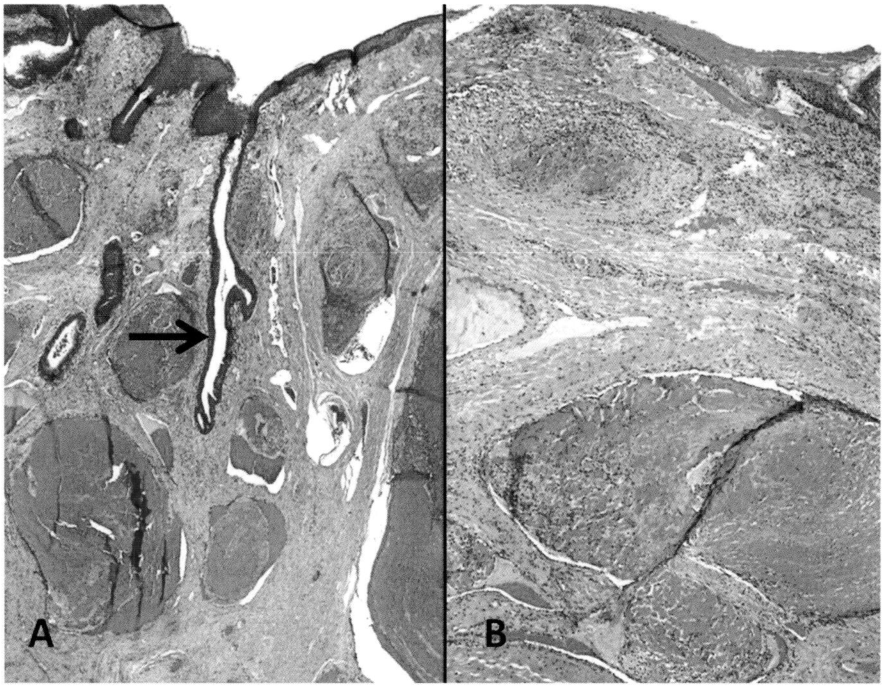

FIGURE 12.4 Hemorrhoids are composed of dilated and blood-filled submucosal vessels that can occur proximal (internal hemorrhoids) or distal (external hemorrhoids) to the dentate line. In (A), a collection of hemorrhoidal vessels underlies the anal squamous mucosa on the right, and the transition zone on the left. Transitional epithelium is seen in the middle of the image (arrow). Hemorrhoids commonly contain evidence of thrombosis and organization (B), where ingrowth of fibroblasts is seen at the periphery of several vessels.

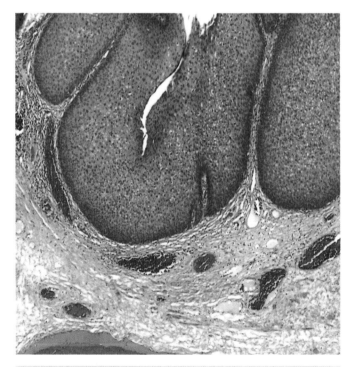

FIGURE 12.5 Other conditions affecting the anal canal can complicate or be superimposed on hemorrhoids. In this case, a dilated hemorrhoidal vessel at the bottom of the image is beneath an HPV-related condyloma.

features of hemorrhoids are present. Additional discussion of the various entities that can mimic or complicate hemorrhoids is present in subsequent sections.

Anal Tags/Fibroepithelial Polyps

These benign lesions consist of polypoid protrusions of anal squamous epithelium and underlying fibrovascular tissue, and are commonly confused with hemorrhoids on clinical examination. They are also known as "hypertrophied anal papillae." These lesions consist of hyalinized subepithelial connective tissue with overlying squamous epithelium (Figure 12.6A–B). They lack the characteristic dilated submucosal vessels of hemorrhoids, and can have reactive-appearing myofibroblasts in their stroma. Anal tags are essentially identical to cutaneous fibroepithelial polyps (also known as acrochordons).

SQUAMOUS DYSPLASIA

Epidemiology and Pathogenesis

Squamous dysplasia of the anus is relatively uncommon compared to the incidence in the female genital tract, but its incidence has risen over recent decades. There is a

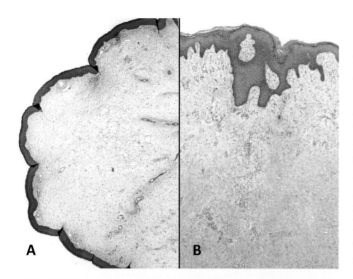

FIGURE 12.6 Anal tags are histologically identical to fibroepithelial polyps in the skin, with a core of fibrovascular tissue that varies from loose and myxoid (A) to more dense and hyalinized (B). There is often overlying squamous epithelium that may have hyperparakeratosis associated with mechanical irritation, as in (B).

slight female predominance overall, but the incidence of anal condylomas, other forms of intraepithelial neoplasia, and squamous cell carcinoma are much higher in homosexual men who practice anal receptive intercourse and/or are HIV positive. In addition, these lesions can complicate other processes found in the anus, such as hemorrhoids or anal tags. Its recognition as a sexually transmitted process related to HPV infection has shed new light on its diagnosis, and has resulted in attempts at screening programs such as anal Pap smears for high-risk populations, including immunosuppressed patients such as those with HIV, and patients with other sexually transmitted infections. Patients with HPV-related disease in the genital region, including the vulva and cervix, are at high risk for anal neoplasia as well.

As with genital HPV-related disease, certain HPV genotypes are considered "high-risk" for inducing the development of anal neoplasms. The most common genotypes infecting this region are 6, 11, 16, and 18, and types 16 and 18 are the most commonly encountered high-risk types. Other high-risk genotypes include 31, 33, and 35. Although these genotypes have the highest likelihood of leading to anogenital neoplasia, the majority of infected patients do not go on to develop squamous carcinoma. Instead, cell-mediated immunity keeps the infection in check for most patients, and a humoral immune response provides permanent immunity. In recent years, this fact has been exploited to develop vaccines against the common high-risk genotypes of HPV. "Low-risk" types, such as 6 and 11, are associated with squamous dysplasia but have a much lower risk of progression to malignancy.

The pathogenesis of HPV-related squamous disease involves direct effects of the virus on patients' genomes, with integration of HPV DNA into the host genetic material in cases related to high-risk genotypes that ultimately lead to malignancy. Low-risk types may remain unintegrated in host cells as episomes. The HPV-associated oncoproteins E5, E6, and E7 are thought to be involved in malignant transformation, via inactivation of the tumor suppressor proteins p53 (by E6) and pRb (by E7). E5 may have an effect on growth factor receptors, further promoting proliferation. The upregulation of p16 that results from pRb inactivation underlies the use of p16 immunohistochemistry in the diagnosis of HPV-related squamous dysplasia and neoplasia, with "block-like" p16 positivity considered a surrogate marker for HPV (Figure 12.7).

Terminology

The terminology of anogenital squamous lesions has historically been confusing and nonstandardized, ranging from terms originally employed in the context of cervical Pap smear cytology and later carried over to biopsy pathology, to language adapted from squamous skin cancer and applied to anogenital mucosae. In 2012, a project jointly undertaken by the College of American Pathologists (CAP) and the American Society for Colposcopy and Cervical Pathology (ASCCP) recommended a standardized terminology for anogenital squamous lesions. This CAP–ASCCP Lower Anogenital Squamous Terminology (LAST) project recommends dividing anal squamous dysplasias into a two-tiered naming/grading convention,

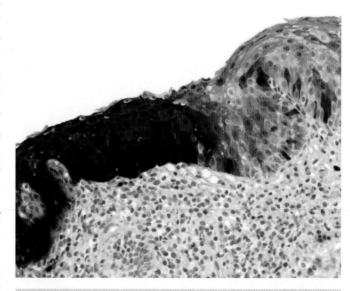

FIGURE 12.7 Immunohistochemistry for p16 is useful as a surrogate marker for HPV-driven squamous dysplasia in the anal canal. Dense, block-like nuclear and cytoplasmic positivity as in the left half of the image is indicative of HPV-related dysplasia.

based on the presence of low-grade or high-grade dyspla-sia. Low-grade squamous intraepithelial neoplasia (LSIL) is most often related to low-risk HPV genotypes such as 6 and 11, while its high-grade counterpart (high-grade squamous intraepithelial neoplasia [HSIL]) and invasive squamous carcinoma tend to be associated with the high-risk types including 16 and 18. The LAST project also provides recommendations on how and when to use p16 immunohistochemistry in the diagnosis and grading of these lesions.

While anal dysplasias are currently divided into low- and high-grade tiers, the older terminology of "anal intraepithelial neoplasia" (AIN) and "perianal intraepi-thelial neoplasia" (PAIN) linger in the system of nomen-clature recommended by the LAST project. The former is used for lesions in squamous mucosa of the anal canal itself, while the latter refers to lesions affecting the peri-anal skin within 5 cm of the anal verge. These older terms reflect a division of squamous dysplasia into three tiers or grades, with LSIL encompassing grade 1 and HSIL grades 2 and 3. According to the LAST criteria, anal squamous lesions are to be reported using the LSIL/HSIL nomen-clature, followed by the P/AIN grade in parenthesis; for example, "LSIL (AIN1)." Histologically, P/AIN1 is charac-terized by squamous atypia and dysmaturation restricted to the basal 1/3 of the epithelium, and P/AIN2 to roughly the lower 2/3. P/AIN3 demonstrates full-thickness atypia/dysplasia, effectively "carcinoma in situ." The designation of HSIL (AIN3) subsumes the now-out-of-date term of "Bowen's disease."

Clinical and Macroscopic Features

Patients typically present with bleeding, pain, and itching. In addition to the macroscopic appearance of condylo-mata, squamous lesions of the anus may present clinically as white, pigmented, or erythematous areas. There may also be papules or scaly plaques. As in the cervix, acetic acid may be used to highlight the lesions, imparting an "acetowhite" appearance that may help in clinical iden-tification. Biopsies from anal tags, hemorrhoids, or other protrusions in the anal canal may come with a request to "rule out condyloma," and these may either mimic or hide true HPV-related dysplasia.

Microscopic Features

The dysplastic cells in these cases are characterized by nuclear irregularity, hyperchromasia, enlargement, and pleomorphism (Figure 12.8A–D). In addition, particu-larly in examples of LSIL, there may be histologic evi-dence of HPV infection in the form of koilocytic changes.

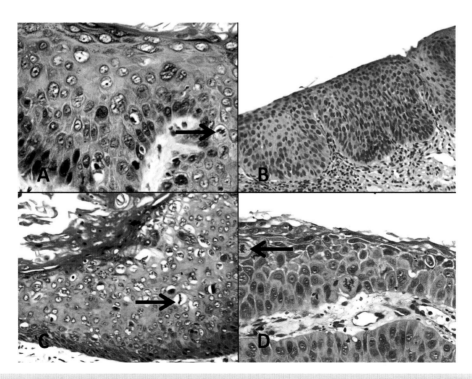

FIGURE 12.8   As in other sites invested with squamous epithelium, dysplasia in the anal canal is characterized by disorganized, immature cells that have pleomorphic and hyperchromatic nuclei (A). Mitotic figures (arrow), normally restricted to the basal layer of proliferative cells, are easily identifiable above the basal layer. In high-grade squamous intraepithelial lesions (HSIL), there is full-thickness atypia and a lack of maturation toward the surface of the epithelium (B). HSIL comprises anal intraepithelial neoplasia grades 2 (C) and 3 (D), where immature cells and mitotic activity (arrows) reach the middle third and upper third of the epithelium, respectively.

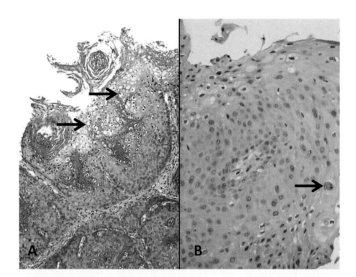

FIGURE 12.9 Low-grade squamous intraepithelial lesion (LSIL; AIN1) is characterized by the presence of koilocytes (A, arrows), which are a hallmark of HPV infection. Koilocytic changes include hyperchromatic, wrinkled, or "raisinoid" nuclei that are surrounded by a sharply demarcated clear cytoplasmic halo. In addition, there is cytologic immaturity and mitotic activity that is limited to the basal third of the epithelium, along with individually dyskeratotic cells (B, arrow).

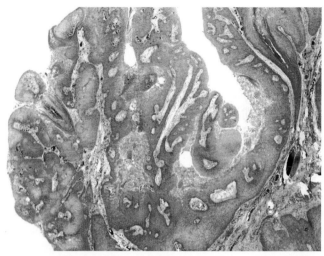

FIGURE 12.10 The term "condyloma acuminatum" refers to a grossly visible, warty squamous proliferation projecting above the surrounding mucosa. Condylomata can have quite complex architecture and are now considered to harbor, by definition, low-grade squamous dysplasia (AIN1; LSIL).

The characteristic features of koilocytes include nuclear "crinkling" or a "raisinoid" appearance, a sharply demarcated perinuclear clearing or halo and, often, binucleation (Figure 12.9A–B). In the past, lesions with koilocytes and squamous hyperplasia or acanthosis that appear as grossly visible lesions have been termed "condylomata acuminata" (singular, *condyloma acuminatum*), a moniker still often used clinically. These anogenital "warts" (Figure 12.10) are now classified, according to the LAST project criteria, to harbor low-grade dysplasia, and are included in the category of LSIL.

Diagnostic Challenges

Glycogenated squamous cells can mimic koilocytes, and inflamed squamous mucosa and/or skin may have reactive atypia that mimics dysplasia (Figure 12.11A–B). Finally, as mentioned in the Introduction, the anal transition zone is lined by a "hybrid" epithelium that is stratified and that can undergo squamous metaplasia. As with metaplasia in the uterine cervix, this can impart an appearance that strongly mimics HSIL (Figure 12.12).

The distinction between anal squamous dysplasia and inflammatory and/or metaplastic atypia can be aided using p16 immunohistochemistry as a surrogate marker for HPV infection. Strong, block-like p16 positivity should push one toward a diagnosis of true dysplasia, while a weak, patchy, or negative result suggests reactive atypia

(Figure 12.13). In addition, the LAST recommendations indicate that p16 should be used when the hematoxylin and eosin (H&E) diagnosis is HSIL (P/AIN2), in order to make a more definite diagnosis of either P/AIN3 (in the setting of strong, block-like positivity) or LSIL (P/AIN1) if the staining is not strong (Figure 12.14). The rationale behind this is the known risk of P/AIN3 as a "precancerous" lesion associated with high-risk HPV, while LSIL is

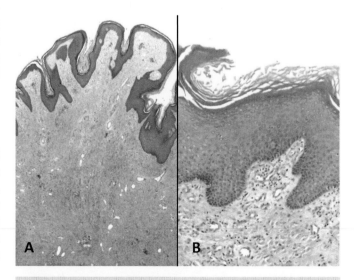

FIGURE 12.11 Not every squamous proliferation in the anal canal is a condyloma. In this case, a vaguely warty-appearing squamous-lined nodule (A) could be misconstrued as a condyloma, but closer inspection of the epithelium (B) reveals only reactive changes with overlying hyperkeratosis, suggesting a prolapse-related phenomenon.

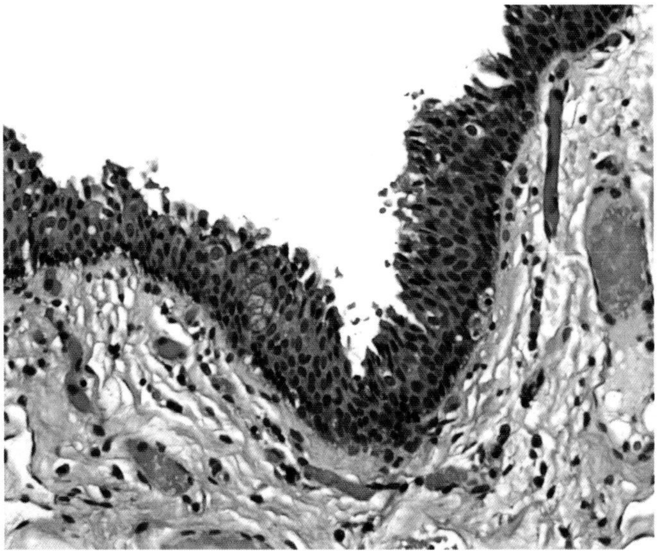

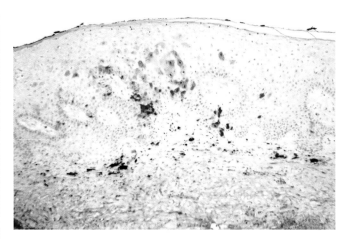

FIGURE 12.14   Patchy weak staining with p16 is characteristic of LSIL/AIN1 as in this case, and should prompt downgrading to that diagnosis if one is contemplating a diagnosis of HSIL/AIN2 (courtesy of Keith K. Lai, MD).

FIGURE 12.12   The anal transitional mucosa can undergo squamous metaplasia, with loss of the characteristic mucus-producing cells. Like immature squamous metaplasia in the uterine cervix, this appearance can be mistaken for high-grade dysplasia/HSIL.

more likely to be associated with low-risk genotypes; histologic P/AIN2 lesions that are p16 positive are thought to behave more like bona fide P/AIN3 lesions. Finally, p16 use is recommended in cases of professional disagreement between observers, when the differential diagnosis includes HSIL. The use of p16 immunostaining is recommended *against* when the histologic findings are thought to be diagnostic of LSIL (P/AIN1) or HSIL (P/AIN3), as an unexpected positive or negative result, respectively, may simply confuse the issue.

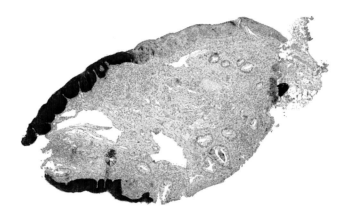

FIGURE 12.13   At very low magnification, the characteristic block-like p16 positivity of HSIL on the left contrasts with patchy, weak positivity on the right. The latter pattern points toward reactive atypia and away from HPV-related dysplasia.

As suggested in the previous paragraph, HSIL lesions are thought to be precursors to invasive squamous cell carcinoma, although the rate of progression in the anus is controversial. In addition, progression of LSIL to HSIL is also thought to be possible, though there is conflicting evidence in the literature. There is some thought that LSIL lesions with block-like p16 positivity may have the highest likelihood for progression, though this somewhat belies the LAST project recommendation that p16 immunohistochemistry be avoided in lesions thought to be diagnostic of LSIL on H&E alone. Therapy for dysplastic squamous lesions in the anus is similar to that in the genitalia, and centers on eradication of the dysplastic process prior to the development of invasive cancer. Local ablation or surgical excision with the aim of achieving negative margins is standard.

INVASIVE SQUAMOUS CELL CARCINOMA

Epidemiology and Pathogenesis

Squamous cell carcinoma (SCC) is the most common primary anal neoplasm, though it is still relatively rare in comparison to other lower GI neoplasms, accounting for less than 5% of large bowel malignancies. As with the "precancerous" dysplastic lesions discussed in the previous section, most are now believed to be related to underlying HPV infection, particularly those arising below the dentate line. The risk factors for SCC parallel those for anal squamous dysplasia, including other sexually transmitted infections, immunosuppression (including HIV), and cigarette smoking. In the past, female patients vastly outnumbered males, but this has equalized somewhat in recent decades.

Clinical and Macroscopic Features

Patients may present with anal pain, with or without discharge; bleeding; pruritus; or a palpable mass. Lymphadenopathy may be present, reflecting spread to regional nodes. Early lesions are often small and verrucoid, whereas later lesions may consist of ulcers, a palpable nodule, or a large fungating mass.

Microscopic Features and Variants

These carcinomas can have a variety of morphologies, including large and very well-differentiated verrucous carcinomas (formerly known as "giant condyloma of Buschke–Lowenstein"), basaloid squamous carcinomas (referred to as "cloacogenic carcinoma" in the past), and typical, keratinizing squamous cell carcinomas identical to those seen elsewhere in the GI tract and on the skin.

Basaloid SCC often arises proximal to the dentate line, and can be difficult to recognize as a squamous-derived tumor based on H&E histology alone. These tumors consist of nests of basophilic cells with relatively scant cytoplasm and peripheral palisading (Figure 12.15A–B). This type of carcinoma can mimic the much rarer basal cell carcinoma (arising in the perianal skin) as well as neuroendocrine carcinomas, another rare tumor that usually occurs in the rectum rather than the anus. Compared to true basal cell carcinomas, basaloid SCCs have more cytologic pleomorphism and often have areas with more recognizable squamous differentiation such as keratinization. Their heritage can also be confirmed using markers of squamous differentiation such as p63 immunostaining.

Conventional SCC arises most often distal to the dentate line, although it can sometimes present when it involves the rectal mucosa. As with other conventional SCCs, it may vary from well- to poorly differentiated (Figure 12.16A–D), and can extend proximally into the rectum and/or make large, obstructive, ulcerating masses. In poorly differentiated tumors, finding foci of keratinization, intercellular bridges/desmosomes, and p63 immunohistochemistry can be helpful in recognizing squamous differentiation.

Verrucous SCC is typically macroscopically impressive, reflected in its older name of "giant condyloma." This name also reflects the difficulty in recognizing that verrucous tumors are truly invasive, due to their wide, pushing front rather than infiltrating borders. These tumors can be very large and, although they are also HPV-related, features of both viral infection and dysplasia are typically difficult to find histologically (Figure 12.17A–B), which also adds to the difficulty in diagnosing malignancy. These tumors often have extensive surface maturation,

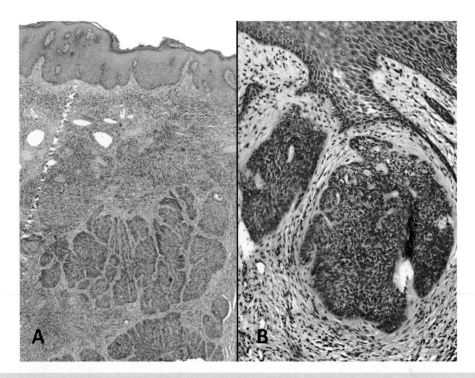

FIGURE 12.15 Basaloid squamous cell carcinoma of the anus has an appearance at low magnification (A) that strongly resembles basal cell carcinoma (BCC) of the skin, with nests of hyperchromatic cells that have peripheral palisading. At higher magnification (B), however, the cells are more pleomorphic than true BCC, often with brisk mitotic activity. These tumors can also resemble high-grade neuroendocrine carcinomas that may extend from the rectum to involve the anal canal.

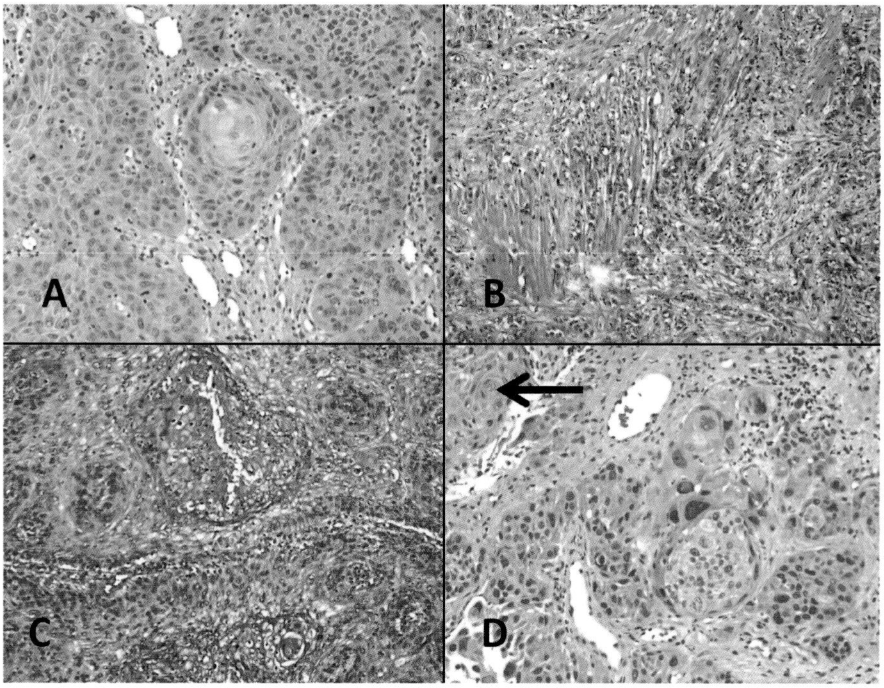

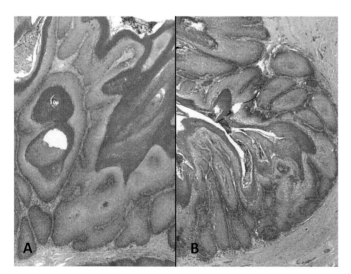

FIGURE 12.16 Conventional anal squamous cell carcinoma, almost always arising in the setting of HPV infection, varies from well-differentiated (A) with cells that have abundant, pale eosinophilic cytoplasm, to very poorly differentiated (B) with cells that are essentially unrecognizable without ancillary studies such as p63 immunostaining. Intercellular bridges (desmosomes) and keratinization (C) are good morphologic clues to squamous differentiation. Some examples (D) are quite pleomorphic, yet can have areas of keratinization (arrow).

FIGURE 12.17 Verrucous carcinomas of the anus are very bulky, deceptively well-differentiated masses that can grow to be very large (A). As in other sites, the determination of malignancy in such lesions can be difficult, particularly if only the superficial part of the process is sampled. Such tumors, however, have a broad, pushing invasive front (B) and can be very locally destructive, as in this tumor that invades into muscle.

and superficial biopsies may only sample benign-appearing, hyperparakeratotic epithelium, leading to a benign diagnosis that is at odds with the clinically impressive and worrisome appearance. While the tumor invasion is broad and pushing rather than infiltrative, verrucous SCC are aggressive neoplasms, invading local structures and sometimes involving the deep soft tissues of the pelvis. There is some evidence that these deceivingly well-differentiated carcinomas are more closely related to low-risk HPV genotypes, in contrast to conventional SCC.

Staging

Regardless of subtype, anal SCC is staged according to the conventions of the AJCC/UICC TNM manual, seventh edition, which currently uses tumor size as the main criterion. The staging scheme is summarized in brief:

- pTx: primary tumor cannot be assessed
- pT0: no evidence of primary tumor
- pTis: carcinoma in situ (includes HSIL and AIN23)
- pT1: tumor 2 cm or less in the greatest dimension
- pT2: tumor more than 2 cm but not more than 5 cm in the greatest dimension
- pT3: tumor more than 5 cm

- pT4: tumor of any size that invades adjacent organs (eg, vagina, urethra, bladder). Of note, direct invasion of rectal wall, perirectal skin, subcutaneous tissues, or anal sphincter muscles is not classified as a T4 lesion.

Tumors arising above the dentate line tend to metastasize to pelvic, perirectal, and para-aortic/paravertebral lymph nodes, while those arising distally metastasize to inguinal nodes. Metastasis in perirectal lymph nodes is classified as N1, whereas metastasis in unilateral internal iliac and/or inguinal lymph nodes is classified as N2. Metastasis in perirectal and inguinal nodes and/or bilateral internal iliac and/or inguinal nodes is classified as N3. Current therapy centers on chemoradiation, with radical (abdominoperineal) resection generally reserved for cases that fail this therapeutic approach. In general, anal SCC has a better prognosis than other primary anal tumors.

ANAL ADENOCARCINOMA

Epidemiology and Pathogenesis

Primary anal adenocarcinoma is very rare. When an adenocarcinoma is found to involve the anal canal, the most likely explanation is distal extension from a primary rectal tumor, which is the main differential diagnosis for primary anal adenocarcinoma. Potential sites for primary anal adenocarcinoma to arise include the mucus-producing epithelial cells of the anal transition zone, as well as the glandular epithelium of the perianal glands/ducts. Assessment of risk factors and etiologic issues is difficult given the rarity of these cancers, but there is some evidence associating anal (and even distal colorectal) adenocarcinomas with HPV.

Clinical and Macroscopic Features

These tumors typically present in older adults (60–70 years of age), and there is a male predominance. Patients often have a painful buttock mass and/or a mucinous anal discharge, and bleeding is less frequently a presenting symptom than in squamous cell carcinoma. These tumors are aggressive, and patients are at high risk for both local and distant recurrences; the overall 5-year survival rate is 30%. Prognosis is stage dependent, however, and staging is similar to anal squamous cell carcinoma.

Macroscopically, anal adenocarcinomas arise within the deep soft tissues of the anal region, and intraluminal anal canal growth is rare.

Microscopic Features

Primary anal gland/duct carcinoma has been described as having one of two morphologic patterns. The first is an infiltrative process composed of small, angulated tubules lined by malignant epithelial cells with very little luminal material (Figure 12.18A–B). Alternatively, these carcinomas may have a "colloid" appearance, with clusters of

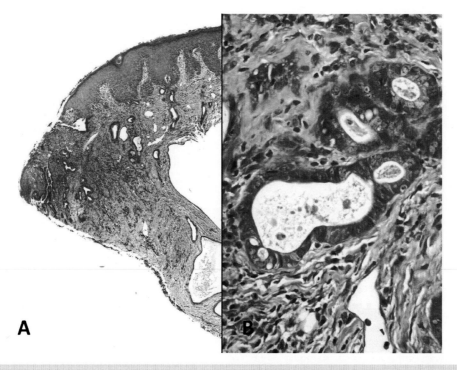

FIGURE 12.18 One form of anal gland/duct carcinoma is characterized by predominantly small, angulated tubules that contain very little luminal material. At low magnification (A), these can be seen infiltrating beneath the overlying squamous epithelium. At high magnification (B), the neoplastic tubules are lined by pleomorphic cells and contain only scant luminal debris.

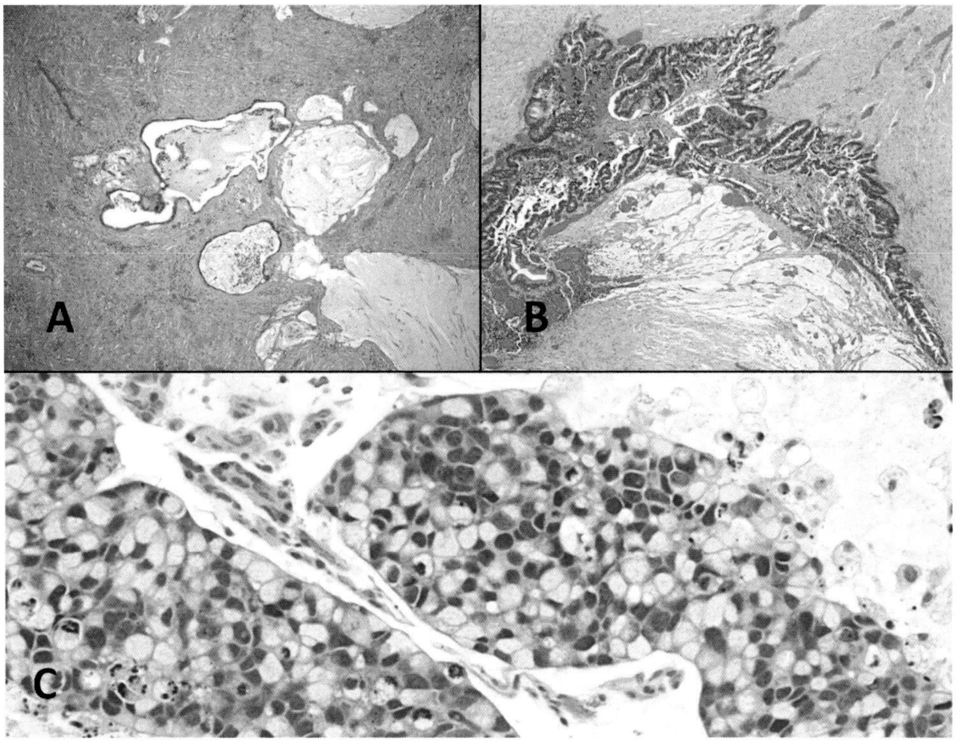

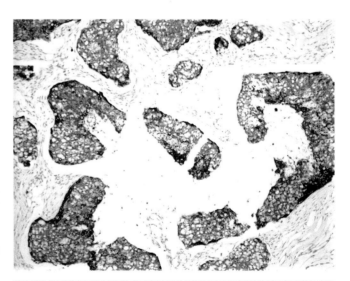

FIGURE 12.19   Another morphologic pattern of anal gland/duct adenocarcinoma consists of large, irregular tubules and/ or paucicellular mucin pools, the so-called "colloid" pattern (A). The neoplastic cells can be reminiscent of colorectal cancer (B) and/or have a signet ring pattern (C).

malignant cells associated with large pools of paucicellular mucin (Figure 12.19A–C).

Diagnostic Challenges

Anal gland/duct carcinomas have an immunophenotype that helps distinguish them from primary rectal tumors that invade the anus. Whereas rectal tumors tend to express cytokeratin (CK)20 and CDX2, primary anal adenocarcinoma expresses CK7 and is usually CDX2 negative (Figure 12.20). Additionally, anal adenocarcinomas express MUC5AC, whereas rectal tumors are more likely to express the intestinal mucin phenotype of MUC2.

Primary anal adenocarcinoma may have associated individual invasive cells within the squamous epithelium of the distal anal canal and the perianal skin, termed "pagetoid" spread (Figure 12.21). It shares this feature with rectal carcinomas, and both are part of the differential diagnosis of so-called "(peri)anal Paget disease," which will be discussed in the next section. The prognosis of primary anal adenocarcinoma is quite poor, and therapy centers on neoadjuvant chemoradiation followed by resection.

FIGURE 12.20   Anal gland/duct carcinoma can usually be distinguished from colorectal carcinoma by its immunostaining pattern, which is characterized by diffuse CK7 positivity (illustrated here), with negativity for CK20 and CDX2. Colonic adenocarcinoma typically has the opposite pattern.

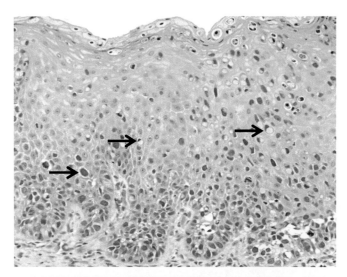

FIGURE 12.21 Anal gland/duct adenocarcinoma is one (rare) cause of pagetoid tumor cell spread into the overlying anal squamous epithelium. In this high-magnification view, individual malignant cells, many with mucin vacuoles (arrows), are scattered throughout the squamous epithelium overlying a carcinoma.

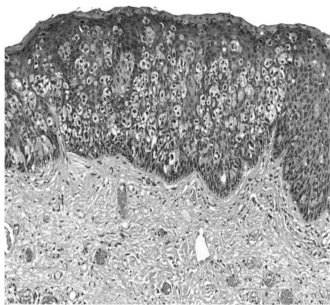

FIGURE 12.22 Perianal Paget disease, in either its primary or secondary form, is characterized by individually infiltrating malignant cells in the anal squamous mucosa. At low magnification, a large number of these pale-staining cells can be seen within the darker-staining squamous epithelium in this case.

(PERI)ANAL PAGET DISEASE

Etiology

Paget disease involving the anus can present a diagnostic challenge. It is important to recognize that the histologic features diagnostic of this entity can arise either as an anal primary ("primary anal/perianal Paget disease") or from neoplasms that are centered in the rectum, from which individual cells infiltrate distally to involve the anal mucosa ("secondary anal/perianal Paget disease"). Primary Paget disease is much less common than the secondary form, reflecting the common occurrence of colorectal adenocarcinoma in general. The primary form is similar to that seen in the vulva and perineum, though it can occur in both men and women. Primary Paget disease is believed to arise from neoplastic cells of either apocrine or eccrine origin.

Clinical and Macroscopic Features

This disease affects both men and women, and typically occurs in patients in the fifth to eight decades. Patients typically present with pruritus and bleeding. Typical lesions consist of crusty, scaly, or ulcerated patches located anywhere between the dentate line and perianal skin.

Microscopic Features

In either of its forms, Paget disease involving the anus is characterized by scattered individual epithelioid cells that infiltrate the squamous epithelium of the anal canal and/or perianal skin, termed "pagetoid spread" (Figure 12.22). The cells have a frankly malignant appearance, with ample pale cytoplasm, and often contain recognizable mucin vacuoles (Figure 12.23A–B). Some may have the appearance of signet ring cells, and mucin-containing examples can be highlighted using cytochemical stains such as mucicarmine and/or immunohistochemical markers of mucin production. The infiltrative nature of the process often incites reactive changes in the adjacent squamous epithelium, including hyperparakeratosis, acanthosis, and basal atypia. In addition to individual cells, small clusters and even tubular structures may be found among the squamous cells (Figure 12.24). Macroscopically, the involved mucosa and skin may be erythematous, excoriated, or ulcerated.

Identification of Paget disease, as well as the differential diagnosis between the two forms, can be aided by immunohistochemistry. It is important to distinguish between the two types of Paget disease, because secondary Paget disease may be the presenting sign of a rectal neoplasm and its identification must prompt a clinical search for the underlying carcinoma. As expected, secondary Paget disease has an immunophenotype consistent with colonic adenocarcinoma, expressing CK20, CDX2, and MUC2 (Figure 12.25A–B); as with other carcinomas of the distal colon, there may be some CK7 positivity, too. In contrast, primary Paget disease has a phenotype identical

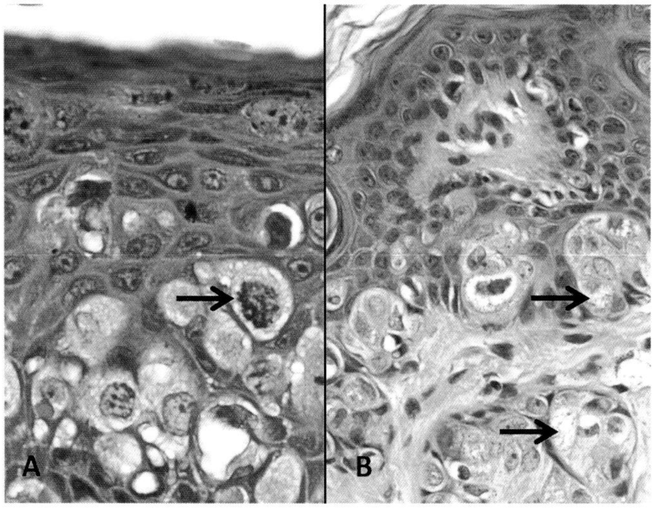

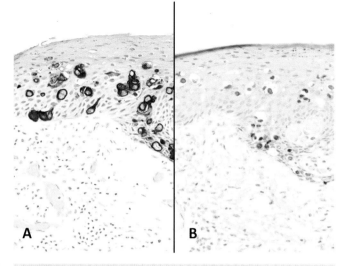

FIGURE 12.23   Perianal Paget disease is characterized by cells with ample, pale cytoplasm and a frankly malignant appearance (A). Mitotic activity is often apparent (arrow, A). The malignant cells may also contain mucin vacuoles (arrow, B), indicative of their adenocarcinoma phenotype.

FIGURE 12.25   Secondary perianal Paget disease most often results from distal extension of a rectal adenocarcinoma and shares the typical immunophenotype of colon cancer, with CK20 (A) and CDX2 (B) positivity.

to that seen in cases involving the vulva, which is much more analogous to mammary carcinoma. Specifically, CK7 (Figure 12.26) and GCDFP-15 are positive, as is MUC5AC, while CK20 and CDX2 are negative. GCDFP-15 (for "gross cystic disease fluid protein") is a marker of apocrine differentiation that is also expressed by many breast carcinomas, and may suggest an apocrine origin for Paget disease as well.

Diagnostic Challenges

In addition to the two types of Paget disease, cells from other tumors arising in and around the anus may spread in a pagetoid fashion. Specifically, adenocarcinomas from the anal glands/ducts, discussed earlier, and melanomas, discussed in the next section, may have this appearance in the squamous epithelium adjacent to the main tumor. The immunophenotype of anal gland/duct carcinoma

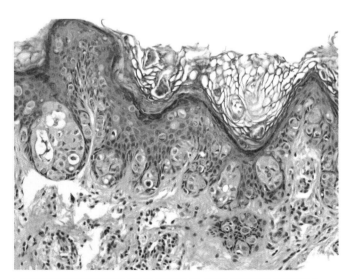

FIGURE 12.24   In addition to individual infiltration, the malignant cells of perianal Paget disease may form small clusters or even tubular structures, which can also contain mucin.

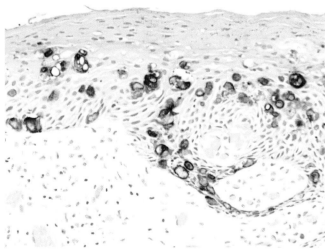

FIGURE 12.26   Primary perianal Paget disease has a unique immunophenotype that is most analogous to that of breast carcinoma. Such cases are positive for CK7, illustrated here, and the mammary marker GCDFP-15.

has overlap with that of primary Paget disease, so an index of suspicion and correlation with clinical findings such as an underlying mass are necessary to differentiate between these diagnoses. In the case of melanoma, the pagetoid cells contain no mucin and express typical melanocyte markers such as S100, HMB-45, and/or melan-A. Even squamous cell carcinomas may occasionally send individual malignant cells into surrounding epithelium in a pagetoid fashion. These express markers of squamous differentiation such as p63, and p16 may be positive in cases associated with HPV.

The therapy and prognosis of Paget disease of the anus depends on the specific type. For primary cases, local therapy is aimed at wide excision, though the condition has a propensity to recur and achievement of negative margins can be problematic. Extensive primary cases or those associated with an anal gland/duct carcinoma may require abdominoperineal resection.

Secondary cases with underlying rectal cancer must be treated with a plan centered on that primary diagnosis. Prognosis in these latter cases depends on the stage of the underlying adenocarcinoma, but is usually poor.

MELANOMA

Epidemiology

Primary anal melanoma is quite rare, even in comparison to some of the other tumors discussed here, and accounts for only 1% to 3% of all melanomas. Normal melanocytes do exist in the anal squamous mucosa and the anal transition zone, and are thought to be the precursors to these tumors. Primary anal melanoma tends to center on the region of the dentate line and, like other tumors discussed in this chapter, can mimic hemorrhoids or anal tags. Thus, it is fairly common for these malignancies to present at a high stage due to lack of suspicion for a malignancy.

Pathologic Features

Anal melanoma typically manifests as a polypoid mass. Pigment is variably present. The overlying mucosa is often ulcerated, and tumors are often large at presentation. Anal melanomas may occur in the anal canal, at the anal verge, or in the rectum.

Anal melanoma is histologically identical to its counterparts in the skin, with characteristic collections of large, epithelioid, and very pleomorphic cells (Figure 12.27A–B). Pigment may or may not be present and, given the relatively unusual location, simply including melanoma in the differential diagnosis can be half the battle. Once the diagnosis is considered, using S100, HMB-45, and/or melan-A to confirm the diagnosis is usually relatively straightforward (Figure 12.28). There are reports of other subtypes of melanoma occurring in the anus as well, including desmoplastic/

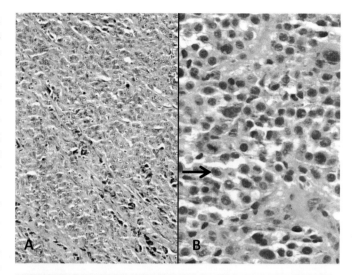

FIGURE 12.27   While most melanomas in the GI tract are metastatic, primary malignant melanomas can occur in the anus. These tumors are morphologically similar to those seen in the skin, with sheets of very pleomorphic malignant cells with variably present pigment (A). At high magnification (B), the typical "dusty" cytoplasm and prominent macronucleoli (arrow) are visible. Pigment is variably present.

sarcomatoid variants. These can be more difficult to recognize, but S100 expression remains fairly sensitive even when other typical melanoma markers are negative. As discussed in the previous section, pagetoid spread by malignant melanocytes (Figure 12.29) can be confused with bona fide Paget disease, but immunohistochemistry is helpful in recognizing these cases for what they are.

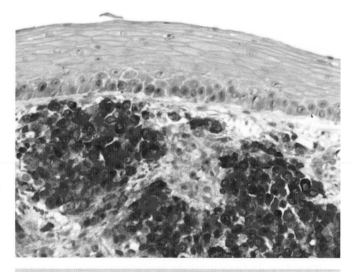

FIGURE 12.28   As in other sites, melanocytic markers such as melan-A (MART-1) highlight the malignant melanoma cells.

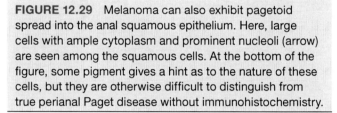

FIGURE 12.29 Melanoma can also exhibit pagetoid spread into the anal squamous epithelium. Here, large cells with ample cytoplasm and prominent nucleoli (arrow) are seen among the squamous cells. At the bottom of the figure, some pigment gives a hint as to the nature of these cells, but they are otherwise difficult to distinguish from true perianal Paget disease without immunohistochemistry.

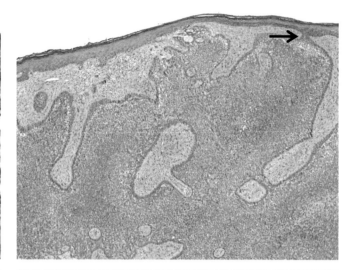

FIGURE 12.30 The perianal skin can give rise to basal cell carcinomas identical to their counterparts elsewhere in the skin. At low magnification, this carcinoma has the characteristic palisading of cells at the periphery of the malignant nests, and can be seen to emanate from the overlying epidermis in one focus (arrow).

The prognosis for anal melanoma is poor, even in cases that seem clinically amenable to resection. Furthermore, radical attempts at resection such as abdominoperineal resection do not appear to improve clinical outcomes. While some cutaneous melanomas have been found to harbor KIT mutations that allow therapy with tyrosine kinase inhibitors, the evidence in anal cases is sparse at this point.

BASAL CELL CARCINOMA

Basal cell carcinoma (BCC), a cutaneous neoplasm that is rarely encountered in perianal skin, is primarily presented here because it can resemble some of the other entities previously discussed in the section on squamous cell carcinoma. Some patients who develop perianal BCC have a genetic predilection such as the basal cell nevus (Gorlin) syndrome or xeroderma pigmentosum. These tumors develop at or below the anal verge in hair-bearing skin, in contrast to basaloid squamous cell carcinomas that involve the anal canal itself. As in the skin elsewhere, BCCs have a nodular, pearly gross appearance, and can be misidentified as anal tags or hemorrhoids in the clinical setting. Histologically, they are composed of nodules of basaloid cells with prominent peripheral palisading, and they can sometimes be seen "budding" from the basal surface of the epidermis (Figure 12.30). Retraction artifact may be prominent around the neoplastic nests, and there may be microcystic spaces filled with mucoid material or foci of abrupt keratinization (Figure 12.31A–B). In contrast to basaloid squamous cell carcinoma, true BCCs

tend to have less pleomorphism and less mitotic activity. Immunohistochemistry for EPCAM/BerEp4 can be of further help in distinguishing the two, as it tends to be positive in BCC and negative in basaloid squamous cell carcinoma. Wide excision is the therapy of choice.

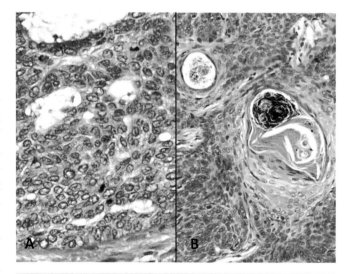

FIGURE 12.31 Most basal cell carcinomas are relatively easy to recognize and to distinguish from basaloid squamous cell carcinomas, because they tend to be less pleomorphic. Potentially confusing histologic features in basal cell carcinoma include microcystic spaces that can contain mucoid material (A), and foci of abrupt keratinization (B) that suggest follicular differentiation.

OTHER UNUSUAL ENTITIES

In addition to basal cell carcinoma of the perianal skin, other tumors arising in dermal appendages and mesenchymal structures can affect the perianal region. These are very rare, and include apocrine adenocarcinomas, Merkel cell carcinomas, smooth muscle neoplasms, granular cell tumors, and others. Analogous to primary perianal Paget disease, other mammary analog tumors such as sclerosing adenosis-like proliferations can appear in this area as well. Finally, similar to other apocrine-gland-containing areas, the perianal region can suffer the effects of hidradenitis suppurativa, which produce a mass lesion in some cases.

SELECTED REFERENCES

General

Bosman FT, Carneiro F, Hruban RH, Theise ND, eds. *WHO Classification of Tumours of the Digestive System.* 4th ed. Lyon, France: IARC Press, 2008.

Fargo MV, Latimer KM. Evaluation and management of common anorectal conditions. *Am Fam Physician.* 2012;85:624–630.

Flejou JF. An update on anal neoplasia. *Histopathology.* 2015;66(1): 147–160.

Kazakov D, Spagnolo DV, Kacerovska D, Michal M. Lesions of anogenital mammary-like glands: an update. *Adv Anat Pathol.* 2011;18:1–28.

Klein JW. Common anal problems. *Med Clin North Am.* 2014;98(3):609–623.

Leonard D, Beddy D, Dozois EJ. Neoplasms of anal canal and perianal skin. *Clin Colon Rectal Surg.* 2011;24(1):54–63.

Longacre TA, Kong CS, Welton ML. Diagnostic problems in anal pathology. *Adv Anat Pathol.* 2008;15:263–278.

Shia J. An update on tumors of the anal canal. *Arch Pathol Lab Med.* 2010;134(11):1601–1611.

Inflammatory/Non-Neoplastic Lesions

Chetty R, Rhathal PS, Slavin JL. Prolapse-induced inflammatory polyps of the colorectum and anal transition zone. *Histopathology.* 1993;23:63–67.

Ganz RA. The evaluation and treatment of hemorrhoids: a guide for the gastroenterologist. *Clin Gastroenterol Hepatol.* 2013;11:593–603.

Mathialagan R, Turner MJ, Gorard DA. Inflammatory cloacogenic polyp mimicking anorectal malignancy. *Eur J Gastroenterol Hepatol.* 2000;12:247–250.

Squamous Dysplasia and Carcinoma

Daling JR, Madeleine MM, Johnson LG, et al. Human papillomavirus, smoking, and sexual practices in the etiology of anal cancer. *Cancer.* 2004;101:270–280.

Darragh TM, Colgan TJ, Cox JT, et al. The lower anogenital squamous terminology standardization project for HPV-associated lesions: background and consensus recommendations from the College of American Pathologists and the American Society for Colposcopy and Cervical Pathology. *Arch Pathol Lab Med.* 2012;136(10):1266–1297.

Maniar KP, Nayar R. HPV-related squamous neoplasia of the lower anogenital tract: an update and review of recent guidelines. *Adv Anat Pathol.* 2014; 21(5):341–358.

Pirog EC, Quint KD, Yantiss RK. P16/CDKN2A and Ki-67 enhance the detection of anal intraepithelial neoplasia and condyloma and correlate with human papillomavirus detection by polymerase chain reaction. *Am J Surg Pathol.* 2010;34:1449–1455.

Rousseau DL Jr., Thomas CR Jr., Petrelli NJ, Kahlenberg MS. Squamous cell carcinoma of the anal canal. *Surg Oncol.* 2005;14:121–132.

Smyczek P, Singh AE, Romanowski B. Anal intraepithelial neoplasia: a review and recommendations for screening and management. *Int J STD AIDS.* 2013;24:843–851.

Wong AK, Chan RC, Aggarwal N, et al. human papillomavirus genotypes in anal intraepithelial neoplasia and anal carcinoma as detected in tissue biopsies. *Mod Pathol.* 2010;23:144–150.

Anal Adenocarcinoma

Jensen SL, Shokouh-Amiri MH, Hagen K, et al. Adenocarcinoma of the anal ducts. A series of 21 cases. *Dis Colon Rect.* 1988;31:268–272.

Meriden Z, Montgomery EA. Anal duct carcinoma: a report of 5 cases. *Hum Pathol.* 2012;43:216–20.

Paget Disease of the Anus

De Nisi MC, D'Amuri A, Toscano M, et al. Usefullness of CDX2 in the diagnosis of extramammary Paget disease associated with malignancies of intestinal type. *Br J Dermatol.* 2005;153;677–679.

Goldblum JR, Hart WR. Perianal Paget's disease: a histologic and immunohistochemical study of 11 cases with and without associated rectal adenocarcinoma. *Am J Surg Pathol.* 1998;22:170–179.

Regauer S. Extramammary Paget's disease: a proliferation of adnexal orgin? *Histopathology.* 2006;48:723–729.

Tulchinsky H, Zmora O, Brazowski E, et al. Extramammary Paget's disease of the perianal region. *Colorectal Dis.* 2004;6:206–209.

Primary Anal Melanoma

Felz MW, Winburn GB, Kallab AM, Lee JR. Anal melanoma: an aggressive malignancy masquerading as hemorrhoids. *South Med J.* 2001;94:880–885.

Heyn J, Placzek M, Ozimek A, et al. Malignant melanoma of the anal region. *Clin Exp Dermatol.* 2007;32:603–607.

Kanaan Z, Mulhall A, Mahid S, et al. A systematic review of prognosis and therapy of anal malignant melanoma: a plea for more precise reporting of location and thickness. *Am Surg.* 2012;78:28–35.

Perianal Basal Cell Carcinoma

Nagendra Naidu DV, Rajakumar V. Perianal basal cell carcinoma-an unusual site of occurrence. *Indian J Dermatol.* 2010;55:178–180.

Patil DT, Goldblum JR, Billings SD. Clinicopathologic analysis of basal cell carcinoma of the anal region and its distinction from basaloid squamous cell carcinoma. *Mod Pathol.* 2013;26:1382–1389.

Wang SQ, Goldberg LH. Multiple polypoid basal cell carcinomas on the perineum of a patient with basal cell nevus syndrome. *J Am Acad Dermatol.* 2007;57(Suppl 2): S36–S37.

13

Applications of Diagnostic Immunohistochemistry

ANDREW M. BELLIZZI

INTRODUCTION

It is fair to say that as of today no special technique has influenced the way that pathology is practiced as profoundly as immunohistochemistry, or has come even close to it.

—Juan Rosai

The ability to visualize antigen expression in the context of tissue morphology is incredibly powerful, allowing us to literally differentiate the undifferentiated. In addition to familiar diagnostic applications including diagnosis of broad tumor class, discernment of carcinoma type, and determination of site of origin, immunohistochemistry (IHC) applications are increasingly prognostic and predictive. Next-generation IHC takes advantage of discoveries in developmental biology and molecular genetics; mining of that literature has revealed lineage-restricted transcription factors, biomarkers identified by gene expression profiling, and protein correlates of molecular genetic events. This chapter will follow the outline of this entire book, proceeding from more general, approach-oriented applications to organ-specific ones.

APPROACH TO EPITHELIAL NEOPLASMS

Immunohistochemistry often plays a critical role in defining tumor type, especially in poorly differentiated neoplasms, and helps assign the primary site of origin in tumors presenting as metastases. In the gastrointestinal (GI) tract, it may be challenging to distinguish an adenocarcinoma of GI origin from a metastasis or another tumor type. When initially evaluating a malignant neoplasm of uncertain type, a useful immunohistochemical screening panel includes a broad-spectrum keratin, S100, and leukocyte common antigen (LCA; also known as CD45), to recognize carcinoma, melanoma, and hematolymphoid neoplasms, respectively.

Keratins represent the principal structural protein of epithelia. Fifty-four human keratins have been described, with most epithelia expressing keratins 4 to 8. Stratified epithelia also highly express keratins 1 to 6 and 9 to 17, while simple epithelia express combinations of keratins 7, 8, 18, 19, and 20, among others. Broad-spectrum keratin immunostains recognize multiple keratins, and commercially available clones including AE1/AE3, OSCAR, MAK-6, MNF116, and CAM5.2 are helpful in diagnosing poorly differentiated carcinomas. Other broad-spectrum epithelial markers include monoclonal antibodies to EPCAM (eg, MOC-31, BerEp4), MUC1 (more commonly referred to as EMA), and claudin-4. As a note of caution, broad-spectrum epithelial markers are occasionally expressed by nonepithelial tumors including select sarcomas (especially epithelioid sarcomas), hematolymphoid neoplasms (especially anaplastic large cell lymphoma and plasma cell neoplasms), melanomas (up to 20% of metastatic tumors), and, of course, mesothelioma (keratin and EMA-positive, while MOC-31 and claudin-4-negative).

S100 expression is very sensitive for a diagnosis of melanoma, but the protein is fairly widely expressed (eg, Schwann cells, adipocytes, chondrocytes, dendritic cells, Langerhans cells, myoepithelial cells), and positivity has been reported in over a third of adenocarcinomas. The melanoma markers melan-A and HMB-45 are more

331

specific, though less sensitive. The transcription factor SOX10, combining superior sensitivity and specificity, is becoming more widely used diagnostically; in addition to melanoma, it is expressed by nerve sheath and myoepithelial tumors and some gliomas.

Among the "big three" of keratin, S100, and LCA, LCA is the most specific, although some lymphoid neoplasms are negative for LCA (eg, plasmablastic lymphoma and some anaplastic large cell lymphomas). For this reason, it is reasonable to add immunostains for CD79a, MUM1, ALK, and CD30 in keratin/S100/LCA "triple-negative" tumors in which a hematolymphoid neoplasm remains a diagnostic consideration morphologically.

There is no broad-spectrum marker specific for mesenchymal tumors. Although vimentin is widely utilized as such a marker, it is also highly expressed by melanoma, lymphoma, and some carcinomas (eg, endometrial and kidney, as well as sarcomatoid carcinomas from any site). CD34 is often expressed by sarcomas, especially vascular and fibroblastic tumors, but also occasionally by less differentiated tumors. As it is only exceptionally expressed by carcinomas, the demonstration of CD34 expression in a poorly differentiated malignant neoplasm of uncertain type is useful to reasonably exclude a diagnosis of carcinoma.

Broad tumor classes and immunostains useful in the diagnosis of poorly differentiated examples are summarized in Table 13.1.

Primary Versus Metastatic Carcinomas in the GI Tract

Squamous cell carcinomas typically produce keratin, and have demonstrable intercellular bridges corresponding to desmosomes. p63 and cytokeratin (CK)5/6 are highly sensitive and moderately specific for the squamous and transitional cell carcinomas (Figure 13.1A–D) as well as for metastatic squamous cell carcinoma.

Urothelial (transitional cell) carcinomas have considerable morphologic overlap with squamous cell carcinomas, and may show foci of overt squamous differentiation. Approximately half of urothelial carcinomas coexpress CK7/CK20, while squamous cell carcinomas are CK7 variable/CK20-negative. The transcription factor

GATA3 is highly expressed by urothelial carcinoma; it is also occasionally expressed by squamous cell carcinoma, in particular those of genitourinary or cutaneous origin, although expression in squamous cell carcinoma is typically weaker than that seen in urothelial carcinoma.

Carcinomas composed of large polygonal cells give rise to a different set of diagnostic considerations, including hepatocellular carcinoma (HCC), renal cell carcinoma (RCC), and adrenal cortical carcinoma. These three tumor types are typically negative for both CK7 and CK20. Key diagnostic markers for these tumors include Hep Par 1 and glypican-3 (HCC); PAX8 (RCC); and melan-A, inhibin, and, more recently, the transcription factor steroidogenic factor 1 (SF1) for adrenal cortical carcinoma. Of note, it is the melan-A clone A103 that reacts with adrenal cortical carcinoma, while other clones (eg, M2-7C10) may only react with melanoma. Adrenal cortical carcinoma also frequently expresses synaptophysin (50%–75%), (but not chromogranin), which may lead to an incorrect diagnosis of a neuroendocrine tumor (NET).

The neuroendocrine neoplasms occurring in the GI tract, both primary and metastatic, include well-differentiated NETs and poorly differentiated neuroendocrine carcinomas (NECs). The presence of neuroendocrine differentiation can be confirmed with the general neuroendocrine markers chromogranin A and synaptophysin, while the Ki-67 proliferation index is useful for assigning grade (see also Chapter 3). An approach to the distinction of carcinoma types is presented in Algorithm 13.1.

Well- and moderately differentiated adenocarcinomas are usually readily recognized based on gland/papillae formation and/or mucin production. However, the distinction between primary and metastatic adenocarcinomas in the GI tract may be challenging. Patterns of coordinate CK7 and CK20 expression (see Table 13.2), supplemented by more specific differentiation markers (see Table 13.3), are useful in assigning the site of origin in adenocarcinomas as well as the large polygonal cell tumors mentioned in the preceding paragraphs (Figure 13.2A–E). Overall, most adenocarcinomas are CK7+/CK20-; urothelial carcinomas, upper GI tract adenocarcinomas, and mucinous ovarian neoplasms are often CK7/CK20 "double positive;" and colon and Merkel cell carcinomas are typically

TABLE 13.1   Useful Immunostains in Poorly Differentiated Malignant Neoplasm

Tumor Type	Useful Immunostains
Carcinoma	Broad-spectrum keratins (eg, AE1/AE3, OSCAR, MAK-6, MNF116, CAM 5.2), EMA
Melanoma	S100, melan-A/MART-1, HMB-45, MiTF, SOX10
Hematolymphoid neoplasm	CD45/LCA; (CD43, CD79a, MUM1, ALK, CD30 if LCA-negative)
Sarcoma	CD34; MDM2/CDK4 (dedifferentiated liposarcoma); additional based on morphology
Mesothelioma	WT-1 (nuclear), calretinin, CK5/6, D2-40
Germ cell tumor	SALL4, PLAP
Neuroendocrine	Chromogranin, synaptophysin

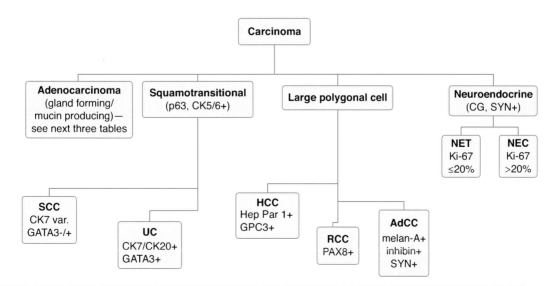

FIGURE 13.1   This essentially undifferentiated anal canal tumor has a syncytial quality and contains frequent tumor infiltrating lymphocytes (A). p63 is diffusely, strongly expressed, supporting a diagnosis of squamous cell carcinoma (B). CDX2 is not expressed (C). p16 demonstrates diffuse, strong expression, suggesting an etiologic association with high-risk human papillomavirus (see later discussion) (D). This squamous cell carcinoma variant has been referred to as lymphoepithelioma-like carcinoma.

ALGORITHM 13.1   Immunohistochemical Approach to Carcinoma Type.

Abbreviations: AdCC, adrenal cortical carcinoma; CG, chromogranin; GPC3, glypican-3; HCC, hepatocellular carcinoma; NEC, neuroendocrine carcinoma; NET, neuroendocrine tumor; RCC, renal cell carcinoma; SCC, squamous cell carcinoma; SYN, synaptophysin; UC, urothelial carcinoma.

TABLE 13.2 Broad Patterns of CK7/CK20 Coordinate Expression

Site	CK7	CK20
Prostate, HCC, RCC, AdCC	–	–
Lung (adenocarcinoma), breast, Müllerian, upper GI, pancreatobiliary	+	–
Bladder (UC), upper GI, pancreatobiliary, mucinous ovarian	+	+
Colon, Merkel cell carcinoma	–	+

CK7-/CK20+. In addition, as noted previously, HCC, RCC, and adrenal cortical carcinoma, along with prostate cancer, are CK7/CK20 "double negative." Transcription factors are increasingly utilized as differentiation markers for the site of origin as well. CDX2 is a key GI differentiation marker, and other emerging markers of intestinal differentiation include SATB2 and CDH17.

There is greater diversity of CK7/CK20 expression in GI tract adenocarcinomas than is generally appreciated. Esophageal adenocarcinomas are most commonly CK7+/CK20-; gastric cancers are fairly evenly split between the four combinations of CK7/CK20 expression; and small intestinal carcinomas are more commonly CK7/CK20 "double positive." Pancreatobiliary adenocarcinomas are nearly always strongly CK7-positive, and 40% to 60% are CK20-positive, though the positivity often manifests as only rare immunoreactive cells. Most colon cancers are CK7-/CK20+, though about 10% are "double positive" and 10% are "double negative." CK7+/CK20+ tumors are common in the rectum, where they comprise up to 25% of adenocarcinomas. CK20-negative tumors tend to be poorly differentiated and/or demonstrate high-level microsatellite instability (MSI-H). The frequencies of the various patterns of CK7/CK20 coordinate expression in the GI tract are presented in Table 13.4.

There is also variation in CDX2 expression in the GI tract. Most upper tubal gut adenocarcinomas are CDX2-positive (up to 80%), though expression tends to be weak to moderate and somewhat patchy (ie, heterogeneous) (Figure 13.3A–B). CDX2 is expressed by 20% of pancreatobiliary tract adenocarcinomas, again typically in a heterogeneous fashion. In colon cancer, expression is usually diffuse and strong (ie, homogeneous) (Figure 13.3C–D). As mentioned in the preceding paragraphs, MSI-H tumors are more likely to be CK20-negative than microsatellite stable (MSS) tumors, and CDX2 may also be weak to negative in this circumstance. Abnormal mismatch repair (MMR) protein IHC may be useful in this setting to secure the diagnosis (Figure 13.4).

In the ovary, metastatic GI adenocarcinoma must be distinguished from mucinous tumors of ovarian origin. Mucinous ovarian neoplasms are generally strongly CK7-positive, while CK20 and CDX2, when expressed, tend to be heterogeneous. This phenotype overlaps with that seen in the upper GI tract and pancreatobiliary adenocarcinomas. Loss of SMAD4 expression supports a pancreatic primary (seen in 50%), while PAX8 expression supports an ovarian primary (seen in 20%–40%). Primary disease tends to be unilateral and quite large (ie, greater than 13 cm), while metastatic disease is more likely to be bilateral.

APPROACH TO NEUROENDOCRINE NEOPLASMS

Neuroendocrine epithelial neoplasms are characterized by expression of general neuroendocrine markers and keratins, as well as production of peptide hormones and/or biogenic amines. In the current WHO classification,

TABLE 13.3 Immunohistochemistry to Assign Adenocarcinoma Site of Origin: Differentiation Markers

Marker	Specificity	Transcription Factor
CDX2	Enteric differentiation	Yes
TTF-1	Lung, thyroid	Yes
ER	Breast, Müllerian	Yes
PR	Breast, Müllerian	Yes
PAX8	Kidney, Müllerian, thyroid	Yes
p53	Serous carcinoma	Yes
WT-1 (nuclear)	Serous carcinoma, mesothelioma	Yes
GATA3	Breast (also urothelial carcinoma, paraganglioma/pheochromocytoma, choriocarcinoma, yolk sac tumor)	Yes
Napsin A	Lung, papillary renal cell carcinoma, Müllerian clear cell carcinoma	No
PSA	Prostate	No
PSAP	Prostate	No
Thyroglobulin	Thyroid	No
GCDFP-15	Breast	No
Mammaglobin	Breast	No

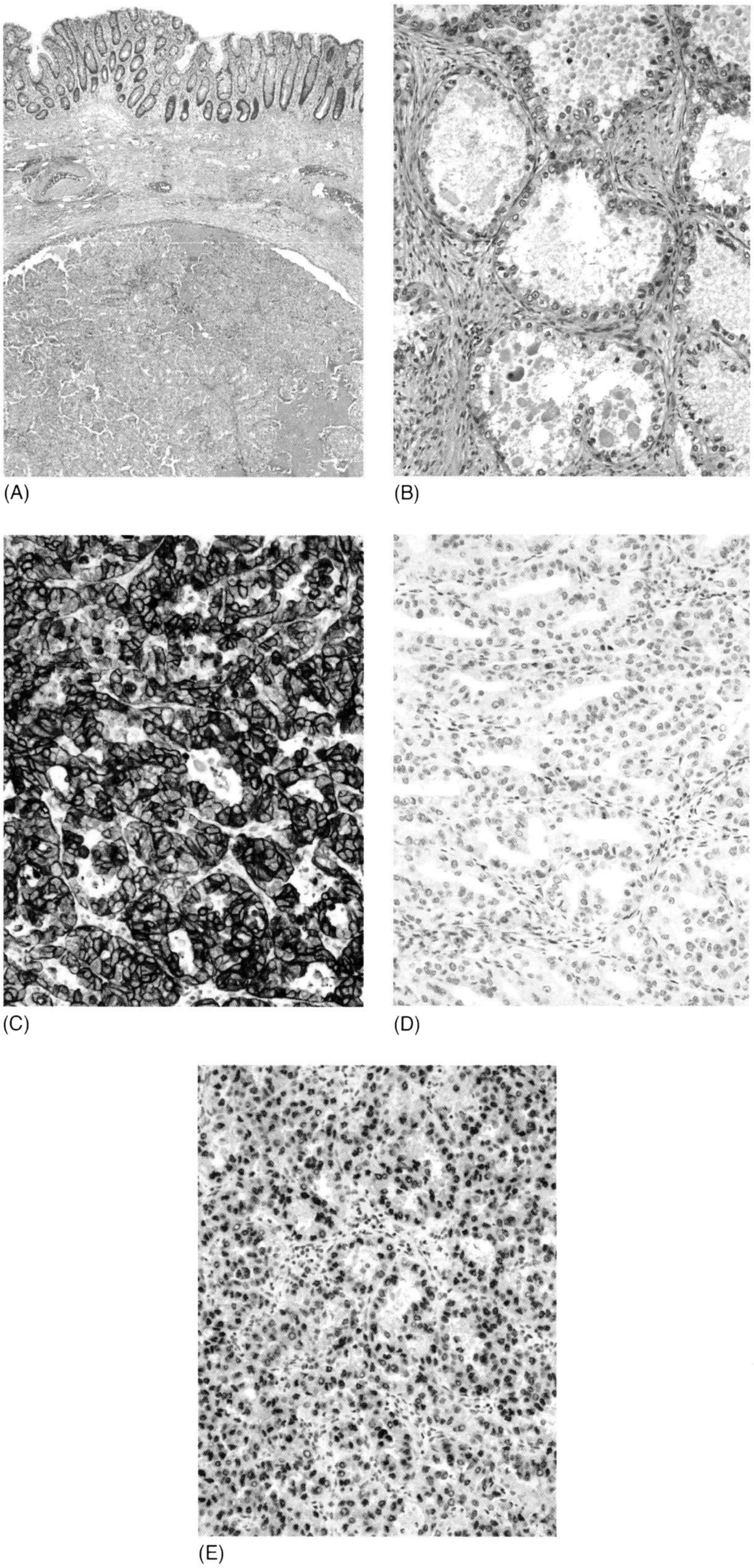

FIGURE 13.2   This tumor, which exhibits tubulopapillary architecture, involves the rectum in an "outside-in"/mural-based fashion, sparing the mucosa (A). At higher power the tumor is composed of clear to eosinophilic cells, which "hobnail" and are associated with flocculent eosinophilic secretions (B). The tumor expresses CK7 (C) but not CK20 (D); CDX2 and WT-1 were also negative, while the transcription factor PAX8 (E) is diffusely, strongly expressed. This morphology and immunophenotype support a diagnosis of involvement by Müllerian clear cell carcinoma and argue against a GI primary.

TABLE 13.4   CK7/CK20 Coordinate Expression in Gastroenteropancreatobiliary Adenocarcinomas

	CK7–/CK20–	CK7+/CK20–	CK7+/CK20+	CK7–/CK20+
Esophagus	8% (7/85)	74% (63/85)	15% (13/85)	2% (2/85)
Stomach	14% (5/37)	19% (7/37)	32% (27/37)	35% (13/37)
Small intestine	0% (0/24)	33% (8/24)	67% (16/24)	0% (0/24)
Pancreas	3% (1/36)	28% (10/36)	64% (23/36)	6% (2/36)
Biliary tree	7% (1/14)	50% (7/14)	43% (6/14)	0% (0/14)
Colon	10% (6/60)	0% (0/60)	8% (5/60)	82% (49/60)

Sources: Wang NP, Zee S, Zarbo RJ, Bacchi CE, Gown AM. Coordinate expression of cytokeratins 7 and 20 defined unique subsets of carcinomas. *Appl Immunohistochem.* 1995;3(2):99–107; Chu P, Wu E, Weiss LM. Cytokeratin 7 and cytokeratin 20 expression in epithelial neoplasms: a survey of 435 cases. *Mod Pathol.* 2000;13(9):962–72; Taniere P, Borghi-Scoazec G, Saurin JC, Lombard-Bohas C, Boulez J, Berger F, et al. Cytokeratin expression in adenocarcinomas of the esophagogastric junction: a comparative study of adenocarcinomas of the distal esophagus and of the proximal stomach. *Am J Surg Path.* 2002;26(9):1213–1221; Chen ZM, Wang HL. Alteration of cytokeratin 7 and cytokeratin 20 expression profile is uniquely associated with tumorigenesis of primary adenocarcinoma of the small intestine. *Am J Surg Path.* 2004;28(10):1352–1359.

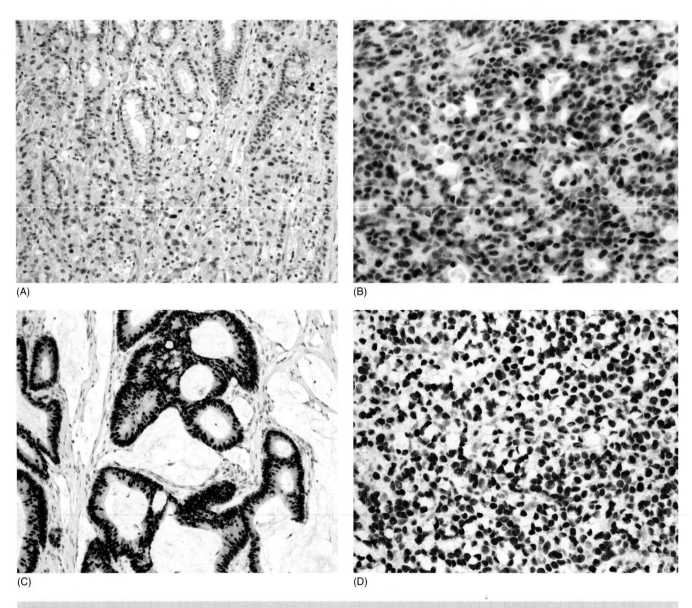

(A)

(B)

(C)

(D)

FIGURE 13.3   Weak, patchy CDX2 expression in a primary diffuse-type gastric cancer (A). Somewhat stronger, more diffuse CDX2 positivity in an esophageal adenocarcinoma (B). Diffuse, strong (homogeneous) CDX2 expression is seen in a colonic adenocarcinoma with mucinous features (C) and a rectal signet ring cell adenocarcinoma (D). Staining that is less than diffuse and strong is referred to as heterogeneous, which is more consistent with upper GI, pancreatobiliary, or mucinous ovarian origin.

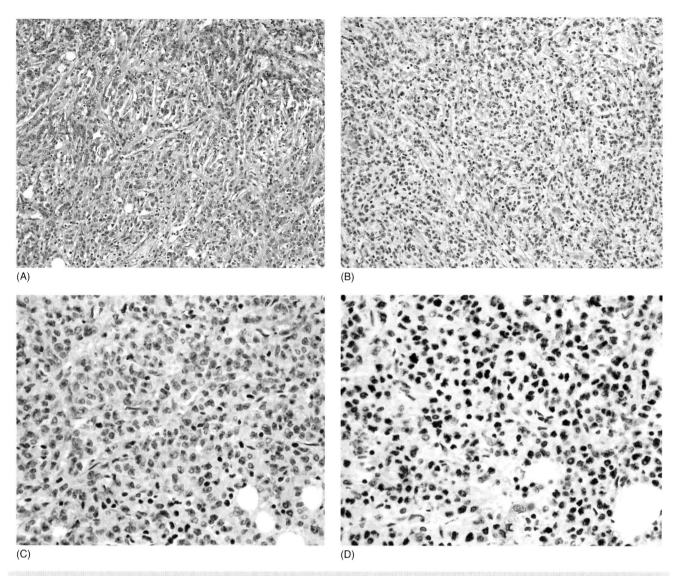

FIGURE 13.4   This tumor in the right colon is composed of cords of large cells with frequent tumor infiltrating lymphocytes (A). The tumor does not express CK7, CK20, or CDX2 (B) and was originally interpreted as a metastasis. MLH1 (C) and PMS2 are absent in tumor cells (note intact staining in intraepithelial lymphocytes), while MSH2 (D) and MSH6 expression are intact. Undifferentiated, microsatellite unstable colon cancer is referred to as medullary carcinoma, and it frequently deviates from the typical CK7-/CK20+/CDX2+ CRC immunophenotype.

well-differentiated examples are referred to as neuroendocrine tumors (NETs) and poorly differentiated examples as neuroendocrine carcinomas (NECs). IHC has several applications regarding the recognition and classification of neuroendocrine epithelial neoplasms (see also Chapter 3), specifically:

- Preferred status of chromogranin A and synaptophysin over other markers in determining the presence of neuroendocrine differentiation
- Importance of Ki-67 in accurately grading neoplasms
- Utility of IHC panels to assign the site of origin of neoplasms of unknown origin

In terms of differentiating primary GI NECs from metastases, 90% or greater of pulmonary small cell carcinomas express TTF-1, while CK20 is rarely expressed. Merkel cell carcinoma (primary NEC of the skin) has the inverse immunophenotype, and CK20 often shows a characteristic "dot-like" pattern of positivity. Extrapulmonary visceral small cell carcinomas often express TTF-1 as well (40%–50%), while CK20 is again rarely expressed. Aside from these two markers, IHC has a limited role in assigning the site of origin, with NECs frequently expressing multiple transcription factors regardless of the site of origin (so-called "transcription factor infidelity").

In contrast, NETs demonstrate fairly characteristic protein expression patterns, as determined by the site of origin (Figure 13.5). This is useful, as 10% to 20% of NETs (13% in a recent analysis of Surveillance, Epidemiology, and End Results data from 35,825 tumors) present as

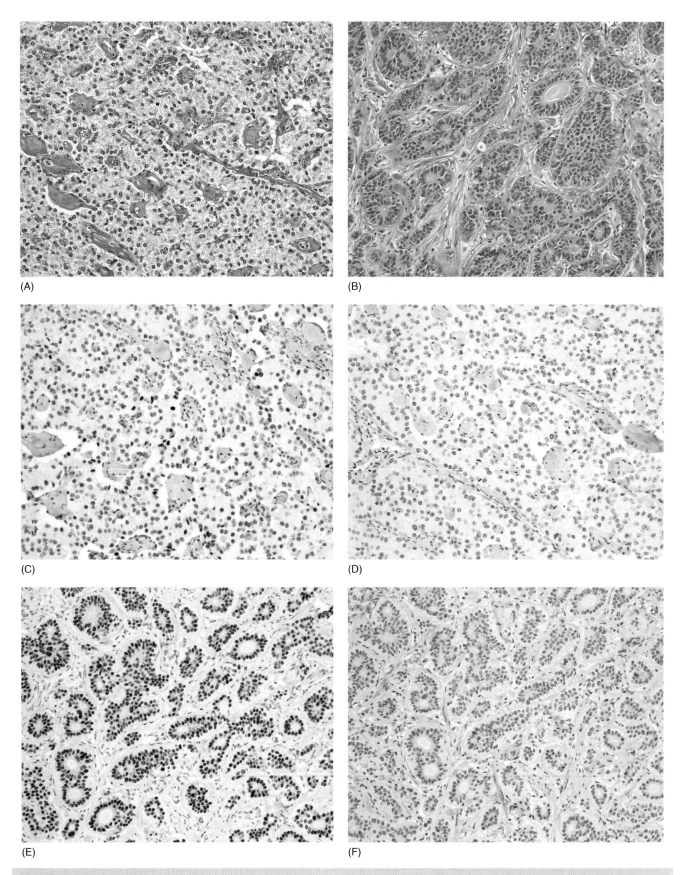

FIGURE 13.5 This patient presented with synchronous neuroendocrine tumors in the pancreas (A) and ileum (B). The pancreatic tumor expresses ISL1 (C) but not CDX2 (D). The ileal tumor demonstrates the inverse immunophenotype—CDX2 positivity (E) and ISL-1 negativity (F)—supporting the presence of two independent primaries rather than a metastasis.

metastases of unknown primary site, and medical and surgical therapeutic decision making is heavily influenced by the primary site. TTF-1 expression is specific for a bronchopulmonary origin, although the sensitivity of this marker is only 30% to 40%. Gastric tumors often demonstrate a "null" transcription factor immunophenotype. Pancreatic and duodenal tumors are not readily separable, with characteristic markers including polyclonal PAX8, monoclonal PAX6, Islet 1, PR, PDX1, and NESP55. Eighty to ninety percent of midgut (ie, jejunoileal and appendiceal) tumors express CDX2, which is typically diffuse and strong; about half express prostatic acid phosphatase (PrAP). Rectal tumors have an overlapping immunophenotype with pancreaticoduodenal tumors, with frequent expression of polyclonal PAX8, monoclonal PAX6, and Islet 1; they are distinguished by frequent expression of PrAP and SATB2. Of all these anatomic sites, jejunoileal (especially) and pancreatic tumors are most likely to present as metastases of occult origin.

Maxwell and colleagues recently evaluated the usefulness of an IHC panel in determining NET site of origin. Given the epidemiology of metastatic NETs of unknown origin, the approach in Algorithm 13.2 was developed to specifically assign a midgut or pancreatic origin. Their approach was 94% accurate in a set of 123 tumors (86 primary, 37 metastatic). Tumors are first stained with antibodies to CDX2, PAX6, and Islet 1. Tumors with strong CDX2 expression in the absence of PAX6 or Islet 1 expression are assigned a jejunoileal origin, while tumors with any PAX6 and/or Islet 1 expression are classified as pancreatic in origin (regardless of CDX2 expression, which is known to occur at varying intensity in 15% of pancreatic NETs). CDX2/PAX6/Islet 1 "triple negative" tumors further undergo testing for PR, PDX1, NESP55, and PrAP expression. PrAP-positive tumors are of suspected jejunoileal origin, while tumors expressing PR, PDX1, and/or NESP55 are of suspected pancreatic origin. Four percent of the tumors in this study were "pan-negative" for all 7 markers; interestingly, these tumors were all jejunoileal.

APPROACH TO HEMATOLYMPHOID TUMORS

The GI tract is the most common site for extranodal lymphomas (see also Chapter 4). At least half of these occur in the stomach, with diffuse large B-cell lymphoma (DLBCL) and extranodal marginal zone lymphoma of mucosa-associated lymphoid tissue (MALT lymphoma) occurring at similar frequencies. Throughout the entire GI tract, DLBCL accounts for almost half of all lymphomas, with MALT lymphoma next most frequent at 20%. The differential immunophenotype of the hematolymphoid neoplasms most commonly encountered in the tubal gut is summarized in Table 13.5.

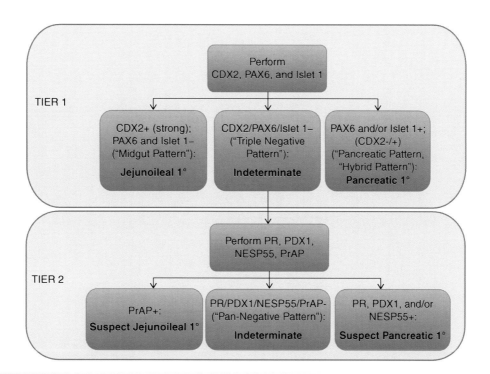

ALGORITHM 13.2 Approach to Assigning Site of Origin in a Neuroendocrine Tumor of Unknown Origin.

Abbreviation: PrAP, prostatic acid phosphatase.

Source: Maxwell JE, Sherman SK, Stashek KM, O'Dorisio TM, Bellizzi AM, Howe JR. A practical method to determine the site of unknown primary in metastatic neuroendocrine tumors. *Surgery*. 2014 Dec;156(6):1359–1366.

TABLE 13.5 Immunophenotype of GI Hematolymphoid Neoplasms

Tumor Type	Most Common Location(s)	CD20 CD79a PAX5	CD10 Bcl-6	CD5	CD43	Cyclin D1	Bcl-2	Other Useful Markers/Notes
Tumors Composed of Small Cells								
Extranodal marginal zone lymphoma of mucosa-associated lymphoid tissues (MALT lymphoma)	Stomach	+	–	–	Occ. (30%)	–	Var.	Kappa/lambda light chain restriction (occ.); keratins to highlight lymphoepithelial lesions
Mantle cell lymphoma	Colon, small intestine	+	–	+	+	+	+	Ki-67 proliferation index >40%–60% associated with poor prognosis; rarely CD5 or cyclin D1-
Follicular lymphoma	Small intestine	+	+	–	–	–	+	Higher-grade tumors more likely to show aberrant immunophenotype (eg, CD10- or CD43+)
Chronic lymphocytic leukemia/small lymphocytic lymphoma	Peri-tubal gut/mesenteric lymph nodes	+	–	+	+	–	+	CD23+
Enteropathy-associated T-cell lymphoma, Type II	Small intestine	–	–	–	+	–	+	CD3+, CD7+, CD4–, CD8+, CD56+
Tumors Composed of Intermediate/Large Cells								
Diffuse large B-cell lymphoma	Anywhere	+	CD10 Var. (30%–60%) Bcl-6+ (60%–90%)	Rare (10%)	Occ. (25%)	–	Var.	MUM1 (35%–65%)
Burkitt lymphoma	Ileocecal region	+	+	–	+	–	–	Ki-67 proliferation index approaches 100%; TdT-; c-Myc+; Bcl-2 occ. weak+
Plasmablastic lymphoma	Rectum	CD20/ PAX5- CD79a+ (50%–85%)	+	–	+	–	+	EBV EBER (60% –75%); CD45-; MUM1/ CD138/ CD38+; EMA/CD30 var.; association with HIV
Granulocytic sarcoma	Lymph nodes (in GI tract)	–	–	–	+	–	–	CD68/KIT/CD99/ CD34/TdT Var.
B-lymphoblastic lymphoma	Liver, lymph nodes (in GI tract)	CD20 Var. (25%–50%) CD79a+ PAX5+	CD10+ (60%) Bcl-6-	–	+ (67%)	–	+	TdT (95%), CD34/CD99+; CD13/CD33 Occ.
T-lymphoblastic lymphoma	Liver, lymph nodes (in GI tract)	CD20/ PAX5- CD79a Rare (5%–10%)	CD10 Var. Bcl-6-	Var.	+ (90%)	–	+	TdT (95%), CD3/CD99+; CD4/CD8 double+ (70%); CD1a (67%); CD34 Var.; CD13/ CD33 Occ.
Enteropathy-associated T-cell lymphoma, Type I	Small intestine	–	–	–	+	–	+	CD3+, CD7+, CD4–, CD8–/+; association with celiac disease

Key: Rare, ≤10%; Occ., >10% and <30%; Var. ≥30% and <60%.

Pathologists typically encounter GI tract lymphomas in two main morphologic contexts. The first is the presence of a small lymphocytic infiltrate, which may present diffusely, as an intraepithelial lymphocytosis, and/or as nodules. The second is an infiltrate of atypical intermediate to large cells. In the first instance, lymphomas composed of small lymphocytes must be distinguished from inflammatory conditions (eg, *Helicobacter pylori* gastritis in the stomach) and exuberant responses to physiologic antigenic stimulation (eg, Peyer's patches in the ileum). In the second instance, cancer should be strongly suspected, and lymphoma must be distinguished from other high-grade malignancies including carcinoma, melanoma, sarcoma, and germ cell neoplasm.

When contemplating the differential diagnosis of a lymphoma composed of small lymphocytes versus an inflammatory/reactive condition, morphologic features favoring lymphoma include effacement and infiltration of the normal architecture by the infiltrate, monotonous cytomorphology, and the inability to identify normal germinal centers (Figure 13.6A–B). Screening IHC may include the pan-B-cell marker CD20 and the pan-T-cell marker CD3 (Figure 13.6C–D). The vast majority of lymphomas in this setting are B-cell lymphomas,

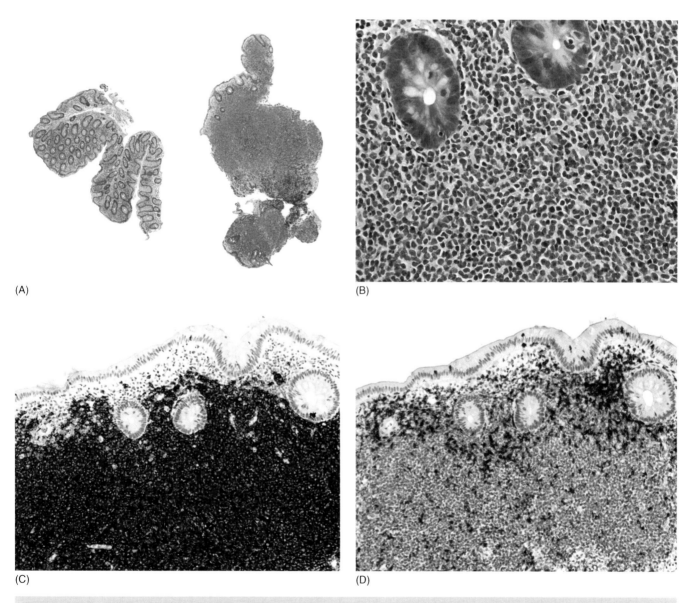

(A)

(B)

(C)

(D)

FIGURE 13.6 These mucosal biopsies were taken at screening colonoscopy, in which a few small polyps were found (A). The fragment on the right demonstrates architectural effacement by a diffuse, small-blue-cell process. At higher power, a monotonous infiltrate of small lymphocytes with somewhat irregular nuclear contours is evident (B). CD20 is diffusely, strongly expressed (C), while CD3 highlights scattered T-cells (D), supporting a diagnosis of a low-grade B-cell lymphoma. This tumor was further shown to coexpress CD5 and cyclin D1 and was thus interpreted as mantle cell lymphoma.

with the CD20 and CD3 staining revealing "too many small B-lymphocytes." CD10 and BCL6 may be useful to highlight germinal center cells, while CD21, CD23, or CD35 may be applied to identify follicular dendritic meshworks.

The principal considerations when diagnosing a lymphoma composed of small lymphocytes in the GI tract include MALT lymphoma, mantle cell lymphoma (MCL), follicular lymphoma (FL), and chronic lymphocytic leukemia/small lymphocytic lymphoma (CLL/SLL) (see also Chapter 4). Useful markers in this context, in addition to those already mentioned, include the pan-B-cell markers CD79a and PAX5 (especially in the setting of rituximab-treated tumors, in which CD20 expression is often abolished), CD5 (expressed by MCL and CLL/SLL), CD43 (aberrantly coexpressed by MCL, CLL, and up to 30% of MALT lymphomas), and cyclin D1 (essentially diagnostic of MCL). Although immunostains for Bcl-2 are often applied, this marker is most useful in the setting of a nodular lymphoid proliferation, where expression favors FL over reactive follicular hyperplasia. Other markers may also be useful in select settings. For example, kappa or lambda light chain restriction (detectable by IHC or in situ hybridization) is occasionally seen in MALT lymphomas with plasmacytic differentiation, and keratin staining may be useful to highlight lymphoepithelial lesions in MALT lymphoma. In MCL, Ki-67 IHC may be applied, as higher proliferation indices appear prognostically adverse. CD23 coexpression may be helpful to secure a diagnosis of CLL/SLL. The details of the less commonly encountered immunohistochemical diagnosis of T-cell lymphomas in the GI tract are discussed in Chapter 4, but summarized in Table 13.5.

When faced with an intermediate to large cell process, the first order of business is to distinguish hematolymphoid malignancies from other high-grade tumors. As previously discussed in the approach to epithelial neoplasms section, important screening markers include LCA, a broad-spectrum keratin, and S100. Some high-grade lymphomas are typically LCA-negative (eg, plasmablastic lymphoma), and when faced with an LCA/keratin/S100-negative tumor, application of additional pan-B-cell (PAX5, CD79a), T-cell (CD3), and plasmacytic markers (CD38, CD138, MUM1) should be considered. As a note of caution, CD138 (also known as syndecan-1) is frequently expressed by carcinomas.

As noted in the preceding paragraphs, most hematolymphoid neoplasms in the GI tract composed of intermediate to large cells are DLBCLs. Additional diagnostic considerations include Burkitt lymphoma (BL), plasmablastic lymphoma, granulocytic sarcoma, B- and T-lymphoblastic lymphoma, and, rarely, type I EATL. In DLBCL, IHC may be applied to determine whether a tumor is of germinal center or activated-B-cell type, as the latter designation is prognostically adverse. In this setting,

useful markers include the germinal center markers CD10 and BCL6, and the activated B-cell marker MUM1, among others.

Burkitt lymphoma is characterized by monomorphous cytomorphology, a germinal center phenotype (CD10/BCL6+), and a Ki-67 proliferation index approaching 100% (Figure 13.7). Diffuse, strong nuclear expression of c-Myc can serve as an IHC surrogate of a MYC translocation. TdT-negativity distinguishes this tumor from lymphoblastic lymphoma, and Bcl-2 is usually not expressed (and if expressed should not be more than weakly positive).

Plasmablastic lymphoma has an association with human immunodeficiency virus. Most cases are LCA, CD20, and PAX5-negative, though CD79a is usually expressed, as are markers of plasmacytic differentiation. In most cases (60% to 75%) Epstein–Barr virus (EBV)-encoded RNA (EBER) expression can be detected by in situ hybridization. The most consistent markers of granulocytic sarcoma include LCA and CD43, with CD68, KIT, CD99, CD34, and TdT variably expressed. Lymphoblastic lymphomas nearly always express TdT, with CD99 also consistently expressed, and CD34 more often expressed in B-lymphoblastic lymphoma than T-lymphoblastic lymphoma. CD79a and PAX5 are often positive in B-lymphoblastic lymphoma, while T-lymphoblastic lymphoma is usually CD3-positive, often CD4/CD8-"double positive," and CD1a-positive.

Post-transplant lymphoproliferative disorders also involve the GI tract, as well as lymph nodes, lungs, liver, or the allograft itself (Figure 13.8). Most cases are EBV-driven, and thus EBER-positive. The morphologic spectrum includes polymorphic and monomorphic disorders, generally of B-cells. Most monomorphic examples resemble DLBCL.

APPROACH TO MESENCHYMAL TUMORS

Mesenchymal tumors involve the tubal gut more than any other visceral organ. Gastrointestinal stromal tumor (GIST) is recognized as the most common mesenchymal tumor of the GI tract and should always be considered in the differential of both spindle cell and epithelioid tumors. At the turn of the century, with the discovery of KIT and PDGFRA activating mutations, availability of KIT IHC, and recognition of the efficacy of imatinib, awareness of this entity increased rapidly. That being said, there are a number of non-GIST GI mesenchymal tumors, several of which demonstrate significant morphologic and immunophenotypic overlap with GIST (see also Chapter 5). The differential immunophenotype of GI mesenchymal tumors is summarized in Table 13.6, and some specific examples by site are discussed directly below.

In the esophagus, leiomyomas are the most common mesenchymal tumor, where they tend to arise in the

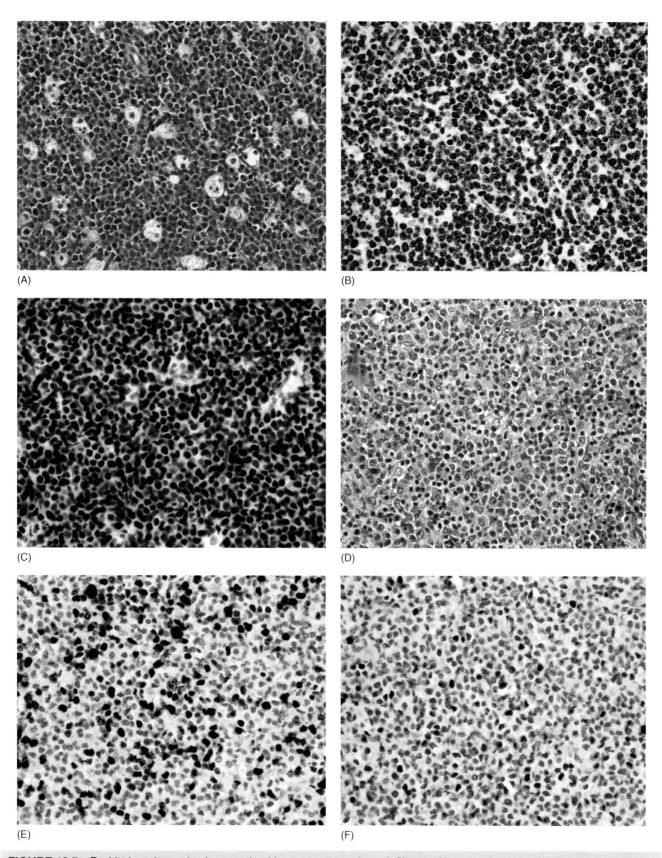

FIGURE 13.7 Burkitt lymphoma is characterized by a monomorphous infiltrate of intermediate-sized cells with a "starry sky" appearance due to admixed tingible-body macrophages (A). The Ki-67 proliferation index approaches 100% (B) in these tumors, and there is diffuse, strong c-Myc expression, in keeping with *MYC* activation (C). In contrast, diffuse large B-cell lymphoma demonstrates greater variation in cell size/shape and nuclear contours (D), more variable Ki-67 proliferation indices, in this case 40% to 50% (E), and only patchy staining for c-Myc (F).

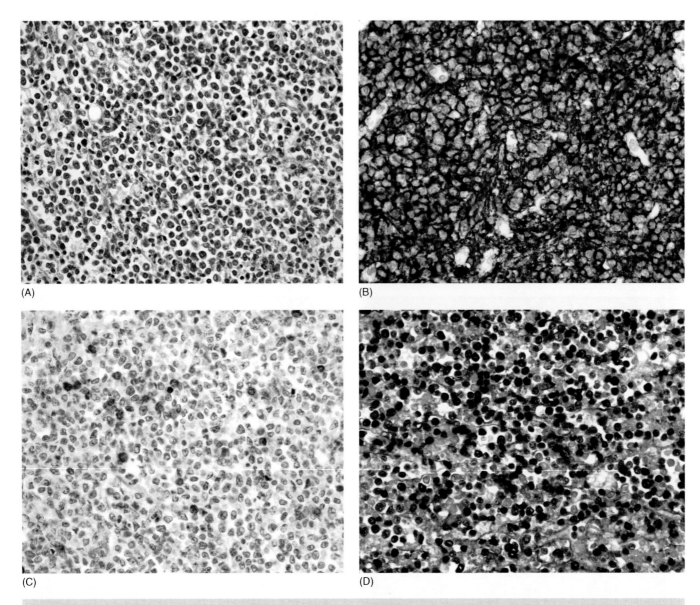

FIGURE 13.8 This patient was 4 months status post kidney transplant and presented with dysphagia. A biopsy demonstrates sheets of large cells (A), which express CD20 (B) but not CD3 (C). In situ hybridization for EBV-encoded RNA (EBER) is strongly positive (D). This monomorphic PTLD demonstrates diffuse large B-cell lymphoma histology. Of note, this EBV-negative recipient received a kidney from an EBV-positive donor.

muscularis propria (as opposed to the colon, where they typically involve the muscularis mucosae). Expression of the muscle markers SMA and desmin is the rule (Figure 13.9A–B). In the esophagus, in particular around the gastroesophageal junction, leiomyomas frequently contain large numbers of KIT-positive non-neoplastic mast cells and interstitial cells of Cajal (the latter are also DOG1-positive), which occasionally leads to a misdiagnosis of GIST (Figure 13.9C). Attention to the distinctive cytomorphology of leiomyoma should guard against this diagnostic error, and, of note, desmin is only exceptionally expressed by GIST.

The esophagus is also the most common site in the tubal GI tract for granular cell tumors. They express S100

and MiTF (though not HMB-45 and only rarely melan-A). The tumor's granular cytoplasm is attributable to massive numbers of lysosomes, and thus CD68 is also expressed.

The most common mesenchymal tumor in the stomach is GIST. Gastrointestinal stromal tumors may demonstrate spindle cell (70% overall), epithelioid (20% overall; relatively overrepresented in the stomach), or mixed spindle cell/epithelioid cytomorphology (10% overall). KIT is expressed by over 90% of GISTs and is nearly always positive in those with spindle cell morphology (Figure 13.10). Tumors that stain weakly for KIT, or are KIT-negative, usually have *PDGFRA* mutations and tend to have epithelioid cytomorphology (Figure 13.11). Up to half of KIT-negative GISTs express the calcium-activated chloride

TABLE 13.6   Immunophenotype of GI Mesenchymal Tumors

Tumor type	Most Common Location(s)	KIT	DOG1	CD34	SMA	Desmin	S100	Other Useful Markers
Relatively Common								
GIST (total)		+ (92%)	+ (95%)	+ (85%)	Occ. (20%)	Rare (5%)	Rare (<1%)	
GIST, spindle cell type	Stomach > small intestine > colon > other	+ (98%)	+ (97%)	+ (93%)	Occ. (20%)	Rare (2%)	Rare (<1%)	
GIST, epithelioid type	Stomach > other sites	+ (86%)	+ (92%)	+ (70%)	Occ. (20%)	Rare (10%)	Rare (<1%)	SDHB (deficient in a subset)
Leiomyoma	Esophagus (muscularis propria) > colon (muscularis mucosae)	–	–	–	+	+	–	
Mucosal perineurioma	Colon (left)	–	–	Occ.	–	–	–	EMA+ (typically weak); claudin-1 (50%)
Mucosal Schwann cell hamartoma	Colon (left)	–	–	–	–	–	+	
Less Common		**KIT**	**DOG1**	**CD34**	**SMA**	**Desmin**	**S100**	
Granular cell tumor	Esophagus	–	–	–	–	–	+	CD68+; MiTF+
Schwannoma	Stomach (corpus) > colon	–	–	Rare (10%)	–	–	+	GFAP (var.)
Plexiform fibromyxoma	Stomach (antrum)	–	–	–	+	Var. (40%)	–	
Glomus tumor	Stomach (antrum)	–	–	Occ. (20%)	+	–	–	
Inflammatory fibroid polyp	Small intestine > stomach (antrum)	–	–	+ (85%)	Occ. (20%)	Rare (5%)	–	PDGFRA+
Kaposi sarcoma	Upper > lower GI tract	Var.	–	+	Var.	–	–	HHV8+; CD31+; ERG+
Desmoid-type fibromatosis	Mesentery	Var.	–	Rare	Var.	–	–	Nuclear β-catenin (70%)
Rare		**KIT**	**DOG1**	**CD34**	**SMA**	**Desmin**	**S100**	
Gastroblastoma	Stomach	Occ. (20%)*	–	–	–	–	–	Keratins+ (epithelial component); CD10+ (stromal component)
Synovial sarcoma	Stomach	–	10%	–	Occ. (20%)	–	Occ. (30%)	Keratins/EMA+; TLE1+; t(X;18) FISH
Follicular dendritic cell sarcoma	Stomach, colon	–	–	–	–	–	Occ.	CD35+; CD21+; CD23 var.; EMA var.
Clear cell sarcoma-like tumor of the GI tract	Small intestine > stomach/colon	–	–	–	–	–	+	SOX10+; other melanocytic markers-; synaptophysin (50%); *EWSR1* FISH
PEComa	Colon	Rare	Rare	–	Var.	Var.	Occ. (20%, focal)	HMB-45+ more often than melan-A/ tyrosinase/ MiTF/TFE3
Inflammatory myofibroblastic tumor	Colon, small intestine	–	–	Rare	+ (90%)	+ (60%)	–	ALK (50%); MDM2 Occ.; keratins (30%, focal)
Leiomyosarcoma	Colon > small intestine/ esophagus	–	–	Occ.	+	+ (75%)	–	Keratins (30%–40%)

Abbreviation: GIST, gastrointestinal stromal tumor.
Key: * in the epithelial component; Rare, ≤10%; Occ., >10% and <30%; Var. ≥30% and <60%.

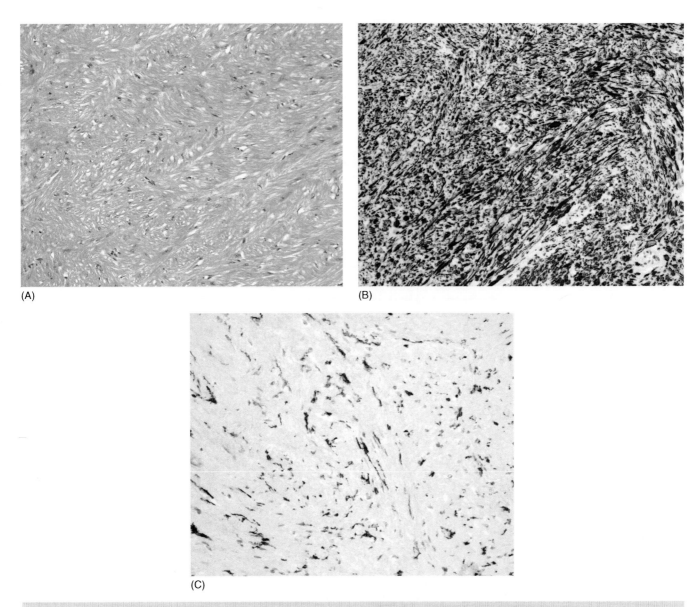

FIGURE 13.9 Leiomyomas are characterized by fascicles of brightly eosinophilic spindle cells with sharp cell borders (A), and consistently express smooth muscle markers including desmin (B). Tumors around the gastroesophageal junction typically contain large numbers of KIT-staining mast cells and interstitial cells of Cajal, which occasionally leads to an incorrect interpretation of gastrointestinal stromal tumor (C).

channel DOG1 (also known as ANO1). This marker is highly specific for GIST among spindle cells tumors, with infrequent and rare positivity reported in synovial sarcoma and leiomyosarcoma, respectively. CD34 is also frequently positive in GIST, especially in spindle cell tumors, although it is also expressed by vascular and some fibroblastic tumors.

Eighty percent of GISTs possess *KIT*-activating mutations, and another 5% demonstrate *PDGFRA*-activating mutations. The remaining 15% are referred to as "wild-type." These wild-type tumors show strong KIT expression immunophenotypically. Among the wild-type tumors is a group characterized by female predominance, gastric location, epithelioid cytomorphology, and a distinctive

multinodular or plexiform growth pattern, which demonstrate functional deficiency of the Krebs cycle enzyme succinate dehydrogenase (SDH) (Figure 13.12). SDH-deficient GISTs occur in four main clinical settings:

- 85% of pediatric GISTs
- Carney triad (ie, paraganglioma, pulmonary chondroma, GIST)
- Carney–Stratakis syndrome (ie, paraganglioma–GIST dyad)
- 7.5% of nonsyndromic adult gastric GISTs

Recognition is important because these tumors frequently metastasize (irrespective of traditional risk assessment based on location, tumor size, and mitotic rate), do not respond

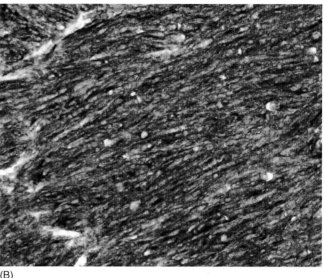

(A)

(B)

FIGURE 13.10 Classic spindle cell GISTs are disposed as fascicles of palely eosinophilic cells with indistinct cell borders; gastric examples often exhibit perinuclear vacuoles (A). KIT is nearly always expressed by spindle cell GISTs (B).

to imatinib, and may have syndromic associations. SDH is composed of four protein subunits (SDHA, SDHB, SDHC, SDHD). Carney–Stratakis syndrome is autosomal dominant, due to an SDH subunit germline mutation; in the other three settings, the basis of SDH-deficiency has been linked to SDHC promoter methylation. While SDH is normally ubiquitously expressed, loss of SDHB expression by IHC can be used to identify SDH-deficient tumors (Figure 13.12C).

In the stomach, the closest histologic mimic of GIST is schwannoma. As elsewhere, schwannomas demonstrate diffuse, strong S100 expression, while GFAP is variably expressed. Other gastric mesenchymal tumors in the differential diagnosis with GIST include plexiform fibromyxoma and glomus tumor (see also Chapter 5). Plexiform fibromyxoma demonstrates myofibroblastic differentiation, and, as such, expresses SMA, while desmin is variably expressed. Glomus tumors demonstrate strong SMA expression, useful in securing the diagnosis. Both of these tumors are KIT negative, as are schwannomas.

Inflammatory fibroid polyps are likely to be encountered in the small intestine as well as the gastric antrum. Investigators have recently identified *PDGFRA*-activating

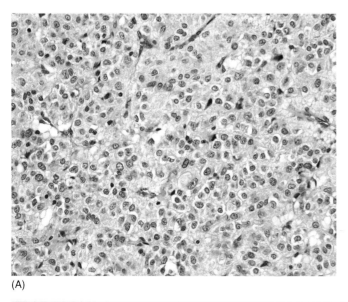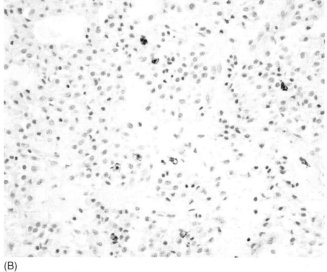

(A)

(B)

FIGURE 13.11 Five percent of GISTs possess *PDGFRA* activating mutations. These tumors tend to be epithelioid (A), and are often KIT-negative or weakly positive (note KIT staining in mast cells) (B).

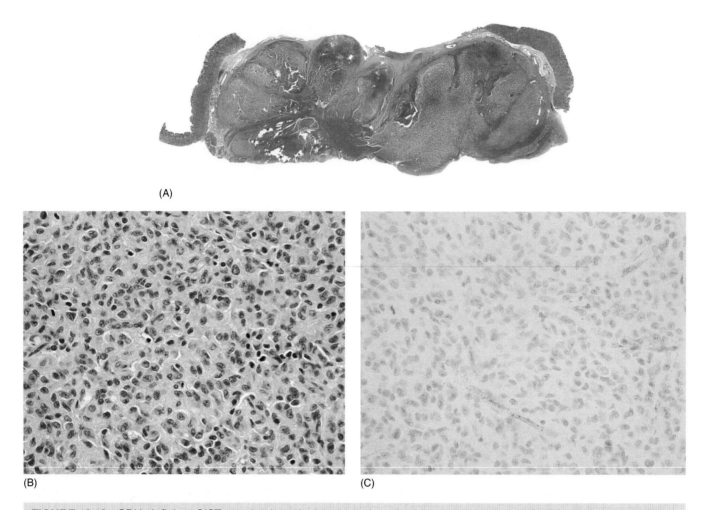

(A)

(B)   (C)

FIGURE 13.12 SDH-deficient GISTs predominate in the stomach and exhibit a distinctive plexiform/multinodular growth pattern (A) and epithelioid morphology (B). SDH-deficiency is confirmed with an SDHB immunostain (note intact staining in endothelium) (C).

mutations in this tumor, supporting its neoplastic nature. Lesional cells are CD34-positive in 85% of cases, while SMA is occasionally expressed and desmin is rarely expressed. If available, PDGFRA IHC is positive, though it is nonspecific (also positive in GISTs, especially *PDGFRA*-mutant tumors, and some sarcomas and carcinomas).

Kaposi sarcoma, when involving the tubal gut, predominates in the small and large intestine. These tumors express HHV8, as well as vascular endothelial markers including CD31, CD34, and ERG. Variable KIT staining has been described, and is especially frequent with antigen retrieval, in which case the lesion is especially apt to be mistaken for GIST (Figure 13.13).

Desmoid fibromatosis may arise intra-abdominally (ie, mesentery or pelvis), within the abdominal wall, or extra-abdominally (in somatic soft tissues at any site). Tumors may arise sporadically (85% of which show *CTNNB1* activating mutations) or in association with familial adenomatous polyposis and related syndromes (due to *APC* mutations). The tumors show fibroblastic/myofibroblastic

differentiation and, as such, demonstrate variable SMA positivity. Seventy percent of desmoid tumors show β-catenin nuclear accumulation, as a consequence of either *CTNNB1* or *APC* mutations (Figure 13.14). Similar to Kaposi sarcoma, variable KIT staining has been described in desmoid-type fibromatosis.

In the colon, mucosal perineurioma and mucosal Schwann cell hamartoma are small, benign spindle cell lesions of essentially no clinical significance. Their recognition is important in that the diagnostically unaware may mistake them for ganglioneuroma or neurofibroma, lesions associated with MEN2B and NF1, respectively. Mucosal perineuriomas express EMA (albeit usually quite weakly) (Figure 13.15) and claudin-1 (in 50%); CD34 is occasionally expressed. Mucosal Schwann cell hamartomas strongly and diffusely express S100, in keeping with the presence of schwannian differentiation (Figure 13.16).

There are several other rare mesenchymal tumors that may enter into the morphologic and immunophenotypic differential diagnosis in the GI tract. Gastroblastoma is

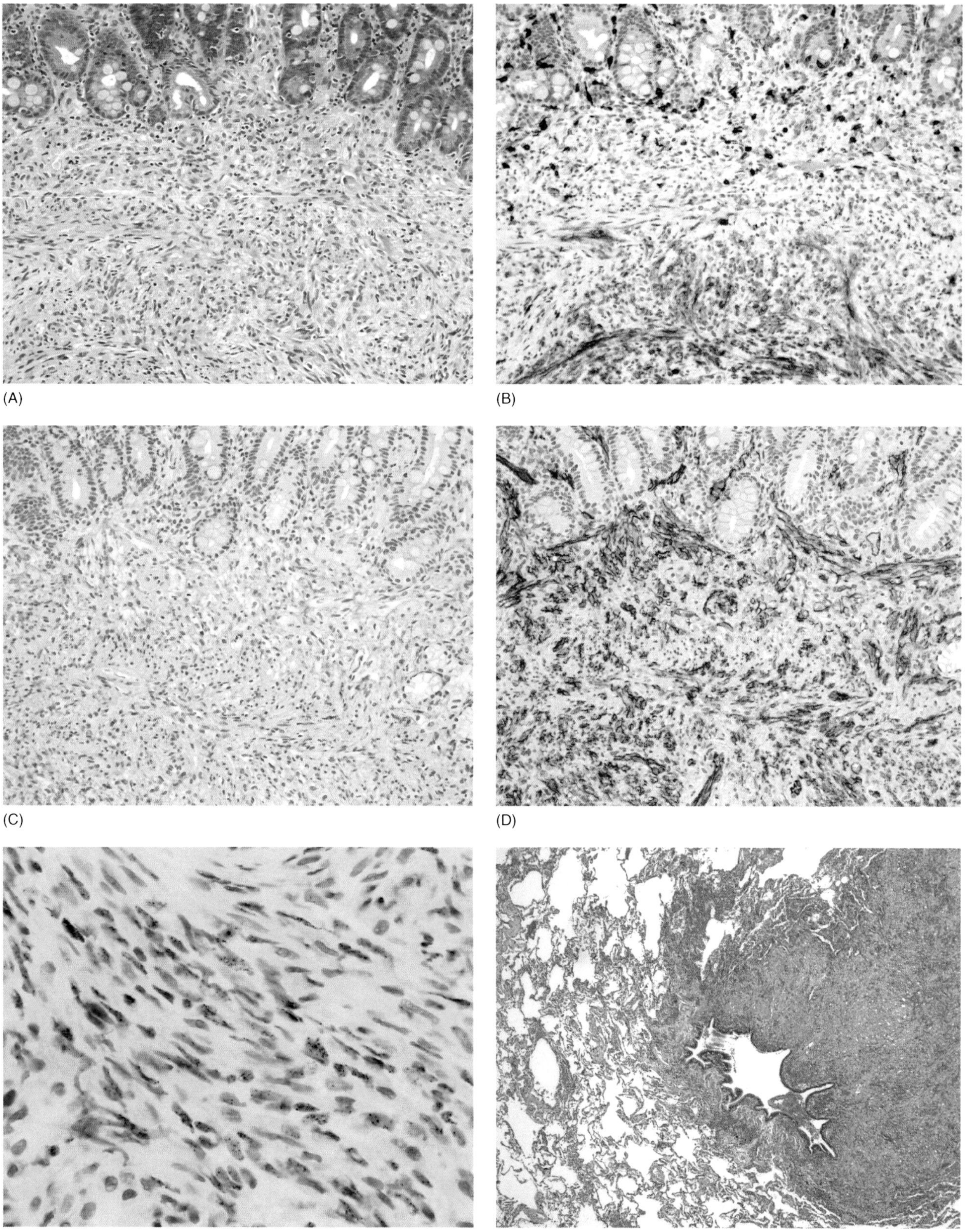

FIGURE 13.13   This bland spindle cell lesion in the duodenum obscures the muscularis mucosae and infiltrates the lamina propria; note also the extravasated erythrocytes (A). Based on the presence of KIT staining, this lesion was originally interpreted as a GIST (B), but DOG1 staining was negative (C). CD31 staining confirms the endothelial nature of this lesion (D), and punctate nuclear HHV8 staining supports the diagnosis of KS (E). A week later, a wedge resection from the lung demonstrated similar lesions (F). Based on the diagnosis of KS, the patient was tested and found to have HIV.

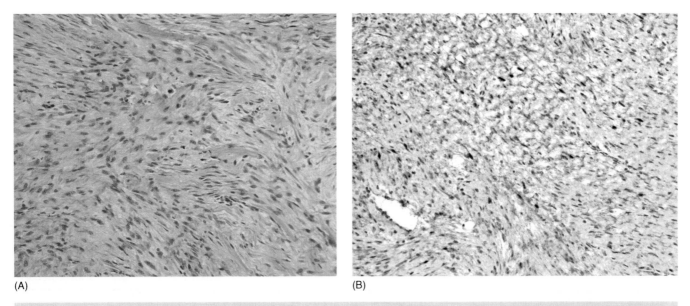

(A)   (B)

FIGURE 13.14 Desmoid tumors are bland spindle cell lesions with collagenous stroma (A); β-catenin nuclear accumulation is detected in 70% of desmoids, distinguishing this tumor from histologic mimics (B).

a recently described biphasic gastric tumor composed of epithelial and stromal elements. The epithelial component expresses keratins but not EMA, while the spindle cell component is CD10-positive. KIT and DOG1-positivity have been described, representing a diagnostic pitfall. Synovial sarcoma is gastroblastoma's closest histologic mimic, though examples in the stomach are quite rare and typically monophasic. In addition to patchy EMA and keratin expression, synovial sarcomas are characterized by diffuse, strong TLE1 expression and *SS18* rearrangement by fluorescence in situ hybridization (FISH).

Follicular dendritic cell sarcoma presents as a monomorphous proliferation of plump spindle cells with moderate amounts of eosinophilic cytoplasm. Tumor cells demonstrate storiform architecture and are arranged syncytially. Frequent tumor-infiltrating lymphocytes are a typical feature. Tumors express markers of follicular dendritic cells including CD35 and CD21, while CD23 is variably expressed.

Clear cell sarcoma-like tumor of the GI tract has recently been separated from conventional clear cell sarcoma. Compared to clear cell sarcoma of tendons and

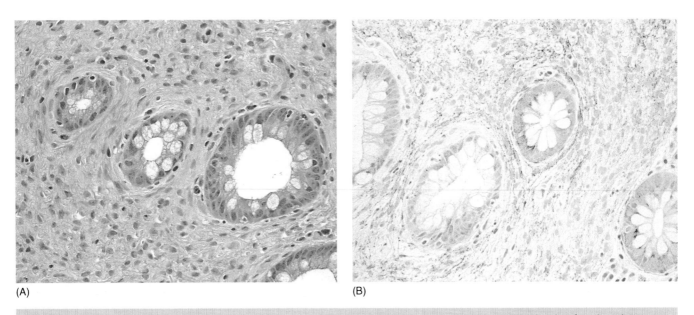

(A)   (B)

FIGURE 13.15 The most consistent marker of mucosal perineurioma (A) is EMA, though expression is often less intense than this (B).

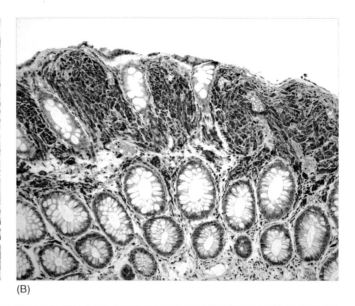

(A)   (B)

FIGURE 13.16 Mucosal Schwann cell hamartomas (A) stain strongly with S100, supporting the schwannian nature of this lesion (B).

aponeuroses, the GI variant typically exhibits sheet-like rather than nested architecture, contains osteoclast-like rather than wreath-like giant cells, and, beyond S100 and SOX10, it does not express more specific melanocytic markers (ie, melan-A, HMB-45, MiTF, tyrosinase); both tumor types contain *EWSR1* rearrangements. Compared to the much more common metastatic melanoma, clear cell sarcoma exhibits relative monomorphism and lacks macronucleoli.

Perivascular epithelioid cell tumor (PEComa) (see also Chapter 5) typically presents as a nested proliferation of epithelioid cells with abundant granular eosinophilic or clear cytoplasm. It demonstrates myomelanocytic differentiation, and thus is characteristically positive for HMB-45, SMA, and calponin. S100 is less likely to be positive than the more specific melanocytic markers. About 10% contain a *TFE3* gene fusion, resulting in strong TFE3 expression. These tumors also occasionally mark with KIT, which may lead to diagnostic confusion, but they do not mark with DOG1.

Inflammatory myofibroblastic tumor is typically composed of long fascicles of spindle cells with a prominent lymphoplasmacytic inflammatory infiltrate. The most characteristic immunohistochemical feature is expression of ALK, corresponding to *ALK* gene rearrangement, though this is seen in only 50% of tumors. Otherwise, tumors usually express SMA (90%) and often express desmin (60%). MDM2 is occasionally expressed, which may lead to confusion with dedifferentiated liposarcoma, though the latter is associated with greater cytologic atypia. Leiomyosarcoma (Figure 13.17) is distinctly uncommon in the GI tract, and most tumors historically

classified as leiomyosarcoma in the tubal gut instead represent GIST. Leiomyosarcomas express SMA and often express desmin. Keratin and EMA expression are seen in 30% to 40%, which represents a diagnostic pitfall.

KIT Immunohistochemistry

Although KIT expression is often considered synonymous with the diagnosis of GIST, it is expressed by several normal cell types, including mast cells, interstitial cells of Cajal, myeloid blasts, germ cells, and melanocytes, as well as several other tumors, especially adenoid cystic carcinoma, myeloid leukemia, seminoma, and some melanomas (25%–35% of metastases; more often in primary tumors) (Figure 13.18; see also Chapter 5). The range of KIT expression is narrow in soft tissue tumors, and it is not expressed by smooth muscle tumors. The list of occasionally KIT-expressing soft tissue tumors includes extraskeletal myxoid chondrosarcoma, Ewing sarcoma/primitive peripheral neuroectodermal tumors, melanotic schwannoma, low-grade fibromyxoid sarcoma, perineurioma, and angiosarcoma.

KIT is extremely sensitive to heat-induced antigen retrieval, and over-retrieval can either decrease expected positive staining or, more commonly, result in high-background staining leading to nonspecific positivity. Rates of KIT-positivity in desmoid fibromatosis have ranged from 0 to 100%, due to variations in IHC experimental conditions. Lucas and colleagues, comparing the performance of two commercially available antibodies at three separate dilutions with and without antigen retrieval, were able to recapitulate this broad range of positivity. While at low titers, both antibodies marked the majority

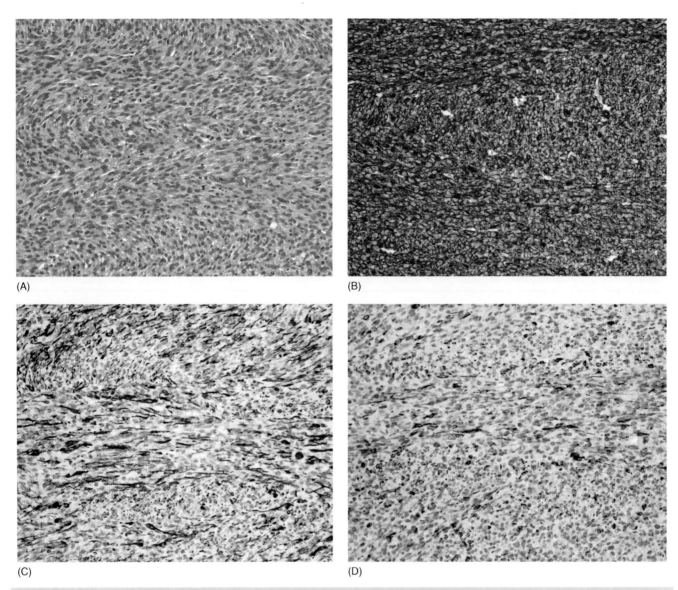

FIGURE 13.17 Leiomyosarcomas are typically overtly malignant fascicular spindle cell tumors with eosinophilic cytoplasm and brisk mitotic activity (A); the presence of smooth muscle differentiation is supported by detection of SMA (B) and desmin expression (C). Keratin is expressed by 30% to 40% of leiomyosarcomas, which occasionally leads to an incorrect diagnosis of sarcomatoid carcinoma (D).

of desmoids (with accompanying nonspecific stromal staining), at higher titers most tumors were negative. The best results were achieved with the rabbit polyclonal antibody A4502 *without* antigen retrieval. Similarly, Parfitt and colleagues, examining GI Kaposi sarcomas, recently reported KIT positivity in 4 of 12 (33%) tumors without and 10 of 12 (83%) with antigen retrieval. Like all immunostains deployed in the clinical laboratory, KIT should be optimized to achieve a high "signal-to-noise ratio," without excessive background staining (Figure 13.19), and antigen retrieval is not required as a matter of course. KIT expression, though characteristic, is not diagnostic of GIST in spindle cell tumors of the GI tract. As discussed above, DOG1 ICH may be complementary in challenging cases.

ORGAN- AND SITUATION-SPECIFIC APPLICATIONS OF IMMUNOHISTOCHEMISTRY IN GI TRACT NEOPLASIA

p53 and Barrett's-Associated Dysplasia and Carcinoma

Esophageal adenocarcinoma arises from Barrett's esophagus (BE) through a metaplasia→dysplasia→carcinoma sequence (see also Chapter 6). Although the risk of developing adenocarcinoma is only on the order of 0.25% per year, patients are typically entered into an endoscopic surveillance program. The risk of progression and the intensity of therapeutic intervention increases significantly given the detection of dysplasia. BE patients with

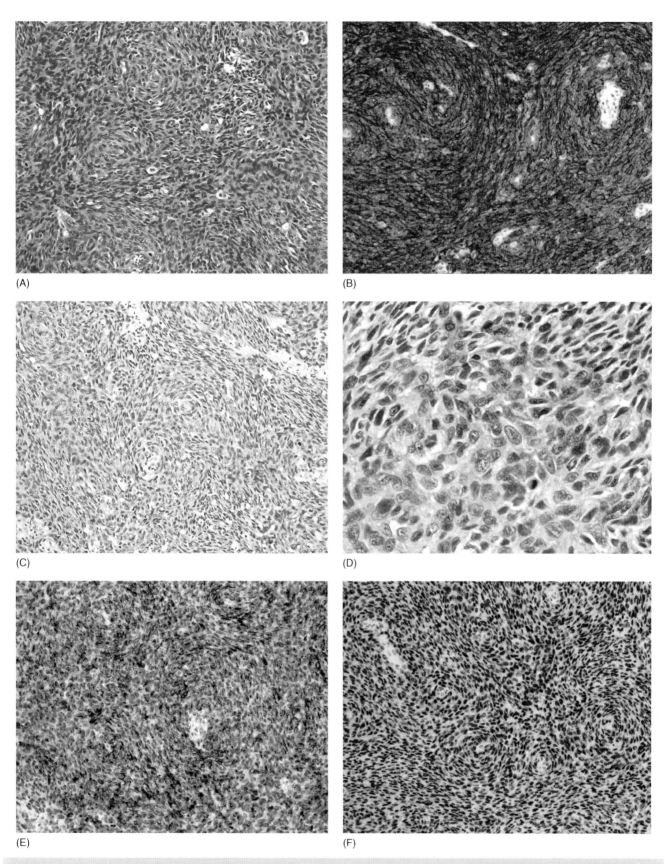

FIGURE 13.18   This ileal spindle cell tumor with perivascular accentuation (A) was originally interpreted as a GIST based on diffuse, strong KIT expression (B). As the morphology was unusual for a spindle cell GIST, additional stains were ordered including S100 (C), which at high power (D) demonstrated focal convincing staining. This result prompted staining for other melanoma markers including HMB-45 (E) and MiTF (F). The patient was subsequently diagnosed with a right forearm melanoma. KIT is not uncommonly expressed by melanoma, presenting a diagnostic pitfall.

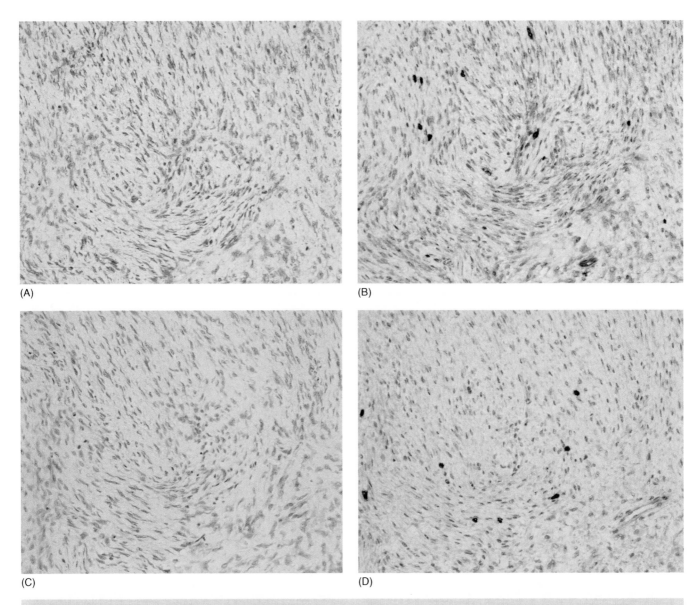

FIGURE 13.19 These four images were taken from a desmoid tumor, which should only rarely, if ever, express KIT. A primary antibody dilution of 1:50 without antigen retrieval results in nonspecific background staining without specific staining of mast cells (A). At 1:50 with antigen retrieval, the staining is even stronger, and mast cell staining is now identified (B). At 1:300 without antigen retrieval there is absolutely no staining (C). Staining is optimized at 1:300 with antigen retrieval, which results in specific mast cell staining and a clean background (D).

no dysplasia undergo surveillance at intervals of every 3 to 5 years. With low-grade dysplasia (LGD), endoscopic follow-up is at 6 to 12 month intervals. In patients with high-grade dysplasia (HGD), eradication (eg, radiofrequency ablation +/− endoscopic mucosal resection) is typically recommended. Thus, the prognosis and management of BE patients clearly hinges on dysplasia assessment.

Unfortunately, however, dysplasia assessment is fraught with difficulty. Because of this, there is ongoing research to discover and validate objective biomarkers that might increase the accuracy and reproducibility of BE dysplasia assessment. Histochemical, immunohistochemical, and molecular markers are all being actively investigated.

p53 IHC is among the most well-vetted biomarkers used in BE dysplasia assessment, and it has the advantage of widespread availability. Historically, the use of p53 in this context was controversial due largely to lack of uniformity as to what constituted an abnormal result. More recently, investigators have focused on patterns of p53 expression correlating with classes of *TP53* abnormalities. Most inactivating mutations lead to a p53 conformational change mitigating protein degradation, leading to high-level nuclear accumulation of a nonfunctioning protein (missense-mutation pattern) (Figure 13.20A–B). Less often, destabilizing mutations or gene deletion leads to the complete absence of p53 expression (null pattern)

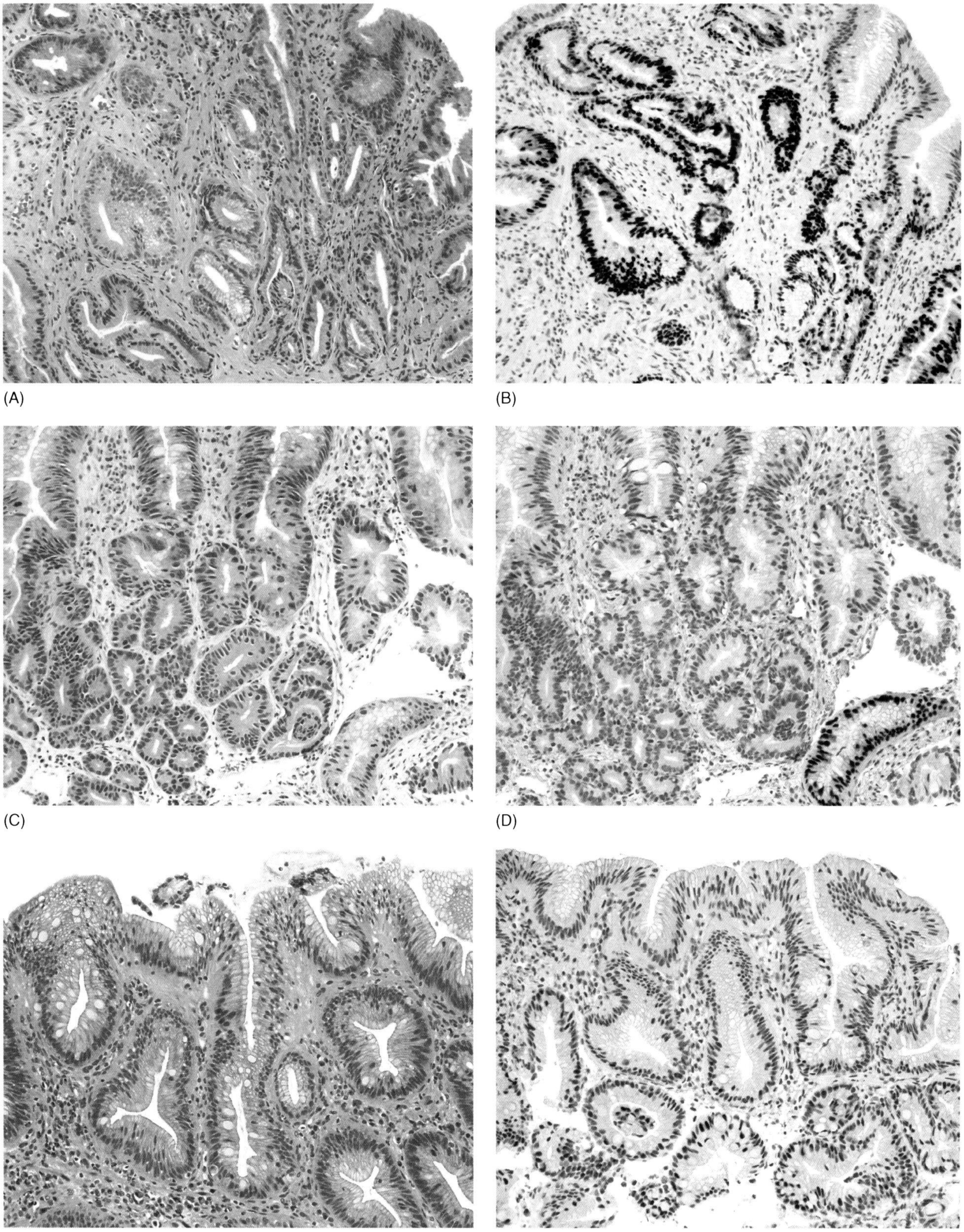

FIGURE 13.20 In each of these cases a differential of indefinite for dysplasia (IND) versus low-grade dysplasia (LGD) was contemplated. Case 1: This patient was rebiopsied after a past diagnosis of IND (A); missense-mutation-pattern p53 staining supports an interpretation of LGD (B). Case 2: In this instance, atypia was largely confined to the crypt compartment (C); null-pattern staining again supports an interpretation of LGD (D). Note the single missense-mutation-pattern staining crypt at the lower right. Case 3: This patient carried a prior diagnosis of LGD (E); wild-type pattern staining neither confirms nor refutes a diagnosis of LGD (F). This biopsy was ultimately considered IND.

TABLE 13.7   Patterns of p53 Expression

Pattern	Description	Biologic Significance	Diagnostic Significance
Missense-mutation pattern	Clonal foci of diffuse, strong staining obscuring nuclear detail	High-level accumulation of inactive p53 due to conformational change that prolongs half-life	Supports a diagnosis of dysplasia
Null pattern	Clonal foci of complete absence of nuclear staining in a background of wild-type pattern staining	Complete absence of expression due to truncating mutations or large deletions	Supports a diagnosis of dysplasia; in the ProBar study null pattern was associated with greater risk of neoplastic progression than missense-mutation pattern
Wild-type pattern	Weak to moderately intense staining, which may be punctuated by scattered darkly staining nuclei	Physiologic p53 accumulation	Does not support, though does not necessarily refute, a diagnosis of dysplasia

(Figure 13.20C–D). Historically, this pattern was likely to be misinterpreted as negative. Finally, p53 has a range of physiologic expression, with increased expression in the setting of cellular stresses (eg, inflammation, DNA damage). This wild-type p53 expression is typically of faint to moderate intensity, occasionally punctuated by more darkly staining nuclei (Figure 13.20E–F). It is occasionally misinterpreted as positive, though it lacks the uniformity of strong nuclear staining and the abrupt/clonal topography of the missense-mutation pattern. These patterns of expression are summarized in Table 13.7.

p53 IHC may be useful in BE cases with atypia in which one is contemplating the differential diagnosis of indefinite for dysplasia versus LGD although its utility in this setting remains somewhat controversial and is not universally accepted. We find it helpful in difficult biopsies, including those with active inflammation, those with atypia confined to the crypts, and those in which the surface is not well-visualized. In this setting, detecting a missense-mutation or null pattern supports a diagnosis of LGD (Algorithm 13.3). In published studies, rates of p53 IHC "positivity" have ranged from 9% to 89%; moreover, HGD and BE-associated adenocarcinomas are usually positive. The wide range of p53 abnormalities in LGD reflects various "thresholds" for LGD diagnosis as

well as application of nonstandardized p53 IHC assessment. The exact frequency of p53 abnormalities remains an open question, though it is suspected that they are quite frequent. Thus, p53 IHC is not useful in distinguishing LGD from HGD. The DO-7 mouse monoclonal antibody for p53, among a host of commercially available antibodies, has been shown to correlate best with *TP53* mutation status.

In a recent prospective case-control study of BE patients in the Netherlands, p53 overexpression was associated with an adjusted relative risk of 5.6 for progression to HGD or adenocarcinoma. Loss of p53 expression (ie, null pattern) was associated with an even higher relative risk of 14.0. It is conceivable that in the future, in addition to its use in assessing difficult biopsies as discussed in the preceding paragraphs, more routine application of p53 IHC for risk stratification may be incorporated in BE surveillance programs. Finally, although there is much less data, we occasionally use p53 IHC in the setting of other inflammation-associated atypias in the tubal gut (ie, those encountered in chronic gastritis and inflammatory bowel disease), and interpret non-wild-type patterns of p53 staining in these cases as evidence of neoplasia (Figure 13.21). As noted previously, however, this practice is somewhat controversial and not universally accepted.

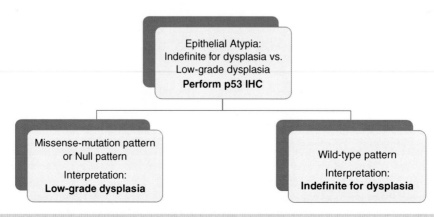

ALGORITHM 13.3   Use of p53 Immunohistochemistry to Adjudicate Epithelial Atypia in BE.

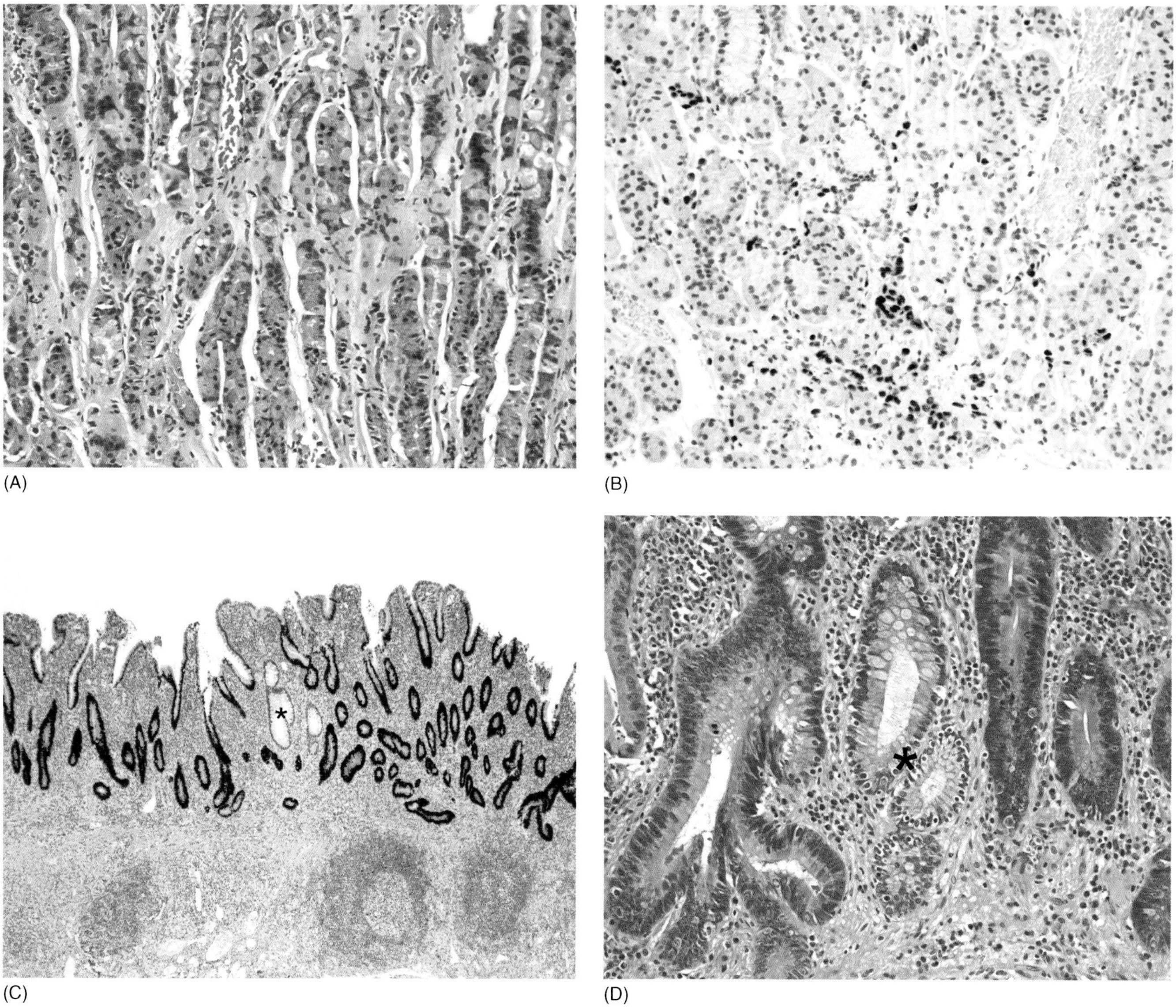

(A)   (B)

(C)   (D)

FIGURE 13.21   Although upper endoscopy demonstrated a linitis-plastica appearance, this biopsy fragment from the corpus appears relatively unremarkable (A). Missense-mutation-pattern p53 staining highlights very subtle involvement by diffuse-type gastric cancer (B). This patient underwent a colectomy for an inflammatory bowel disease-associated adenocarcinoma; p53 staining of the section of distal margin reveals a large field of missense-mutation-pattern staining with rare spared crypts (*) (C). These non-neoplastic crypts (*) are flanked by flat LGD (D).

Poorly Differentiated Esophageal Carcinomas

In the West, most esophageal cancers are BE-associated adenocarcinomas. Poorly differentiated, solid adenocarcinomas may be difficult to distinguish from squamous cell carcinomas, especially in small biopsies. Historically, the distinction of adenocarcinoma from squamous cell carcinoma in the esophagus had no specific bearing on therapy, as clinical trials of locally advanced and metastatic tumors enrolled patients regardless of histologic type. The distinction has become more significant in the era of directed biologic therapy, as only patients with adenocarcinoma are potential candidates for anti-human epidermal growth factor receptor 2 (HER2; see subsequent sections) and anti-VEGF therapy. Also of note, in the seventh edition of the *AJCC Cancer Staging Manual*, esophageal squamous cell carcinoma and adenocarcinoma have separate tumor, node, metastasis (TNM) stage groupings.

NECs represent up to 4% of carcinomas in the esophagus; these are evenly split between those arising de novo and those arising in association with a non-neuroendocrine carcinoma. The treatment paradigm for advanced NECs at this site is similar to that for pulmonary small cell carcinoma.

Several immunohistochemical markers are useful in this situation. Markers of squamous differentiation

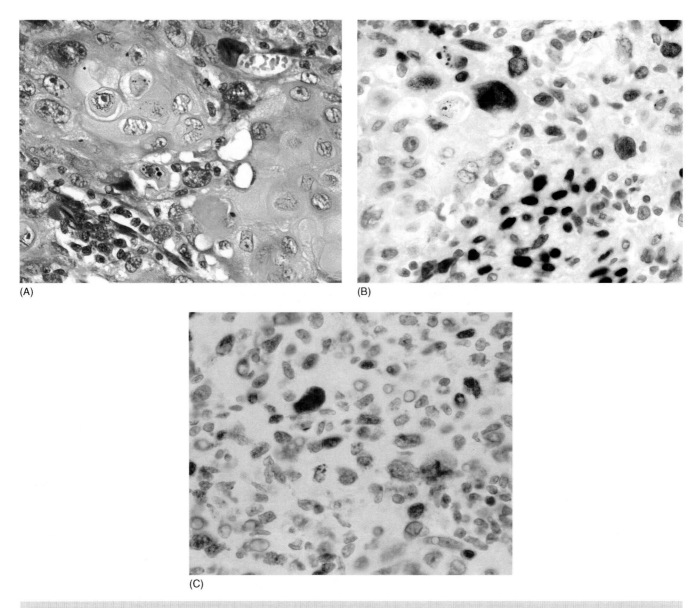

FIGURE 13.22 Squamous cell carcinoma is often recognized based on the presence of keratin formation and intercellular bridges (A). Curiously, up to 20% of esophageal (and anal) squamous cell carcinomas demonstrate CDX2-positivity (B); p63 is often coexpressed (C). MUC5AC is the preferred "adenocarcinoma marker" at this anatomic location.

include p63 and CK5/6. Both are highly sensitive, though not entirely specific, as CK5/6 is noted to be expressed by approximately 20% of esophageal adenocarcinomas. CK7 and CDX2 are often applied as adenocarcinoma markers at this anatomic site as well. As a note of caution, these are expressed by esophageal squamous cell carcinomas in about 30% and 20% of cases, respectively (Figure 13.22). Mucin histochemistry may be helpful, though mucin may be very focal to absent in poorly differentiated tumors. MUC5AC appears to be the most specific adenocarcinoma marker in this setting, though it is only expressed by two-thirds of cases. The embryonic stem cell transcription factor SOX2 can be used as a marker of squamous cell carcinoma, though it is also expressed by the vast majority of NECs (greater than 90%) and up to a third

of adenocarcinomas. MOC-31, a monoclonal antibody to EPCAM, is sometimes mistakenly interpreted as an adenocarcinoma marker in this diagnostic context. Although MOC-31 reliably marks adenocarcinoma, it is expressed by 70% of esophageal squamous cell carcinomas (Figure 13.23) and most (60%) NECs. Expression is of greater extent and intensity in poorly differentiated squamous cell carcinomas.

As at other sites, IHC for the general neuroendocrine markers chromogranin A and synaptophysin can be requested when NEC is a consideration. Scattered positive cells should not be overinterpreted as representing a neuroendocrine component. Instead, areas of diffuse, strong staining should be sought. TTF-1 is expressed by 60% to 70% of esophageal small cell carcinomas.

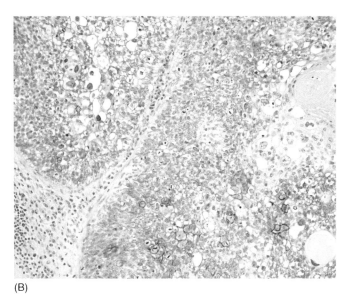

(A)   (B)

FIGURE 13.23 This keratinizing esophageal squamous cell carcinoma (A) demonstrates strong MOC-31 positivity (B), which, contrary to popular belief, does not support a diagnosis of adenocarcinoma. Overall, 40% of squamous cell carcinomas are MOC-31-positive; the rate is even higher in the esophagus.

TABLE 13.8 Immunophenotype of Esophageal Adenocarcinoma Versus Squamous Cell Carcinoma

	Adenocarcinoma (%, n)	Squamous Cell Carcinoma (%, n)
p63	8% (7/92)	99% (66/67)
CK5/6	21% (19/92)	97% (65/67)
CDX2	63% (58/92)	19% (13/67)
CK7	91% (62/68)	34% (14/41)
MUC5AC	64% (44/69)	2% (1/41)
SOX2	29% (27/92)	84% (56/57)

Source: Long KB, Hornick JL. SOX2 is highly expressed in squamous cell carcinomas of the gastrointestinal tract. *Hum Pathol.* 2009;40(12):1768–73; DiMaio MA, Kwok S, Montgomery KD, Lowe AW, Pai RK. Immunohistochemical panel for distinguishing esophageal adenocarcinoma from squamous cell carcinoma: a combination of p63, cytokeratin 5/6, MUC5AC, and anterior gradient homolog 2 allows optimal subtyping. *Hum Pathol.* 2012;43(11):1799–1807.

When facing a poorly differentiated carcinoma in the esophagus, a reasonable immunopanel includes p63 and CDX2 (substituting MUC5AC, if available); additional immunostains, including general neuroendocrine markers, can be added as needed. A comparison of the immunophenotype of esophageal adenocarcinoma and squamous cell carcinoma is presented in Table 13.8.

Poorly Cohesive Gastric Cancer Versus Metastatic Lobular Breast Cancer

Gastric cancer and breast cancer each may present as gland forming or dyscohesive histologic types. Compared to gland-forming tumors, which are more likely to spread hematogenously to the liver and lung, dyscohesive ones have a tendency to spread transperitoneally to involve the tubal gut, peritoneal surfaces, and ovaries. Invasive lobular carcinoma symptomatically involves the GI tract in 0.5% of cases, while in autopsy series metastases to the tubal gut can be found in around half of patients. Any segment of the tubal gut may be involved, but there is a special predilection for the stomach, followed by the large intestine. Clinically evident GI metastases present, on average, 7 to 10 years after the initial presentation in the breast. Metastasis to the GI tract is occasionally the initial clinical presentation of breast cancer, though, and metastases have been reported as far as 30 years out. Endoscopically, metastatic lobular breast cancer often results in a linitis-plastica-like appearance, identical to that produced by diffuse-type gastric cancer; and metastatic lobular breast cancer and diffuse-type gastric cancer are not readily distinguished on H&E evaluation. Thus, it is mandatory to consider a breast metastasis when faced with a diffuse-type anywhere in the tubal gut, but especially in the stomach (Figure 13.24A). Background findings such as *H. pylori* gastritis, intestinal metaplasia, or epithelial dysplasia in the stomach support a diagnosis of gastric adenocarcinoma.

There are several useful immunohistochemical markers applicable to this differential diagnosis (Figure 13.24B–C). An initial primary immunopanel often includes CDX2 and ER. CDX2 is expressed by most gastric cancers, although typically in fewer cells and of less intensity than in colon cancer, while it is not expressed

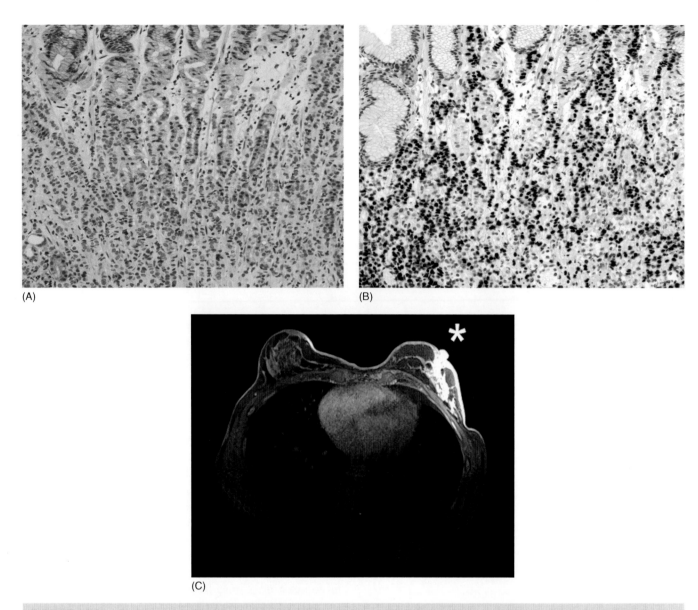

(A)

(B)

(C)

FIGURE 13.24 This 53-year-old woman presenting with nausea, vomiting, and fatigue was found to have a hemoglobin of 5.3. Gastric biopsy demonstrates involvement by a poorly cohesive carcinoma (A). The tumor was found to express ER (B) and not CDX2, consistent with spread from breast. The patient had a negative mammogram, and there was concern over whether or not this represented a breast primary. The tumor was subsequently shown to express GATA3, and a fat-saturated T1-weighted MRI revealed extensive nonmass enhancement of the left breast (C, *) measuring 6 cm and involving the nipple.

by lobular breast cancer. ER is usually positive in lobular breast cancer, and contemporary clones including 1D5, 6F11, and SP1 are almost never positive in gastric cancer. In CDX2/ER "double-negative" cases, additional markers can be applied including the gastric cancer markers Hep Par 1, MUC2, MUC5AC, and CK20, and the breast cancer markers gross cystic disease fluid protein-15 (GCDFP-15) and mammaglobin. Recently, GATA3 has emerged as a very useful breast cancer marker, and one might consider adding it to the initial CDX2/ER panel or substituting it for ER. GATA3 is less likely to be positive in ER-negative than in ER-positive breast cancers, though in our experience it is expressed by 70% to 80% of the former (and all

of the latter). Miettinen and colleagues reported GATA3 positivity in 5% of 133 gastric cancers, with diffuse-type tumors uniformly negative. A comparison of the immunophenotype of poorly cohesive gastric cancer and metastatic lobular breast cancer is presented in Table 13.9.

HER2 Assessment in Gastroesophageal Adenocarcinoma

Numerous factors culminated in an international, phase 3, open-label, randomized controlled trial comparing trastuzumab plus standard chemotherapy (fluoropyrimidine + cisplatin) to chemotherapy alone in advanced

TABLE 13.9 Immunophenotype of Poorly Cohesive Gastric Cancer Versus Metastatic Lobular Breast Cancer

	Poorly Cohesive Gastric Cancer (%, n)	Metastatic Lobular Breast Cancer (%, n)
CDX2	78% (42/54)	0% (0/51)
ER	0% (0/58)	76% (42/55)
Hep Par1	83% (25/30)	0% (0/21)
GCDFP-15	0% (0/28)	76% (26/34)
MUC1	20% (10/51)	100% (27/27)
MUC2	51% (40/79)	13% (8/60)
MUC5AC	54% (43/79)	5% (3/60)
MUC6	35% (17/49)	10% (4/39)
CK7	66% (38/58)	100% (21/21)
CK20	53% (31/58)	5% (1/20)
E-cadherin (intact)	57% (17/30)	29% (6/21)
GATA3	0% of diffuse-type tumors 5% overall (6/133) including intestinal-type tumors[a]	71% (867/1229)[b]

Source: Chu PG, Weiss LM. Immunohistochemical characterization of signet-ring cell carcinomas of the stomach, breast, and colon. *Am J Clin Pathol*. 2004;121(6):884–892; O'Connell FP, Wang HH, Odze RD. Utility of immunohistochemistry in distinguishing primary adenocarcinomas from metastatic breast carcinomas in the gastrointestinal tract. *Arch Pathol Lab Med*. 2005;129(3):338–347; Nguyen MD, Plasil B, Wen P, Frankel WL. Mucin profiles in signet-ring cell carcinoma. *Arch Pathol Lab Med*. 2006;130(6):799–804; [a]Miettinen M, McCue PA, Sarlomo-Rikala M, et al. GATA3: a multispecific but potentially useful marker in surgical pathology: a systematic analysis of 2500 epithelial and nonepithelial tumors. *Am J Surg Pathol*. 2014;38(1):13–22; [b]Ordonez NG. Value of GATA3 immunostaining in tumor diagnosis: a review. *Adv Anat Pathol*. 2013;20(5):352–360.

(ie, locally advanced, metastatic, or recurrent) gastric and gastroesophageal junction (GEJ) adenocarcinomas, known as the Trastuzumab for Gastric Cancer (ToGA) trial. These factors included an observed rate of HER2 overexpression in gastric cancer similar to that seen in breast cancer; the efficacy of trastuzumab (Herceptin®) in preclinical models of gastric cancer; and a paucity of effective therapies in advanced gastric cancer. For the purpose of the trial, cases were tested by both IHC and FISH. Patients with an IHC score of 3+ and/or with a FISH HER2:CEP17 ratio of >/=2 were considered positive. Among 3,807 tumors screened for enrollment, HER2-positivity was seen in 20.9% of gastric and 33.2% of gastroesophageal junction tumors. Histologic type influenced expression, with positivity in 32.2% of intestinal, 20.4% of mixed, and only 6.1% of diffuse tumors. The addition of trastuzumab in HER2-positive patients improved median overall survival by 2.7 months (13.8 months vs. 11.1 months). This "positive" study has resulted in the assessment of HER2 in advanced gastric and gastroesophageal adenocarcinomas becoming the standard of care. The National Comprehensive Cancer Network (NCCN) has further extended this recommendation to patients with esophageal adenocarcinoma. In the near future, it is anticipated that anti-HER2 therapy in HER2-positive tumors will be explored in clinical trials as a component of neoadjuvant regimens.

There are two key differences between HER2 IHC testing in gastroesophageal cancer and breast cancer. These are based, in part, on observations made in the context of a validation study performed in anticipation of the ToGA trial. More frequent HER2 heterogeneity (areas of positive and negative staining) was observed in gastroesophageal tumors than had been seen in breast tumors (Figure 13.25). Also, several cases with basolateral (U-shaped) or lateral membrane staining (rather than complete membrane staining) were observed, and some of these were HER2-amplified by FISH. Because of heterogeneity, there are different scoring criteria for gastroesophageal biopsies and resections, with any amount of 2+ or 3+ staining in a biopsy considered equivocal or positive, respectively (one group has alternatively suggested the need for at least five cells that stain—key difference 1). Because cases with basolateral and lateral membrane staining may be HER2-amplified, the strict requirement for "complete membrane staining" that applies in breast cancer is relaxed (key difference 2). GI HER2 scoring criteria are summarized in Table 13.10 and illustrated in Figure 13.26.

In the ToGA trial, the survival benefit from trastuzumab was greatest in patients with IHC 3+ or IHC 2+/FISH-positive tumors (4.2 months), while patients with HER2 amplification in the absence of protein overexpression (IHC 0/1+) derived no survival benefit. This latter group constituted 22% of all HER2-positive cases. Based on this result, many laboratories have established HER2 IHC as the first-line test, with FISH principally reserved for HER2 2+ (equivocal) cases. Other laboratories have taken the stance that the biology of HER2 IHC-negative/FISH-positive cases is still an open question and either perform IHC and FISH in parallel or reflex HER2 0 and 1+ (in addition to 2+) cases to FISH.

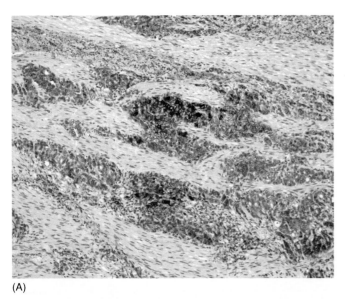

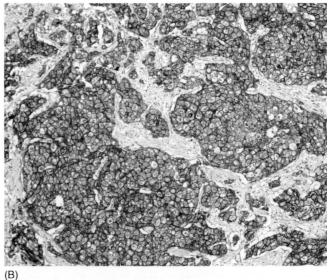

(A)   (B)

FIGURE 13.25 Gastroesophageal adenocarcinomas occasionally demonstrate HER2 heterogeneity, as seen in this example where there are areas of 3+, 2+, and 1+ staining in the same tissue section (A), while breast tumors, if positive (3+), tend to be uniformly so (B). This heterogeneity in GI tumors is the basis of separate scoring criteria in biopsies and resections and repeating HER2 testing on resection specimens from patients who have had negative results on biopsy.

At our institution, we perform HER2 testing on all advanced esophageal, gastroesophageal junction, and gastric adenocarcinomas, and some perform testing on nonadvanced cases as well. Potential specimens include endoscopic mucosal biopsies, resection specimens, and biopsies of metastatic sites. Studies of matched endoscopic mucosal biopsies and resection specimens and matched primary and metastatic tumors have reported concordances of 75% to 95%. Given an initially negative result, it may be prudent to test more than one specimen, particularly if a biopsy from a metastatic site becomes available, as metastatic tumors have been reported to convert to HER2-positive 10% of the time. Similar to breast cancer specimens, it is recommended that samples be placed in 10% neutral buffered formalin within 1 hour and fixed for 6 to 72 hours, with the fixation time documented in the pathology report. Although

the ToGA trial screened tumors with the Food and Drug Administration (FDA)-approved Dako HercepTest™ (rabbit polyclonal), the 4B5 antibody (rabbit monoclonal) has been shown to produce equivalent results. The College of American Pathologists provides proficiency testing for GI HER2 IHC.

MISMATCH REPAIR PROTEIN IMMUNOHISTOCHEMISTRY

Malignant neoplasms are characterized by genomic instability, which takes two main forms (see also Chapter 14). Colorectal cancers can be divided into those demonstrating chromosomal instability (85%) and those demonstrating microsatellite instability (MSI; 15%). MSI occurs due to

TABLE 13.10 HER2 Immunohistochemistry Scoring Criteria for Resections and Biopsies

Biopsy	Resection	Score	Interpretation	Action
No reactivity	No reactivity or reactivity in <10% of tumor cells	0	Negative	Some laboratories will reflex to HER2 FISH
Tumor cell cluster with faint/barely perceptible reactivity (ie, discernible at 400x)	Faint/barely perceptible reactivity in ≥10% of tumor cells	1+	Negative	Some laboratories will reflex to HER2 FISH
Tumor cell cluster with weak to moderate reactivity (ie, discernible at 100–200x)	Weak to moderate reactivity in ≥10% of tumor cells	2+	Equivocal	Reflex to HER2 FISH
Tumor cell cluster with strong reactivity (ie, visible with naked eye or discernible at 20–40x)	Strong reactivity in ≥10% of tumor cells	3+	Positive	Consider anti-HER2 therapy

Note: Significant reactivity includes complete, lateral, or basolateral membrane staining; in one study, a tumor cell cluster was defined as five or more cells.
Abbreviation: FISH, fluorescence in situ hybridization.

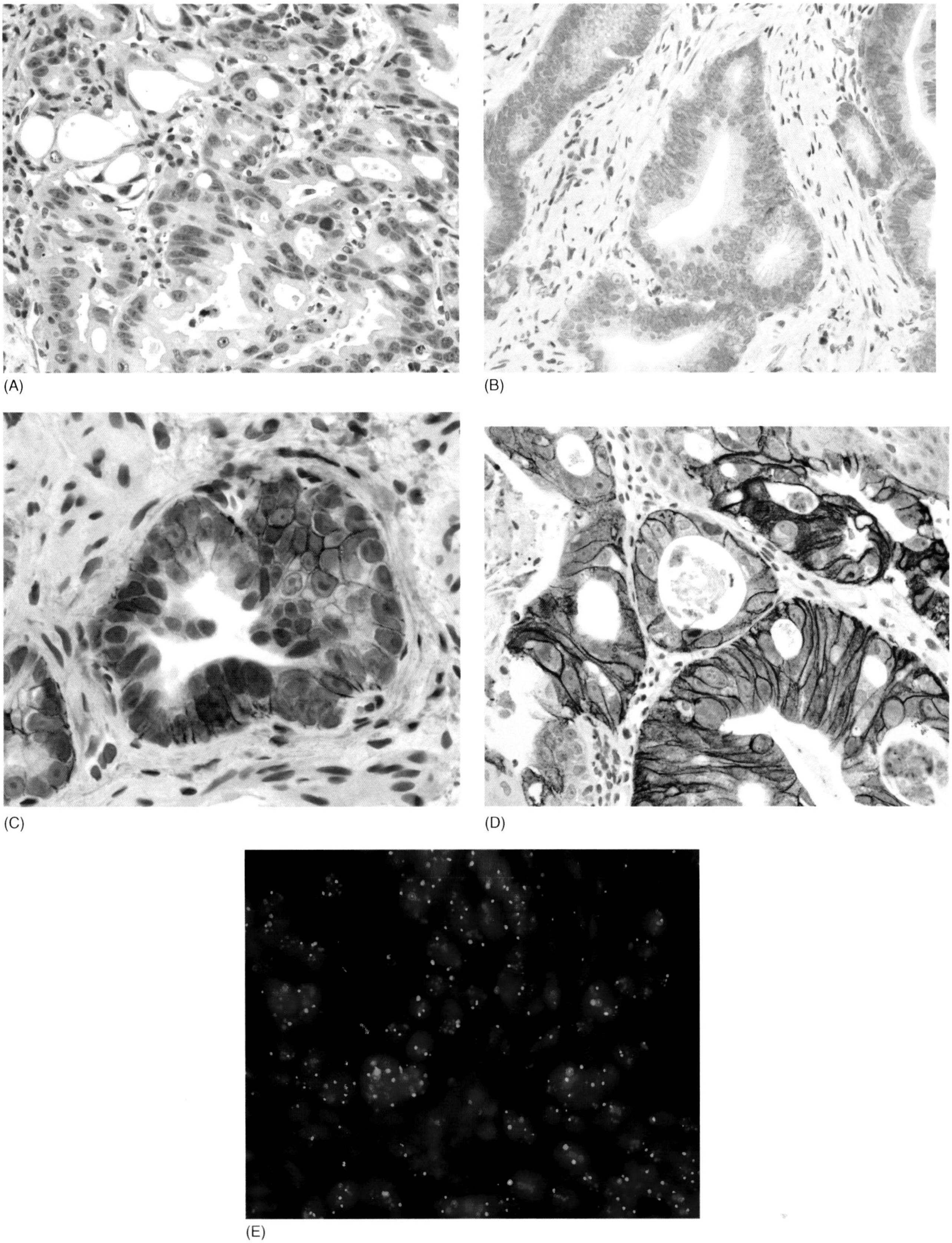

FIGURE 13.26   In gastroesophageal adenocarcinomas, a score of zero equals no reactivity (A); 1+: faint/barely perceptible reactivity (B); 2+: weak to moderate reactivity (C); 3+: strong reactivity (D). The 2+ biopsy illustrated in "C" was reflexed to FISH, which demonstrates a HER2 (orange) to CEP17 (green) ratio of 3.0 (ie, amplified) (E). Note that in the 1+ to 3+ cases, staining is predominantly lateral or basolateral, generally sparing the apical surface.

deficient DNA mismatch repair (dMMR) function, which may arise sporadically (typically due to methylation of the *MLH1* promoter and seen in up to 15% of colon cancers) or in the setting of germline mutations (ie, Lynch syndrome). The identification of colon cancers with dMMR/MSI-H is desirable to identify Lynch syndrome (2–4% of colon cancers) but also because this phenotype is prognostically favorable stage for stage and predicts a relative lack of benefit from 5-FU-based chemotherapy. Either polymerase chain reaction (PCR)-based MSI testing or MMR protein IHC may be used as screening tests for the dMMR/MSI-H phenotype, with highly concordant results. MMR IHC offers the advantages of widespread availability and rapid turnaround time, and, when abnormal, it directs the next steps in the patient's evaluation and plan for therapy.

Although age, clinical history, and histology-based strategies to identify which tumors to screen for dMMR/MSI-H may be employed, there has been a trend toward more intensive, if not universal, screening. The Centers for Disease Control and Prevention (CDC)-sponsored Evaluation of Genomic Applications in Practice and Prevention (EGAPP) working group and the Association for Molecular Pathology (AMP) Mismatch Repair-Defective CRC working group have endorsed universal screening. The most recent NCCN Guidelines recommend (a) testing tumors in patients aged 70 and less, as well as those above 70 who meet Bethesda guidelines or (b) universal testing. The NCCN guidelines also suggest that testing may be helpful in patients with stage II colon cancer, in which the result influences the decision as to whether to pursue adjuvant chemotherapy.

The DNA MMR apparatus is one of several DNA repair mechanisms. It specifically recognizes mispaired bases and insertion–deletion loops, which, if unrepaired, would lead to missense and frameshift mutations, respectively. The system functions as two heterodimers, with MSH2 pairing with MSH6 to recognize the errors and MLH1 pairing with PMS2 to direct the repair. Each heterodimer is composed of a dominant (expressed regardless of the status of its partner) and dependent (not expressed in the absence of its partner) protein; MLH1 and MSH2 are dominant, while PMS2 and MSH6 are dependent. Biallelic *MLH1* promoter methylation silences MLH1 (and PMS2) expression. In Lynch syndrome, a germline mutation and a somatic "second hit" silences expression of one or more proteins in ~95% of cases. There are five main patterns of MMR protein expression seen in tumors:

1. All four proteins expressed
2. Loss of MLH1/PMS2; intact MSH2/MSH6
3. Loss of MSH2/MSH6; intact MLH1/PMS2
4. Loss of MSH6; intact MLH1/PMS2/MSH2
5. Loss of PMS2; intact MLH1/MSH2/MSH6

We perform MMR IHC on biopsies (if available) rather than resections because patients with colon cancer due to Lynch syndrome are typically counseled to undergo subtotal rather than segmental colectomy due to a substantial (~40%) risk of metachronous tumors. In 80% to 85% of colon cancer cases, all four proteins are normally expressed (pattern 1). Because in rare Lynch syndrome patients a nonfunctioning protein is still expressed, complementary MSI testing may be considered in patients with normal IHC but clinical suspicion of Lynch syndrome. Loss of MLH1 and PMS2 is seen in 15% of cases (pattern 2). This is usually due to *MLH1* promoter methylation and is less often due to *MLH1* germline mutation. *BRAF V600E* and/or *MLH1* promoter methylation testing can be pursued in this setting to distinguish sporadic from hereditary cases. In tumors with wild-type *BRAF* and/or without demonstrable *MLH1* promoter methylation, *MLH1* germline mutation testing is then undertaken. Until recently, patterns 3 to 5 were considered tantamount to a diagnosis of Lynch syndrome, with germline mutation testing directed by the specific result of the IHC.

In at least 30% of patients with suspected Lynch syndrome (abnormal MMR IHC and/or MSI-H in whom a sporadic tumor due to *MLH1* promoter methylation has been excluded), a germline mutation is not detected. This had been ascribed to the relative insensitivity of germline mutation testing. Several groups have recently shown that in up to two-thirds of these cases biallelic inactivation of an MMR gene arises somatically (ie, only within the tumor). These cases have been referred to as "Lynch-like" or "pseudo-Lynch" syndrome. Family members of patients with Lynch-like syndrome have a risk of colon cancer intermediate between that seen in families with Lynch syndrome and those in which colon cancer appears to have arisen sporadically, and Lynch-like syndrome is *not* associated with the typical Lynch-associated extracolonic tumors (eg, carcinomas of the endometrium, ovary, stomach, and upper urinary tract).

Historically, patients with abnormal MMR IHC and/or MSI testing that remained "unexplained" (ie, *BRAF* wild-type, *MLH1* promoter methylation negative, germline DNA MMR mutation negative) were followed as if they had Lynch syndrome (ie, intensive colonoscopy, endometrial sampling, transvaginal ultrasound, urine cytology). Because potentially affected family members could not be effectively evaluated for Lynch syndrome due to the lack of an identifiable mutation, they too, were often placed into intensive surveillance. The identification of Lynch-like syndrome, by testing the tumors of patients with unexplained MMR IHC and/or MSI results for somatic DNA MMR gene mutations, promises to be cost-effective, sparing patients and their family members the expense of Lynch-syndrome-specific surveillance. Patterns of MMR protein IHC and their frequency, interpretation, and follow-up are summarized in Table 13.11.

TABLE 13.11 Patterns of Mismatch Repair Protein Expression

Immunohistochemistry Result	Frequency	Interpretation	Action(s)
All four proteins intact	80%–85%	Normal MMR function Unlikely Lynch syndrome	Consider follow-up microsatellite instability testing to confirm normal result Refer to *Cancer Genetics* if clinically appropriate
MLH1/PMS2 lost MSH2/MSH6 intact	15%	Abnormal MMR function Likely sporadic dMMR due to *MLH1* promoter methylation Less likely Lynch syndrome due to *MLH1* (usually) or *PMS2* (rarely) mutation	*BRAF V600E* and/or *MLH1* promoter methylation testing If *BRAF V600E* and/or *MLH1* promoter methylation testing are normal: Refer for genetics evaluation *MLH1* germline mutation testing (followed by *PMS2* if needed) Consider tumor mutation testing if germline mutation not detected
MSH2/MSH6 lost MLH1/PMS2 intact	1%–2%	Abnormal MMR function Possibly Lynch syndrome due to *MSH2* (usually) or *EPCAM* deletion or *MSH6* mutation (rarely)	Refer for genetics evaluation *MSH2* germline mutation testing (followed by *EPCAM* and *MSH6* if needed) Consider tumor mutation testing if germline mutation not detected
MSH6 lost MLH1/PMS2/MSH6 intact	Up to 0.5%	Abnormal MMR function Possibly Lynch syndrome due to *MSH6* (usually) or *MSH2* (rarely) mutation	Refer for genetics evaluation *MSH6* germline mutation testing (followed by *MSH2* if needed) Consider tumor mutation testing if germline mutation not detected
PMS2 lost MLH1/MSH2/MSH6 intact	up to 0.5%	Abnormal MMR function Possibly Lynch syndrome due to *PMS2* (usually) or *MLH1* (rarely) mutation	Refer for genetics evaluation *PMS2* germline mutation testing (followed by *MLH1* if needed) Consider tumor mutation testing if germline mutation not detected

Abbreviations: dMMR, deficient mismatch repair function; MMR, mismatch repair.

Investigators have noted several potential pitfalls in the interpretation of MMR IHC. A determination of loss of protein expression can only be made in the setting of intact staining in internal control lymphocytes and stroma. MMR protein expression may be difficult to detect (including in internal control tissue) with some fixatives other than formalin (Figure 13.27A). Protein expression may be heterogeneous, especially in resections as compared to biopsies (attributed to delays in fixation or under/overfixation) (Figure 13.27B–C), and after neoadjuvant chemoradiotherapy (MSH6 is especially prone to this, and may demonstrate a peculiar nucleolar pattern of expression; Figure 13.27D–E). In general, MMR IHC should only be considered abnormal in the setting of complete absence of one or more proteins. Rarely, one or more proteins demonstrate diffuse, weak staining, which is weaker than associated internal control tissue (Figure 13.27F–G). These cases may cautiously be interpreted as abnormal, likely due to mutations that abrogate protein function and diminish, although not entirely silence, protein expression. MSH6 has microsatellites in its coding region, and it is occasionally silenced as a secondary event in dMMR/MSI-H tumors (ie, MSH6 loss, which may be block-like/clonal rather than diffuse, may accompany loss of MLH1/PMS2 or loss of PMS2; Figure 13.27H). Loss of the other MMR proteins may rarely show similar block-like/clonal loss, corresponding to the unusually late acquisition of the second hit to an MMR gene at the carcinoma stage.

EPCAM Immunohistochemistry

Recently, large deletions in the 3' end of *EPCAM* have been found to account for about 20% of Lynch syndrome cases in patients with loss of MSH2/MSH6 expression without identifiable *MSH2* germline mutations. *EPCAM* lies directly upstream of *MSH2*, and these large deletions lead to *MSH2* promoter methylation and transcriptional silencing. There is loss of EPCAM expression in affected tumors, with intact expression in non-neoplastic crypts. The monoclonal antibody BerEp4 recognizes EPCAM and may be used to identify MSH2/MSH6-deficient tumors due to *EPCAM* mutation.

BRAF V600E Mutation-Specific Immunohistochemistry

A BRAF V600E mutation-specific monoclonal antibody has recently become commercially available. Several groups have published near-perfect to perfect sensitivity and specificity for this antibody in, collectively, several

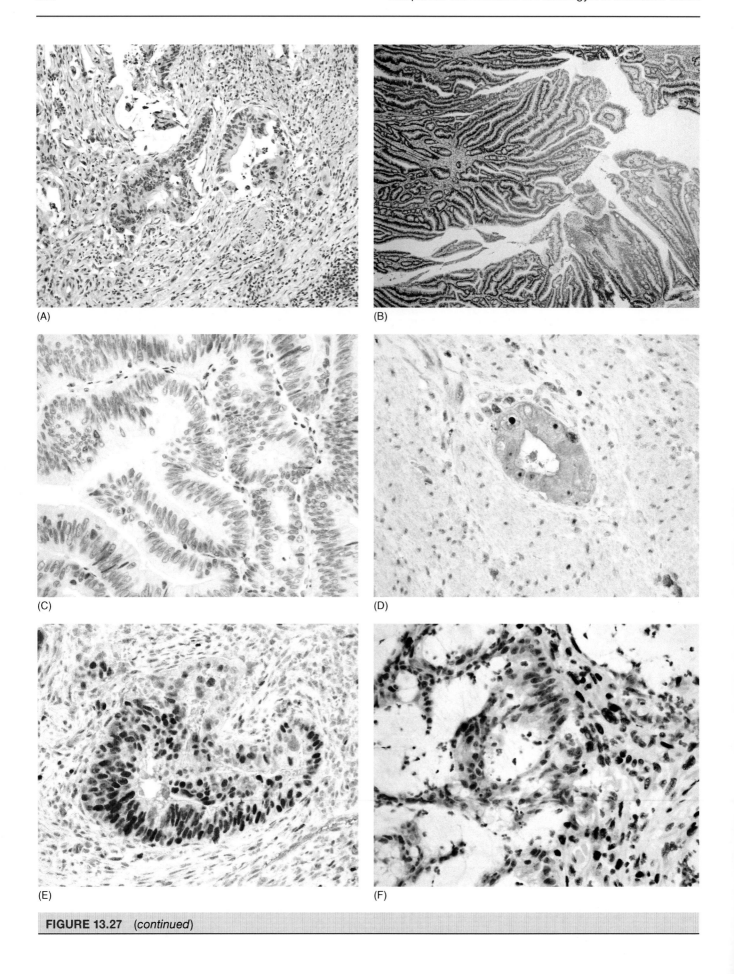

FIGURE 13.27 (*continued*)

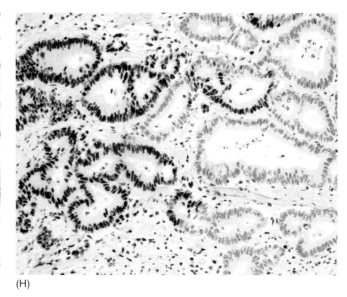

(G)

(H)

FIGURE 13.27   Absent internal control staining with use of a nonformalin, glyoxal-based fixative; this result is uninterpretable (A). Variation in staining is not unusual in resection specimens (B), including areas of very focal and weak, though intact, staining (C). Reduced staining intensity and peculiar nucleolar localization may be seen after neoadjuvant chemoradiotherapy; MSH6 is preferentially affected (D); MSH6 staining in a matched pretreatment biopsy is clearly intact (E). This tumor demonstrates uniform weak MSH6 staining in tumor (left side), relative to strongly staining internal control (right side) (F), while MSH2 staining intensity is similar in tumor and internal control (G); this tumor was subsequently shown to be MSI-H. Clonal loss of MSH6 as a secondary event in a tumor that was uniformly MLH1/PMS2-deficient (H).

thousand colon cancers. Of note, the assay appears most likely to achieve these superior test characteristics when run on Ventana automated immunostainers. In contrast, a group using manual staining reported a sensitivity and specificity of only 71% and 74%, respectively, in a cohort of 52 tumors, and another group, using a Leica Bond-Max autostainer found moderate to strong staining with the antibody to be 85% sensitive and 68% specific in a group of 113 colon cancer patients. BRAF V600E IHC may substitute for *BRAF* mutation analysis in the evaluation of MLH1-deficient colon cancers, but the assay must be carefully validated, and it may not achieve acceptable test characteristics on some testing platforms. Interestingly, papillary thyroid cancers and melanomas may not be susceptible to the same platform-specific variability.

Mismatch Repair Immunohistochemistry in Colon Polyps

Patients with Lynch syndrome inherit one defective copy of a DNA MMR gene. The second hit occurs in adenomatous polyp tissue sometime after polyp initiation, and has nearly always occurred by the time cancer develops. MMR protein deficiency (or MSI-H) may be detected in 60% to 80% of adenomas from patients with Lynch syndrome (Figure 13.28). Although larger polyps and those harboring HGD are more likely to demonstrate abnormal MMR

IHC, even small polyps with LGD are often abnormal. Testing adenomatous polyps may be useful in patients with family histories compelling for Lynch syndrome in whom cancer tissue is unavailable, as an abnormal result is fairly sensitive and highly specific for Lynch syndrome. However, routine testing of adenomatous polyps in patients without any clinical or family history that is compelling for Lynch syndrome is not recommended.

Sporadic MSI-H colon cancers due to *MLH1* promoter methylation are characterized by loss of MLH1/PMS2 expression. These tumors arise from sessile serrated polyps, which develop cytologic dysplasia before becoming invasive cancer. While sessile serrated polyps without cytologic dysplasia demonstrate intact MLH1/PMS2 protein expression, loss is demonstrated in most foci of superimposed HGD. The frequency of protein loss in sessile serrated polyp with LGD is not well-established, but, in our experience, it is relatively infrequent (Figure 13.29).

ANAL SQUAMOUS INTRAEPITHELIAL LESIONS/INTRAEPITHELIAL NEOPLASIA (SIL/AIN)

Anogenital squamous cell carcinoma is etiologically linked to high-risk human papillomavirus. Neoplastic progression is driven, in part, by production of the E6

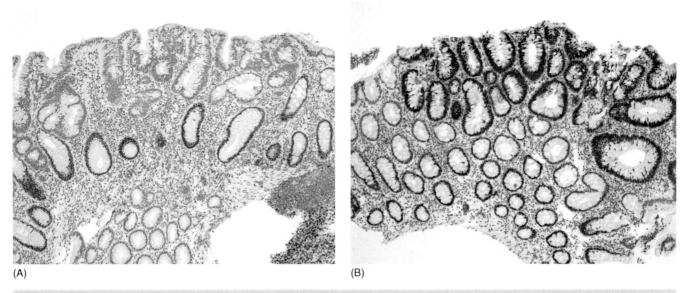

(A)   (B)

FIGURE 13.28 Loss of MSH2 (A) and MSH6 expression in a small adenoma from a woman with a history of endometrial cancer and sebaceous adenoma. Intact mismatch repair protein expression (B, MSH2) in the same patient in a separate polyp from the same colonoscopy.

and E7 oncoproteins, the latter of which inactivates the tumor suppressor retinoblastoma protein (pRb). p16 is upregulated in the face of pRb inactivation, and p16 IHC is therefore widely used as a surrogate marker of high risk HPV-driven squamous lesions (eg, in the uterine cervix, oropharynx, and anus) (see also Chapter 12).

p16 has been shown to be overexpressed in 76% to 100% (median 86%) of high-grade squamous intraepithelial lesions (HSIL; encompassing AIN2 and AIN3). Positive staining is "block-like" (diffuse, strong), rather than weak

and/or "spotty." Block-like staining has been described in 0% to 21.4% (median 9.5%) of cases of AIN1. Although AIN1 is typically associated with low-risk HPV, some of these p16-positive cases have been shown to harbor high risk HPV.

In addition to distinguishing HSIL from AIN1, p16 IHC is also useful in separating HSIL from anal transitional zone (ATZ) mucosa. Although the anal squamocolumnar junction may be abrupt, stretches of a multilayered epithelium, four to nine cells thick, often with a fairly high nucleus–cytoplasm ratio, and variously composed

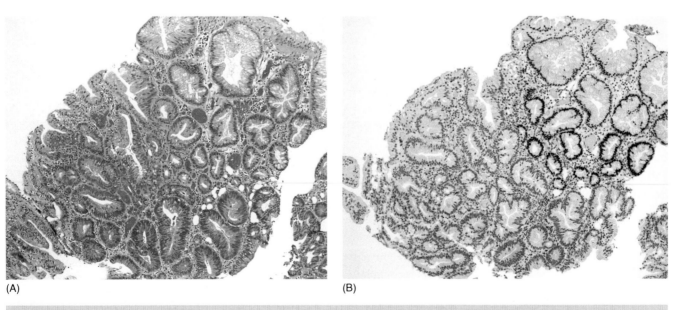

(A)   (B)

FIGURE 13.29 Sessile serrated polyp (upper right) with superimposed low-grade cytologic dysplasia (lower left) (A); MLH1 immunostain demonstrates loss of expression in the area of cytologic dysplasia (B).

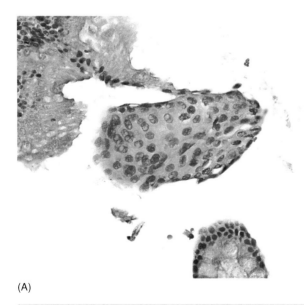

FIGURE 13.30   Anal transitional zone mucosa, given the often moderately high nucleus:cytoplasm ratio, is occasionally overinterpreted as HSIL (A). p16-negativity argues against the diagnosis of HGSIL (B).

of squamous, transitional, and mucous cells, may be mistaken for HSIL (Figure 13.30A). Two studies have shown ATZ mucosa to be p16-negative (Figure 13.30B); it is also CK7-positive, while HSIL rarely is.

Several studies have also evaluated the efficacy of Ki-67 IHC, generally in concert with p16, to adjudicate anal squamous lesions. Various definitions of "positive" have been used, including staining of greater than one third or greater than one half of the lesional epithelial

thickness. Ki-67 performs similarly, though not quite as well, as p16, because inflammatory/reactive changes sometimes stain in a pattern that may be interpreted as "positive." In noninflamed ATZ mucosa, staining is characteristically confined to the basal layer.

We typically perform p16 IHC (sometimes along with Ki-67) in small biopsies in which we are uncertain on the H&E as to whether HSIL is present. Block-like staining supports a diagnosis of HSIL (Figure 13.31).

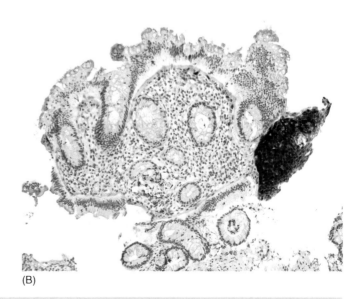

FIGURE 13.31   This patient had a history of squamous cell carcinoma in situ of the anus, which had been irradiated. Follow-up biopsy contained extremely scant squamous epithelium (A), which demonstrated block-pattern p16 staining (B, right side of biopsy), supporting the diagnosis of HSIL.

Pagetoid Tumors of the Anal Canal

In 1874, the English surgeon and pathologist James Paget reported an association between chronic nipple ulceration and the subsequent development of breast cancer. It was later shown that these nipple–areolar changes were neoplastic, rather than inflammatory, and in fact an underlying in situ or invasive carcinoma is identified in more than 95% of patients with Paget disease of the nipple. Histologically, Paget disease is characterized by intraepidermal involvement by cytologically malignant cells, singly and in small groups, which tend to predominate at the base and disperse toward the epithelial surface (so-called "upward spread"). This histologic appearance is referred to as "pagetoid" (Figure 13.32A).

Extramammary Paget disease is a histologically similar lesion, often presenting in the anogenital region. In contrast to mammary Paget disease, it often represents a primary intraepithelial adenocarcinoma, which rarely invades (see also Chapter 12). Primary anogenital Paget disease must be distinguished from secondary involvement of anogenital epithelium by an underlying visceral malignancy (eg, anal duct, colorectal, or genitourinary). The differential diagnosis of pagetoid lesions also includes melanoma in situ/superficial spreading melanoma and some examples of squamous cell carcinoma in situ.

In challenging cases, this differential diagnosis may be readily solved immunohistochemically (Figure 13.32B–D). Primary Paget disease of the anus reliably expresses CK7,

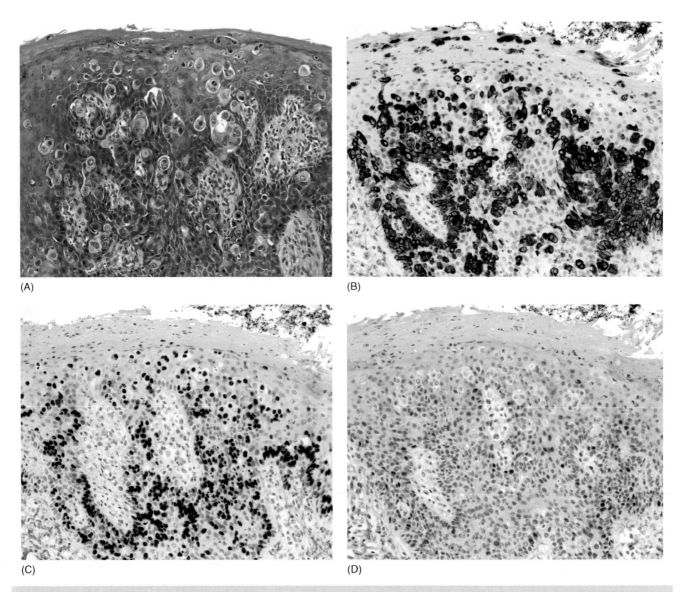

(A)

(B)

(C)

(D)

FIGURE 13.32 Malignant-appearing cells with abundant eosinophilic cytoplasm involve the anal squamous epithelium singly and in small groups (A); the neoplastic population expresses CK20 (B) and CDX2 (C), but not GATA3 (D; note weak expression in the squamous epithelium, however). This immunophenotype suggests pagetoid involvement of the anal canal mucosa by a lower GI tract adenocarcinoma.

TABLE 13.12 Immunophenotype of Neoplasms Involving Perianal Area in Pagetoid Fashion

Neoplasm	Positive Stains	Comments
Extramammary Paget disease	CK7, GATA3, HER2 (var.), GCDFP-15 (var.), androgen receptor (var.)	Reportedly rarely may be CK20+
Colorectal adenocarcinoma involving anal mucosa/perianal skin in pagetoid fashion	CK20, CDX2	May be CK7+
Pagetoid squamous cell carcinoma in situ	p63, CK5/6, p16	May be CK7+
Melanoma in situ/superficial spreading melanoma	S100, melan-A/MART-1, HMB-45, MiTF, SOX10, tyrosinase	

while HER2, GCDFP-15, and androgen receptor are variably expressed. Recently, in two small studies published in abstract form, GATA3 was shown to be uniformly expressed by extramammary Paget disease. Rare CK20-positive examples of extramammary Paget disease have been published, although it is possible that in these instances an underlying colorectal carcinoma escaped clinical detection. Although mucin histochemistry distinguishes extramammary Paget disease from melanocytic and squamous examples, it will not distinguish it from secondary involvement by an underlying adenocarcinoma. Colorectal adenocarcinomas will generally express CK20 and CDX2 (80%–90%), and aside from expressing CK7 in up to 25% of cases, they would not be expected to express any of the other "extramammary Paget disease-specific" markers. Pagetoid squamous cell carcinoma in situ expresses p63 and CK5/6, and rare examples have been shown to express CK7, leading to diagnostic confusion with extramammary Paget disease. Melanocytic lesions express the array of melanocyte markers including S100, melan-A/MART-1, and HMB-45.

Our primary immunopanel, given a pagetoid neoplasm at the anal margin, includes CK7, CK20, CDX2, p63, and S100. Additional markers can be added, as needed. Given recent findings, we would consider substituting GATA3 for CK7. The immunophenotype of neoplasms involving the perianal area in pagetoid fashion is summarized in Table 13.12.

Basaloid Squamous Cell Carcinoma Versus Basal Cell Carcinoma at the Anal Margin

Rarely, we have encountered small biopsies in which the distinction of basaloid squamous cell carcinoma from basal cell carcinoma (BCC) has proven challenging (see also Chapter 12). The distinction is clinically significant, because invasive anal squamous cell carcinoma is treated with radiation and chemotherapy (eg, 5-FU), while BCC is treated with wide local excision. Of note, BCC only rarely arises at this anatomic location but it does occur. A recent study examined the ability of histologic features and a panel of immunohistochemical stains to distinguish these tumors. There was substantial morphologic overlap, with the only statistically significant distinguishing morphologic features being retraction of nests of tumor from the adjacent stroma (BCC) and the presence of atypical mitotic figures (basaloid squamous cell carcinoma). Basaloid squamous cell carcinomas expressed p16 and SOX2, while BCCs did not; BerEp4 and Bcl-2 were more frequently expressed in BCCs; and p63 and CK5/6 were frequently expressed by both tumor types (see Table 13.13 and Figure 13.33).

TABLE 13.13 Immunophenotype of Anal Region Basaloid Squamous Cell Carcinoma Versus Basal Cell Carcinoma

	Basaloid Squamous Cell Carcinoma (%, n)	Basal Cell Carcinoma (%, n)
p16	93% (14/15)	0% (0/9)
SOX2	93% (14/15)	0% (0/9)
BerEp4	40% (6/15)	100% (9/9)
Bcl-2	33% (5/15)	100% (9/9)
p63	87% (13/15)	100% (9/9)
CK5/6	80% (12/15)	100% (9/9)

Source: Patil DT, Goldblum JR, Billings SD. Clinicopathological analysis of basal cell carcinoma of the anal region and its distinction from basaloid squamous cell carcinoma. *Mod Pathol.* 2013;26(10):1382–1389.

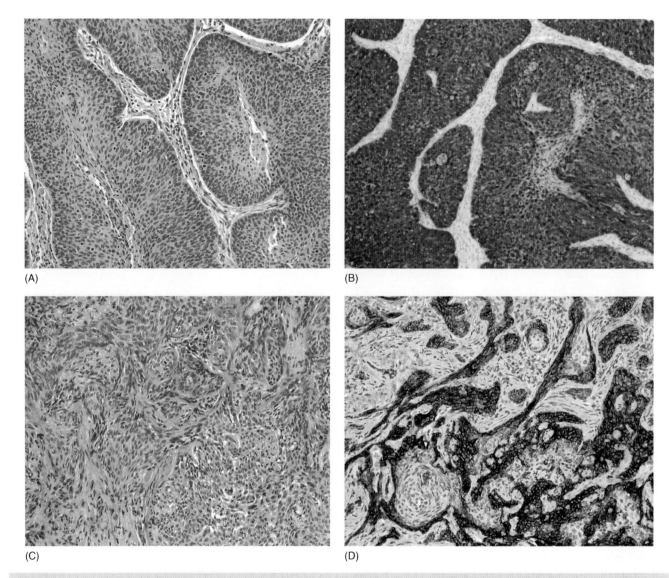

FIGURE 13.33 Basaloid squamous cell carcinoma presents as nests of cells with a high nucleus:cytoplasm ratio and brisk mitotic activity (A); diffuse, strong p16 expression, etiologically linked to high-risk human papillomavirus, confirms the morphologic impression (B). Characteristic retraction artifact is inconspicuous in this infiltrative BCC of the perianal skin (C); BerEp4 positivity is typical, though it may also be seen in anogenital squamous cell carcinomas (D).

SELECTED REFERENCES

Approach to Epithelial Neoplasms

Adams H, Schmid P, Dirnhofer S, Tzankov A. Cytokeratin expression in hematological neoplasms: a tissue microarray study on 866 lymphoma and leukemia cases. *Path Res Prac.* 2008;204(8):569–573.

Chen ZM, Wang HL. Alteration of cytokeratin 7 and cytokeratin 20 expression profile is uniquely associated with tumorigenesis of primary adenocarcinoma of the small intestine. *Am J Surg Pathol.* 2004;28(10):1352–1359.

Chu P, Wu E, Weiss LM. Cytokeratin 7 and cytokeratin 20 expression in epithelial neoplasms: a survey of 435 cases. *Mod Pathol.* 2000;13(9):962–972.

Chu PG, Schwarz RE, Lau SK, Yen Y, Weiss LM. Immunohistochemical staining in the diagnosis of pancreatobiliary and ampulla of Vater adenocarcinoma: application of CDX2, CK17, MUC1, and MUC2. *Am J Surg Pathol* 2005;29(3):359–367.

Goldstein NS, Bassi D. Cytokeratins 7, 17, and 20 reactivity in pancreatic and ampulla of vater adenocarcinomas. Percentage of positivity and distribution is affected by the cut-point threshold. *Am J Clin Pathol.* 2001;115(5):695–702.

Gustmann C, Altmannsberger M, Osborn M, Griesser H, Feller AC. Cytokeratin expression and vimentin content in large cell anaplastic lymphomas and other non-Hodgkin's lymphomas. *Am J Pathol.* 1991;138(6):1413–1422.

Herrera GA, Turbat-Herrera EA, Lott RL. S-100 protein expression by primary and metastatic adenocarcinomas. *Am J Clin Pathol.* 1988;89(2):168–176.

Ji H, Isacson C, Seidman JD, Kurman RJ, Ronnett BM. Cytokeratins 7 and 20, Dpc4, and MUC5AC in the distinction of metastatic mucinous carcinomas in the ovary from primary ovarian mucinous tumors: Dpc4 assists in identifying metastatic pancreatic carcinomas. *Int J Gyn Pathol.* 2002;21(4):391–400.

Laury AR, Perets R, Piao H, et al. A comprehensive analysis of PAX8 expression in human epithelial tumors. *Am J Surg Pathol.* 2011;35(6):816–826.

Logani S, Oliva E, Arnell PM, Amin MB, Young RH. Use of novel immunohistochemical markers expressed in colonic adenocarcinoma to distinguish primary ovarian tumors from metastatic colorectal carcinoma. *Mod Pathol.* 2005;18(1):19–25.

Lugli A, Tzankov A, Zlobec I, Terracciano LM. Differential diagnostic and functional role of the multi-marker phenotype CDX2/CK20/CK7 in colorectal cancer stratified by mismatch repair status. *Mod Pathol.* 2008;21(11):1403–1412.

Magnusson K, de Wit M, Brennan DJ, et al. SATB2 in combination with cytokeratin 20 identifies over 95% of all colorectal carcinomas. *Am J Surg Pathol.* 2011;35(7):937–948.

Nonaka D, Chiriboga L, Rubin BP. Sox10: a pan-schwannian and melanocytic marker. *Am J Surg Pathol.* 2008;32(9):1291–1298.

Ordonez NG. Broad-spectrum immunohistochemical epithelial markers: a review. *Human Pathol.* 2013;44(7):1195–1215.

Ozcan A, Shen SS, Hamilton C, et al. PAX 8 expression in non-neoplastic tissues, primary tumors, and metastatic tumors: a comprehensive immunohistochemical study. *Mod Pathol.* 2011;24(6):751–764.

Panarelli NC, Yantiss RK, Yeh MM, Liu Y, Chen YT. Tissue-specific cadherin CDH17 is a useful marker of gastrointestinal adenocarcinomas with higher sensitivity than CDX2. *Am J Clin Pathol.* 2012;138(2):211–222.

Saad RS, Silverman JF, Khalifa MA, Rowsell C. CDX2, cytokeratins 7 and 20 immunoreactivity in rectal adenocarcinoma. *Appl Immunohistochem Mol Morphol.* 2009;17(3):196–201.

Tacha D, Zhou D, Cheng L. Expression of PAX8 in normal and neoplastic tissues: a comprehensive immunohistochemical study. *Appl Immunohistochem Mol Morphol.* 2011;19(4):293–299.

Taniere P, Borghi-Scoazec G, Saurin JC, et al. Cytokeratin expression in adenocarcinomas of the esophagogastric junction: a comparative study of adenocarcinomas of the distal esophagus and of the proximal stomach. *Am J Surg Pathol.* 2002;26(9):1213–1221.

Vang R, Gown AM, Wu LS, et al. Immunohistochemical expression of CDX2 in primary ovarian mucinous tumors and metastatic mucinous carcinomas involving the ovary: comparison with CK20 and correlation with coordinate expression of CK7. *Mod Pathol.* 2006;19(11):1421–1428.

Wang NP, Zee S, Zarbo RJ, Bacchi CE, Gown AM. Coordinate expression of cytokeratins 7 and 20 defined unique subsets of carcinomas. *Appl Immunohistochem.* 1995;3(2):99–107.

WHO Classification of Tumours of Soft Tissue and Bone. 4th ed. Lyon: IARC; 2013.

Winn B, Tavares R, Fanion J, et al. Differentiating the undifferentiated: immunohistochemical profile of medullary carcinoma of the colon with an emphasis on intestinal differentiation. *Hum Pathol.* 2009;40(3):398–404.

Yemelyanova AV, Vang R, Judson K, Wu LS, Ronnett BM. Distinction of primary and metastatic mucinous tumors involving the ovary: analysis of size and laterality data by primary site with reevaluation of an algorithm for tumor classification. *Am J Surg Pathol.* 2008;32(1):128–138.

Approach to Neuroendocrine Neoplasms

Bellizzi AM. Assigning site of origin in metastatic neuroendocrine neoplasms: a clinically significant application of diagnostic immunohistochemistry. *Adv Anat Pathol.* 2013;20(5):285–314.

Fischler DF, Bauer TW, Tubbs RR. Tissue reactivity of anti-Leu19. *Histopathology.* 1992;21(6):563–567.

Maxwell JE, Sherman SK, Stashek KM, O'Dorisio TM, Bellizzi AM, Howe JR. A practical method to determine the site of unknown primary in metastatic neuroendocrine tumors. *Surgery.* 2014;156(6):1359–1365; discussion 65–66.

Rindi G, Arnold R, Bosman FT, Capella C, Klimstra DS, Kloppel G, et al. Nomenclature and classification of neuroendocrine neoplams of the digestive system. In: Bosman FT, Carneiro F, Hruban RH, Theise ND, eds. *World Health Organization Classification of Tumours WHO Classification of Tumours of the Digestive System.* 4th. ed. Lyon: IARC; 2010:13–14.

van Velthuysen ML, Groen EJ, van der Noort V, van de Pol A, Tesselaar ME, Korse CM. Grading of Neuroendocrine Neoplasms: Mitoses and Ki-67 both Essential. Neuroendocrinology. 2014;100(2–3):221–227.

Approach to Hematolymphoid Tumors

Bagdi E, Diss TC, Munson P, Isaacson PG. Mucosal intra-epithelial lymphocytes in enteropathy-associated T-cell lymphoma, ulcerative jejunitis, and refractory celiac disease constitute a neoplastic population. *Blood.* 1999;94(1):260–264.

Chan JK, Chan AC, Cheuk W, Wan SK, Lee WK, Lui YH, et al. Type II enteropathy-associated T-cell lymphoma: a distinct aggressive lymphoma with frequent gammadelta T-cell receptor expression. *Am J Surg Pathol.* 2011;35(10):1557–1569.

Chu PG, Chen YY, Molina A, Arber DA, Weiss LM. Recurrent B-cell neoplasms after Rituximab therapy: an immunophenotypic and genotypic study. *Leuk Lymphoma.* 2002;43(12):2335–2341.

Dong HY, Scadden DT, de Leval L, Tang Z, Isaacson PG, Harris NL. Plasmablastic lymphoma in HIV-positive patients: an aggressive Epstein-Barr virus-associated extramedullary plasmacytic neoplasm. *Am J Surg Pathol.* 2005;29(12):1633–1641.

Dreyling M, Ferrero S, Vogt N, Klapper W. New paradigms in mantle cell lymphoma: is it time to risk-stratify treatment based on the proliferative signature? *Clin Cancer Res.* 2014;20(20):5194–5206.

Lai R, Weiss LM, Chang KL, Arber DA. Frequency of CD43 expression in non-Hodgkin lymphoma. A survey of 742 cases and further characterization of rare CD43+ follicular lymphomas. *Am J Clin Pahtol.* 1999;111(4):488–494.

Menasce LP, Banerjee SS, Beckett E, Harris M. Extra-medullary myeloid tumour (granulocytic sarcoma) is often misdiagnosed: a study of 26 cases. *Histopathology.* 1999;34(5):391–398.

O'Malley DP, Goldstein NS, Banks PM. The recognition and classification of lymphoproliferative disorders of the gut. *Hum Pathol.* 2014;45(5):899–916.

Oschlies I, Burkhardt B, Chassagne-Clement C, d'Amore ES, Hansson U, Hebeda K, et al. Diagnosis and immunophenotype of 188 pediatric lymphoblastic lymphomas treated within a randomized prospective trial: experiences and preliminary recommendations from the European childhood lymphoma pathology panel. *Am J Surg Pathol.* 2011;35(6):836–844.

Rubio-Tapia A, Murray JA. Classification and management of refractory coeliac disease. *Gut.* 2010;59(4):547–557.

Ruzinova MB, Caron T, Rodig SJ. Altered subcellular localization of c-Myc protein identifies aggressive B-cell lymphomas harboring a c-MYC translocation. *Am J Surg Pathol.* 2010;34(6):882–891.

Smith LB, Owens SR. Gastrointestinal lymphomas: entities and mimics. *Arch Pathol Lab Med.* 2012;136(8):865–870.

Swerdlow SH, Yang WI, Zukerberg LR, Harris NL, Arnold A, Williams ME. Expression of cyclin D1 protein in centrocytic/mantle cell lymphomas with and without rearrangement of the BCL1/cyclin D1 gene. *Hum Pathol.* 1995;26(9):999–1004.

Wu TT, Swerdlow SH, Locker J, Bahler D, Randhawa P, Yunis EJ, et al. Recurrent Epstein-Barr virus-associated lesions in organ transplant recipients. *Hum Pathol.* 1996;27(2):157–164.

Approach to Mesenchymal Tumors

Arber DA, Tamayo R, Weiss LM. Paraffin section detection of the c-kit gene product (CD117) in human tissues: value in the diagnosis of mast cell disorders. *Hum Pathol.* 1998;29(5):498–504.

Bhattacharya B, Dilworth HP, Iacobuzio-Donahue C, et al. Nuclear beta-catenin expression distinguishes deep fibromatosis from other benign and malignant fibroblastic and myofibroblastic lesions. *Am J Surg Pathol.* 2005;29(5):653–659.

Carlson JW, Fletcher CD. Immunohistochemistry for beta-catenin in the differential diagnosis of spindle cell lesions: analysis of a series and review of the literature. *Histopathology.* 2007;51(4):509–514.

Coffin CM, Watterson J, Priest JR, Dehner LP. Extrapulmonary inflammatory myofibroblastic tumor (inflammatory pseudotumor). A clinicopathologic and immunohistochemical study of 84 cases. *Am J Surg Pathol.* 1995;19(8):859–872.

Cook JR, Dehner LP, Collins MH, et al. Anaplastic lymphoma kinase (ALK) expression in the inflammatory myofibroblastic tumor: a comparative immunohistochemical study. *Am J Surg Pahtol.* 2001;25(11):1364–1371.

Deshpande A, Nelson D, Corless CL, Deshpande V, O'Brien MJ. Leiomyoma of the gastrointestinal tract with interstitial cells of Cajal: a mimic of gastrointestinal stromal tumor. *Am J Surg Pathol.* 2014;38(1):72–77.

Doyle LA, Hornick JL, Fletcher CD. PEComa of the gastrointestinal tract: clinicopathologic study of 35 cases with evaluation of prognostic parameters. *Am J Surg Pathol.* 2013;37(12):1769–1782.

Espinosa I, Lee CH, Kim MK, et al. A novel monoclonal antibody against DOG1 is a sensitive and specific marker for gastrointestinal stromal tumors. *Am J Surg Pathol.* 2008;32(2):210–218.

Foo WC, Cruise MW, Wick MR, Hornick JL. Immunohistochemical staining for TLE1 distinguishes synovial sarcoma from histologic mimics. *Am J Surg Pathol.* 2011;135(6):839–844.

Gibson JA, Hornick JL. Mucosal Schwann cell "hamartoma": clinicopathologic study of 26 neural colorectal polyps distinct from neurofibromas and mucosal neuromas. *Am J Surg Pathol.* 2009;33(5):781–787.

Gill AJ, Chou A, Vilain R, et al. Immunohistochemistry for SDHB divides gastrointestinal stromal tumors (GISTs) into 2 distinct types. *Am J Surg Pathol.* 2010;34(5):636–644.

Hollowood K, Stamp G, Zouvani I, Fletcher CD. Extranodal follicular dendritic cell sarcoma of the gastrointestinal tract. Morphologic, immunohistochemical and ultrastructural analysis of two cases. *Am J Clin Pathol.* 1995;103(1):90–97.

Hornick JL, Fletcher CD. Immunohistochemical staining for KIT (CD117) in soft tissue sarcomas is very limited in distribution. *Am J Clin Pathol.* 2002;117(2):188–193.

Hornick JL, Fletcher CD. Intestinal perineuriomas: clinicopathologic definition of a new anatomic subset in a series of 10 cases. *Am J Surg Pathol.* 2005;29(7):859–865.

Hornick JL, Fletcher CD. Validating immunohistochemical staining for KIT (CD117). *Am J Clin Pathol.* 2003;119(3):325–327.

Iwata J, Fletcher CD. Immunohistochemical detection of cytokeratin and epithelial membrane antigen in leiomyosarcoma: a systematic study of 100 cases. *Pathol Int.* 2000;50(1):7–14.

Killian JK, Miettinen M, Walker RL, Wang Y, Zhu YJ, Waterfall JJ, et al. Recurrent epimutation of SDHC in gastrointestinal stromal tumors. *Sci Transl Med.* 2014;6(268):268ra177.

Lasota J, Wang ZF, Sobin LH, Miettinen M. Gain-of-function PDGFRA mutations, earlier reported in gastrointestinal stromal tumors, are common in small intestinal inflammatory fibroid polyps. A study of 60 cases. *Mod Pathol.* 2009;22(8):1049–1056.

Lee CH, Liang CW, Espinosa I. The utility of discovered on gastrointestinal stromal tumor 1 (DOG1) antibody in surgical pathology-the GIST of it. *Adv Anat Pathol* 2010;17(3):222–232.

Liu TC, Lin MT, Montgomery EA, Singhi AD. Inflammatory fibroid polyps of the gastrointestinal tract: spectrum of clinical, morphologic, and immunohistochemistry features. *Am J Surg Pathol.* 2013;37(4):586–592.

Lopes LF, West RB, Bacchi LM, van de Rijn M, Bacchi CE. DOG1 for the diagnosis of gastrointestinal stromal tumor (GIST): Comparison between 2 different antibodies. *Appl Immunohistochem Mol Morphol.* 2010;18(4):333–337.

Lucas DR, al-Abbadi M, Tabaczka P, Hamre MR, Weaver DW, Mott MJ. c-Kit expression in desmoid fibromatosis. Comparative immunohistochemical evaluation of two commercial antibodies. *Am J Clin Pathol.* 2003;119(3):339–345.

Makhlouf HR, Ahrens W, Agarwal B, et al. Synovial sarcoma of the stomach: a clinicopathologic, immunohistochemical, and molecular genetic study of 10 cases. *Am J Surg Pathol.* 2008;32(2):275–281.

Medeiros F, Corless CL, Duensing A, et al. KIT-negative gastrointestinal stromal tumors: proof of concept and therapeutic implications. *Am J Surg Pathol.* 2004;28(7):889–894.

Miettinen M, Dow N, Lasota J, Sobin LH. A distinctive novel epitheliomesenchymal biphasic tumor of the stomach in young adults ("gastroblastoma"): a series of 3 cases. *Am J Surg Pathol.* 2009;33(9):1370–1377.

Miettinen M, Furlong M, Sarlomo-Rikala M, Burke A, Sobin LH, Lasota J. Gastrointestinal stromal tumors, intramural leiomyomas, and leiomyosarcomas in the rectum and anus: a clinicopathologic, immunohistochemical, and molecular genetic study of 144 cases. *Am J Surg Pathol.* 2001;25(9):1121–1233.

Miettinen M, Kopczynski J, Makhlouf HR, et al. Gastrointestinal stromal tumors, intramural leiomyomas, and leiomyosarcomas in the duodenum: a clinicopathologic, immunohistochemical, and molecular genetic study of 167 cases. *Am J Surg Pathol.* 2003;27(5):625–641.

Miettinen M, Makhlouf HR, Sobin LH, Lasota J. Plexiform fibromyxoma: a distinctive benign gastric antral neoplasm not to be confused with a myxoid GIST. *Am J Surg Pathol.* 2009;33(11):1624–1632.

Miettinen M, Paal E, Lasota J, Sobin LH. Gastrointestinal glomus tumors: a clinicopathologic, immunohistochemical, and molecular genetic study of 32 cases. *Am J Surg Pathol.* 2002;26(3):301–311.

Miettinen M, Sarlomo-Rikala M, Sobin LH, Lasota J. Gastrointestinal stromal tumors and leiomyosarcomas in the colon: a clinicopathologic, immunohistochemical, and molecular genetic study of 44 cases. *Am J Surg Pathol.* 2000;24(10):1339–1352.

Miettinen M, Virolainen M, Maarit Sarlomo R. Gastrointestinal stromal tumors—value of CD34 antigen in their identification and separation from true leiomyomas and schwannomas. *Am J Surg Pathol.* 1995;19(2):207–216.

Miettinen M, Wang ZF, Lasota J. DOG1 antibody in the differential diagnosis of gastrointestinal stromal tumors: a study of 1840 cases. *Am J Surg Pathol.* 2009;33(9):1401–1408.

Miettinen M, Wang ZF, Sarlomo-Rikala M, Osuch C, Rutkowski P, Lasota J. Succinate dehydrogenase-deficient GISTs: a clinicopathologic, immunohistochemical, and molecular genetic study of 66 gastric GISTs with predilection to young age. *Am J Surg Pathol.* 2011;35(11):1712–1721.

Miettinen M. Immunoreactivity for cytokeratin and epithelial membrane antigen in leiomyosarcoma. *Arch Pathol Lab Med.* 1988;112(6):637–640.

Miselli F, Millefanti C, Conca E, Negri T, Piacenza C, Pierotti MA, et al. PDGFRA immunostaining can help in the diagnosis of gastrointestinal stromal tumors. *Am J Surg Pathol.* 2008;32(5):738–743.

Montgomery E, Torbenson MS, Kaushal M, Fisher C, Abraham SC. Beta-catenin immunohistochemistry separates mesenteric fibromatosis from gastrointestinal stromal tumor and sclerosing mesenteritis. *Am J Surg Pathol.* 2002;26(10):1296–1301.

Montone KT, van Belle P, Elenitsas R, Elder DE. Proto-oncogene c-kit expression in malignant melanoma: protein loss with tumor progression. *Mod Pathol.* 1997;10(9):939–944.

Parfitt JR, Rodriguez-Justo M, Feakins R, Novelli MR. Gastrointestinal Kaposi's sarcoma: CD117 expression and the potential for misdiagnosis as gastrointestinal stromal tumour. *Histopathology.* 2008;52(7):816–823.

Pileri SA, Grogan TM, Harris NL, et al. Tumours of histiocytes and accessory dendritic cells: an immunohistochemical approach to classification from the International Lymphoma Study Group based on 61 cases. *Histopathology.* 2002;41(1):1–29.

Prevot S, Bienvenu L, Vaillant JC, de Saint-Maur PP. Benign schwannoma of the digestive tract: a clinicopathologic and immunohistochemical study of five cases, including a case of esophageal tumor. *Am J Surg Pathol.* 1999;23(4):431–436.

Sarlomo-Rikala M, Kovatich AJ, Barusevicius A, Miettinen M. CD117: a sensitive marker for gastrointestinal stromal tumors that is more specific than CD34. *Mod Pathol.* 1998;11(8):728–734.

Shin DH, Lee JH, Kang HJ, et al. Novel epitheliomesenchymal biphasic stomach tumour (gastroblastoma) in a 9-year-old: morphological, ultrastructural and immunohistochemical findings. *J Clin Pathol.* 2010;63(3):270–274.

Singhi AD, Montgomery EA. Colorectal granular cell tumor: a clinicopathologic study of 26 cases. *Am J Surg Pathol.* 2010;34(8):1186–1192.

Stockman DL, Miettinen M, Suster S, Spagnolo D, Dominguez-Malagon H, Hornick JL, et al. Malignant gastrointestinal neuroectodermal tumor: clinicopathologic, immunohistochemical, ultrastructural, and molecular analysis of 16 cases with a reappraisal of clear cell sarcoma-like tumors of the gastrointestinal tract. *Am J Surg Pathol.* 2012;36(6):857–868.

Terry J, Saito T, Subramanian S, et al. TLE1 as a diagnostic immunohistochemical marker for synovial sarcoma emerging from gene expression profiling studies. *Am J Surg Pathol.* 2007;31(2):240–246.

Wong NA, Campbell F, Shepherd NA. Abdominal monophasic synovial sarcoma is a morphological and immunohistochemical mimic of gastrointestinal stromal tumour. *Histopathology.* 2015;66(7):974–981.

Yamamoto H, Oda Y, Saito T, et al. p53 Mutation and MDM2 amplification in inflammatory myofibroblastic tumours. *Histopathology.* 2003;42(5):431–439.

Barrett's Associated Dysplasia and Carcinoma

Baas IO, Mulder JW, Offerhaus GJ, Vogelstein B, Hamilton SR. An evaluation of six antibodies for immunohistochemistry of mutant p53 gene product in archival colorectal neoplasms. *J Pathol.* 1994;172(1):5–12.

Fels Elliott DR, Fitzgerald RC. Molecular markers for Barrett's esophagus and its progression to cancer. *Curr Opin Gastroenterol.* 2013;29(4):437–445.

Finlay CA, Hinds PW, Tan TH, Eliyahu D, Oren M, Levine AJ. Activating mutations for transformation by p53 produce a gene product that forms an hsc70-p53 complex with an altered half-life. *Mol Cell Biol.* 1988;8(2):531–539.

Kastelein F, Biermann K, Steyerberg EW, et al. Aberrant p53 protein expression is associated with an increased risk of neoplastic progression in patients with Barrett's oesophagus. *Gut.* 2013;62:1676–1683.

Kaye PV, Haider SA, Ilyas M, et al. Barrett's dysplasia and the Vienna classification: reproducibility, prediction of progression and impact of consensus reporting and p53 immunohistochemistry. *Histopathology.* 2009;54(6):699–712.

Kaye PV, Haider SA, James PD, et al. Novel staining pattern of p53 in Barrett's dysplasia—the absent pattern. *Histopathology.* 2010;57(6):933–935.

Poorly Differentiated Esophageal Carcinoma

DiMaio MA, Kwok S, Montgomery KD, Lowe AW, Pai RK. Immunohistochemical panel for distinguishing esophageal adenocarcinoma from squamous cell carcinoma: a combination of p63, cytokeratin 5/6, MUC5AC, and anterior gradient homolog 2 allows optimal subtyping. *Hum Pathol.* 2012;43(11):1799–1807.

Huang Q, Wu H, Nie L, et al. Primary high-grade neuroendocrine carcinoma of the esophagus: a clinicopathologic and immunohistochemical study of 42 resection cases. *Am J Surg Pathol.* 2013;37(4):467–483.

Long KB, Hornick JL. SOX2 is highly expressed in squamous cell carcinomas of the gastrointestinal tract. *Hum Pathol.* 2009;40(12):1768–1773.

Pai RK, West RB. MOC-31 exhibits superior reactivity compared with Ber-EP4 in invasive lobular and ductal carcinoma of the breast: a tissue microarray study. *Appl Immunohistochem Mol Morphol.* 2009;17(3):202–206.

Distinguishing Poorly Cohesive Gastric Cancer From Metastatic Lobular Breast Cancer

Chu PG, Weiss LM. Immunohistochemical characterization of signet-ring cell carcinomas of the stomach, breast, and colon. *Am J Clin Pathol.* 2004;121(6):884–892.

Harris M, Howell A, Chrissohou M, Swindell RI, Hudson M, Sellwood RA. A comparison of the metastatic pattern of infiltrating lobular carcinoma and infiltrating duct carcinoma of the breast. *Br J Cancer.* 1984;50(1):23–30.

McLemore EC, Pockaj BA, Reynolds C, et al. Breast cancer: presentation and intervention in women with gastrointestinal metastasis and carcinomatosis. *Ann Surg Oncol.* 2005;12(11):886–894.

Miettinen M, McCue PA, Sarlomo-Rikala M, et al. GATA3: a multispecific but potentially useful marker in surgical pathology: a systematic analysis of 2500 epithelial and nonepithelial tumors. *Am J Surg Pathol.* 2014;38(1):13–22.

Nazareno J, Taves D, Preiksaitis HG. Metastatic breast cancer to the gastrointestinal tract: a case series and review of the literature. *World J Gastroenterol.* 2006;12(38):6219–6224.

Nguyen MD, Plasil B, Wen P, Frankel WL. Mucin profiles in signet-ring cell carcinoma. *Arch Pathol Lab Med.* 2006;130(6):799–804.

O'Connell FP, Wang HH, Odze RD. Utility of immunohistochemistry in distinguishing primary adenocarcinomas from metastatic breast carcinomas in the gastrointestinal tract. *Arch Pathol Lab Med.* 2005;129(3):338–347.

Ordonez NG. Value of GATA3 immunostaining in tumor diagnosis: a review. *Adv Anat Pathol.* 2013;20(5):352–360.

HER2 Assessment in Gastroesophageal Adenocarcinoma

Bang YJ, Van Cutsem E, Feyereislova A, Chung HC, Shen L, Sawaki A, et al. Trastuzumab in combination with chemotherapy versus chemotherapy alone for treatment of HER2-positive advanced gastric or gastro-oesophageal junction cancer (ToGA): a phase 3, open-label, randomised controlled trial. *Lancet.* 2010;376(9742):687–697.

Bozzetti C, Negri FV, Lagrasta CA, Crafa P, Bassano C, Tamagnini I, et al. Comparison of HER2 status in primary and paired metastatic sites of gastric carcinoma. *Br J Cancer.* 2011;104(9):1372–1376.

Hofmann M, Stoss O, Shi D, et al. Assessment of a HER2 scoring system for gastric cancer: results from a validation study. *Histopathology.* 2008;52(7):797–805.

Lee S, de Boer WB, Fermoyle S, Platten M, Kumarasinghe MP. Human epidermal growth factor receptor 2 testing in gastric carcinoma: issues related to heterogeneity in biopsies and resections. *Histopathology.* 2011;59(5):832–840.

Perrone G, Amato M, Callea M, et al. HER2 amplification status in gastric and gastro-oesophageal junction cancer in routine clinical practice: which sample should be used? *Histopathology.* 2012;61(1):134–135.

Ruschoff J, Dietel M, Baretton G, et al. HER2 diagnostics in gastric cancer-guideline validation and development of standardized immunohistochemical testing. *Virchows Arch.* 2010;457(3):299–307.

Ruschoff J, Hanna W, Bilous M, et al. HER2 testing in gastric cancer: a practical approach. *Mod Pathol.* 2012;25(5):637–650.

Mismatch Repair Protein Immunohistochemistry

Bao F, Panarelli NC, Rennert H, Sherr DL, Yantiss RK. Neoadjuvant therapy induces loss of MSH6 expression in colorectal carcinoma. *Am J Surg Pathol.* 2010;34(12):1798–1804.

Bellizzi AM, Frankel WL. Colorectal cancer due to deficiency in DNA mismatch repair function: a review. *Adv Anat Pathol.* 2009;16(6):405–417.

Boland CR. The mystery of mismatch repair deficiency: lynch or lynch-like? *Gastroenterology.* 2013;144(5):868–870.

Carethers JM. Differentiating Lynch-like from Lynch syndrome. *Gastroenterology*. 2014;146(3):602–604.

Engstrom PF, Arnoletti JP, Benson AB 3rd, et al. NCCN Clinical Practice Guidelines in Oncology: Colon Cancer. J Natl Compr Canc Netw. 2009;7(8):778–831. http://www.nccn.org/professionals/physician_gls/pdf/colon.pdf

Evaluation of Genomic Applications in Practice and Prevention (EGAPP) Working Group. Recommendations from the EGAPP Working Group: genetic testing strategies in newly diagnosed individuals with colorectal cancer aimed at reducing morbidity and mortality from Lynch syndrome in relatives. *Genet Med*. 2009;11(1):35–41.

Fadhil W, Field J, Cross G, Kaye P, Ilyas M. Immunostaining in the context of loss mismatch repair function: interpretive confounders and cautionary tales! *Histopathology*. 2012;61(3):522–525.

Funkhouser WK, Jr., Lubin IM, Monzon FA, et al. Relevance, pathogenesis, and testing algorithm for mismatch repair-defective colorectal carcinomas: a report of the association for molecular pathology. *J Mol Diagn*. 2012;14(2):91–103.

Hampel H. NCCN increases the emphasis on genetic/familial high-risk assessment in colorectal cancer. J Natl Compr Canc Netw. 2014;12(5):829–831. http://www.nccn.org/professionals/physician_gls/pdf/genetics_colon.pdf

Haraldsdottir S, Hampel H, Tomsic J, et al. Colon and endometrial cancers with mismatch repair deficiency can arise from somatic, rather than germline, mutations. *Gastroenterology*. 2014;147(6):1308–1316.

Hyde A, Fontaine D, Stuckless S, et al. A histology-based model for predicting microsatellite instability in colorectal cancers. *Am J Surg Pathol*. 2010;34(12):1820–1829.

Jenkins MA, Hayashi S, O'Shea AM, et al. Pathology features in Bethesda guidelines predict colorectal cancer microsatellite instability: a population-based study. *Gastroenterology*. 2007;133(1):48–56.

Mensenkamp AR, Vogelaar IP, van Zelst-Stams WA, et al. Somatic mutations in MLH1 and MSH2 are a frequent cause of mismatch-repair deficiency in Lynch syndrome-like tumors. *Gastroenterology*. 2014;146(3):643–646.

Radu OM, Nikiforova MN, Farkas LM, Krasinskas AM. Challenging cases encountered in colorectal cancer screening for Lynch syndrome reveal novel findings: nucleolar MSH6 staining and impact of prior chemoradiation therapy. *Hum Pathol*. 2011;42(9):1247–1258.

Rodriguez-Soler M, Perez-Carbonell L, Guarinos C, et al. Risk of cancer in cases of suspected lynch syndrome without germline mutation. *Gastroenterology*. 2013;144(5):926–932.

Shia J, Stadler Z, Weiser MR, et al. Immunohistochemical staining for DNA mismatch repair proteins in intestinal tract carcinoma: how reliable are biopsy samples? *Am J Surg Pathol*. 2011;35(3):447–454.

Sourrouille I, Coulet F, Lefevre JH, et al. Somatic mosaicism and double somatic hits can lead to MSI colorectal tumors. *Fam Cancer*. 2013;12(1):27–33.

EPCAM Immunohistochemistry

Huth C, Kloor M, Voigt AY, et al. The molecular basis of EPCAM expression loss in Lynch syndrome-associated tumors. *Mod Pathol*. 2012;25(6):911–916.

Kloor M, Voigt AY, Schackert HK, Schirmacher P, von Knebel Doeberitz M, Blaker H. Analysis of EPCAM protein expression in diagnostics of Lynch syndrome. *J Clin Oncol*. 2011;29(2):223–227.

Musulen E, Blanco I, Carrato C, et al. Usefulness of epithelial cell adhesion molecule expression in the algorithmic approach to Lynch syndrome identification. *Hum Pathol*. 2013;44(3):412–416.

BRAF V600E Mutation-Specific Immunohistochemistry

Adackapara CA, Sholl LM, Barletta JA, Hornick JL. Immunohistochemistry using the BRAF V600E mutation-specific monoclonal antibody VE1 is not a useful surrogate for genotyping in colorectal adenocarcinoma. *Histopathology*. 2013;63(2):187–193.

Affolter K, Samowitz W, Tripp S, Bronner MP. BRAF V600E mutation detection by immunohistochemistry in colorectal carcinoma. *Genes Chromosomes Cancer*. 2013;52(8):748–752.

Capper D, Voigt A, Bozukova G, et al. BRAF V600E-specific immunohistochemistry for the exclusion of Lynch syndrome in MSI-H colorectal cancer. *Int J Cancer*. 2013;133(7):1624–1630.

Kuan SF, Navina S, Cressman KL, Pai RK. Immunohistochemical detection of BRAF V600E mutant protein using the VE1 antibody in colorectal carcinoma is highly concordant with molecular testing but requires rigorous antibody optimization. *Hum Pathol*. 2014;45(3):464–472.

Lasota J, Kowalik A, Wasag B, et al. Detection of the BRAF V600E mutation in colon carcinoma: critical evaluation of the imunohistochemical approach. *Am J Surg Pathol*. 2014;38(9):1235–1241.

Sinicrope FA, Smyrk TC, Tougeron D, et al. Mutation-specific antibody detects mutant BRAFV600E protein expression in human colon carcinomas. *Cancer*. 2013;119(15):2765–2770.

Mismatch Repair Immunohistochemistry in Colon Polyps

Halvarsson B, Lindblom A, Johansson L, Lagerstedt K, Nilbert M. Loss of mismatch repair protein immunostaining in colorectal adenomas from patients with hereditary nonpolyposis colorectal cancer. *Mod Pathol*. 2005;18(8):1095–1101.

Sheridan TB, Fenton H, Lewin MR, et al. Sessile serrated adenomas with low- and high-grade dysplasia and early carcinomas: an immunohistochemical study of serrated lesions "caught in the act". *Am J Clin Pathol*. 2006;126(4):564–571.

Walsh MD, Buchanan DD, Pearson SA, et al. Immunohistochemical testing of conventional adenomas for loss of expression of mismatch repair proteins in Lynch syndrome mutation carriers: a case series from the Australasian site of the colon cancer family registry. *Mod Pathol*. 2012;25(5):722–30.

Anal Squamous Intraepithelial Lesions/ Intraepithelial Neoplasia (SIL/AIN)

Bala R, Pinsky BA, Beck AH, Kong CS, Welton ML, Longacre TA. p16 is superior to ProEx C in identifying high-grade squamous intraepithelial lesions (HSIL) of the anal canal. *Am J Surg Pathol*. 2013;37(5):659–668.

Bean SM, Eltoum I, Horton DK, Whitlow L, Chhieng DC. Immunohistochemical expression of p16 and Ki-67 correlates with degree of anal intraepithelial neoplasia. *Am J Surg Pathol*. 2007;31(4):555–561.

Bernard JE, Butler MO, Sandweiss L, Weidner N. Anal intraepithelial neoplasia: correlation of grade with p16INK4a immunohistochemistry and HPV in situ hybridization. *Appl Immunohistochem Mol Morphol*. 2008;16(3):215–220.

Pirog EC, Quint KD, Yantiss RK. P16/CDKN2A and Ki-67 enhance the detection of anal intraepithelial neoplasia and condyloma and correlate with human papillomavirus detection by polymerase chain reaction. *Am J Surg Pathol*. 2010;34(10):1449–1455.

Walts AE, Lechago J, Bose S. P16 and Ki67 immunostaining is a useful adjunct in the assessment of biopsies for HPV-associated anal intraepithelial neoplasia. *Am J Surg Pathol*. 2006;30(7):795–801.

Approach to Tumors Presenting in a Pagetoid Fashion in the Anal Canal

Diaz de Leon E, Carcangiu ML, Prieto VG, et al. Extramammary Paget disease is characterized by the consistent lack of estrogen and progesterone receptors but frequently expresses androgen receptor. *Am J Clin Pathol*. 2000;113(4):572–575.

Fogel BJ, Lai KK, Lindberg MR, Lamps LW, Quick CM. Pathologic Features Differentiating High-Grade Anal Squamous Intraepithelial Lesions from Reactive Transition Zone. *Mod Pathol*. 2014;27(Suppl 2):173A.

Goldblum JR, Hart WR. Perianal Paget's disease: a histologic and immunohistochemical study of 11 cases with and without associated rectal adenocarcinoma. *Am J Surg Pathol*. 1998;22(2):170–179.

Goyal A, Zhang G, Yang B. Immunohistochemical Expression of GATA3 in Primary Extramammary Paget Disease of the Vulva. *Mod Pathol*. 2014;27(Suppl 2):284A.

Nowak MA, Guerriere-Kovach P, Pathan A, Campbell TE, Deppisch LM. Perianal Paget's disease: distinguishing primary and secondary lesions using immunohistochemical studies including gross cystic disease fluid protein-15 and cytokeratin 20 expression. *Arch Pathol Lab Med*. 1998;122(12):1077–1081.

Ohnishi T, Watanabe S. The use of cytokeratins 7 and 20 in the diagnosis of primary and secondary extramammary Paget's disease. *Br J Dermatol*. 2000;142(2):243–247.

Ramalingam P, Hart WR, Goldblum JR. Cytokeratin subset immunostaining in rectal adenocarcinoma and normal anal glands. *Arch Pathol Lab Med*. 2001;125(8):1074–1077.

Sah SP, Kelly PJ, McManus DT, McCluggage WG. Diffuse CK7, CAM5.2 and BerEP4 positivity in pagetoid squamous cell carcinoma in situ (pagetoid Bowen's disease) of the perianal region: a mimic of extramammary Paget's disease. *Histopathology*. 2013;62(3):511–514.

Zeng HA, Cartun R, Ricci A, Jr. Potential diagnostic utility of CDX-2 immunophenotyping in extramammary Paget's disease. *Appl Immunohistochem Mol Morphol*. 2005;13(4):342–346.

Zhou L, Rao X, Jia L, et al. GATA3 is Expressed in Vulvar Paget's Disease. *Mod Pathol*. 2014;27(Suppl 2):314A.

Basaloid Squamous Cell Carcinoma Versus Basal Cell Carcinoma at the Anal Margin

Patil DT, Goldblum JR, Billings SD. Clinicopathological analysis of basal cell carcinoma of the anal region and its distinction from basaloid squamous cell carcinoma. *Mod Pathol*. 2013;26(10):1382–1389.

14

Applications of Molecular Pathology

RHONDA K. YANTISS

INTRODUCTION

Gastrointestinal carcinomas account for more cancer-related deaths than those of any other organ system. Recent discoveries have uncovered key genetic, epigenetic, and post-transcriptional regulatory mechanisms underlying their development, some of which may be exploited for diagnostic and therapeutic purposes. Detection of tumor suppressor or mismatch repair deficiencies may identify patients and family members with heritable cancer risk, whereas elucidation of cellular signal transduction pathways continues to uncover proteins involved in cell survival and proliferation. Many of these molecules represent predictors of response to, or potential targets of, directed medical therapies.

Although a comprehensive discussion of the molecular abnormalities of all types of gastrointestinal malignancy is beyond the scope of this chapter, its purpose is to discuss molecular changes that are important for pathologists to understand as they participate in the care of cancer patients, both in terms of diagnosis, risk assessment, and emerging treatment strategies (see Table 14.1). In addition, the majority of the prognostic and therapeutic molecular assays discussed in this chapter are now considered the standard of care for patient management.

TERMINOLOGY

Oncogenes

Proto-oncogenes encode regulatory proteins important to embryogenesis, proliferation, differentiation, and apoptosis.

They include a variety of growth factors, growth factor receptors, members of signal transduction pathways, and transcription factors that are normally produced in small quantities and rapidly degraded. Proto-oncogenes are classified as oncogenes when genetic alterations, such as point mutations, chromosomal translocations, and amplification, lead to dysregulation of their protein products and an overall "gain of function." Alterations of only one allele are generally sufficient to cause oncoprotein dysregulation. A number of oncogenes have been implicated in the pathogenesis of gastrointestinal malignancies and are routinely evaluated in clinical situations, namely *HER2, EGFR, KIT, KRAS,* and *BRAF.*

Tumor Suppressor Genes

Tumor suppressor genes are highly conserved across species and encode proteins that suppress transcription of proto-oncogenes. They can be inactivated through mutations, translocations, loss of heterozygosity (LOH), and promoter hypermethylation that silences transcription. One functional allele is generally sufficient to regulate proto-oncogenes, so dysregulation usually requires inactivation of both tumor suppressor gene alleles. Most heritable cancer syndromes result from germline mutations affecting tumor suppressor genes, in which case each cell harbors one dysfunctional allele. Inactivation of the second allele may result from a second mutation, but more often reflects hypermethylation of its promoter region. The *APC* gene is one example of a tumor suppressor gene important to colorectal carcinogenesis; others include *MUTYH, MLH1, PMS2, MSH2,* and *MSH6.*

TABLE 14.1 Summary of Diagnostic, Therapeutic, and Predictive Molecular Tests in Gastrointestinal Neoplasia

Molecular Feature Assessed	Methodology	Clinical Scenario
HER2	In situ hybridization (ISH), fluorescence in situ hybridization (FISH), immunohistochemistry	Adenocarcinoma of the esophagus, stomach, and gastroesophageal junction
CDH1	Germline testing	Suspected hereditary diffuse gastric cancer
APC	Germline testing	Suspected familial adenomatous polyposis
MUTYH	Germline testing	Suspected familial adenomatous polyposis, but APC wild-type
SMAD4	Germline testing	Suspected juvenile polyposis syndrome
BMPR1A	Germline testing	Suspected juvenile polyposis syndrome
LKB1/STK11	Germline testing	Suspected Peutz–Jeghers polyposis syndrome
PTEN	Germline testing	Suspected PTEN hamartoma tumor syndrome
SDHB and SDHD	Germline testing	Suspected PTEN hamartoma tumor syndrome, but wild-type PTEN in some reports
DNA Mismatch Repair Mechanisms	Microsatellite instability (MSI) Immunohistochemistry for MLH1, MSH2, PMS2, MSH6 Germline MLH1, MSH2, PMS2, or MSH6 based on results of immunohistochemistry	Suspected Lynch syndrome
BRAF	Mutational testing in tumor	Suspected Lynch syndrome; loss of MLH1/PMS2 with BRAF mutation is virtually diagnostic of sporadic tumor
KRAS	Mutational testing in tumor	Management of advanced colorectal carcinoma
KIT	Mutational testing in tumor	Gastrointestinal stromal tumor
PDGFRA	Mutational testing in tumor	Gastrointestinal stromal tumor with wild-type KIT
SDHA and SDHB	Immunohistochemistry mutational testing in tumor based on results of immunohistochemistry	Gastrointestinal stromal tumor; immunohistochemistry used to screen for tumors with succinate dehydrogenase deficiency Mutations occur in KIT/PDGFRA wild-type tumors

MicroRNAs

MicroRNAs comprise a recently recognized class of molecules involved in the post-transcriptional regulation of protein expression. These short, noncoding sequences are part of complexes that bind to mRNA strands and prevent their translation. MicroRNAs may have either growth promoting or tumor suppressor activity. Some microRNAs normally suppress translation of oncogenic mRNA transcripts, thus negatively regulating cell proliferation. Decreased expression of these microRNA species promotes cell proliferation by removing their inhibitory effects. Conversely, abnormally increased expression of microRNAs that prevent translation of tumor suppressor gene transcripts further diminish their capacity to regulate cell growth. Data from preliminary studies indicate that microRNAs may be of predictive value or represent attractive therapeutic targets among gastrointestinal malignancies. Several agents that inhibit microRNAs show some promise as therapeutic agents in vitro and in animal studies. Antisense oligonucleotides comprise one class of such molecules that competitively inhibit microRNAs, whereas microRNA sponges consist of synthetic polynucleotides that contain multiple tandem sequences complementary to specific miRNAs. These sponges act as decoy transcripts to sequester miRNA complexes and prevent their binding to mRNA transcripts. Some investigators have also developed techniques to introduce deficient microRNAs into tumor cells. Clinical applications of microRNA technology are at an early stage of development and none are currently utilized in the management of cancer patients.

KEY MOLECULAR FEATURES OF GASTROINTESTINAL MALIGNANCIES

Barrett Esophagus and Associated Adenocarcinoma

Overview

Adenocarcinomas of the distal esophagus and proximal stomach (ie, cardia) share similar epidemiologic and histologic features (see also Chapters 7 and 8). Most are associated with gastroesophageal reflux disease and intestinal metaplasia, although some tumors arising in the cardia develop in association with *Helicobacter pylori* related pangastritis and display epidemiologic features typical of distal gastric carcinomas. Metaplastic epithelium in this location is genetically unstable and prone to accumulate molecular changes, even in the absence of dysplasia. The acquisition of genetic events confers a growth advantage to clonal subpopulations, leading to the evolution of low-grade dysplasia, high-grade dysplasia, and, ultimately, invasive carcinoma. The overall cancer risk of Barrett esophagus is relatively low (less than 2%), but increases among patients with low-grade (10%) and high-grade dysplasia (25%). Cancer risk among patients with intestinal metaplasia limited to the gastric cardia is even lower than that of Barrett esophagus, presumably reflecting the smaller surface area affected by metaplasia.

Molecular Alterations

Specific molecular changes in nondysplastic epithelium may predict subsequent cancer risk among patients with intestinal metaplasia of the esophagus and gastroesophageal junction. Abnormal DNA content and LOH at 17p (*TP53*) and 9p, as well as overexpression of cyclins D1 and E, are strongly associated with the development of esophageal adenocarcinoma. Messenger RNA levels of inducible nitric oxide synthase progressively increase among patients with gastroesophageal reflux disease, Barrett esophagus, and esophageal adenocarcinoma. This enzyme facilitates production of free nitric oxide radicals, which generate reactive oxygen and nitrogen species that promote DNA alterations, post-translational modification of TP53, and oxidization of thiols, all of which contribute to carcinogenesis. Finally, the NF (nuclear factor)-κB signaling cascade plays an important role in stress responses, immune cell activation, apoptosis, proliferation, and differentiation. Increased NF-κB levels also show an inverse correlation with a robust pathologic response to neoadjuvant therapy, suggesting that this marker may be of predictive value among patients with adenocarcinomas of the distal esophagus and gastroesophageal junction.

In addition to the above-mentioned features, most adenocarcinomas of the esophagus and gastroesophageal junction show alterations in tumor suppressor genes, oncogenes, growth factor receptors, or enzymes involved in cell signaling. Common mechanisms of dysregulation include chromosomal instability, amplification, and epigenetic modification of key genes. Alterations of *TP53* resulting from mutations and LOH are detected in up to 80% of cases. Amplification of chromosomes 7p (*EGFR*), 8q (*MYC*), and 17q (*ERBB2*) are detected in more than 40% of cases. Hypermethylation, or LOH, involving *CDKN2A/p16* is detected in up to 80% of cases and occurs early in cancer development. Promoter methylation of *CDH1*, *APC*, *MGMT*, and *TMEFF2/HPP1* is also common.

Epidermal growth factor receptor (EGFR) is one member of the HER family of tyrosine kinase receptors and has been implicated in the pathogenesis of several types of gastrointestinal cancer. This receptor has an extracellular ligand binding domain, a transmembrane region, an intracellular domain with tyrosine kinase activity, and a tail of tyrosine residues responsible for downstream signaling. Ligand binding induces dimerization of the receptor with another tyrosine kinase receptor of the same (homodimerization) or different (heterodimerization) class, followed by internalization of the receptor and autophosphorylation of tyrosine kinase domains. Autophosphorylation of internal domains initiates intracellular signaling of key regulatory pathways, including the Ras/Raf/mitogen-activated protein kinase, PI3K/AKT, and signal transducers and activators of transcription (STAT) signaling pathways, which promote cell proliferation and prolong cell survival. Approximately 30% to 60% of esophageal and gastroesophageal junctional adenocarcinomas show amplification of EGFR, which is associated with a negative clinical outcome (see also Chapter 13). Amplification of chromosome 17q21 is seen in 25% to 30% of cases. This region contains *ERBB2*, which encodes HER2. Importantly, HER2 is the preferred heterodimerization partner of other members of the family and, when present in high concentrations, it can spontaneously dimerize in the absence of ligand binding. For these reasons, HER2 represents the most important target of directed therapy in the tyrosine kinase receptor family.

Targeted Molecular Therapies

Cetuximab is a chimeric monoclonal antibody that binds to EGFR and inhibits ligand-induced dimerization of the receptor. Although initial data suggested potential benefits of cetuximab in the management of advanced stage esophageal and gastroesophageal junctional adenocarcinomas, several phase II and III trials have yielded only modest results when the drug is used in combination with conventional chemotherapy. Cetuximab as a second-line, single agent has essentially no efficacy when used in the management of patients with metastatic disease and, unlike carcinomas of the colorectum, the likelihood of response to inhibitor therapy is not clearly linked to the presence of mutations in *KRAS*, *BRAF*, *PI3KCA*, or *PTEN*. Trastuzumab is a humanized monoclonal antibody that binds the HER2 extracellular domain and prevents activation of its intracellular tyrosine kinase. Data from several studies clearly show that this agent prolongs survival among patients with advanced adenocarcinomas of the distal esophagus and gastroesophageal junction that display moderate to strong basolateral or membranous staining for HER2 by immunohistochemistry (see also Chapter 13), or show gene amplification by in situ hybridization (Figure 14.1). Other growth factor receptor inhibitors targeting EGFR (eg, matuzumab, panitumumab, and nimotuzumab) or showing anti-vascular endothelial growth factor (VEGF) activity (eg, bevacizumab, sunitinib, and sorafenib) are currently under investigation.

Tyrosine kinase inhibitors represent a second class of agents that showed promise in cell line studies and early clinical trials of patients with carcinoma of the upper gastrointestinal tract. Agents under investigation include gefitinib, erlotinib, and lapatinib, an orally administered

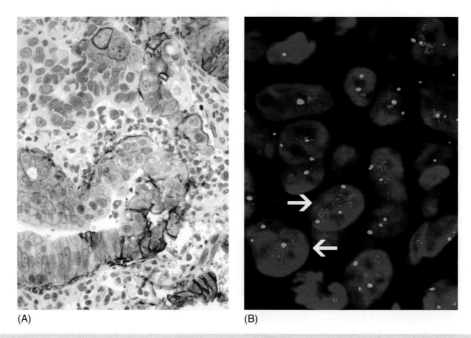

FIGURE 14.1 Immunohistochemical staining for HER2 is often patchy, and this pattern is considered a positive result. This case was associated with amplification by in situ hybridization. Discontinuous, predominantly basolateral staining of the cell membrane is present in approximately 50% of the tumor cells (A). Amplification of *ERBB2* results in overexpression of HER2 receptor. Several tumor cells contain multiple copies denoted by red signals in this in situ hybridization assay (arrow). The green signals represent chromosome 17 centromeric signals (B, courtesy of Dr. Shivakumar Subramaniyam).

small molecule tyrosine kinase inhibitor that targets HER2 and EGFR. Unfortunately, most compounds evaluated to date have shown disappointing results when used to treat patients with esophageal and gastroesophageal junctional adenocarcinomas.

Gastric Adenocarcinoma

Overview

Gastric adenocarcinoma is a major cause of global cancer-related morbidity and mortality. Most (greater than 80%) cases are sporadic and develop in patients with long-standing chronic gastritis and mucosal atrophy due to a variety of etiologies, including chronic *H. pylori* infection, autoimmune gastritis, Ménétrier disease, and long-standing chemical gastropathy, especially in patients who have undergone distal gastrectomy and a Billroth II procedure (see also Chapter 8). Strains of *H. pylori* that express vacuolating cytotoxin (VacA) and cytotoxin-associated antigen A (CagA) are more closely linked to cancer risk because they elicit a robust inflammatory response and promote carcinogenesis through a variety of mechanisms. Infection promotes expression of inducible nitric oxide synthetase and oxidative stress in epithelial stem cells, resulting in elaboration of free radicals and active oxygen species that cause DNA damage. The organism also facilitates binding of activator protein-1, c-Jun, and c-Fos to the promoter region of *EGFR*, indirectly activates NF-kB-mediated transcription, and induces TNF (tumor necrosis factor)-α.

Hypermethylation of *MGMT*, a DNA repair gene, is associated with infection by CagA-positive strains of *H. pylori* and is a common feature of gastric carcinomas.

Molecular Alterations

The molecular features of gastric carcinoma are variable and related to tumor morphology. Intestinal-type carcinomas generally display molecular alterations similar to those of colorectal carcinomas, namely LOH or mutations affecting *APC* (30%–40%), *DCC* (60%), *KRAS* (up to 30%), and *TP53* (25–40%), whereas abnormalities affecting these genes are detected in less than 2% of diffuse-type carcinomas. Epigenetic alterations and promoter methylation are also more common among intestinal-type gastric adenocarcinomas. Up to one-third of tumors show methylation of the *CDKN2A* promoter and nearly two-thirds show hypermethylation of the retinoic acid receptor-β (*RARB*). High-frequency microsatellite instability (MSI-H) is more frequently encountered in intestinal-type carcinomas (15%–40%) compared to diffuse-type tumors (5%–10%). Virtually all sporadic carcinomas with MSI-H develop via hypermethylation of the *MLH1* promoter, similar to MSI-H colon cancers, although gastric carcinomas may also represent a manifestation of hereditary nonpolyposis colon cancer (HNPCC). Morphologic features linked to MSI-H gastric adenocarcinomas include tumor heterogeneity, abundant lymphoid stroma with intraepithelial lymphocytes (ie, medullary carcinoma), and mucinous differentiation. Some gastric adenocarcinomas, particularly those of intestinal-type, show increased expression of receptor kinases. Up to 20% of cases show increased *EGFR* copy number by in situ hybridization, reflecting gene amplification or polysomy of chromosome 7. Approximately 25% of intestinal-type tumors overexpress HER2 compared to 5% of diffuse-type carcinomas and 10% of tumors containing intestinal and diffuse areas.

The molecular features of purely diffuse-type carcinomas have not been as extensively studied as those with an intestinal phenotype, although these tumors do show some distinct alterations. More than 50% of diffuse-type gastric adenocarcinomas show diminished E-cadherin expression, reflecting abnormalities of *CDH1* located on chromosome 16q22. This calcium-dependent transmembrane glycoprotein normally interacts with either β-catenin or γ-catenin to facilitate cell–cell adhesion. Slightly more than half of sporadic tumors harbor *CDH1* mutations, or LOH, in a single allele and show promoter hypermethylation of the other allele, indicating that hypermethylation represents the "second hit" responsible for completely suppressed E-cadherin expression in these tumors.

Epstein–Barr virus (EBV) is important to the development of up to 10% of gastric cancers, particularly those containing abundant lymphoid stroma or developing in the remnant stomach following a Billroth II procedure. The background mucosa is frequently inflamed or atrophic, suggesting a role of chronic injury in the development of EBV-related gastric cancers. Mechanisms underlying virally induced oncogenesis are not entirely clear, but such tumors often show epigenetic DNA hypermethylation of promoter regions in tumor suppressor genes, such as *MGMT, MINT2, PTEN,* and *RASSF1A.* These tumors also show loss of cell cycle regulation with increased cyclin D1 and decreased p16 expression.

Hereditary Diffuse Gastric Cancer

Hereditary diffuse gastric cancer is an autosomal dominant cancer syndrome characterized by signet ring cell carcinoma of the stomach, often in combination with lobular breast carcinoma. Families with the syndrome are defined by the presence of two or more documented cases of diffuse gastric cancer in first- or second-degree relatives, at least one of whom is diagnosed before age 50; or three or more cases of diffuse gastric cancer in first- or second-degree relatives, regardless of age. The presence of either of these features, a diagnosis of diffuse gastric cancer at a young age (less than 40 years), or a family history of both lobular breast cancer and diffuse gastric cancer should prompt evaluation for germline *CDH1* mutations, as they underlie a substantial proportion (30%–40%) of cases. Truncating mutations that produce a premature stop codon are most commonly identified (75%–80%

of cases), whereas the remaining 20%–25% of cases are due to missense mutations. Unlike sporadic diffuse-type gastric cancers that show clustering of mutations around exons 7 and 8, germline mutations can occur over a large part of the gene of the affected allele. Thus, screening of all 16 exons is generally necessary when a potential diagnosis of hereditary diffuse gastric cancer is considered. Of note, both familial and sporadic diffuse gastric cancers may show decreased, or absent, E-cadherin immunoexpression, so this technique cannot be reliably used to identify patients with germline mutations. Patients with suspected hereditary diffuse gastric cancer require evaluation of peripheral blood DNA, usually in the form of direct sequencing.

Targeted Molecular Therapies

As is the case in adenocarcinomas of the esophagus and gastroesophageal junction, trastuzumab improves survival of patients with advanced gastric cancers that overexpress HER2 when used in combination with conventional chemotherapy. Although data from the ToGA trial suggested that immunohistochemical overexpression of HER2 correlates with the response to trastuzumab better than in situ hybridization, several studies since have shown comparable predictive values of these assays and many laboratories now use either immunohistochemistry, in situ hybridization, or both to determine whether patients with advanced gastric cancer should receive trastuzumab (see also Chapter 13).

Ramucirumab is a fully human monoclonal antibody directed against vascular endothelial growth factor receptor 2 (VEGFR2). It functions as a receptor antagonist to competitively inhibit binding of VEGF and prevent angiogenesis and proliferation. This agent was recently approved as a second-line therapy in the management of advanced gastric cancer. It is the first biologic treatment shown to be of survival benefit when administered as a single agent to patients with metastatic gastric cancer.

Unfortunately, most other targeted molecular therapies analyzed to date are of limited value in the management of gastric carcinoma, or are in preliminary stages of development. Cetuximab, an EGFR inhibitor, was initially reported to improve survival in patients with advanced gastric cancer, but the efficacy of this agent has not borne out in recent phase III clinical trials. Tyrosine kinase inhibitors have minimal activity against gastric carcinomas. Several other agents show promising antitumor effects in preclinical studies, including inhibitors of insulin-like growth factor-1 receptor, fibroblast growth factor receptor, and c-Met signaling. Histone deacetylase inhibitors represent potentially valuable agents, as they can theoretically promote re-expression of previously silenced tumor suppressor genes.

Colorectal Cancer

Overview

Colorectal cancer is the third most common cause of cancer-related mortality in the United States. It is now largely considered to be a genetic disease driven by a complex array of genetic and epigenetic alterations. Early mutations in cancer cells affect genomic stability and propagate additional alterations that facilitate cell proliferation. Two major types of genomic instability occur in colorectal carcinoma: chromosomal instability and microsatellite instability (MSI). Both of these mechanisms occur in sporadic colorectal carcinomas as well as in association with familial syndromes, namely familial adenomatous polyposis and Lynch syndrome (hereditary nonpolyposis colorectal cancer), respectively (see also Chapters 6 and 11). Study of these familial cancers has facilitated our understanding of the mechanisms underlying sporadic tumors and aided recognition of several clinically important molecular aberrations. Mutations in tumor suppressor and DNA repair genes aid identification of patients and family members with heritable cancer risk, whereas others have prognostic and therapeutic implications.

Molecular Alterations

APC/Wnt Signaling and Chromosomal Instability

Most sporadic colorectal carcinomas, and all tumors that develop in association with familial adenomatous polyposis, display chromosomal instability and biallelic *adenomatous polyposis coli (APC)* inactivation. Mutations in *APC* are either nonsense mutations that introduce a premature stop codon or frameshift mutations resulting from insertions or deletions. Tumors with chromosomal instability are characterized by gains and losses of large amounts of genetic material (ie, LOH) that results in karyotypic variability among tumor cells. Patients with familial adenomatous polyposis generally have at least one mutation between codons 1250 and 1450. Germline mutations in this region are followed by mutations in the second allele that result in complete loss of the gene, whereas germline mutations outside this region are associated with somatic mutations between codons 1250 and 1450. Selection for at least one mutation in this region ensures that mutant APC retains some capacity to bind β-catenin and provides enough Wnt/β-catenin signaling to promote tumor formation. Importantly, some patients with a clinical phenotype suggesting familial adenomatous polyposis have biallelic inactivating mutations of *MUTYH,* a base excision repair gene, rather than germline *APC* mutations. This gene is located at 1p32-34 and contains mutational hot spots at Y165C and G382D. Patients with inactive *MUTYH* acquire somatic *APC* mutations as a consequence of impaired base excision repair function.

Inactivation of *APC* occurs early in the progression of adenomas to adenocarcinomas. The *APC* protein product is normally expressed in nonproliferating colorectal epithelium and is essential for regulating cell growth and differentiation. Loss of *APC* affects the Wnt signaling pathway, which is an evolutionarily conserved mechanism important to colorectal neoplasia. In the absence of Wnt signaling, the APC–axin–GSK3ß cytoplasmic complex sequesters β-catenin and targets it for destruction. However, activation of Wnt signaling interferes with the APC–axin–GSK3ß cytoplasmic complex and prevents phosphorylation and ubiquitination of β-catenin, resulting in its accumulation within the cytoplasm. Excess β-catenin translocates to the nucleus where it forms a complex with T cell factor and lymphoid enhancer factor that promotes expression of several important cell cycle regulating genes. Thus, APC negatively regulates Wnt signaling via participation in the APC–axin–GSK3ß destruction complex that promotes β-catenin degradation.

The antitumorigenic effects of APC are not limited to β-catenin degradation. It also acts on promoters of Wnt-responsive genes and shuttles β-catenin out of the nucleus for destruction. It binds microtubules and F-actin to negatively regulate cell cycling and direct cell migration, and interferes with microtubule dynamics that directly affect mitosis. Cells containing mutant *APC* are predisposed to mitotic errors and aneuploidy due to defects in mitotic spindles. Inactivation of *APC* also promotes chromosomal alterations involving *KRAS2* (12p12), chromosome 18q, and *TP53* (17q13).

Microsatellite Instability

Microsatellite instability is a term used to describe expansion or contraction of short nucleotide repeats (microsatellites), which are prone to replication errors because DNA polymerase frequently slips over repetitive sequences. Slippage of the DNA strand creates insertion–deletion loops and single base pair mismatches that are normally recognized and corrected by the mismatch repair system. Dysfunctional mismatch repair mechanisms result in a failure to correct these errors and their propagation during the second round of replication. Both insertion–deletion loops and single base pair mismatches alter the lengths of microsatellites in the DNA of tumor cells compared to those of non-neoplastic tissues. Microsatellites are more numerous in noncoding regions of the genome, although alterations in those that occur in coding regions can lead to downstream nonsense mutations. Single base pair mismatches result in point mutations and insertion–deletion loops cause frameshift mutations in the defective daughter strand.

MSI is seen in two clinical contexts. This mechanism accounts for nearly all tumors associated with Lynch syndrome (see also Chapters 6 and 11) as well as the development of 10% to 15% of sporadic colorectal cancers. Tumors that occur in association with Lynch syndrome generally result from a germline mutation in one of four mismatch repair genes: *MLH1*, *MSH2*, *MSH6*, or *PMS2*. Sporadic microsatellite unstable tumors usually display acquired hypermethylation of the *MLH1* promoter, which suppresses its transcription, although biallelic inactivation of any mismatch repair gene can occur via a combination of somatic mutations and methylation.

Tumors are evaluated for MSI using polymerase chain reaction (PCR) to amplify a panel of five microsatellite repeats. The Bethesda panel consists of two mononucleotide repeats (eg, AAAAAAAAA) and three dinucleotide repeats (eg, CACACACACA). Tumors are classified as MSI-H if two or more repeats showed instability, MSS (microsatellite stable) if no repeats are unstable, and MSI-low if one repeat is unstable. The biologic significance of the latter category is controversial, but is probably irrelevant to the detection of Lynch syndrome. As it turns out, mononucleotide repeat instability is more sensitive and specific for mismatch repair deficiency than instability at dinucleotide repeats and, thus, commercially available panels that employ five mononucleotide repeats without any dinucleotide repeats have increasingly replaced the Bethesda panel in clinical practice. Instability at two or more mononucleotide repeats is classified as MSI-H and no instability is considered to be MSS (Figure 14.2). Instability in one repeat is classified as indeterminate rather than MSI-low because this finding may reflect underlying mismatch repair deficiency.

Results of immunohistochemistry for mismatch repair proteins correlate well with those of MSI testing by PCR of microsatellite repeats. Colorectal cancers normally display nuclear staining of all four mismatch repair proteins, whereas loss of staining of one or more of these proteins implies mismatch repair deficiency (see also Chapters 11 and 13). The pattern of staining reflects the tendency of mismatch repair proteins to form heterodimers. Tumors deficient in MLH1 show loss of MLH1 and PMS2 staining because these proteins form a heterodimer that stabilizes PMS2. Similarly, tumors deficient in MSH2 show loss of MSH2 and MSH6 because the MSH2/MSH6 heterodimer stabilizes MSH6. In contrast, both MLH1 and MSH2 staining are preserved when either PMS2 or MSH6 is lost, probably reflecting the capacities of MLH1 and MSH2 to bind other partners.

There are several caveats to the interpretation of immunohistochemical stains for mismatch repair proteins. Tumor staining should only be evaluated in areas that show staining of internal control cells, such as lymphocytes or fibroblasts; negative tumor staining in areas without internal control staining is not interpretable. One important exception to this rule is the patient with constitutional mismatch repair deficiency. Tumors from these patients show an absence of staining for mismatch repair proteins in both tumor and normal tissues. However, the constellation of clinical features is an important clue to

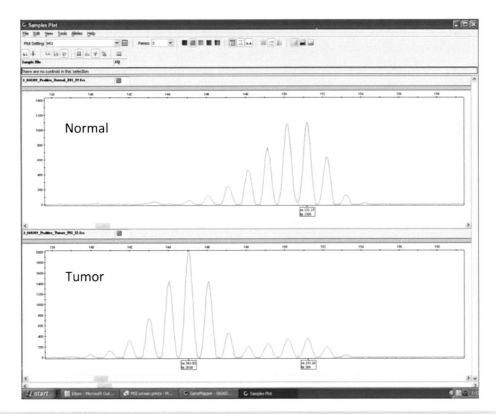

FIGURE 14.2 Microsatellite instability is present in the BAT-25 mononucleotide repeat. DNA from a colonic adenocarcinoma with MSI shows left-shifted peaks in this microsatellite relative to the non-neoplastic tissue from the same patient (courtesy of Dr. Wade Samowitz).

the underlying diagnosis. Missense changes in a protein that destroy its function may have preserved antigenicity that leads to a false negative immunohistochemical result. Abnormal immunohistochemical staining is usually manifest as complete loss of nuclear staining, although weak nuclear staining, rather than complete loss, may rarely reflect the presence of a germline mutation. Combined loss of MLH1 and PMS2 staining usually reflects deficient MLH1, which may reflect a germline *MLH1* mutation (Lynch syndrome) or acquired *MLH1* hypermethylation in sporadic tumors. Distinction between Lynch-associated tumors with defective MLH1 and sporadic cancers is facilitated by assessment for the presence of the Val600Glu (V600E) mutation in *BRAF* and *MLH1* methylation. More than 50% of sporadic MSI-H colorectal cancers harbor *BRAF* mutations. This alteration has not been described in Lynch-related tumors with *MLH1* mutations, but rarely occur in those with *PMS2* mutations that show a different immunohistochemical staining profile (ie, isolated loss of PMS2 staining). Hypermethylated *MLH1* is characteristic of sporadic MSI-H tumors, but may also be seen in occasional Lynch-associated tumors, so this feature is less reliable than a *BRAF* mutation in distinguishing sporadic and syndromic carcinomas.

Other types of genetic alterations may underlie rare cases of Lynch syndrome. Some patients with phenotypic Lynch syndrome have heritable epigenetic inactivation of *MLH1*, or *MLH1* constitutional epimutation, in which case the germline defect is promoter methylation of *MLH1*. Other patients with loss of MSH2 and MSH6 by immunohistochemistry have germline deletions affecting the polyadenylation site located in exon 9 of *epithelial cell adhesion molecule* (*EPCAM*), which is located upstream of *MSH2*. Deletion of this region results in loss of the *EPCAM* stop codon and subsequent CpG methylation in *MSH2* or formation of *EPCAM–MSH2* fusion transcripts, both of which abrogate the function of MSH2.

The CpG Island Methylator Phenotype

There are several types of epigenetic alteration that regulate gene expression. These include DNA hypermethylation, DNA hypomethylation, post-translational histone modification, and chromatin looping. Methyltransferases add methyl groups to the carbon 5 position of cytosine residues located 5′ to guanine. Subsequent methyl cytosines are clustered in regions rich in cytosine (C) and guanine (G) dinucleotides (ie, CpG islands) that are present in the promoter regions of up to 50% of mammalian genes. Promoter methylation in this fashion suppresses gene transcription by inhibiting binding of transcription factors, affecting histone acetylation, and altering conformations to effectively block access of transcriptional machinery to the gene. Epigenetic hypermethylation of genes prevents their transcription and may account for the first, second, or both hits in silencing tumor suppressor genes.

Tumors that show DNA hypermethylation at multiple promoters are classified as showing the CpG Island Methylator Phenotype (CIMP). They frequently display MSI-H and wild-type *TP53*, as well as *BRAF* mutations and methylation of *MINT1*, *MLH1*, *RIZ1*, and *TIMP3*. Higher levels of DNA methylation are associated with *BRAF* mutations compared with *KRAS* mutations among colorectal cancers, whereas tumors wild-type for both *BRAF* and *KRAS* show essentially no methylation. Colorectal carcinomas with CIMP tend to occur in the proximal colons of older women and are associated with a history of cigarette smoking. They frequently harbor *BRAF* mutations and show methylation of *MLH1* resulting in MSI-H in up to 70% of cases.

Targeted Molecular Therapies

Cetuximab and panitumumab are monoclonal antibodies against EGFR that are used to treat metastatic colorectal cancer. Drug efficacy is unrelated to EGFR expression by immunohistochemistry and *EGFR* mutations are infrequently encountered in colorectal carcinoma. Thus, evaluation of colorectal cancers for EGFR expression is of no clinical value at this time. However, mutations affecting genes in signaling pathways downstream of EGFR predict a lack of response to EGFR antagonists. Oncogenic activation of these downstream genes leads to activation of cell signaling despite pharmacologic inhibition of EGFR binding to its ligand. For this reason, these agents are not effective against tumors that harbor mutations affecting cell signaling downstream of EGFR. For example, colorectal cancers with mutations in codons 12 and 13 of *KRAS* show a lack of, or diminished, response to cetuximab and panitumumab. These monoclonal antibodies are very expensive therapeutic agents and may cause severe toxicities, so it is understandable that the Food and Drug Administration now mandates mutational evaluation of these *KRAS* codons before therapy with such agents is initiated (Figure 14.3).

Several other types of mutation may abrogate the efficacy of cetuximab and panitumumab. Oncogenic *KRAS* mutations in codons 61, 117, and 146 decrease the efficacy of cetuximab and similar agents, as do mutations in *NRAS*, another member of the Ras family. Mutations in *BRAF* would also be predicted to activate this pathway independent of EGFR and certainly *BRAF*-mutated MSS colorectal cancers are associated with decreased survival, but it is not clear whether this observation reflects a lack of response to EGFR inhibitor therapy or the inherently aggressive nature of *BRAF*-mutated MSS cancers. Mutations in exon 20 of *PIK3CA* affect the PIK3CA–AKT–mTor pathway downstream of EGFR and are associated with a lack of responsiveness to cetuximab. Loss of PTEN, an inhibitor of PIK3CA, also serves to activate the PIK3CA–AKT–mTor pathway and is associated with a lack of responsiveness to EGFR antagonists. Cetuximab and similar agents are most likely to be beneficial among

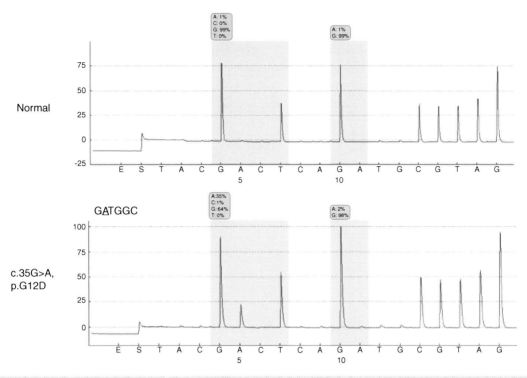

FIGURE 14.3 Pyrosequencing detects a 35G>A p.G12D mutation in *KRAS* in a colorectal carcinoma. Results of DNA analysis of the normal tissue are provided for comparison (courtesy of Dr. Wade Samowitz).

patients with tumors that are wild-type *KRAS*, wild-type *BRAF*, wild-type *PIK3CA*, and maintained PTEN expression (ie, quadruple negative carcinomas).

Gastrointestinal Stromal Tumors

Overview

Gastrointestinal stromal tumors (GISTs) are biologically aggressive mesenchymal neoplasms characterized by *KIT* mutations in approximately 80% of cases (see also Chapter 5). This gene encodes the KIT tyrosine kinase receptor, which is a membrane-associated member of the type III tyrosine kinase family. The receptor consists of five loops in its extracellular domain that are connected to the cytoplasmic domain via a transmembrane region. The cytoplasmic domain contains a juxtamembrane region and a split tyrosine kinase domain with two components: an adenosine triphosphate (ATP) binding region (kinase I) and a phosphotransferase region (kinase II). Binding of stem cell factor induces KIT dimerization followed by phosphorylation of tyrosine residues in the cytoplasmic domain, the latter of which activates several signal transduction pathways that drive cell proliferation.

Molecular Alterations

Oncogenic *KIT* mutations impair regulation of receptor activation or alter enzymatic function of tyrosine kinases. Most occur in exon 11, promoting constitutive kinase activity by changing the conformation of the intracellular juxtamembrane. Mutation types affecting exon 11 include in-frame deletions, single-nucleotide substitutions, duplications, and insertions. Deletions are associated with a poorer prognosis than those with single nucleotide substitutions, whereas duplications in the 3' region are associated with a better prognosis than other changes. Approximately 10% of GISTs have mutations in exon 9 that affect the extracellular domain, whereas mutations affecting kinase I (exon 13) and kinase II (exon 17) are less frequent. Exon 9 mutations are more common among small bowel tumors than those of gastric origin.

Although *KIT* mutations are found in most GISTs, up to 20% of tumors contain wild-type *KIT*. Of these, nearly 10% harbor mutations in platelet-derived growth factor receptor alpha polypeptide (*PDGFRA*), particularly tumors of the stomach and proximal small bowel. This gene also encodes a tyrosine kinase receptor mapping to chromosome 4q11-q12, which is highly homologous to *KIT* and shows a parallel distribution of functional mutations. Mutations in *PDGFRA* usually occur in exon 18 and result in conformational changes in the ATP-binding pocket that promote kinase activation. Exon 12 mutations affecting the juxtamembrane domain and those of exon 14 encoding kinase I are less common. Monosomy, or partial loss, of chromosome 14q occurs in two-thirds of GISTs and 50% show chromosome 22 losses. Losses affecting 1p, 9p, and 11p, and gains involving 8q and 17q are associated with aggressive biologic behavior.

GISTs that develop in pediatric patients or in association with type 1 neurofibromatosis generally lack both *KIT* and *PDGFRA* mutations. Tumors developing in Carney–Stratakis syndrome (ie, GISTs and paragangliomas) frequently show mutations in subunits B, C, or D of *SDH*, which encode succinate dehydrogenase. Sporadic GISTs that affect children also contain *SDH* mutations. They show a predilection for females and usually develop in the stomach or omentum. Tumors deficient in succinate dehydrogenase are often resistant to imatinib, but may show some response to therapy with sunitinib.

Targeted Molecular Therapies

Imatinib is a tyrosine kinase inhibitor that competes with ATP for its binding site to kinase I and prevents phosphorylation of cellular substrates. It is highly effective as a first-line agent against most advanced GISTs and is associated with therapeutic response rates up to 90%. Some tumors show diminished response to therapy over time, reflecting acquisition of additional *KIT* or *PDGFRA* mutations that affect imatinib binding to the ATP pocket of the KIT receptor. Sunitinib is a second-line agent currently approved in patients with imatinib-resistant GISTs. This agent can bind to KIT and PDGFRA, but also shows affinity for VEGFR. Mutational analyses of GISTs are increasingly used to guide patient management. Tumors with exon 11 *KIT* mutations respond best to imatinib therapy, followed by those that are *KIT/PDGFRA* wild-type. GISTs with exon 9 *KIT* mutations may respond to a higher dose of imatinib or standard dosing with sunitinib.

SUMMARY AND CONCLUSIONS

Intensive research and technological advances have enabled investigators to begin unraveling genetic, epigenetic, and post-translational regulatory mechanisms that facilitate carcinogenesis in the gastrointestinal tract. Efforts to elucidate cellular signal transduction pathways continue to unravel relationships between proteins promoting cell survival and proliferation, many of which represent potential targets for directed medical therapies. Membrane-bound receptor kinases are important candidates for inhibitor therapies. Inhibitors of HER-2, EGFR, KIT, and other receptor kinases are effective in the treatment of patients with specific gastrointestinal malignancies. Future management strategies will likely include the use of these agents, as well as other therapies aimed at specific molecular alterations.

SELECTED REFERENCES

General

Tanzer M, Liebl M, Quante M. Molecular biomarkers in esophageal, gastric, and colorectal adenocarcinoma. *Pharmacol Ther.* 2013;140(2):133–147.

Vogelstein B, Kinzler KW. Cancer genes and the pathways they control. *Nat Med.* 2004;10(8):789–799.

Barrett Esophagus and Adenocarcinoma

Chandra S, Gorospe EC, Leggett CL, Wang KK. Barrett's esophagus in 2012: updates in pathogenesis, treatment, and surveillance. *Curr Gastroenterol Rep.* 2013;15(5):322.

Gibson MK, Dhaliwal AS, Clemons NJ, et al. Barrett's esophagus: cancer and molecular biology. *Ann NY Acad Sci.* 2013;1300:296–314.

Kordes S, Cats A, Meijer SL, van Laarhoven HW. Targeted therapy for advanced esophagogastric adenocarcinoma. *Crit Rev Oncol Hematol.* 2014;90(1):68–76.

Lennerz JK, Kwak EL, Ackerman A, et al. MET amplification identifies a small and aggressive subgroup of esophagogastric adenocarcinoma with evidence of responsiveness to crizotinib. *J Clin Oncol.* 2011;29(36):4803–4810.

Mayne GC, Hussey DJ, Watson DI. MicroRNAs and esophageal cancer—implications for pathogenesis and therapy. *Curr Pharm Des.* 2013;19(7):1211–1226.

Norguet E, Dahan L, Seitz JF. Targeting esophageal and gastric cancers with monoclonal antibodies. *Curr Top Med Chem.* 2012;12(15):1678–1682.

Okines AF, Gonzalez de Castro D, Cunningham D, et al. Biomarker analysis in oesophagogastric cancer: Results from the REAL3 and TransMAGIC trials. *Eur J Cancer.* 2013;49(9):2116–2125.

Poehlmann A, Kuester D, Malfertheiner P, Guenther T, Roessner A. Inflammation and Barrett's carcinogenesis. *Pathol Res Pract.* 2012;208(5):269–280.

Powell SM, Petersen GM, Krush AJ, et al. Molecular diagnosis of familial adenomatous polyposis. *N Engl J Med.* 1993;329(27):1982–1987.

Rajendra S, Sharma P. Barrett's Esophagus. *Curr Treat Options Gastroenterol.* 2014;12(2):169–182.

Thompson SK, Sullivan TR, Davies R, Ruszkiewicz AR. Her-2/neu gene amplification in esophageal adenocarcinoma and its influence on survival. *Ann Surg Oncol.* 2011;18(7):2010–2017.

Wainberg ZA, Lin LS, DiCarlo B, et al. Phase II trial of modified FOLFOX6 and erlotinib in patients with metastatic or advanced adenocarcinoma of the oesophagus and gastro-oesophageal junction. *Brit J Cancer.* 2011;105(6):760–765.

Winberg H, Lindblad M, Lagergren J, Dahlstrand H. Risk factors and chemoprevention in Barrett's esophagus—an update. *Scand J Gastroenterol.* 2012;47(4):397–406.

Gastric Adenocarcinoma

Bang YJ, Van Cutsem E, Feyereislova A, et al. Trastuzumab in combination with chemotherapy versus chemotherapy alone for treatment of HER2-positive advanced gastric or gastro-oesophageal junction cancer (ToGA): a phase 3, open-label, randomised controlled trial. *Lancet.* 2010;376(9742):687–697.

Bornschein J, Malfertheiner P. Helicobacter pylori and Gastric Cancer. *Dig Dis.* 2014;32(3):249–264.

Camargo MC, Kim WH, Chiaravalli AM, et al. Improved survival of gastric cancer with tumour Epstein-Barr virus positivity: an international pooled analysis. *Gut.* 2014;63(2):236–243.

Chen S, Duan G, Zhang R, Fan Q. Helicobacter pylori cytotoxin-associated gene A protein upregulates alpha-enolase expression via Src/MEK/ERK pathway: Implication for progression of gastric cancer. *Int J Oncol.* 2014;45(2):764–770.

Hirahashi M, Koga Y, Kumagai R, Aishima S, Taguchi K, Oda Y. Induced nitric oxide synthetase and peroxiredoxin expression in intramucosal poorly differentiated gastric cancer of young patients. *Path Int.* 2014;64(4):155–163.

Martinez-Lopez JL, Torres J, Camorlinga-Ponce M, Mantilla A, Leal YA, Fuentes-Panana EM. Evidence of Epstein-Barr virus association with gastric cancer and non-atrophic gastritis. *Viruses.* 2014;6(1):301–318.

Nishikawa J, Yanai H, Hirano A, et al. High prevalence of Epstein-Barr virus in gastric remnant carcinoma after Billroth-II reconstruction. *Scand J Gastroenterol.* 2002;37(7):825–829.

Okada T, Nakamura M, Nishikawa J, et al. Identification of genes specifically methylated in Epstein-Barr virus-associated gastric carcinomas. *Cancer Sci.* 2013;104(10):1309–1314.

Ruschoff J, Hanna W, Bilous M, et al. HER2 testing in gastric cancer: a practical approach. *Mod Pathol.* 2012;25(5):637–650.

Shimizu T, Marusawa H, Matsumoto Y, et al. Accumulation of Somatic Mutations in TP53 in Gastric Epithelium with Helicobacter pylori infection. *Gastroenterology.* 2014;147(2):407–17.

Watari J, Chen N, Amenta PS, et al. associated chronic gastritis, clinical syndromes, precancerous lesions, and pathogenesis of gastric cancer development. *World J Gastroenterol.* 2014;20(18):5461–5473.

Colorectal Cancer

Albuquerque C, Breukel C, van der Luijt R, et al. The 'just-right' signaling model: APC somatic mutations are selected based on a specific level of activation of the beta-catenin signaling cascade. *Hum Mol Genet.* 2002;11(13):1549–1560.

Boland CR, Goel A. Microsatellite instability in colorectal cancer. *Gastroenterology.* 2010;138(6):2073–2087 e3.

Boland CR, Thibodeau SN, Hamilton SR, et al. A National Cancer Institute Workshop on Microsatellite Instability for cancer detection and familial predisposition: development of international criteria for the determination of microsatellite instability in colorectal cancer. *Cancer Res.* 1998;58(22):5248–5257.

Douillard JY, Oliner KS, Siena S, et al. Panitumumab-FOLFOX4 treatment and RAS mutations in colorectal cancer. *N Engl J Med.* 2013;369(11):1023–1034.

Durno CA, Holter S, Sherman PM, Gallinger S. The gastrointestinal phenotype of germline biallelic mismatch repair gene mutations. *Am J Gastroenterol.* 2010;105(11):2449–2456.

Kane MF, Loda M, Gaida GM, et al. Methylation of the hMLH1 promoter correlates with lack of expression of hMLH1 in sporadic colon tumors and mismatch repair-defective human tumor cell lines. *Cancer Res.* 1997;57(5):808–811.

Lamlum H, Ilyas M, Rowan A, et al. The type of somatic mutation at APC in familial adenomatous polyposis is determined by the site of the germline mutation: a new facet to Knudson's 'two-hit' hypothesis. *Nat Med.* 1999;5(9):1071–1075.

Lefevre JH, Colas C, Coulet F, et al. MYH biallelic mutation can inactivate the two genetic pathways of colorectal cancer by APC or MLH1 transversions. *Fam Cancer.* 2010;9(4):589–594.

Liao X, Lochhead P, Nishihara R, et al. Aspirin use, tumor PIK3CA mutation, and colorectal-cancer survival. *N Engl J Med.* 2012;367(17):1596–1606.

Ligtenberg MJ, Kuiper RP, Chan TL, et al. Heritable somatic methylation and inactivation of MSH2 in families with Lynch syndrome due to deletion of the 3' exons of TACSTD1. *Nat Genet.* 2009;41(1):112–117.

Samowitz WS. The CpG island methylator phenotype in colorectal cancer. *The J Mol Diag.* 2007;9(3):281–283.

Shen L, Toyota M, Kondo Y, et al. Integrated genetic and epigenetic analysis identifies three different subclasses of colon cancer. *Proc Natl Acad Sci U S A.* 2007;104(47):18654–18659.

Spirio LN, Samowitz W, Robertson J, et al. Alleles of APC modulate the frequency and classes of mutations that lead to colon polyps. *Nat Genet.* 1998;20(4):385–388.

Gastrointestinal Stromal Tumors

Barnett CM, Corless CL, Heinrich MC. Gastrointestinal stromal tumors: molecular markers and genetic subtypes. *Hematol Oncol Clin North Am.* 2013;27(5):871–888.

Beadling C, Patterson J, Justusson E, et al. Gene expression of the IGF pathway family distinguishes subsets of gastrointestinal stromal tumors wild type for KIT and PDGFRA. *Cancer Med.* 2013;2(1):21–31.

Demetri GD, Benjamin R, Blanke CD, et al. NCCN Task Force report: optimal management of patients with gastrointestinal stromal tumor (GIST)—expansion and update of NCCN clinical practice guidelines. *J Natl Compr Canc Netw.* 2004;2 Suppl 1:S-1–S-26.

Demetri GD, Benjamin RS, Blanke CD, et al. NCCN Task Force report: management of patients with gastrointestinal stromal tumor (GIST)—update of the NCCN clinical practice guidelines. *J Natl Compr Canc Netw.* 2007;5 Suppl 2:S1–S29.

Espinosa I, Lee CH, Kim MK, et al. A novel monoclonal antibody against DOG1 is a sensitive and specific marker for gastrointestinal stromal tumors. *Am J Surg Pathol.* 2008;32(2):210–218.

Heinrich MC, Maki RG, Corless CL, et al. Primary and secondary kinase genotypes correlate with the biological and clinical activity of sunitinib in imatinib-resistant gastrointestinal stromal tumor. *J Clin Oncol.* 2008;26(33):5352–5359.

Janeway KA, Liegl B, Harlow A, et al. Pediatric KIT wild-type and platelet-derived growth factor receptor alpha-wild-type gastrointestinal stromal tumors share KIT activation but not mechanisms of genetic progression with adult gastrointestinal stromal tumors. *Canc Res.* 2007;67(19):9084–9088.

Lasota J, Corless CL, Heinrich MC, et al. Clinicopathologic profile of gastrointestinal stromal tumors (GISTs) with primary KIT exon 13 or exon 17 mutations: a multicenter study on 54 cases. *Mod Pathol.* 2008;21(4):476–484.

Mason EF, Hornick JL. Succinate dehydrogenase deficiency is associated with decreased 5-hydroxymethylcytosine production in gastrointestinal stromal tumors: implications for mechanisms of tumorigenesis. *Mod Pathol.* 2013;26(11):1492–1497.

Pantaleo MA, Astolfi A, Urbini M, et al. Analysis of all subunits, SDHA, SDHB, SDHC, SDHD, of the succinate dehydrogenase complex in KIT/PDGFRA wild-type GIST. *Eur J Hum Genet.* 2014;22(1):32–39.

Vadakara J, von Mehren M. Gastrointestinal stromal tumors: management of metastatic disease and emerging therapies. *Hematol Oncol Clin North Am.* 2013;27(5):905–920.

Index